DR. SUSAN LOVE'S
BREAST BOOK

THIRD EDITION
FULLY REVISED

DR. SUSAN LOVE'S BREAST BOOK

THIRD EDITION
FULLY REVISED

Susan M. Love, M.D.

with Karen Lindsey

Illustrations by Marcia Williams

A MERLOYD LAWRENCE BOOK

PERSEUS PUBLISHING

Cambridge, Massachusetts

This book is meant to educate and should not be used as an alternative to appropriate medical care. The authors have exerted every effort to ensure that the information presented is accurate up to the time of publication. However, in light of ongoing research and the constant flow of information it is possible that new findings may invalidate some of the data presented here.

Table 14-1, page 217, is used with the kind permission of Elsevier Science Publishing Company, Inc.

Table 14-2, page 218, is used with the kind permission of the American Cancer Society.

Table 14-3, page 218, is used with the kind permission of J.B.Lippincott/ Harper & Row.

A CIP record for this book is available from the Library of Congress.

ISBN 0–7382–0235–5

Perseus Publishing is a member of the Perseus Books Group.

Find us on the World Wide Web at http://www.perseuspublishing.com

Perseus Publishing books are available at special discounts for bulk purchases in the U.S. by corporations, institutions, and other organizations. For more information, please contact the Special Markets Department at HarperCollins Publishers, 10 East 53rd Street, New York, NY 10022, or call 1–212–207–7528.

Text design by Anna George

First printing, August 2000

2 3 4 5 6 7 8 9 10—03 02 01 00

*This book is dedicated
to the memory of Verna and Watson Lindsey,
to Helen and Katie with all my love,
and to all of the women over the years
who have given me the honor of caring for them
and learning from them.*

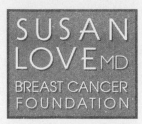

Education · Research
Advocacy

THE SUSAN LOVE, M.D. BREAST CANCER FOUNDATION

As you can tell from this book and especially Chapter 17, I think the intraductal approach to the breast has the potential to revolutionize our approach to breast cancer. However, much more needs to be learned for it to complete our mission of eradicating breast cancer so that our daughters and granddaughters never live in fear of this disease. The answers are within our reach.

The Susan Love, M.D. Breast Cancer Foundation is dedicated to realizing this vision. We support investigators doing research on the intraductal approach to breast cancer and conduct an international scientific conference to foster communication among researchers, breast cancer advocacy organizations and medical professionals. We also focus on education and advocacy.

I have donated a percentage of my royalties on this book to support the Foundation, so that no one will ever again have to hear the words, "You have breast cancer."

For more information about supporting the programs of the Susan Love, M.D. Breast Cancer Foundation, visit our website at www.susan lovemd.com, or call 805-963-2877.

ABOUT THE AUTHORS

Susan Love MD, MBA, is an author, surgeon, activist and mother. She is Adjunct Professor of Surgery at UCLA, Founder and Director of the National Breast Cancer Coalition and author of *Dr. Susan Love's Breast Book* and *Dr Susan Love's Hormone Book*. In December 1998 President Clinton appointed her to the National Cancer Advisory Board. In addition to her media appearances, speaking and political activities, she has found time to do research, in particular on a new intraductal approach to screening for changes that could lead to breast cancer. She is co-founder of a medical device company, ProDuct Health, Inc. which is developing the equipment needed to implement this approach. Her website, www.susanlovemd.com is designed as the site where midlife women can find answers to all their health care questions. She shares her home in Southern California with her life partner, Helen Cooksey MD, their daughter Katie, and their companions, a dog and two cats.

Karen Lindsey is the author of *Divorced, Beheaded, Survived: A Feminist Reinterpretation of the Wives of Henry VIII, Friends as Family*, and *Falling Off the Roof*; and co-author of *Dr. Susan Love's Hormone Book* and, with Dr. Daniel Tobin, *Peaceful Dying*. Her articles have appeared in *Ms, The Women's Review of Books, Sojourner, International Figure Skating*, and many other publications and anthologies. She teaches women's studies at the University of Massachusetts/Boston, and writing at Emerson College.

Contents

Acknowledgments

Completing this third edition as always has involved an orchestra of people. There are the researchers and others over the years who have worked with me on the intraductal approach to breast cancer: Margaret Lawler, Maggie Gibbons, Jean Chou, La Leche League, Sanford Barsky, Sharon Hirschowitz, Stella Grosser, Regina Offodile, DaWanda Pesicka, Julian Nikolchev, Howard Palefsky, Lori Palomares, Linda Gont, Xuamin He, Shawn O'Leary, David Hung, Angela Soito, Mary Alpaugh, and all the women who bravely volunteered to participate. In addition we had financial support from the Revlon UCLA Women's Cancer Fund, the Department of Defense, and ProDuct Health.

Then there are the scientists and clinicians and other experts who carefully read various chapters for me to make sure I had it all right. If there are errors in the book, they are all mine; if it is accurate it is thanks to the generosity of these people. My thanks go to: Sanford Barsky MD, Larry Bassett MD, Leslie Bernstein Ph.D., Al Butner MD, Betsy Carpenter, Anne Coscarelli Ph.D., Nikki DeBruhl MD, Kay Dickersin Ph.D., Carol Fred MD, Silvia Formenti MD, Irene Gage MD, Patti Ganz MD, Sherry Goldman RNP, Jay Harris MD, Judi Hirshfield-Bartek RN, Craig Henderson MD, David Hung MD, Barbara Kalinowski RN, Ellen Mahoney MD, Nick Petrakis Ph.D., Marcie Richardson MD, Joyce O'Shaughnessy MD, William Shaw MD, Mel

Silverstein MD, Sara Sukumar Ph.D., Susan Troyan MD, Margaret Wrensch Ph.D., Fran Visco JD. I would also like to thank Pat Waring and Ewa Witt for all their help organizing the research.

Throughout the editions, many women have been willing to share their experiences with breast disease, and their concerns, with us. These interviews have shown, as nothing else could, the effects of what the book addresses. I thank them all. In this edition, I wish to thank Betsy Carpenter, Sara Furrer, Mary Smith, Karen Aleckson and the women from Breast Health Access for Women with Disabilities.

I am grateful to all the people who have worked with me this past year at SusanLoveMD.com, often competing with "the book" for my attention: Beverly Merz, Gail Carpenter, John Carpenter, Karen Meryash, Brett Butler, Sherry Goldman, Judi Hirshfield Bartek, and Barbara Kalinowski.

Within the orchestra there are always the soloists: my wonderful agent Jill Kneerim who is always ready to hear my latest greatest new idea. Karen Lindsey who has worked on all my books with me, knows just how to capture my voice and just when to say "Huh? What does that mean?. . . ." Her patience and diligence are overwhelming. Marcia Williams has also worked on all three editions, brilliantly translating my ideas into concrete illustrations that add much to the book's accessibility. Connie Long who has been my right hand person and office goddess for seven years is also an essential part of this volume and the soloist team. From Perseus there is my terrific editor Merloyd Lawrence and the wonderful managing editor Chris Coffin, as well as Elizabeth Carduff and Lissa Warren, who worked on getting the word out. The newcomer John Carter has done a fantastic job in organizing the book tour and keeping all the stakeholders happy.

Finally there is my family. Helen Sperry Cooksey is still the love of my life after 18 years. Katie, our twelve year old, keeps saying: "If you hate writing a book so much why do you keep doing more of them?" I hope the process doesn't scare her from sharing her own prodigious literary talents as she gets older. Brownie, our faithful cocker spaniel, sits patiently at my feet well into the night keeping watch and listening carefully to all my rambling.

I am honored to have so much help. And I am especially humbled by all the women with breast cancer and their families who have found this book useful over the years. It is a true honor to be able to help you understand a bit better what happens to this organ called the breast.

Introduction
to the Third Edition

It has been a decade since the first edition of *Dr. Susan Love's Breast Book* was published. The major theme of this third edition is that all of medicine and science, and especially the study of the breast, is a work-in-progress. At any stage, we are only making our best guess at that moment, and because of the enormous amount of research going on, we are likely to have a new guess soon. Very often we present new data as if they were the whole answer, when they're actually only a piece of the puzzle—and we can't even be sure how important a piece. It's like the fable of the blind men describing an elephant. One was examining its tail and said triumphantly: "An elephant is long and stringy." The second, feeling around the trunk, said, "What do you mean? It's a long cylindrical animal with hot air coming out of its center." The third, who had grasped the foot, said, "You're both crazy! It has a tough rubbery exterior with hard bones inside." All were correct, and yet, since none of them had the whole picture, they were also all incorrect.

In medicine, we are often describing very accurately one hair in the elephant's tail. This is very useful when we understand what it is that we have—one piece of information that can help lead us to the next piece. The problem comes when we try to extrapolate a description of the whole animal from the one hair. As long as we keep collecting observations and trying to figure out breast cancer, we will have new approaches and new theories. Someday we will have figured out the whole animal.

The most exciting news in the field, and thus in this book, is the shift in science's approach to breast cancer. We are moving from an emphasis on diagnosing an existing tumor toward an ability to predict who is likely to get breast cancer, and thus to prevention. Ductal lavage and the intraductal approach to the disease are real breakthroughs for the study of the earliest signs of oncoming breast cancer, and promise to revolutionize the way we approach this disease. The usefulness of such techniques is magnified because we now have proven means of risk reduction—in tamoxifen and prophylactic mastectomy—and other prevention forms are on the way. We are finally going beyond imaging techniques like mammography that show the presence of an already existing cancer and into techniques that find what is happening in the cells where cancer might be likely to begin.

The other big shift is in our approach to treatment. We have always talked about breast cancer in militaristic words—the "war on cancer," "she lost her battle with cancer." This comes from approaching cancer as if it were a foreign invader attacking a woman's body, and our job is to kill every last cancer cell. Surgery, radiation therapy, and chemotherapy, (slash, burn and poison) are very crude treatments, attempts to blast away cancer cells while hoping we don't kill too many healthy cells in the process. But, in reality, cancer cells aren't foreign invaders; they're your own cells. They've gone crazy and lost their regulatory controls, and we've begun to understand that it's possible to create new regulatory controls, alter the environment around the cells, and thus change their behavior.

Mina Bissel, a researcher in Berkeley, California, has done studies in which she has taken cells that have the mutations of cancer, grown them on normal breast tissue, and found that they behave normally. This, as well as the concept of tumor dormancy (the behavior of a cancer cell that exists peacefully in the body), leads us to believe that we don't always have to kill cancer cells. At least in some cases controlling them or reversing them may be better.

This new approach has in many cases led us away from high-dose chemotherapy to hormones. In this approach we have come full circle. The earliest systemic treatment for breast cancer was oophorectomy (removal of the ovaries); now, after a chemotherapy diversion, we are back on that track, at least for certain types of tumors. Furthermore, we're starting to go beyond one-size-fits-all treatment to targeted therapy aimed at correcting the key defects in that particular cancer cell.

In this third edition we have once again altered almost every chap-

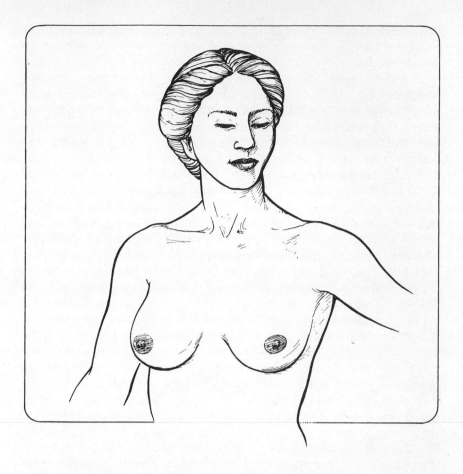

ter. In fact, we have even changed the anatomy chapter. In the introduction to the second edition I wrote, "The only chapter that remains untouched is Chapter 1 on anatomy. (The breast, I'm glad to report, is still located on the chest!)" Well, the breast hasn't relocated, but our understanding of its internal workings turns out to be far more important than we ever realized. New studies on the ductal systems, which we present in Chapter 17 on the intraductal approach, hold great promise for the approach to early diagnosis and treatment. We are learning to think medically not of two breasts, but of two sets of between six and nine ductal systems.

The identification of BRCA1 and 2 and the ability to test for mutations have made progress since the last edition. The state of cells known as *atypical hyperplasia* has taken on new importance as a potentially reversible precancerous condition. The possibility of prevention has grown with the recent reports that the hormone tamoxifen can re-duce the risk in women with a strong chance of getting breast cancer. This is just the first of many such developments.

Many of the new therapies are based on the genetics and molecular biology of the cell. We have included a whole chapter on molecular biology for those who want a deeper understanding of what this means. With access to the ductal cells in high-risk women, I predict that by the fourth edition we will have the genetic defects that lead to breast cancer worked out fairly well.

Treatments too have changed. We now have less-invasive biopsies, the sentinel node biopsy to augment or replace the removal of many lymph nodes under the arm, and skin-sparing mastectomies. We have better kinds of radiation and new chemotherapy drugs such as Tax-otere and Taxol. We have many more hormonal approaches to the dis-ease, and many more options for women with metastatic disease.

All these new technologies have allowed more women with breast cancer to survive, and even women with metastatic disease are living longer than before. So we are finally paying more attention to the *quality* of life after breast cancer. Although the studies reported here on symptoms such as bone loss and fuzzy thinking caused by chemother-apy are preliminary, there is a great deal of interest in what our treat-ments do to the quality of women's lives. One of the major side effects of chemotherapy is that it can throw women into premature meno-pause, adding further stress and confusion to the physical and emo-tional devastation of the disease itself. For these women, as well as for those healthy menopausal women who are nervous about the dangers of prolonged hormone therapy use, we have added a whole chapter on menopause and its symptoms. The politics of breast cancer, nonexis-tent at the time of the first edition of the book, has at least partially moved into the mainstream, while bone marrow transplant, a great hope at the time of the second edition, has proved a disappointment. The changes are constant as we try to describe more and more parts of our elephant. Although my new website (www.SusanLoveMD.com) can help you keep up with them, it is important to pause and capture where we are in a book. Our dreams for the eradication of breast can-cer remain alive and well. We think we are closer than ever before. We can only keep working, in the labs, in the clinics, and politically, so that this particular work-in-progress will reach a conclusion.

PART ONE

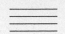

THE HEALTHY BREAST

1

The Breast and Its
Development

Few women know what "normal" breasts look like. Most of us haven't seen many other women's breasts, and since childhood we've been exposed to the "ideal" image of breasts that permeates our society. But few of us fit that image, and there's no reason why we should. The actual range of size and shape of breasts is so wide that it's hard to say what's "normal." Not only are there very large and very small breasts, but in most women one breast is slightly larger than the other. Breast size is genetically determined—depending chiefly on the percentage of fat to other tissue in the breasts. Usually about a third of the breast is composed of fat tissue; the rest is breast tissue. The amount of fat varies as you gain or lose weight; the amount of breast tissue remains constant. A "flat-chested" woman's breasts will grow as she gains weight, just as her stomach and thighs do; if she loses that weight, she'll also lose her larger breasts.

Breast size has nothing to do with capacity to make milk, or with vulnerability to cancer or other breast disease. Very large breasts, however, can be physically uncomfortable, and, like very small or very uneven breasts, they can be emotionally uncomfortable as well. We'll discuss this at length in Chapter 4.

Usually the breast itself is tear-shaped (Fig. 1-1). There's breast

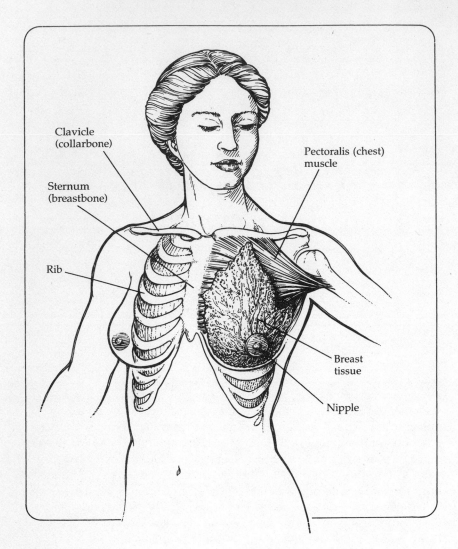

Clavicle
(collarbone)

Sternum
(breastbone)

Rib

Pectoralis (chest)
muscle

Breast
tissue

Nipple

FIGURE 1-1

tissue from the collarbone all the way down to the last few ribs, and from the breastbone in the middle of the chest to the back of the armpit. Most of the breast tissue is toward the armpit and upper breast, while the fat is chiefly in the middle and lower part of the breast. Your ribs lie behind the breast, and sometimes they can feel hard and lumpy. When I was in medical school I embarrassed myself horribly when I found a "lump" in my breast, and frantically ran to one of the older doctors to find out if I had cancer. I found out I had a rib.

Often there's a ridge of fat at the bottom of the breast—the *infra-mammary ridge.* This ridge is perfectly normal. Because we walk upright, our breasts fold over themselves, creating the ridge of fat.

The *areola* is the darker area of the breast surrounding the nipple (Fig. 1-2). Its size and shape vary from woman to woman, and its color varies according to complexion. In blondes it tends to be pink, in brunettes it's browner, and in dark-skinned people it's brown to black. In most women it gets darker after the first pregnancy. Its color also changes during the various stages of sexual arousal and orgasm.

Many women find their nipples don't face front; they stick out slightly toward the armpits. There's a reason for this. Picture yourself holding a baby you're about to nurse. The baby's head is held in the crook of your arm—a nipple pointing to the side is comfortably close to the baby's mouth (Fig. 1-3).

There are hair follicles around the nipple, so most women have at least some nipple hair. It's perfectly natural, but if you don't like it, don't worry. You can shave it off, pluck it out, use electrolysis, or get rid of it any sensible way you want—it's just like leg or armpit hair. And, as with leg or armpit hair, if it doesn't bother you, you can just ignore it. You may also notice little bumps around the areola that look like goose pimples. They're little glands known as *Montgomery's glands.* The nipple also has sebaceous glands, which I talk about later on in this chapter.

Sometimes nipples are "shy": when they're stimulated they retreat into themselves and become temporarily inverted. This is nothing to worry about; it has no effect on milk supply, breast feeding, sexual

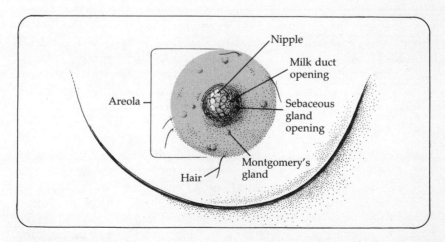

Nipple

Milk duct opening

Areola —

Sebaceous gland opening

Montgomery's gland

Hair

FIGURE 1-2

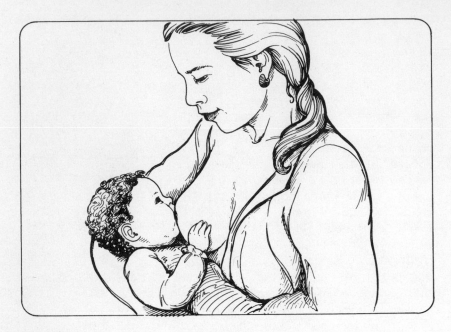

FIGURE 1-3

pleasure, or anything else. (Permanently inverted nipples are discussed in Chapters 4 and 5.)

Inside, as I noted before, the breast is made up primarily of fat and breast tissue (Fig. 1-4). The breast tissue is sandwiched between layers of fat, behind which is the chest muscle. The fat has some give to it, which is why we bounce. The breast tissue is firm and rubbery. One of my patients told me while I was operating on her that she thought the breast was constructed like a woman—soft and pliant on the outside, and tough underneath. The breast also has its share of the connective tissue that holds the entire body together. This material creates a solid structure—like gelatin—in which the other kinds of tissues are loosely set.

Like the rest of the body the breast has arteries, veins, and nerves. As you probably know, the arteries carry blood rich with oxygen and fuel to the cells, while the veins carry the depleted blood full of carbon dioxide back to the lungs. What you may not know is that there is another, almost parallel, network of vessels called the lymphatic system, or *lymphatics*. These vessels are like recyclers. They collect the garbage from the cells and strain it through the lymph nodes found scattered in nests throughout the body; they then send the filtered fluid back into the bloodstream to be reused (Fig. 1-5). They do more than just recycle, however. In the process of filtering the discarded fluid, they register

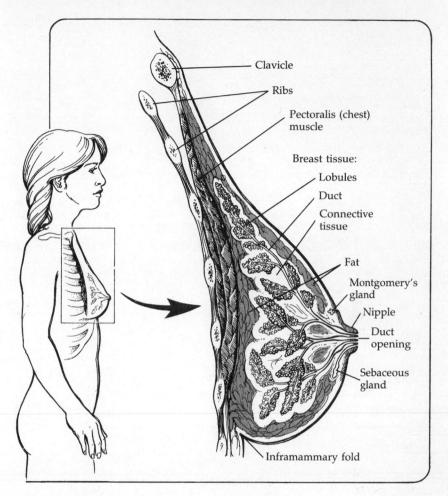

FIGURE 1-4

what is in it. If there is anything threatening—a bacterial cell, a piece of suture material, or a virus—they hold on to it and use it to develop an immune response. They send cells to the site to identify the invader and make antibodies to combat it. This is the reason the lymph nodes are important when we talk about breast cancer later in the book. It is crucial to identify which lymphatic and which lymph node is draining a particular area of the breast so that the correct lymph nodes can be removed and examined for signs of cancer.

There's very little muscle in the breast. There's a bit of muscle in the areola, which is why it contracts and stands out with cold, sexual stimulation, and, of course, breast feeding. This too makes sense: if the nipple stands out, it's easier for the baby's mouth to get a good grip on

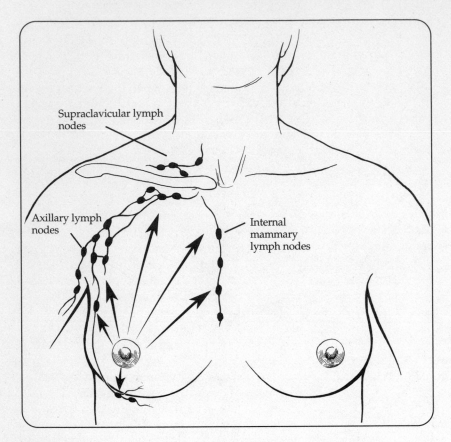

FIGURE 1-5

it. There are also tiny muscles around the lobules that help deliver milk, as we will discuss in Chapter 3. But the major muscle in the area is behind the breasts—the pectorals. Because of this, the idea that you can grow larger breasts through exercise is false. You can grow stronger pectorals—like bodybuilders do—but all that means is that your breasts will rest on an expanded chest.

THE DUCTAL ANATOMY

All of this structure is really there to surround and support the critical ductal system. Although the ducts and lobules are the main "business" part of the breast, their anatomy has largely been ignored.

Years ago, when I began my own research, I was amazed to find how little information there was on the milk ducts—how many there were, where they were, which little holes in the nipple were ducts and which weren't. The only study I could find was done in 1839, by Sir Astley Cooper.[1] Experimenting on cadavers, he injected soft wax into the ducts through the nipple, and made casts when the wax hardened. He discovered that the ducts did not connect to one another, that there were separate ductal systems. Though he mentioned that the nipple contained between 15 and 20 holes, he found that he could only get into between five and eight milk duct openings.

From then on all the textbooks dutifully reported that there were 15 to 20 ductal systems. No one followed up on Dr. Cooper's research, and no one thought to investigate the issue further.

So I began to explore the possibility of an intraductal approach to the detection of precancerous cells (see Chapter 17). I had to start at the beginning. My team and I tried to figure out an easy way to determine how many holes there were in the nipple. One of my research assistants, Jean Chou, came up with a wonderful idea: we could undoubtedly see the ductal openings best when women were breast-feeding, so why not go to meetings of La Leche League? This organization promotes breast feeding, and with their help Jean was able to examine the women who were breast-feeding and map the holes in the nipple that were squirting milk.

She examined the breasts of 219 amiable women who had agreed to have their breasts catalogued by a stranger. Examining both breasts, she mapped out the openings. She found that there were about six to eight, arranged in a fairly consistent pattern. It's possible that she missed a few. If you've ever breast-fed, you know that once the milk starts coming out, it's like a watering can—and of course it immediately becomes one big blob of milk on your nipple. Still, if she was undercounting, it was probably by two or three, not by 10 or more.

Usually, we learned, there are two or three milk duct orifices in the center of the nipples, with others scattered around them (Fig. 1-6). The middle ones were consistent in all the women we examined. The number and placement of the openings around the periphery tended to be more variable: one woman might have three on the outside, and another, five. However, they never varied in an individual woman: if she had three in her left breast, she had three in her right breast.

What, then, were those other holes that Dr. Cooper found back in 1839—the ones that everybody's been calling "ducts" ever since? They're little glands that make a sebaceous material—a white, oily, cheesy substance. These *sebaceous glands* are found all over the body. We don't know what they're for, or why there are so many around the nipple. My own theory is that the body produces them to provide a coating and protection for the skin—sort of your own little skin-care

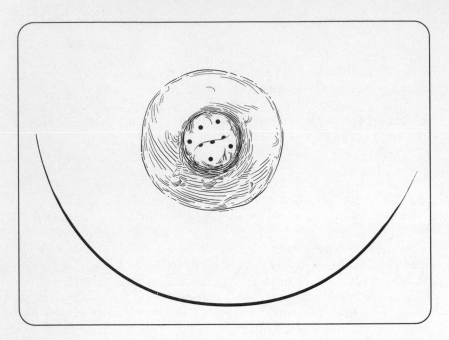

FIGURE 1-6

system. The nipple, designed to be sucked on, is especially vulnerable to getting chapped and sore, so it makes sense that it would have a lot of these glands.

We then explored the anatomy beyond the nipple by studying cadavers and breasts that had been removed by mastectomy. We learned that the duct opening in the nipple leads into the breast in a straight line for a very short distance—only about a centimeter. It has a small amount of keratin—dead skin—that forms a kind of plug. There's a little sphincter muscle here that prevents a breast-feeding woman from having milk spill out when she's not actually in the process of feeding her baby. Behind that is a little antechamber called the *lactiferous sinus*. From there, the ductal system, like a tree, breaks up into little branches, which go all the way to the back of the breast. These branches are the ducts. Leafing out at the end of each branch are the lobules, which make the breast milk and then send it through the ducts to the nipple. Each ductal system is independent of all the others; each creates milk separately. They coexist, but they don't connect with one another.

We explored the pattern of the ducts themselves. In the '70s and '80s Dr. Otto Sartorius, a breast surgeon in Santa Barbara, did many ductograms—a procedure in which he put a tiny catheter into a woman's nipple, ran dye through it, then took x rays. He did about 2,000 of these

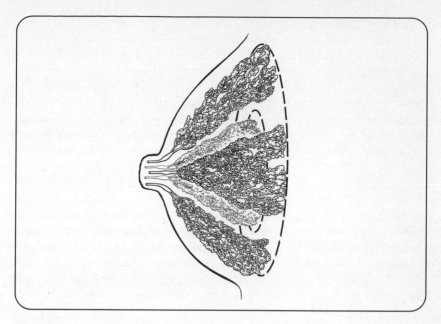

FIGURE 1-7

procedures. When he died in 1994 I inherited these x rays and continued his work. My research team and I analyzed the x rays, which gave us a good idea of where ducts tended to be within the breast. We discovered a few surprises. Until now, we've visualized the breast as though it were pie-shaped. Finally, the obvious occurred to us— the breast isn't two-dimensional! Anatomy exists in three dimensions, though it appears two-dimensional in photographs and x-ray images. The breast is in reality shaped more like a giant gumdrop. What this means is that the ductal systems go from the nipple toward the chest wall (Fig. 1-7). One system might cover the whole upper part of the breast, or perhaps two or three ducts cover that area. In addition, the ductal systems run throughout the breast, often as far up as the collarbone or as far down as the lower ribs. Our x-ray studies of the ducts matched the findings from La Leche League, even though they involved different patients. Medically, then, it may be that we should be thinking not of a breast, but of six to nine ductal systems.

HOW THE BREAST DEVELOPS

To understand how the breast typically develops, we need to know what it's for. The breast is an integral part of a woman's reproductive

11

system. It actually defines our biological class: mammals derive their name from the fact that they have mammary glands, and feed their young at their breasts. Different mammals have different numbers and sizes of breasts, but the most interesting, and probably the most significant, difference between human females and the other mammals is that we're the only ones to develop full breasts long before they're needed to feed our young. Humans are also the only animals who are actively sexual when we're not fertile. This suggests that our breasts have an important secondary function as contributors to our sensual pleasure.

It's also worth noting that although women have traditionally been thought of as "other" (to use Simone de Beauvoir's word) in our male-dominated culture, biologically we're the norm. The genitalia of all embryos are female. When the hormone testosterone is produced at the direction of the Y chromosome, the fetus starts to develop male genitalia. If the testes are destroyed early in fetal development, the male fetus will develop breasts and retain female genitalia. It makes sense to ask whether the basis of "mankind" is, in fact, woman.

Early Development

Human breast tissue begins to develop remarkably early—in the sixth week of fetal life. It develops across a line known as the *milk ridge,* which runs from the armpit all the way down to the groin (Fig. 1-8). In most cases the milk ridge soon regresses, and by the ninth week it's just in the chest area. (Other mammals retain the milk ridge, which is why they have multiple nipples.) So you already have breast tissue at birth, and it's sensitive to hormones even then (your mother's sex hormones have been circulating through her placenta). Infants may even have nipple discharge. This "witch's milk," as it's called, goes away in a couple of weeks, because the infant is no longer getting the mother's hormones. Between 80 and 90 percent of all infants of both genders have this discharge on the second or third day after birth.

Dr. Nicholas Petrakis, a researcher in San Francisco, has been studying infants' breast tissue.[2] He is looking at the possibility that it's a sign of how much estrogen the fetus is exposed to *in utero.* With a group of women in mainland China and a group in San Francisco, he is comparing the amount of breast tissue in babies in the neonatal nurseries, to see if the exposure that leads to cancer actually begins in the mother's uterus. There is a very low incidence of breast cancer in mainland China, a very high incidence among white women in San Francisco, and a moderate incidence among Chinese women who have migrated

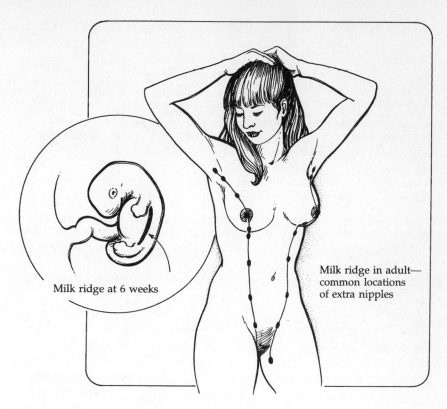

Milk ridge at 6 weeks

Milk ridge in adult—
common locations
of extra nipples

FIGURE 1-8

to San Francisco. If indeed it proves that the babies of the women in China have less breast tissue, it could be an early tip-off about those infants who might be at higher risk as they grow older.

If your baby has a lot of breast tissue, however, don't panic. Dr. Petrakis himself isn't even sure his theory is correct: it's simply an area worth studying. Even if he finds a big difference in the amount of breast tissue that has witch's milk, it wouldn't prove a correlation with cancer. It would simply mean this warrants further study. In any case, many other factors are involved.

Puberty

After early infancy, not much happens to the breast until puberty (Fig. 1-9). Then the ductal tissue begins to grow and create the beginnings of

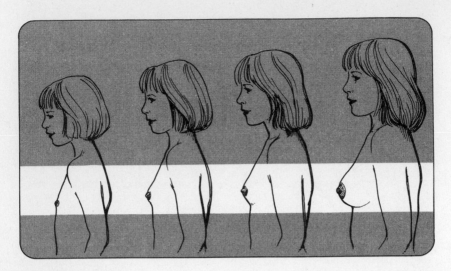

FIGURE 1-9

ducts. Though they aren't yet capable of making milk, the general out-line of the ductal system is there. The cells that make this happen are called *stem cells*—cells capable of turning into other cells. They're sort of great-grandmother progenitor cells that can become a lot of things. The stem cells can become duct cells or lobular cells growing along the ductile system.

Soon after the pubic hair begins to grow, the breasts start respond-ing to the hormonal changes in the girl's body. (Typically, her period won't start until a year or two after her breasts have begun growing.) They begin with a little bud of breast tissue under the nipple—it can be itchy, and sometimes a bit painful. The rudimentary ducts begin to grow, and the breasts expand more and more until they've reached their full growth—usually by the time menstruation begins. One little girl quoted in *Breasts,* a book of photos and text about women's rela-tionship to their breasts, described it beautifully: "At first they were flat, then all of a sudden the nipples came out like mosquito bites. And three or four days ago I noticed that my breasts were coming out from the sides. When I first started they were just little lumps by the nipple."[3]

The first tiny breasts can be confusing to children, and to their par-ents as well. One of my patients was an 11-year-old girl whose mother had breast cancer, and they found what they were sure was a lump un-der the girl's nipple. I was certain it was just the beginning of her breast development, but everyone, including the child, was so upset I did a needle aspiration just to reassure them. It's never advisable in a situation like that to remove this newly forming breast tissue, since it won't grow back, and the child will never have that breast.

The rate at which breasts grow varies greatly from girl to girl; some start off very "flat-chested" and end up with large breasts; others have large breasts at an early age. Often one breast grows more quickly than the other. (We'll discuss this and other variations in breast development in Chapter 4.)

The emotional confusion around all of puberty can be intensified for the girl growing up in a society that both mystifies and obsesses about breasts. For the adolescent girl, the growth of her breasts can be a source of extreme pleasure or extreme dismay—and often both at once. In a 1980 British survey researchers learned that 56 percent of the women they questioned had been pleased with their breast development, while 33 percent were shy and 24 percent, embarrassed. Ten percent had been "worried" or "unhappy."[4] I did an informal survey among my own patients, with similar results. Of 165 patients who filled out a questionnaire in my office, 70 recalled having been happy or proud of their budding breasts; 61 had been embarrassed and angry; 20, confused; and 9, ambivalent. One had been "amazed." Not surprisingly, only four were "indifferent."

I also talked with a number of my patients about their memories of how they felt when their breasts began to develop. Again, I found a range of feelings. Two of my youngest patients had opposite reactions to their breasts' growth. One, 13, said that when her breasts began to grow, "I felt older and I felt mature, that I was becoming a woman." She was proud of her new breasts: "I think that for my age, my boobs are just right," she said. But a 16-year-old patient told me she was embarrassed when her breasts began to grow, because she "always felt as if people were staring at me and talking about me." She didn't like her breasts, which she saw as "too hard and lumpy, and triangular, not round."

Similar differences of attitude appeared in the recollections of my older patients. One 48-year-old recalled the first day she wore her bra to school: "I was so proud—I was the second girl in the sixth grade to have one. All the other girls gathered around me and I showed them my bra." A 44-year-old remembered "anticipating with joy and awe that my body was changing, and the blossoming of my breasts was such a delightful, exciting period for me. I was becoming a woman!" Others were less delighted. A 39-year-old remembered thinking, "Oh, shit, now I'm supposed to be a girl!" To her, developing breasts represented confusion and "the world getting much worse." Another, 45, hated her new breasts so much that she would fantasize about ways "to cut them off with my grandmother's long, thin embroidery scissors." She was ashamed of them, and angry at her mother for making her drink milk, which she was convinced had caused her breasts to grow. A 65-year-old patient said that she hadn't been "ready for this sign of growing up. It was like going down a roller coaster and not being able to stop it." A middle-aged mother recalled that for many years she wore overlarge sweaters to hide the breasts that embarrassed her. "My teenage daughter does the same thing now," she said, "and it makes me a bit sad to remember that stage of my life." For many women, breasts represented enforced femininity: they could no longer play ball with the boys, and felt they had lost forever a kind of freedom little boys still had.

On the other hand, a delay in the appearance of breasts can be equally upsetting. One of my friends, whose breasts didn't begin developing until her midteens, recalled her feelings of inadequacy. "I was so upset," she said. "My grandmother had told me that I'd get breasts if I rubbed cocoa butter on my chest. So for months, every night, before I went to sleep, I rubbed cocoa butter on my flat little chest, hoping I'd wake up with breasts."

Sometimes, because of their hormonal development, adolescent boys develop a condition called *gynecomastia*—which translates to "breasts like a woman." For obvious reasons, the boys' reactions don't parallel the ambivalence of the developing girls—for them, breast development is uniformly embarrassing. I remember my seventh-grade boyfriend was so humiliated by it that he paid another boy to push him into the swimming pool: that way, he didn't have to take off his shirt to swim, and didn't have to explain to the other kids why he was swimming with his shirt on. I occasionally have had patients suffering from gynecomastia, and their mental anguish, as well as their acute embarrassment at having to show me their chests, is really painful to see. Fortunately the condition usually regresses on its own in about 18 months; if it doesn't, it can easily be helped through surgery.

The Menstruating Years

A girl's initial breast development is soon followed by the establishment of the menstrual cycle as her body begins to prepare for reproduction. Hormones play a crucial part in this development, as they do in all aspects of reproductive growth. On the ovary are follicles with eggs encased in their developmental sacs (Fig. 1-10). These, stimulated by FSH (follicle stimulating hormone) in the pituitary gland, produce estrogen. The resulting high levels of estrogen in the blood tell the pituitary to turn off the FSH and start secreting LH (luteinizing hormone). When the estrogen and LH are both at their peak, you *ovulate*— the follicle bursts and releases its egg into the fallopian tube.

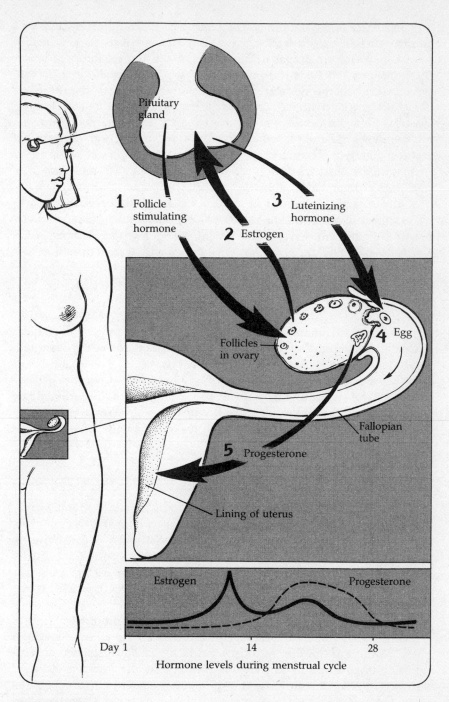

FIGURE 1-10

The follicle is now an empty sac, but it still has a job to do: it becomes what is known as the *corpus luteum,* and it starts producing *progesterone,* which prepares the lining of the uterus for pregnancy ("progesterone" means "pro-pregnancy"). Normally, the egg *doesn't* get fertilized: the progesterone level falls off, the lining of the uterus is shed, and you start all over again. If the egg *is* fertilized, it starts to produce HCG (human choriogonadotropin), which maintains the progesterone level until the placenta takes over the production, and you're well on your way to a baby.

In addition to maintaining fertility, these cyclical hormones are preparing the breast for a potential pregnancy each month. In a very general sense, estrogen causes the increase of ductal tissue in the breast, and progesterone causes the increase in lobular tissue. This obviously has something to do with the cyclical changes women's breasts go through—swelling, pain, tenderness—but exactly how it does it is still unclear.

Breast Feeding

Breast feeding, as I've mentioned before, is what the breast is designed for. In a purely technical sense, your breast isn't fully mature until—or unless—you've given birth and your body has begun to produce milk. The breasts of women who do not give birth remain in the earlier stage of development until menopause. Because breast feeding is so complex, and so central, I've given it a chapter of its own (Chapter 3).

Menopause

We've got the menstruating years figured out, but our understanding of the process is a little fuzzier when we come to the end of the fertile years. The standard line in the textbooks is that when you run out of eggs and you're no longer ovulating, your body stops making estrogen. This causes your FSH to go up as your pituitary tries to kickstart the ovary into producing more eggs. When that doesn't work, everything just shuts down.

Yet often the symptoms of perimenopause (right before menopause)—breast tenderness, headaches, increased vaginal lubrication—are not symptoms of low estrogen, but rather of *high* estrogen. Sometimes your estrogen levels are high and your progesterone is low, and you might get symptoms of PMS (premenstrual syndrome), while other times your estrogen levels shift and you get hot flashes. Then for several months you're back to normal. So the common explanation is wrong: your symptoms aren't due to low estrogen. They're caused by *fluctuations* of high and low estrogen.

Sometimes doctors test FSH levels in the blood to decide whether you are in menopause. The problem is that just as estrogen and progesterone fluctuate widely so does FSH. It could be high at one time and low a month later. If you've stopped menstruating for several months, the FSH tests might be a little more useful for determining if you've really gone into menopause. But even then, it's not 100 percent accurate. One study found that 20 percent of women who had had no period for three months started having their cycles again.[5] I've had patients with breast cancer who were thrown into menopause by their chemotherapy treatments, missed three or four months of periods, showed high FSH levels—and then got their periods back. There's no foolproof test to determine menopause. The only way we can really do that is the good old-fashioned way. If you haven't menstruated for a year, you're menopausal.

BIOLOGY OF MENOPAUSE:
THE MISUNDERSTOOD OVARY

Throughout most of medical history we have never really understood the ovary. And because we haven't grasped the full complexity of this intricate organ, doctors have assumed that after menopause, when it is no longer capable of making eggs, the ovary shrivels up, dries out, and becomes completely useless.

But egg making isn't the ovary's whole function any more than reproduction is a woman's whole function. The ovary is more than just an egg sack. It's an endocrine organ—one that produces hormones. And it produces them before, during, and after menopause. With menopause, the ovary goes through a shift. It changes from a follicle-rich producer of estrogen and progesterone into a stromal-rich producer of estrogen and androgen (a male hormone). Stroma is the glue that holds all the eggs together. In youth, you have more eggs and less stroma. As time goes on, you have fewer and fewer eggs and more and more stroma. In its hormonal dance with the hypothalamus and pituitary, the postmenopausal ovary continues to respond to the call of the pituitary. It responds to the high levels of FSH and LH with increased production of testosterone as well as lower levels of estrone and estradiol (two forms of estrogen) and androstenedione (a male hormone).[6,7] The hormonal dance doesn't end: the band just strikes up a different tune.

Testosterone, of course, is a male hormone. But don't panic: you're not going to grow a beard. Every human being produces both male and female hormones; the proportion differs according to gender. Much of the testosterone and androstenedione is converted to estrone by fat and muscle. This continued production of hormones varies somewhat from one woman to the next and may well explain some of the individual differences in symptoms after menopause. It also explains why women who have both ovaries removed surgically, losing all of these hormones, have worse symptoms of menopause, and increased vulnerability to cardiovascular disease and osteoporosis.[8]

What all this means is that the ovaries have more than one function. Reproduction is their most dramatic function, but it isn't the only one. These organs have as much to do with the maintenance of the woman's own life as they do with her role in bringing other lives

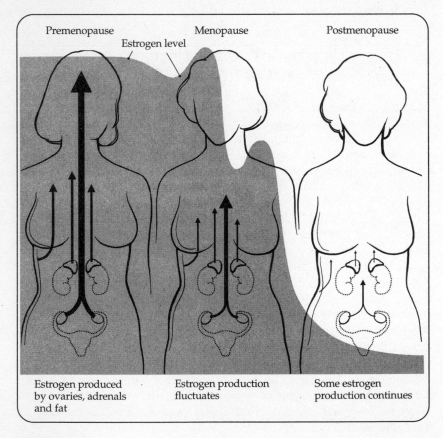

FIGURE 1-11

into the world. The menopausal ovary is neither failing nor useless. It's simply beginning to shift from its reproductive to its maintenance function. It's doing in midlife exactly what many people do—it's changing careers.

As we learn more about the levels of hormones in women after menopause we begin to understand their effects on the breast. We have observed, for example, that women with osteoporosis have 60 percent less breast cancer than women with normal bone density. This is undoubtedly due to natural estrogen levels. If you have relatively high levels of estrogen in your body postmenopausally you will have good bones and bad breasts; on the other hand, if your own estrogen levels are lower you will have good breasts and bad bones.

The postmenopausal breast is even more complex. Giving women hormones postmenopausally increases estrogen (and usually progestins), resulting in hormone sensitive tumors (see Chapter 20). Yet not every woman who takes postmenopausal hormones gets breast cancer. Also, women on postmenopausal hormones often, but not always, experience an increase in breast density, known to be a risk factor for breast cancer (see Chapter 6). It is likely that some women are more sensitive to postmenopausal hormones than others. Which ones and why is a subject of much research. In addition, recent studies have shown that breast tissue itself has the enzyme *aromatase*, which can convert testosterone and androstenedione into estrogen. This means that estrogen levels in the breast may indeed be higher than those in the rest of the body after menopause and may explain the estrogen sensitive cancers that occur at this age. Our increasing understanding of the postmenopausal breast's response to hormones will give us insight into the cause of breast cancer after menopause.

BRAS

In our society breasts and their coverings have become almost a fetish. The bra is a relatively recent invention—it became popular in the 1920s. As a replacement for the uncomfortable and often mutilating corsets of the 19th century, it was certainly an improvement. However, while wearing a bra is never physically harmful, it has no medical necessity whatsoever. Many of my large-breasted patients have found it more comfortable to wear a bra, especially if they run or engage in other athletic activities. As one of my large-breasted patients said, "These babies need all the support they can get!"

Many women, however, find bras uncomfortable. Interestingly, I had one patient who got a rash underneath her breasts when she didn't wear a bra and her breasts sagged, and another who had very sensitive skin and got a rash when she *did* wear a bra, because of the elastic, the stitching, and the metal hooks (she switched to camisoles). Except for the women who find bras especially comfortable or uncomfortable, the decision to wear or not wear one is purely aesthetic—or emotional.

For some women, bras are a necessity created by society. One of my patients told me she enjoyed going without a bra, but, she said, "Men made nasty and degrading comments as I walked down the street." Another patient, a high school teacher, felt obligated to wear a bra, although she described it as "a ritual object, like a dog collar. . . . I take it off immediately after work."

But to other women bras can be enjoyable. Some of my patients like the uplift and the different contours a bra provides. A woman quoted in *Breasts* said she was "crazy about bras—I think of them as jewelry."[9] She and others find them sexy and enjoy incorporating them into their lovemaking rituals.

A mistaken popular belief maintains that wearing a bra strengthens your breasts and prevents sagging. But you sag because of the proportion of fat and tissue in your breasts, and no bra changes that. Furthermore, breast feeding and lactation increase the breast size (see Chapter 3), and when the breast tissue returns to its normal size the skin is still stretched out and saggy. As I noted earlier, except for the small muscles of the areola and lobules, the only breast muscles are behind your breast—muscles that will not be affected by whether or not you wear a bra. If you've been wearing a bra regularly and decide to give it up, you may find that your breasts hurt for a while. Don't be alarmed. The connective tissue in which the ducts and lobules are suspended is suddenly being strained. It's the same tissue that hurts when you jog or run. Once your body adjusts to not wearing a bra, the pain will go away.

No type of bra is better or worse for you in terms of health. Some of my patients who wear underwire bras have been told they can get cancer from them. This is total nonsense. It makes no difference medically whether your bra opens in the front or back, is padded or not padded, is made of nylon, cotton, or anything else, or gives much support or little support. The only time when I would recommend a bra for medical reasons is after any kind of surgery on the breasts. Then the pull from a hanging breast can cause more pain, slow the healing of the wound, and create larger scars. For this purpose, I recommend a firmer rather than a lighter bra.

Otherwise, if you enjoy a bra for aesthetic, sexual, or comfort reasons, by all means wear one. If you don't enjoy it, and job or social pressures don't force you into it, don't bother. Medically, it's all the same.

BREAST SENSITIVITY

Breasts are usually very sensitive—as you'll notice if you get hit in the breasts. It's very painful, but if you've been told being injured in the breast leads to cancer, ignore it. All a bruised breast causes is temporary pain. Similarly, scar tissue that results from an injury to the breast won't cause cancer. The supposed fragility of women's breasts has been used as an excuse to keep girls from playing contact sports. Interestingly, however, the extreme sensitivity of testicles is rarely used to keep men from such sports. Your own pain threshold, plus your enthusiasm for the particular game, should determine whether or not you want to avoid risking pain by playing. A bruised breast will hurt, but so will a bruised shin.

The sensitivity of the breast changes within the menstrual cycle. During the first two weeks of the cycle it's less sensitive; it's very sensitive around ovulation and after, and it's less sensitive again during menstruation.[10] There are also changes during the larger development process. There's little sensitivity before puberty, much sensitivity after puberty, and extreme sensitivity during pregnancy and perimenopause. After menopause, the sensitivity decreases slightly, but never fully vanishes. As in most aspects of the normal breast, sensitivity varies greatly among women. There's no "right" or "healthy" degree of responsiveness.

Breasts also vary greatly in their sensitivity to sexual stimuli. Physiologic changes in the breasts are an integral part of female sexual response. In the excitement phase the nipples harden and become more erect, the breasts plump up, and the areola swells. In the plateau just before orgasm breasts, nipples, and areola get larger still, peaking with the orgasm and then gradually subsiding. For most women, breast stimulation contributes to sexual pleasure. Many enjoy having their breasts stroked or sucked by their lovers, but have been told that this can lead to cancer. It can't. Breasts, after all, are made to be suckled, and your body won't punish you because it's a lover rather than a baby doing it. Some women's breasts are so erogenous that breast stimulation alone can bring them to orgasm; others find breast stimulation uninteresting or even unpleasant. Neither extreme is more "normal": as we know, different people have different sexual needs and respond to different sexual stimuli. Patients ask me whether their lack of sexual excitement around their breasts means something is wrong with them. It doesn't. There is an unfortunate tradition in our culture to label as "frigid" women whose sexual needs don't correspond to those of their (usually) male partners. Ironically, the converse of this still persists in our supposedly liberated era: a woman who is easily sexually stimulated is seen as a "tramp." All such stereotypes are unfortunate and destructive. If your breasts contribute to your sexual pleasure, enjoy it. If not, enjoy what you do like, and don't worry about it.

LUMPINESS

Lumpy breasts have inspired some of the most unfortunate misconceptions about our bodies. Women have been told their lumpy breasts are symptoms of "fibrocystic disease" (see Chapter 6) and have suffered from needless anxiety, fear, and even at times disfiguring surgery.

Lumpy breasts are caused simply by the way the breast tissue forms itself. In some women the breast tissue is fairly fine and thus not perceived as "lumpy." Others clearly have lumpy breasts, which can feel somewhat like cobblestone paving. Still others are somewhere between the extremes—just a bit nodular. There's nothing at all unusual about this—breasts vary as much as any other part of the body. Some women are tall and some short; some women are fair-skinned and some dark; some women have lumpier breasts and some have smoother breasts. There can also be differences within the same woman's breasts. Your breasts might be a little more nodular near your armpit, or at the top, for example, and the pattern may be the same on both breasts, or may occur only in one. You'll find, if you explore your own breasts, that there's a general pattern that stays fairly consistent. As I will discuss in the next chapter, it's important to become acquainted with your breasts and get a sense of what your pattern is.

2

Getting Acquainted with Your Breasts

One of the most useful concepts to come out of the women's health movement in the 1970s was the idea that women should become fully acquainted with their own bodies. This had a twofold purpose. The first was a medical one: if we knew what our bodies normally felt like, we'd be better able to know when something was wrong with them.

The other, more profound purpose was to help us know, accept, and cherish our bodies. In our culture, people, and particularly women, have been taught to feel shame and alienation around their bodies. And we're taught this early in childhood.

Babies, unconditioned as yet by social constrictions, are wiser than their elders. Watch a baby gleefully playing with its toes. We smile at this, without learning its real lesson. Too often we stop smiling when the baby's joyful self-discovery begins to include genitals. Early on, children learn that body parts associated with sexuality are taboo. We need to reverse this process, to teach little children to respect and cherish their bodies. And as adults, we need to reclaim that lesson for ourselves.

This is as true for breasts as for any other part of the body. Little girls should be encouraged to know their breasts, so that when the changes of puberty come about, they can experience their growing breasts with comfort and pride, and continue to do so for the rest of their lives. Most of us have not been raised that way, however, and it's often hard for an adult woman to begin feeling comfortable with her breasts. Yet it's important to become acquainted with your breasts—to know what they feel like, and what to expect from them. No part of your body should be foreign to you.

This chapter helps you to get acquainted with your breasts, and learn how to explore them yourself. It isn't as easy as it might seem because of all the taboos about "erogenous zones." Our culture both overemphasizes and negates sexual arousal, and that makes it difficult to allow yourself to touch your breasts unself-consciously.

There are two things to remember as you read this chapter. One is that breasts are a body part, just as elbows and ribs are, and there's nothing shameful about exploring them. The other is that for many women they are centers of erotic feeling, and in the process of exploring them you might experience some sexual arousal. So what? That's a perfectly reasonable response. We've finally come to realize, in childrearing, that it's a bad idea to teach kids to be ashamed of their sexual feelings, rather than help them to understand and cherish them. Similarly, we need to give ourselves permission to feel the entire range of reactions to our own bodies—sexual as well as nonsexual reactions.

To begin getting acquainted with your breasts, simply look at them. Stand in front of a mirror and look at yourself. See how your breasts hang, and get a sense of how they project. If you're young they'll tend to stick out more; if you're older they'll tend to be more droopy. In Chapter 1 we talked about the inframammary ridge, where the breast actually folds over itself, and the underlying muscles, the pectorals. Look at your nipple—what color is it? Does it have hairs or little bumps on it? If so, that's perfectly normal. You might want to swing your arms around and watch how your breasts move, or don't move, with the motion. Put your hands on your hips; flex your muscles; stretch your arms up. How do your breasts look with each change of position?

It's important to do this nonjudgmentally. You're not evaluating your possibilities of becoming a *Playboy* centerfold; you're learning about your body. Forget everything you've learned about what breasts are supposed to look like. These are your breasts, and they look fine.

Then the next step is to feel the breasts. It's best to do this soaped up in the shower or bath. Your hands slip very easily over your skin. You can put the hand on the side you want to explore behind your head. This shifts the breast tissue that's beneath your armpit to over your chest wall. Since the tissue is sandwiched between your skin and your chest bones you have good access to the tissue. If you're very large breasted you may want to do it lying down, in the bathtub or even in bed. You can then roll on one side and then the other to shift the breast closer to your chest wall so you can get a better feel for it.

Breast tissue generally has a particular texture: it's finely nodular, or granular, like large seeds, or cobblestones. A lot of this more or less bumpy feeling is simply the normal fat that intermingles with the breast tissue.

In the middle part of your chest you can feel your ribs. They jut out from your breastbone. If your ribs are very prominent, you may even feel them under the breast tissue. Many women have congenital deformities in their ribs, which affect the flatness of the rib cage. This can show in different ways. One is the condition called "chicken-breasted" in which the ribs arch outward. Then there's a sunken chest, in which the breastbone is depressed. Women can have either of these conditions and not realize it because their breasts camouflage their chest structure. Sometimes, when I would do a mastectomy, the patient would discover this unusual rib cage formation and think I created it in surgery.

Another common variation in the rib cage occurs with scoliosis. Many women have minor scoliosis and never realize it. As you feel your breast tissue you may notice that your ribs are more prominent on one side or the other. This occurs because your back is not entirely straight. It has no real significance except that it can cause your ribs to be asymmetrical. Like the breasts themselves, everybody's rib cage is a little different, and it affects the feel of the breast area differently in different women.

Usually you'll feel more tissue up toward your armpit than in the middle of the breast. As I said in Chapter 1, the breast is really tear-shaped. The tissue toward the armpit is often the part that tends to get lumpier premenstrually and less lumpy after your period. There are lymph nodes in the armpits, as there are in many other parts of the body, and if you've had any sort of infection you might feel these nodes. The inframammary ridge is an area of thickening, and the older you get, the thicker that area gets. It usually has some fat globules that are larger than in other areas. There's a hollow spot under the nipple, where the ducts all join together to exit the nipple. Around this area is a ridge of tissue—shaped rather like the crater edge of a volcano.

All of this you can easily get to know with the pads of your fingers just by running your hand over your breast area, getting a sense of how it feels (Fig. 2-1). There's no point in grabbing at the breast. You won't get a good idea of its texture because you're pulling it forward into a big wad.

You can squeeze your nipple if you're curious about how that feels. Don't be surprised if there's some discharge—squeezing the nipple can

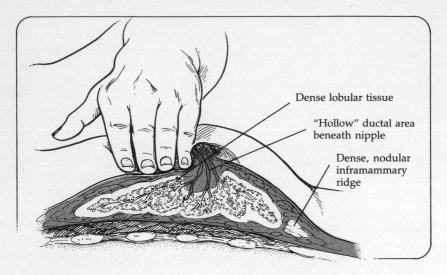

Dense lobular tissue

"Hollow" ductal area beneath nipple

Dense, nodular inframammary ridge

FIGURE 2-1

produce discharge in many women. (If you're concerned about it, see Chapter 7.)

To be thoroughly acquainted with your breasts, explore them during different times of the month. Hormones affect your breasts and they'll feel different at different points in your menstrual cycle. It's interesting to be aware of these changes. Are they lumpier, or more tender, before your period? If you've had a hysterectomy but still have your ovaries, the hormone patterns continue: monitoring your breasts may even help you to know where you would have been in your menstrual cycle. If you're postmenopausal, or if you've had your ovaries out and aren't taking hormones, the changes no longer occur. Your breast tissue in general will be less sore, less full, less lumpy. If you take hormones—Premarin, or Premarin and Provera—postmenopausally, that too will affect your breasts. They often become more sore and bigger although not necessarily firmer. Similarly, if you're on birth control pills, your breasts may respond to those hormonal changes by becoming more sore or less lumpy.

There's a good practical as well as psychological reason for knowing your breasts. Such knowledge can help prevent needless biopsies. In our mobile era, you rarely have the same doctor all your life. If you've got a lump from, say, silicone injections or scar tissue from a previous operation, and you go to a new doctor who doesn't know your medical history, the doctor may well feel a biopsy is necessary. If you can say with conviction, "Yes, I know about that lump: it formed right after my operation ten years ago, and it's been there ever since," the doctor will know the lump is okay. I've often been through this with patients. If a doctor thinks a lump is okay, but the patient doesn't know whether or not it's been there a long while, the doctor has to assume it might be dangerous, and will want to operate. If you know it's an old lump, your doctor won't have to worry.

If the doctor argues with you, argue back. Remember that you are a perfectly valid observer of your own body. You don't need to be a medical expert to know that you've had the same lump in the same place and it hasn't grown at all in 10 years. I had one 80-year-old patient who came to me after her doctors insisted that she'd been wrong about a lump in her breast that looked troublesome on her mammogram. Sexism and ageism can unite into a potent force, and obviously the doctors had decided that the "little old lady" didn't know what she was talking about when she told them her breast had been that way since her last child was born, 50 years earlier. They intimidated her enough so that she decided they must be right and had me do a biopsy. What I found was a congenital condition, perfectly harmless, that she'd probably had all her life and noticed after breast feeding. She knew her body, as her doctors couldn't.

Women with disabilities may have a more difficult time getting to know their bodies. Often, as in the case of one woman we've talked with, they have less mobility and thus don't reach all the areas of their bodies when they bathe. This woman and many others use adaptive equipment to help them bathe—which is wonderful for its purpose, but of course can't feel lumps, the way one's hand does. (For those who wish to do breast self-exam, this is also a problem.) In such cases, more frequent physician examination is a good idea.

Is This Breast Self-Examination?

This may all sound a bit like "breast self-examination," but there's a crucial difference. In breast self-examination (BSE) you're hunting for something. What I'm talking about is very different—knowing your body, apart from anything ominous that may or may not occur there. For example, while advocates of BSE tell you to examine your breasts once a month, at the same time each month, to see if there's a lump, what I'm suggesting is that you check out your breasts at different times of the month to know how they feel at all times. Once you do know, you don't have to keep checking on a rigid schedule every month, unless that pleases you. (Do keep in mind that breasts, like the rest of your body, change over time, so that it's worth exploring your breasts regularly, every couple of months, even after you feel fully acquainted with them. But again, this isn't on any particular timetable.)

As you can see, I am consciously not presenting the idea of getting to know your breasts in terms of breast self-examination. The idea is to become familiar with your breasts as one significant part of your body, and to experience all their variations. Breast self-exam, on the other hand, has been set up as a way to monitor your breasts for cancer. Why am I making such a big point of this? I have very strong feelings about the concept of breast self-exam and its overuse. I think it alienates women from their breasts instead of making them more comfortable with them. It puts you in a position of examining yourself once a month to see if your breast has betrayed you. It becomes you against your breast: can you find the tiniest lump that may be cancer?

Admittedly, breast cancer is scary, and, as I discuss later, it has become almost an epidemic. At the same time, the majority of women will never get breast cancer. To set up this alienation is a mistake. I get particularly alarmed when I hear people talk about teaching breast self-exam in the high schools. This takes young girls just developing breasts and, instead of teaching them to revel in their changing bodies, teaches them to see the breast as an enemy, something alien that has the ability to hurt them. It's a destructive way to define breasts.

Ironically, for all the fuss about breast self-exam, most women don't do it—even women who are at high risk because they have a mother or sister with breast cancer.[1] Only about 30 percent of women do BSE with any regularity. If you talk to women about BSE, most of them say they don't do it because they're scared of what they'll find. Sometimes they have lumpy breasts (see Chapter 8), and they can't tell whether one of their little bumps is actually a lump. But even when they're not doing BSE, it dominates their thinking about their breasts. I keep coming across women in their 30s and 40s who are very fearful of breast cancer—out of proportion to the real risk they face. Some of this comes from having been saturated with the idea of breast self-exam and the "need" to constantly search their bodies for signs of betrayal.

The idea of breast self-exam originated with Cushman Haagensen, who was a breast surgeon at Columbia University in New York in the 1950s, before mammography. Haagensen and his colleagues had women coming in with huge lumps in their breasts, far too big to be removed surgically. This was also an era when women were taught that it was bad to touch themselves "down there"—and "down there" was anyplace below the chin. Haagensen hoped that BSE would encourage women to touch their breasts and find cancerous lumps earlier, when they were still operable.

There are a couple of problems with his thinking, well intentioned though it was. He assumed that most of these women didn't touch their breasts, because they were ashamed to. But that may not have been the case. They may have touched their breasts and found their lumps long before they came to the doctor: shame and fear may have prevented them not from touching their breasts, but from admitting it to the doctor, or from going to a doctor about a problem in that "shameful" area.

Still, in its early days it might have been useful to some women who did indeed feel ashamed to touch themselves without a medical directive. But the idea of BSE soon grew into something more than a permissible way for women to touch their breasts. It became standardized into a technique to find a cancer early, with the implication that this would save lives. That assumption is really not true, as we'll discuss in Chapter 19.

This rigid, standardized technique has become ubiquitous and serves mostly to make women very anxious. They'll read a book or go to a lecture about breast self-examination, and come home and stand in front of a mirror and do the exam. Then they feel these little bumps, and if they've never felt their breasts before, they start to get scared. There are these lumps here, and then they feel the other breast and the bumps are there too, and they think the "cancer" had spread. This gets them so upset they avoid touching their breasts anymore. They feel guilty if they don't keep doing their BSE every month, and scared if they do.

Many women will stop me at this point and tell me that they or their friend found their cancer themselves. This is undoubtedly true: 80 percent of cancers not found on mammography are found by the woman herself. But when I question such women I find that very few actually did a formal breast self-exam, as seen on those shower cards you get from the American Cancer Society. More typically, the woman just rolled over in bed, or felt a lump while soaping up in the shower, or had it pointed out by a lover. This touching and knowing your body is what we are after, not the rigid routine of looking for cancer.

Breast self-exam as currently presented is not a good model. It's important to learn how your breasts feel, but not so you can go on a search-and-destroy mission once a month, cataloguing every grain-sized nodule you feel and deciding that this is the one that is going to kill you. It's important to help give you a good, integrated sense of your body.

This process should start in adolescence. Its side benefits are marvelous—it teaches the girl to be comfortable with her own body, and it can be a pleasing rite-of-passage, a confirmation and exploration of her womanhood. Every woman should continue to explore her breasts periodically for the rest of her life, noting and embracing each change that all the stages of life entail in her breasts, as in the rest of her body. There is a powerful feeling that comes from knowing and becoming comfortable with your body—a feeling and a power that is yours alone, and that no one can take from you.

3

Breast Feeding

The purpose of the breast is to make milk, and your breast doesn't reach its full potential until you've been through a nine-month pregnancy. This stage of the breast's development is evident quite soon after conception. Even before you've missed your period you may notice that your breasts are unusually tender or that your nipples are unusually sore. I've had a few patients coming to me complaining of strange breast pain and I've asked them when their last periods were. "Oh, about four weeks ago," they say—and I say, "Well, you could be pregnant." They either groan or grin, depending on how interested they are in motherhood at that time—and a couple of weeks later they call back to say, "Guess what? I'm pregnant."

Your breasts enlarge rapidly when you're pregnant, and they become very firm. The Montgomery's glands—those little glands around your areola (see Chapter 1)—become darker and more prominent, and the areola itself darkens. The nipples become larger and more erect, preparing themselves for future milk production (Fig. 3-1).

The development of the breast into a milk-producing machine involves orchestration of several hormones, including estrogen and progesterone as well as prolactin and oxytocin. Meanwhile, other hormones are at work—insulin, thyroid, and cortisol, as well as background nutritional hormones. These take part of the food you eat and

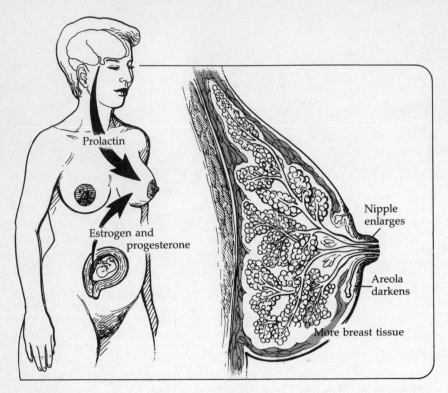

Prolactin

Estrogen and
progesterone

Nipple
enlarges

Areola
darkens

More breast tissue

FIGURE 3-1

remanufacture it in a new way, so that it can become part of the baby's milk (see Figs. 3-2 and 3-3).

Once your baby is born and the placenta has been delivered, your levels of estrogen and progesterone plummet fast, while prolactin levels begin a much slower decline. This is the sign for your breasts to begin producing milk. The milk, however, doesn't come right away. It takes between three and five days, during which time your breasts are making another liquid, a sort of pre-milk called *colostrum,* which the baby can drink instead of the milk it will soon get. Colostrum is filled with antibodies that help the infant fight off infections. Studies suggest that colostrum decreases the baby's chances of later developing allergies and asthma. Soon the baby's own immune system has begun to develop, and it no longer needs the antibodies supplied by colostrum.

While some of the milk is actually sucked out by the baby, some simply gushes into the baby's mouth as it is squeezed out by the tiny muscles lining the lobules. The mother experiences this as "letdown": her milk is literally being let down inside her breasts. The other sur-

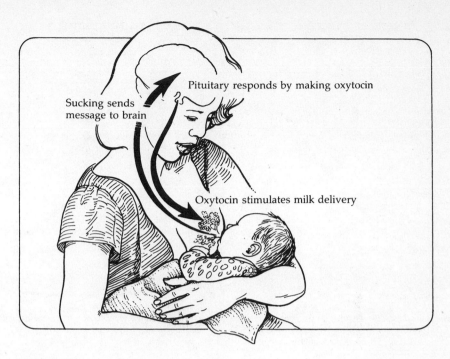

Sucking sends message to brain

Pituitary responds by making oxytocin

Oxytocin stimulates milk delivery

FIGURE 3-2

prise to most new parents is that the milk comes out of many holes in the nipple—like a watering can. These holes are the openings of the six to nine milk ducts and are best seen in the lactating woman (see Chapter 1).

The American Academy of Pediatrics, a staunch supporter of breast feeding, has stated, "Human milk is uniquely superior for infant feeding and is species-specific."[1] They list the benefits to the child with regard to general health, growth, and development, and also cite the significantly decreased risk for a large number of acute and chronic diseases. In addition, there are advantages to the mother, including an earlier return to prepregnant weight, a delay in the return of ovulation (i.e., less likelihood of closely spaced babies), improved bone remineralization after birth, and reduced risk of ovarian cancer and possibly even breast cancer (see Chapter 18). There are guides to the initiation of breast feeding which help women know what to do. They recommend starting nursing within an hour of birth, and nursing on demand. Rather than wait until babies cry, women should offer the breast whenever the babies show signs of hunger, such as increased alertness or activity, mouthing, or rooting. Pediatricians note that crying is a late sign of hunger. They suggest nursing a newborn 8–12 times

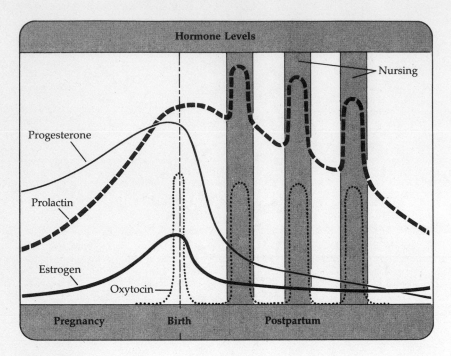

FIGURE 3-3

every 24 hours for about 10–15 minutes per breast. If babies tend to sleep through the night, pediatricians actually advise waking them up to feed every four hours in the beginning few weeks. To encourage nursing, they urge that no supplements (water, sugar water, or formula) be given to newborns unless there's a medical reason. One way women can tell if their newborn is getting enough nutrition is by monitoring what comes out the other end. There should be at least six wet diapers per day and three to four stools per day by five to seven weeks of age.

Breast feeding is a relationship between two people, and each nursing pair is unique. Help and advice are out there to help smooth the way—from nurses and lactation consultants in the hospital and from La Leche League and other nursing support groups. Eventually you'll establish your own pattern and you'll know it's successful because your baby gains weight and thrives.

For the first six months of life breast feeding is all a baby needs. Gradual introduction of iron-enriched solid foods in the second half of the first year should complement the breast milk diet. The Academy recommends that breast feeding be continued for at least 12 months and longer if both mother and child are enjoying it.

In days when breast feeding was unpopular, doctors typically gave new mothers milk-inhibiting drugs such as bromocriptine or DES (diethylstilbesterol). These are rarely used today, partly because social mores have changed—women are much more inclined to breast-feed for a while and then perhaps switch over to bottle feeding—and partly because drugs have serious side effects. Though you often hear that having unused milk in your breasts is extremely painful, it's rarely all that bad. When you don't suckle your newborn, the prolactin doesn't signal your breasts to produce more milk and the milk simply stops: you're likely to be uncomfortable for a day or two and then feel fine. Applying ice to your breasts can help, as can binding your breasts with a tightly pinned towel.

If a new mother is not producing milk within a week of the baby's birth, something is wrong and a clinician should be consulted. Aside from deliberate attempts to inhibit milk, several things can prevent your breasts from producing milk. You may have a problem in your pituitary gland—you might have hemorrhaged into it, or it may be otherwise damaged, and you won't be able to produce the necessary prolactin and oxytocin. Sometimes you'll find that milk has come into your breast, but can't get out. This is caused by damage that's been done to the duct system, usually by surgery around the nipple or perhaps by breast reduction surgery (see Chapter 5). Sometimes the ducts can be unblocked, but often they can't, and in that case you will have to bottle-feed instead of breast-feed. (The milk will be reabsorbed back into your body.) This happened to a patient of mine in the ob/gyn section of the hospital where I worked. I was called in to look at her because her milk had come in, but nothing was coming out of the breast. I tried to probe her ducts, but nothing would pass. I discovered that an operation she'd had on a nipple abscess many years before had caused scarring, sealing off her milk ducts in one breast. Sometimes the baby has a problem coordinating tongue motions, or the shape of a woman's nipples makes it hard for the baby to latch on. Insufficient milk needs to be evaluated by a clinician expert in breast feeding: a pediatrician, family doctor, or lactation consultant.

If you've been breast-feeding and you suddenly stop, your body will stop creating prolactin and oxytocin, so milk isn't being let down and milk production will taper off and stop. For this reason, if you need to stop breast-feeding temporarily—for instance, if you have to travel or are about to be on medication that you don't want the child to consume—you should keep expressing milk manually or with a pump, so that the production continues. Otherwise it may be difficult to resume breast-feeding—the body has to start the whole business over again, and it takes time.

On the other hand, once you've had a baby you can always breast-feed in the future. If, for example, you adopt a child some time after you've breast-fed your biological baby, you can have the new baby suck your breast and, with time, that can eventually start the whole process up again.

Breast milk will look different at each stage of its production. According to standard teaching, colostrum is yellow and clear; early breast milk is bluish-white, mature milk is white and creamy, and late milk, as you begin to breast-feed less and less, is thin-white. But it may vary. I found my own early milk to be white and the later milk to be blue. It was also interesting to me to find that milk left to stand in the refrigerator layered out with the cream at the top. If I skipped a meal there would be less cream—"skim milk." When I ate regular meals, there was more cream. The milk of a premature baby's mother is different from that of a mother whose baby was delivered at full term: the premie's nutritional needs are different, and the mother's body knows this and adjusts the milk to her child's needs. Similarly, if you have twins your body will adjust to that, and provide you with twice as much milk. You can even nurse two consecutive children at the same time, tandem nursing. I discovered something else from my own experience: if you freeze early milk and give it to the baby weeks later, it will put the baby to sleep; it has a natural sedative effect.

Another important fact worth noting: you should alternate breasts and not just feed from one. One of my patients found it comfortable to feed on one breast, and ignored the other—which in turn ignored her and stopped making milk. The result is she now has an asymmetry she never had before.

Though having your first baby late in life can have other effects on your body, it won't affect your breast milk at all: you'll be as able to produce good milk for your child at 40 as you were at 20.

After you've stopped breast-feeding you'll still have some secretions for two or three months, and sometimes as long as a year or two, afterward. Usually you can breast-feed for two or three years. The length of time is up to you. Your child probably won't be traumatized by weaning. My sister decided to stop breast-feeding her daughter after three years. She was sure the child would be shattered, and spent a lot of time working out her explanation. When she broached the subject, my niece's response was a cheerful, "It's okay, Mom, I understand."

Breast feeding has some contraceptive effect, but only in the first three or four months—and even then, it isn't 100 percent effective. Don't assume that because you're breast-feeding you can engage in sexual intercourse without other contraceptives—unless you want to be breast-feeding again in nine months.

If you plan to go back to work while you're still breast-feeding, you can pump your breasts every three or four hours, freeze the milk or just refrigerate it, and use it to feed your baby later. This can be done by manually expressing milk into a sterile container or by using any of the commercially available breast pumps (Figs. 3-4 and 3-5). These come in a number of forms—there are hand pumps, electric pumps, and battery-operated pumps. Depending on the type of pump, it will take 10 to 15 minutes on each side—there is even an extra attachment for the electric pump that will allow you to empty both breasts simultaneously. As one of my busy doctor colleagues says, "Why waste a letdown?" Many workplaces (especially hospitals) have pumps available, and many others will rent one for you. It's certainly worth asking your employer, since it is to their advantage to keep you at work. After my daughter was born, I was explaining to a patient how the breast was a milk factory, and in the middle of my session with her I had to interrupt and go pump my breasts—nicely illustrating my metaphor.

For many working mothers, the special intimacy of breast feeding can soften the blow of having to return to work. The feeling that "only I can nurse my baby" (and I will keep doing it) is a strong antidote to the guilt of having to go back to work.

Sometimes problems in the mother's body interfere with breast feeding. One problem is sore nipples, created by the infant's suckling.

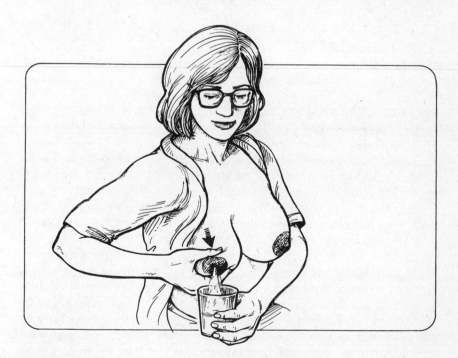

FIGURE 3-4

39

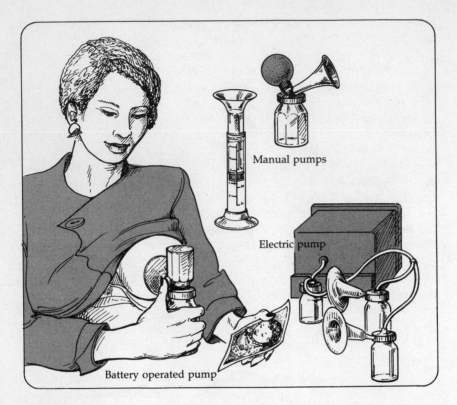

Manual pumps

Electric pump

Battery operated pump

FIGURE 3-5

There is a strong sucking sensation that increases with time and peaks on day four with nipple pain. This pain soon is resolved and women are encouraged to keep on breast feeding for at least 14 days before giving up. Sometimes the nipple soreness can go on to cracks or breaks in the skin, causing bleeding and blistering. This can often be alleviated by alternating the position in which the child is sucking.

It is also important to support your breast in your cupped hand with your thumb on top and your fingers underneath. Do this even if you're small breasted as it allows the baby to latch onto your nipple correctly. In addition, you should make sure the baby opens its mouth wide with its tongue covering the lower gum line. Avoid soaps, which irritate the delicate nipple skin. At the end of feeding express a little colostrum or milk and rub it into your nipple and areola. Allow it to air dry. Human milk contains antibodies that fight infection. The milk also contains fat, which acts as a skin moisturizer. Some of the experts used to suggest toughening up your breast ahead of time by rolling your nipples between your fingers or by sunbathing topless! (Obviously, if

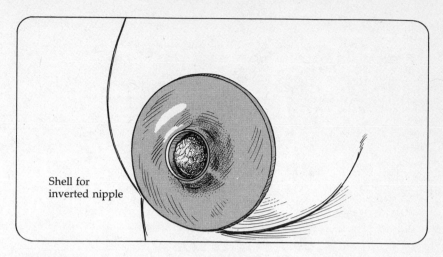

Shell for
inverted nipple

FIGURE 3-6

you're going to try this method, be aware that the law might not agree
with your decision; either find a private place to sunbathe, or be prepared for a court case!) If problems continue, seek help from a lactation
specialist. Breast feeding shouldn't hurt.

Women with inverted nipples can have trouble breast-feeding initially. I discuss this in Chapter 4. If your infant doesn't figure out
how to get the nipple out, there's a shell you can buy and put over
the nipple, squeezing down and making it more available to the child
(Fig. 3-6).

Some women suffer from engorgement of the breasts: they fill up
too fast and don't empty enough, and then the nipple is so stretched
out the child can't get its mouth around it, and the problem gets worse.
This is especially true when the milk first comes in, before the body has
figured out the right amount of milk to produce—the first three or four
days. It can be very uncomfortable, as I learned when my own baby
was born. The best thing to do then is to express a little milk manually
before feedings, and to feed the baby as often as possible. Frequent
massage, hot tubs, and hot showers help to express the milk; ice packs
and aspirin or Tylenol can help relieve the pain. One interesting study
showed that compresses of cooked cabbage leaves relieved the pain of
engorgement. [2]

Sometimes a duct can become blocked (Fig. 3-7). You'll know this
has happened if you find in one segment of the breast a lumpy area
that doesn't go away after breast feeding. It's important to treat it right
away, because it can lead to infection and, in rare cases, the infection
can turn into an abscess. Again, you can treat it with hot soaks, hot

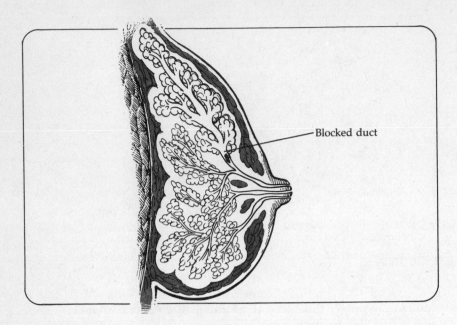

Blocked duct

FIGURE 3-7

showers, and massage; if those don't work, call your doctor. Redness, fever, or flu symptoms might suggest mastitis. There's a detailed description of these problems in Chapter 7.

Some women have too little milk. In most cases this can be alleviated by feeding more often—an every-two-hour-feeding generally helps. If such a rigorous schedule is impossible for you, it may be time to stop breast feeding and turn to formula—or at least combine breast and bottle feeding. Sometimes even frequent feeding doesn't help: for some reason, the woman's body simply doesn't make enough milk, no matter what she does. Many women feel an irrational guilt when this happens, as though they've failed in their "motherly duties." They haven't—it's a biological idiosyncracy, not a cosmic flaw.

At the other extreme is the woman whose body produces too much milk, and she finds herself leaking between feedings, or having her milk squirt out into the baby's face when she starts to nurse. She should avoid expressing the milk between feedings as it will only increase production.

In any case, if you find yourself having physical or emotional problems with any aspect of breast feeding, or just wanting moral support, contact a lactation consultant or La Leche League, or one of the other breast feeding organizations, which offer counseling, peer support groups, and practical advice. (See Appendix B.)

BREAST FEEDING AND LUMPS IN THE BREAST

Pregnancy and lactation don't prevent lumps from occurring: you can get any of the usual fibroadenomas, cysts, or pseudolumps (see Chapter 8). In addition, a nursing mother can get a galactocele, a milk cyst that forms when some of the milk closes off in a sac and ultimately gets thick and cheesy. A needle aspiration can determine if the lump is a galactocele (Fig. 3-8). It's harmless, as is any cyst, but you want to be sure that's what it is. I had one patient with two milk cysts, which had been there for at least two years.

And, of course, you can get a cancerous lump, just as you can when you're not breast-feeding. Any dominant lump that doesn't go away with massage should be checked out. It appears that a woman who gets breast cancer during pregnancy or breast feeding may have a worse prognosis than she would at another time.[3] (See Chapter 24.) In addition, it usually gets diagnosed at a later stage, because a pregnant

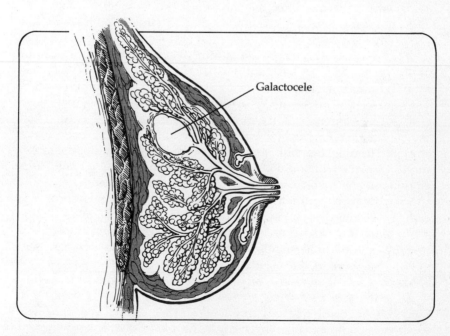

FIGURE 3-8

woman and her doctor are focused on the pregnancy and are not thinking about cancer.[4] It's important to be as aware of the possibility of cancer during pregnancy and lactation as at any other time. Continue to explore your breasts (see Chapter 2), and be aware of the normal changes that pregnancy and breast feeding have created in them. As always, this shouldn't simply be about hunting for cancer. You're having a new and probably wonderful relationship to the breasts that are now feeding your baby, and it's nice to know how your breasts feel during this time. A pregnant breast will feel like a premenstrual breast; it is usually sore and lumpy in the first trimester and less in the second and third; a lactating breast feels both full and lumpy, as if it had cottage cheese inside, because it's filled with fluid.

If you do find a suspicious lump, get it checked out. Should a biopsy be called for, neither pregnancy nor breast feeding need prevent it. When you're pregnant, it's best to have a biopsy done under a local anesthetic, to avoid exposing the fetus to general anesthesia. And a core biopsy (see Chapter 11) may well be easier for both mother and child than an open one.

A nursing mother can have either a general or a local anesthetic. I preferred to operate right after a woman had fed her baby, or expressed the milk. I used the lowest percentage of local anesthetic possible, usually lidocaine, since the child could suck some of it later. It's not terrible for the child to swallow a bit of anesthetic, but it's well that it be as little as possible. I would also advise the mother not to feed the baby from that breast for 12 hours after the surgery, since a gulp of the lidocaine might be harmful. It should be given time to disperse throughout the breast.

It's messier to perform surgery on a lactating woman than on a nonlactating woman; and it's always possible that the operation can create a milk cyst or leakage, but it's no great tragedy if it does. It can temporarily make the milk messy, too, since blood from the operation can mix with the milk. Blood won't hurt your baby, so the problem is really mostly aesthetic.

Some surgeons will tell a lactating woman she has to stop breast-feeding if she needs a biopsy. She doesn't. If your surgeon tells you this at a time when you're thinking of stopping breast-feeding anyway, it's probably a good time to stop. Otherwise, find another surgeon who will operate while you're lactating.

Another breast-feeding worry has been women with silicone implants. Some studies have shown silicone in the breast milk of these women. An interesting study in Canada answered this question.[5] The researchers compared the breast milk and blood of women who had silicone implants and were breast-feeding to those of women without implants who were also breast-feeding. They found no difference in the levels of silicone in the two groups. They then tested cow's milk and formula and found silicone levels 10 times higher in cow's milk than in breast milk of women with implants and even higher in formula. Their conclusion was that lactating women with silicone implants are similar to control women with respect to levels of silicon in their breast milk.

There are some misconceptions about cancer and breast feeding that need to be addressed. The first is that a child who drinks from a cancerous breast will get the cancer. This theory is based on a study of one species of mouse, which does transmit a cancerous virus to its female offspring through breast feeding. At this time, it hasn't been found in any other species of mouse, or any other animal, or in humans.

Another notion is that a baby won't drink milk from a cancerous breast. Normally this isn't so. If a breast has a lot of cancer, it probably won't produce as much milk, so the baby will, quite sensibly, favor the milkier breast. There's nothing wrong with this: in fact, many babies prefer one breast to another even with a very healthy mother.

There is also the question of whether breast feeding helps prevent breast cancer. This discussion often takes on a slightly moralistic tone: if the breast is doing what it's supposed to do, it won't get cancer. As of 1997, more than 40 independent research studies have examined the role of breast feeding in breast cancer risk. The evidence is now convincing, and it is widely accepted that breast feeding reduces the risk of premenopausal breast cancer. But the association of breast feeding with risk of postmenopausal breast cancer remains controversial.[6] In a recent study from Los Angeles, researchers looked again at the relationship between breast feeding and postmenopausal breast cancer.[7] They found that women who breast-fed at least 16 months had 30 percent less pre- and postmenopausal cancer than women who had not breast-fed. Another study showed that the risk of breast cancer of women who first lactated before the age of 20 and breast-fed their infants for a total of six months was half that of women who had been pregnant and had not breast-fed. Unfortunately for most women, *after* age 20 breast feeding demonstrated only a slightly smaller risk of breast cancer.[8] (The age at which you first have a baby does have an effect on your vulnerability to breast cancer—see Chapter 14.) These are interesting findings, but not very useful for most women in our culture.

SEX AND BREAST FEEDING

There's no reason for breast feeding to interfere with an active sex life. Breast stimulation may cause some milk to flow out. Sometimes your lover will actually enjoy sucking at your breast and getting some milk. If this is pleasing to the two of you, it's fine—your lover won't be using up your child's milk, only stimulating the breast to produce more. Orgasm can also cause squirting of milk. If either of you finds stimulation of the breast unappealing at this time, you can adjust your sexual practices accordingly. On the other hand, you may find that your general libido is markedly reduced while you are breast-feeding, and you're not as interested in sex as you usually are. You may also note that the sudden decrease in estrogen has led to vaginal dryness; lubricants like Astroglide can fix this temporary problem. You and your partner should be aware of this possibility, so your partner doesn't feel rejected and you don't feel like you've suddenly become "frigid." In fact, most nursing mothers would much rather sleep than have sex.

Many women feel sexual stimulation during breast feeding, and it's perfectly natural—oxytocin causes the uterus to contract. Don't worry about it: it doesn't mean you're a potential child molester. It's usually a fairly mild form of sexual feeling, and there's no reason not to just enjoy it. (If you don't feel it, don't worry about that either; just enjoy the sensations you do feel.)

BREAST FEEDING WHEN YOU HAVEN'T GIVEN BIRTH

If you've never breast-fed or been pregnant before, you can still do a form of breast feeding. This must be done in conjunction with bottle formula (or milk from another woman's breast, as in the case of lesbians raising the biological child of one partner together). Stimulated by suckling which increases prolactin, the breast will produce a kind of pre-milk fluid, which can provide a small amount of nutrition to the child. Since many women find breast feeding pleasurable and since breast feeding intensifies the bonding of mother and infant, this can be a good idea, as long as the baby is given other forms of nutrition. (Men, by the way, don't have this fluid, since their breasts haven't developed through puberty the way women's have.) This kind of breast feeding can be enhanced by using an invention called a Lactaid kit (Fig. 3-9). It has a bag into which formula (or pumped breast milk) is placed, and a long plastic tube that winds around the breast and ends up at the nipple. The child sucks the milk from a catheter next to the nipple, thus creating the bonding effect of breast feeding.

The kit might also help a woman who has had a baby (or been pregnant for several months) in the past to revive her own milk-producing abilities. In this case she will eventually produce full milk. But the chief virtue of the kit is that it helps you to bond with the child and experience breast feeding, even if your own milk isn't available. Hormones

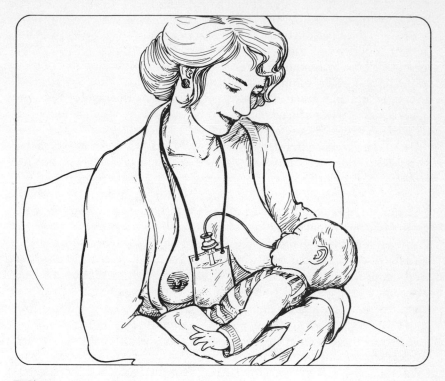

FIGURE 3-9

and other drugs have also been used to stimulate breast feeding, with varying results.

BREAST FEEDING VS. BOTTLE FEEDING

When I was born breast feeding was very unfashionable. Bottle feeding was considered less messy, and it gave mothers more mobility than they had with breast feeding. Since the early '70s, the popularity has continued to rise overall with some waxing and waning. I think it's unfortunate that there are fashions in baby feeding: they tend to include pressures and guilt trips, or the idea that there's a universally correct way to feed your baby, and that there's something odd and probably immoral about doing it any other way. In reality, there are advantages and disadvantages to both methods of baby feeding, and you need to weigh them all before you decide what you want to do.

What are the advantages of breast feeding? Earlier in this chapter I enumerated the benefits cited by the American Academy of Pediatrics.

Probably the most important advantage is the nutritional composition of breast milk. It's tailor-made for the human baby's needs—it's got the perfect combination of water, protein, carbohydrates (mainly lactose), immunoglobin (which helps create immunity against disease), lots of cholesterol (which, though unhealthy for adults, is great for babies), and vitamins and minerals. Cow's milk, on the other hand, is tailor-made for the needs of baby cows, which are obviously somewhat different from those of the human baby.

Formula is our attempt to modify cow's milk to make it as close as possible to human milk. We've done a pretty impressive job, but it's not perfect. For one thing, cow's milk isn't as digestible as human milk: it takes a baby four hours to digest formula, and only two to digest human milk. No formula has been able to duplicate the immunity-providing properties of colostrum.

Breast feeding also creates a unique bonding between mother and infant which some psychologists feel is essential to the child's later well-being. While there are plenty of emotionally healthy people who were bottle-fed, and many neurotics who were breast-fed, it's clear that the particular bonding created by breast feeding can't be wholly duplicated in bottle feeding. Many of my patients have talked with me about the importance of this bonding to them emotionally. "The realization of what breasts are meant for was tremendous," says one, who calls it a "generative experience." Another, who had felt self-conscious about her small breasts, changed her attitude when she realized that "my small breasts nursed three sons." I enjoyed breast-feeding my daughter and found that even pumping milk for her was a pleasant interlude in an otherwise hectic day. I think being able to fill her nutritional needs while working made me feel more connected to her.

On the other hand, breast feeding can create difficulties for the mother that may outweigh the advantages to the child—difficulties that proselytizers for breast feeding sometimes underrate. Breast feeding every two hours may be very difficult for a woman who has a job outside her home, and it's not always that easy for the woman at home who has primary responsibility for raising other children and/or doing housework. Bottle feeding allows the mother to get some rest, and to do other work, while her husband or another member of the household does some of the feeding. Sometimes a combination of breast feeding and bottle feeding (using either formula or breast milk expressed by the mother at an earlier time) can be a useful compromise, but many women still find breast feeding too demanding of time and energy. Also, lactation can cause problems, even for the mother combining breast and bottle feeding. Oxytocin can be produced by emotional as well as direct physical responses to the baby, and many mothers will find to their embarrassment that, while they're thinking about the baby, milk will suddenly begin to flow. A surgeon colleague of mine decided to stop breast feeding when the thought of her baby came to her during an operation and suddenly milk started dripping onto her patient.

Still other women find the idea of breast feeding unpleasant, even repugnant. This isn't an indication that the woman will be a bad mother; reactions to physical experiences vary greatly among human beings. Forcing oneself to go through with an unpleasant experience will be counterproductive to the bonding experience between mother and child. Some women feel more comfortable with bottle feeding because they know how much nutrition the child is getting, since it's premeasured, and the exact amount of breast milk is not something one can know for certain.

There are also women whose own food habits can make breast feeding a problem. It's true that the baby will consume, through your milk, everything you consume, and many women really cherish their cups of coffee or their evening martinis. Although small amounts of liquor and caffeine are probably all right, if you want to breast-feed, you should keep them very limited. A study from the University of Michigan demonstrated a slight decrease in motor development, but not in mental development, in the year-old offspring of mothers who drank one alcoholic beverage per day.[9] Thus, although some data suggest that a glass of beer a day will actually improve your milk production, it probably isn't worth the slight but potentially harmful consequences. And, of course, other recreational drugs are also potentially dangerous. It's probably safest to remain drug- and alcohol-free while breastfeeding. Some women can do this easily, and for them it's worth the sacrifice; for others, it's not, and they may prefer to bottle-feed rather than adopt uncomfortable behaviors. It isn't necessarily "selfish" to take care of your own needs as well as your baby's. Similarly, some mothers are on medication for chronic health problems, and some (though certainly not all) medication will harm a breast-feeding baby. Sacrificing your own health or comfort, again, may not be the best thing for either you or your child.

Yet many women today feel pressured to breast-feed, regardless of their own needs, and often others can play unconsciously into those pressures. A patient once came to see me in her eighth month of pregnancy. She reminded me that, four months earlier, I'd said to her, "I'll see you again toward the end of your pregnancy, and then again when you've finished breast-feeding." She was concerned because she didn't want to breast-feed, and felt I'd been implying that she should.

At the same time, there are still parts of our culture that have retained the old prejudices against breast feeding, and this too can be very damaging to a mother. There's still some feeling that the female breast is a sexual organ and shouldn't be exposed in public. (Some people see men's breasts as erotic, but that doesn't force them to cover their chests.) Thus, a woman who's breast-feeding may find herself pressured to give it up, or to confine it to her own home. I remember going to a wedding and seeing my cousin's wife sitting off in a corner, very discreetly breast-feeding her baby. Some of the other guests were horrified. Feeding your baby is a perfectly natural and sensible thing to do, and you shouldn't be made to feel like some kind of slut for doing it. Obviously, given social mores, it's usually unwise to bare your whole breast in public, but sensibly chosen clothing can allow for discreet feeding anywhere, and you shouldn't feel guilt-tripped by other people's puritanism.

There's another prejudice that can get in the way of breast feeding. The breast-fed baby doesn't gain weight as rapidly as the bottle-fed baby does. That's perfectly fine, except that we've been raised with the image of the chubby, healthy baby. But chubby isn't necessarily healthy, and breast feeding may in fact produce a healthier child. There is some evidence that breast-fed babies are less likely to be obese in later life.

It's important to realize that anti-breast-feeding feelings originated in the early days of formula feeding, and it was very much in the interests of the manufacturers of baby formula. We see this quite tragically in Third World countries, where poor mothers were told that formula was better for their babies than breast milk, then given formula until their own milk dried up, when they were forced to buy more formula at costs they couldn't afford. Many babies died as a result.

Fortunately, most women in the United States are well enough off to be able to choose either breast or bottle feeding. You should make your choice realistically, taking into consideration your own needs and priorities. If the various social criticisms of one mode or the other make sense to you, take them into consideration. If they don't, ignore them. You want to do what's best for you and your baby, and for the relationship that develops between you. Only you can best determine what that is.

4

Variations in Development

Breasts are found in many different shapes and sizes. Medically speaking, a "normal" breast is one that is capable of producing milk, so there's nothing "abnormal" about large, small, or asymmetrical breasts, or about extra nipples.

There are a number of common variations in breast development. They fall into one of two categories: those that are obvious from birth and those that don't show themselves until puberty. The latter are far more common. (There are also variations due to accident or illness, the surgical remedies for which are essentially the same as those used for genetic variations.)

VARIATIONS APPARENT AT BIRTH

The most common variation to appear at birth is *polymastia*—an extra nipple, or nipples. These can appear anywhere along the milk ridge (see Fig. 1-8). Usually the milk ridge—a throwback to the days when we were animals with many nipples—regresses before birth, but in some people it remains throughout their lives. Between 1 and 5 percent of extra nipples are on women whose mothers also had extra nipples. Usually they're below the breast, and often women don't even know they're there, since they look very much like moles. I've frequently pointed out an extra nipple to a patient, and it's the first time she's known about it.

They cause no problems, and because of their size and resemblance to moles they usually don't appear cosmetically unattractive. One of my patients was actually very fond of her extra nipple: she told me that her husband had one too, and that's how they knew they were meant for each other! Men do sometimes have extra nipples, though as far as we know, less frequently than women do. This may be due to some biological factor we don't yet know about, or it may simply be that men and their doctors don't notice the nipples because they're covered by chest hair.

Extra nipples don't cause any problems, though they may lactate if you breast-feed. There's nothing wrong with this, unless it causes you discomfort.

A variation of the extra nipple is extra breast tissue, without a nipple; most often under the armpit. It may feel like hard, cystlike lumps that swell and hurt the way your breasts do when you menstruate. Like extra nipples, this extra breast tissue is often unnoticed by doctor and patient. One of my patients found that, during her second pregnancy, she had swelling under both armpits: it was probably caused by extra breast tissue and it went down again after she finished lactating. The extra tissue is subject to all the problems of normally situated tis-

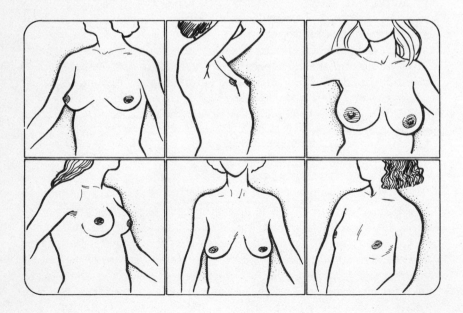

sue. I have had patients with cysts, fibroadenomas, or even cancers in such tissue.

Unless the extra nipple or breast tissue causes you extreme physical discomfort or psychological distress, there's no need to worry about it. If it does bother you, it's easy to get rid of surgically. The nipple can be removed under local anesthetic in your doctor's office, much the way a mole can, and the extra breast tissue can be removed under either local or general anesthetic.

A much rarer condition is *amastia*—being born with breast tissue but no nipple. When it occurs, it's usually associated with problems in the development of the chest bone and muscles, like scoliosis and rib deformities. Aside from whatever medical procedures you may need because of the associated problems, you might want to have a fake nipple created by a plastic surgeon, the same way a nipple is created during reconstruction after a mastectomy. The nipple can be tattooed on or a skin graft can be taken from tissue on the inner thigh. The skin becomes darker after it's grafted and, if it still doesn't match the color of your other nipple, it can be tattooed to a darker shade. Though this artificial nipple will look real, it won't feel completely like a real nipple: there is no erectile tissue, so it won't vary like your other nipple does. It's usually constructed midway between erect and flat. It will have no sensation because it has no nerves. Because it won't have ducts, it can't produce milk. Its advantages are wholly cosmetic.

Some women have practically no breasts at all. This condition is sometimes called Poland's syndrome, and it involves not just the breast but also the pectoralis muscle and the ribs, as well as, in some cases, abnormalities of the arm and side on one side of the body. At times, a woman with Poland's syndrome does have a small but very deformed breast. A recent patient of mine in Los Angeles was doubly unlucky. She had been born with Poland's syndrome and had a very undeveloped breast on one side. She developed breast cancer in the good breast. She was anxious to have a lumpectomy rather than a mastectomy, because she very much wanted to preserve her only functional breast. Some women have permanently inverted nipples (they grow in instead of out)—a congenital condition which usually won't manifest until puberty.

Various kinds of injuries can affect breast development. This may happen surgically or with trauma. If the nipple and breast bud are seriously injured before puberty, the potential adult breast is destroyed as well. Sometimes injuring the skin can limit future breast development. Most commonly this occurs as a result of a severe burn. The resulting scars are so tight that they won't allow the breast tissue to develop. In the past, some congenital conditions such as hemangiomas ("birthmarks") were treated with radiation, which damaged the nipple and breast bud and prevented later growth. Any serious injury to the breast bud can cause this arrested development.

VARIATIONS APPEARING AT PUBERTY

Three basic variations appear when the breasts begin to develop: extremely large breasts, extremely small breasts, and asymmetrical breasts.

Very Large Breasts

Very large breasts can occur early in puberty—a condition known as "virginal hypertrophy." After the breasts begin to grow, the shut-off mechanism, whatever it is, forgets to do its job and the breasts keep on growing. The breasts become huge and greatly out of proportion to the rest of the body. Sometimes the condition runs in families. In very rare instances, virginal hypertrophy occurs in one breast and not the other. It's worth noting here that "large" is both a subjective and a variable term. A five-foot-tall woman with a C cup is very large-breasted; a five-foot-eight woman with a C cup may not feel especially uncomfortable with her size. A five-foot-eight woman with a DD cup is likely to be very uncomfortable.

Large breasts have been a problem for a number of my patients. "I almost never wear a bathing suit," one patient told me, "because people stare at my breasts." Another, at 71, still "hunches over" when she walks to avoid having her breasts stared at.

Huge breasts can be very distressful to a teenage girl. She faces ridicule from her schoolmates, and—unlike the small-breasted girl—extreme physical discomfort as well. She may be unable to participate in sports, and she may have severe backache all the time. She usually needs a bra to hold the breasts in, but the bra, pulled down by the weight of the breasts, can dig painful ridges into her shoulders.

If the breasts cause this much discomfort, the girl might want to have reduction surgery done while she's still in her teens. There are a number of procedures. Though they're all major surgery, because they're done on the body's surface they're less dangerous than other equally complex operations, and the recovery period is speedier. (We'll discuss plastic surgery at length in the next chapter.)

The procedures vary according to the size of the girl's breasts. If they're really huge, the nipple will have to be moved further up on the newly reduced breast. In this case, the ducts may be cut and so breast feeding will be compromised.

For this reason, some mothers refuse to let their daughters have reduction surgery, urging them to wait until they've had their children. This concern must be weighed against the physical and emotional damage the girl will go through first. If she decides to have children, pregnancy itself may worsen her problem. When the breasts become engorged with milk, they become even larger, and thus, in a woman with huge breasts, more uncomfortable. Though it's unfortunate that someone so young is faced with a decision that affects her whole life, it's important to realize that not having the surgery will also affect her life. Many girls of 15 or 16 are mature enough to make their own decisions if all the facts are carefully explained to them, including the possibility of bottle feeding. In any case, the losses and gains of either choice are the girl's, and she should be given the right to decide for herself what to do. She should be encouraged to talk to doctors, mothers of young children, and very large-breasted women; to read all the material she can find about the pros and cons of the procedure and of breast feeding; and to make her decision only when she feels she is fully informed.

Not all problems with huge breasts appear right after puberty. Some comfortably large-breasted women find that their breasts have expanded considerably after pregnancy; others become uncomfortable after their breast size has increased with an overall weight gain. Many surgeons are reluctant to operate in this latter case, preferring to wait till the woman has lost weight. Sometimes, however, this can backfire psychologically: I've known women who were so depressed by their huge breasts that they compensated by overeating, thus intensifying both problems. In such cases, the pleasing appearance of their breasts created by reduction surgery can be a spur to continue self-improvement.

In any case, the decision must be made by the individual woman; she's the one who lives with the problem and she's the one who can best judge its impact on her life. Some women with very large breasts don't mind them. One patient, who admits they cause her discomfort, says that she nonetheless enjoys their size. "They feel feminine and sexy," she says.

Very Small Breasts

The opposite problem is extreme flat-chestedness. Like "large-breasted," the notion of "small-breasted" is subjective and relative, and to some extent culturally determined. Some women, however, have breasts so small that their chests look like men's. This causes no physical or medical problems. Yet it can cause psychological ones, making a woman feel unattractive and sexless. Plastic surgeons often inaccurately call very small breasts a "disease," contributing even further to the woman's lack of comfort with her anatomy.

For many women, these problems are solved simply by the use of "falsies" or padded bras. Others want to have the breasts altered. For years there was nothing that could be done for women who wanted larger breasts. Some surgeons experimented with paraffin injections, with fairly awful results. In the 1960s, the silicone implant and silicone injections were introduced. These implants, their safety, and the surgery involved, are discussed in Chapter 5.

Drs. Andrew and Penny Stanway in their book *The Breast* suggest a somewhat surprising alternative to augmentation surgery—hypnosis and visualization.[1] Visualization is a form of self-hypnosis in which you put yourself in a state of deep relaxation and then see yourself, as vividly as possible, achieving the state you want to be in. (We'll discuss it at greater length in Chapter 23, which talks about nonmedical components of cancer treatment.)

The Stanways describe a study in which volunteers, put into a trance, were asked to visualize a wet, warm towel over their breasts. They were told to concentrate on the warmth of the towel and on the breasts' pulsation. They did this exercise every day for weeks. At the end of that time half the patients reported having to buy bigger bras! The authors suggest that the deep relaxation and visualizing might effect a hormonal change that influences breast size. While the study is hardly conclusive, it's certainly interesting, and you might want to give visualization a try before considering surgery. It's painless, it has no harmful side effects, and it might just produce the results you want in a less expensive and physically invasive way than surgery. (See Appendix B for books on visualization techniques.)

Asymmetrical Breasts

There is a third situation that often occurs in puberty: the breasts grow unevenly. In some cases this is simply a question of the rate of the breasts' growth, and in a year or two the breasts are fairly symmetrical—for example, one breast will be an A cup size, while the other is a B cup size. (Keep in mind that most people's breasts are slightly uneven, as are their feet and hands.) But sometimes the breasts remain extremely asymmetrical. Again, asymmetrical breasts are perfectly "normal" from a medical viewpoint: they can both produce milk. But they can create extreme psychological distress, causing the adolescent girl—

and the grown woman—to feel like a sexual freak. Some girls refuse to date in their teens because they fear their condition will be discovered and ridiculed. (My coauthor had her first date at the age of 20—two weeks after her last silicone injection.) A falsie—or a pile of several falsies—can be worn on one side, of course, but that can still leave a feeling of something ugly and somehow shameful that must be hidden from the world.

For a woman who is bothered by extreme asymmetry, cosmetic surgery can help achieve a reasonable match. Either the larger breast can be reduced or the smaller one augmented—or a combination of both can be done. It's important for the surgeon to discuss these options— often we assume a woman will want her small breast made larger and neglect to suggest the possibility of reducing the larger breast. What a woman decides will depend on the size of both breasts, the degree of asymmetry, and, above all, her own aesthetic judgment.

It's fortunate that plastic surgery techniques exist for women who want them. But don't assume that because you have atypical-looking breasts you have to get them altered. Many women are quite pleased with how their breasts look. Some women with large breasts feel, as did the patient I mentioned earlier, that their breasts are "feminine and sexy." Small breasts, too, have their advantages. One of my patients liked her small breasts because "they're unobtrusive, and they worked well during nursing. Occasionally some male person will intimate that they're less than optimal. That's his problem, not mine." Another likes her tiny breasts ("they're really just enlarged nipples") because they don't get in her way when she engages in sports. A patient with very asymmetrical breasts says she used to feel self-conscious about them, but has "come to terms with them" since she nursed her child.

And another patient tells a wonderful story about a friend of hers who had inverted nipples. "When I was 12 and my cousin was 14, we stood before the bathroom mirror and compared breasts. I noticed how different her nipples were; they didn't protrude, the way mine did. We had this big discussion about whose were 'normal.' I was convinced mine were, but she insisted hers were, and since she was older and, I thought, more knowledgeable, I decided she must be right.

"After she graduated from college and was studying in Paris, she became ill and had to be hospitalized. The doctor who was examining her asked if her nipples 'had always been like that.' That's how she learned that she had inverted nipples—and that mine were the normal ones!"

Obviously, the woman's inverted nipples hadn't caused her any distress. If you don't object to the way your breasts look, don't think about plastic surgery. You're fine as you are.

5

Plastic Surgery

Many women with atypical breasts are perfectly comfortable with them, and never consider having them altered. On the other hand, some women are very unhappy with the way their breasts look. For them, cosmetic surgery is worth thinking about. Women are often made to feel frivolous and vain for having cosmetic surgery, while at the same time they are expected to meet an impossible, Hollywood-style standard of beauty. It's no more vain to alter your breasts than to have a scar removed, or to get a suntan to darken your complexion; it's certainly no more vain than it is for a balding man to get a hair transplant.

Plastic surgery has been done on breasts for a long time. Interestingly, the first recorded breast surgery was done on a man with gynecomastia, in A.D. 625.[1] It was not until more than a thousand years later, in 1897, that they performed mammoplasty on a woman—but we needn't feel too deprived. With the primitive state of surgery in the past, that poor man in the seventh century can't have had too comfortable a time with it.

Good breast reduction techniques have now been with us for decades. Augmentation, as I mentioned earlier, is a much more recent procedure.

From a surgical standpoint the procedures themselves are quite safe. They are often labeled "unnecessary surgery," and of course they *are* unnecessary in the sense that you won't die without them. But for many women the risk is well worth the chance of improved self-image and, in the case of large breasts, increased physical comfort.

Plastic surgery itself has always raised ethical concerns, especially for feminists. We have always been told that we aren't right as we are, that we need to change our looks to please men, or a particular man. Cosmetic surgery is often seen as only a high-tech version of painful assaults on the body which women have experienced for centuries—for example, foot binding, corsets, genital mutilation. Rather than subjecting our bodies to procedures that carry the risk all surgery entails and may cause other health problems as well, many activists in the women's health movement argue, we should change society's approach so that we don't feel the need to have "perfect" or "ideal" bodies.

But that doesn't seem reasonable to me. First of all, it takes a very paternalistic—or maternalistic—view of what's best for other people. Second, some women have very practical needs for bodies that society defines as ideal—like many of the young women I used to meet in my Los Angeles practice who were trying to succeed as actresses and models. Third, even for women whose needs are emotional rather than practical, the feelings are deeply ingrained—they can't just decide not to feel that way. Years of fighting an uphill battle against internalized social expectations can be as devastating as physical illness. A nose job, a face-lift, or enlarged breasts can make a major difference in a woman's life—and whether that would or wouldn't be the case in an ideal world is beside the point.

Not everyone who wants to alter her body is a bimbo. Over the years, I had a range of patients who wanted their breasts augmented. Among them was a gynecologist, married to a surgeon: a well-educated professional, not terribly young, who had silicone implants and said they had made a tremendous difference in her life, and that she'd do it again if she had to make the choice today. Another had gotten her implants in 1980 at the age of 40. "For the first time in my life I was proud of my figure," she told me. "I felt like a new woman." Perhaps it's a pity that society has made these women feel that way, and perhaps we should work to change the way we're taught to view our bodies. But meanwhile, we all have irrational feelings that deeply affect our lives, and none of us needs to be a martyr.

Before we get into the various kinds of plastic surgery, there's a practical consideration you need to address: insurance. You'll need to check with your insurance company about what forms of plastic surgery they will or won't pay for. You'll also want to find out if the insurance company has a disclaimer or exclusion for coverage of future implant-related health problems (medical/surgical). You may have to shoulder the financial responsibility for the procedure yourself.

SILICONE IMPLANT CONTROVERSY

The plastic surgery debate has been kept alive further by the ongoing silicone implant controversy. When silicone was introduced in America in the 1960s as a tool for breast augmentation, it seemed like a godsend. Early experiments with such substances as paraffin, polyurethane foam, and even steel had proved disastrous. But silicone—synthetic plastic composed of the natural material silicon, blended with carbon, hydrogen, and oxygen—is an inert substance, and was perceived at the time as totally harmless. It had been (and continues to be) used in a variety of medical devices: in artificial limbs, in pacemakers, in implants to replace surgically removed testicles, and in penises to make them stiffer.

In its early use for breast augmentation, silicone was given to women in two forms—injections of silicone gel into the breast over a period of weeks, or pockets of silicone gel in a harder, breast-shaped silicone shell implanted surgically into the breast.

Some women have had excellent long-term results from the injections, but many others developed problems. The silicone often traveled through the body, causing unsightly and alarming lumps to form in unexpected spots. The injections were eventually banned, and women wanting their breasts enlarged got the presumably safer implants.

Saline implants were tried very early, but because of leakage, doctors went on to develop the silicone implant, which seemed more appealing at the time. Saline implants work similarly to silicone, except that saline—salt water—is inside the silicone shell instead of silicone gel. Saline implants are no more likely to leak than silicone, but when they leak the saline becomes absorbed by the body fairly quickly so that you realize suddenly that your breast has shrunk. Gel implants, on the other hand, may rupture or leak but the bulk of the material stays together inside the fibrous scar capsule. Therefore the outside appearance may not be changed for some time. Leakage of saline won't cause any medical problems. It has a somewhat less realistic feel than silicone. Dr. William Shaw, a plastic surgeon and one of my former colleagues at UCLA, describes it as feeling "less fleshy than silicone; it's more like a bag of water, particularly when the covering tissue is thin."

Patients with saline implants have complained about problems of capsular contracture, poor aesthetic results, asymmetry, a fluidlike feeling in the breasts, and "rippling" of the breast skin surface due to rippling of the implant shell and capsule. These, however, are all part of the standard issues related to the use of implants; imperfect results occur sometimes. There are no known, specific, documented problems with the saline material itself, compared to gel material. There has been some scandalous speculation of cases of "infection" or fungus growth in the saline of the implant. According to Dr. Shaw, however, these represent isolated cases of positive laboratory culture reports from implants that may be subject to question. There have not been any clinical cases of clinical infection because of bacterial growth inside the implant. The major issues that have been raised regarding silicone gel implants by scientists, consumer groups, regulating agencies, the legal community, the media, and patient support groups center on the harmful effects of implant rupture, the response of human tissue to silicone gel, a possible immune response stimulated by silicone, the development of connective-tissue diseases in patients with implants, and the possible relationship of implants to breast carcinoma.

In 1990, complaints began to be heard from women who were having health problems they were certain were related to silicone implants.[2] In 1992, the FDA banned silicone implants. According to FDA head David Kessler, they did this not because silicone implants were known to pose a risk, but because manufacturers had not fulfilled their legal responsibilities to collect data on the question.

Despite the lack of data, the media reportage of the FDA decision led the public and most judges and juries to believe that there was indeed a connection between the implants and a variety of health problems. Over 18,000 lawsuits were filed against the manufacturers. Three manufacturers of breast implants finally decided, on April 1, 1994, that a global settlement would be the easiest way out, and they set up a fund of $4.2 billion to compensate women with implants who had developed one of eight different diseases.

Under the 1992 FDA ruling, women wishing to have silicone implants can now have them only in conjunction with a long-range study, and only certain categories of women are eligible for these studies. Women with mastectomies, serious injury to the breast, or severe breast abnormality, or those who need new implants due to a rupture in the old one, will be accepted for the study. Women who simply want their breasts enlarged will not be. We'll discuss the implications of all this later in this chapter.

The FDA hearings on the saline implants resulted in a requirement that manufacturers undertake further studies. However, the implants were not taken off the market. Activists are angry that the implants have been used for so long without being studied by manufacturers, scientists, or the FDA. That anger is justified. Women were led to believe by their doctors that the absence of data meant they were safe (much like fertility drugs and postmenopausal hormones today).

As it now exists, I have trouble accepting the FDA ban. We may not have had data showing that implants are safe, but neither do we have data showing that they are dangerous. Despite the testimony of hundreds of women who attributed their health problems to the implants, recent studies have not been able to demonstrate a connection.[3,4]

Even complaints to the FDA suggest that not all women are unhappy with their implants. The FDA reviewed 112 letters received in January 1992.[5] When they analyzed them, they discovered four main themes to the complaints: the women didn't get enough information prior to surgery; they weren't taken seriously by their doctors when they complained of pain; some of them had difficulties carrying on their normal activities; and they had concerns about the future. Most of the complaints were about doctor-patient communication, not medical problems with the implants.

These stories never reached the general population because the media weren't interested in reporting them. Presumably, contented consumers make less exciting copy. When the FDA hearings were going on, a number of people from the press called my office asking to interview some of my patients with silicone implants who were having health problems. I agreed to put them in touch with some patients, as long as they also interviewed other patients who were happy with their implants. They weren't interested. This is shabby, unbalanced journalism, harmful to women with implants who have had no problems but who are now seeing only the horror stories on television. I got calls from some of my scared patients, and I had to reassure them they weren't necessarily going to have problems—that lots of women didn't.

I don't mean to dismiss women's concerns about silicone implants. Larger studies may turn out to validate the suspected links to some diseases. Meanwhile, there are less dramatic but still significant problems for which we do have data.

Implants interfere with how well mammograms can detect tumors in the breast. A study by Mel Silverstein and his colleagues showed that implants create shadows on mammograms, blocking areas from the picture and leading to a decrease in accuracy of a mammogram.[6] It must be remembered, however, that small breasts themselves are hard to visualize on mammogram and that it is not always a surefire way to detect breast cancer. But mammography is still the best tool we have for finding breast cancer before it spreads, and any process that interferes with its effectiveness should be entered into only with great forethought. Women who do have implants need to remember that a normal mammogram cannot be considered reassuring and that they need to take any abnormality seriously.

Furthermore, says Dr. Shaw, silicone isn't the wholly inert substance it was once thought to be, and it always creates some reaction around it. Minuscule amounts of silicone will always leak. The reaction may be something that you'd never notice or be bothered by—the sort of thing that only shows up if the breast is biopsied. Furthermore, he says, "every patient who has an implant develops a capsule around the implant, and the capsule itself is a form of inflammation—like the callous that can develop around a sore spot on your foot after you've stepped on a thorn. And the fact that you have a chronic inflammation can create biological mediators that can, in turn, create some uncomfortable symptoms—soreness around the breast, for example."

Contracture—which means the formation of a thick, spherical scar tissue that causes the breast to be overly firm (Fig. 5-1)—is a real possibility with most implants. It occurs in 1–18 percent of cases in which the implant is under the muscle, and between 18 and 50 percent of cases in which it's between the muscle and breast. This firmness can be so minimal that it's unnoticeable, or it can feel like solid wood—or anything in between. Contracture can be painful, and it can change the appearance of the breast. Contracture, warns Dr. Shaw, may happen to one implant and not the other, or may happen differently in the two implants. "One side is higher, the other lower." Also, the incidence of contracture tends to increase over time. Thus, many results are very good at 5–10 years but may develop progressive distortion and contracture by 15–20 years.

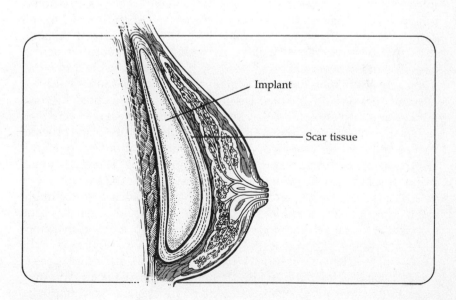

FIGURE 5-1

Failures of reconstruction or augmentation result mostly from surgical problems such as infection, poor healing, and recurrent capsule formation. Some silicone always escapes from the surface of any implant. When levels of silicon ("silicon" is found naturally in everyone's body) are measured in the blood of women with implants, they are significantly higher than in women without implants. In addition, silicone has been found in several other areas of the body, including the skin, pleura (sac surrounding the lungs), chest wall muscles, and lymph nodes. The actual incidence of silicone spread or rupture, however, is unknown. Most of the studies have been on women who were having their implants removed, which is usually done for a reason. This gives us an estimate of rupture in women who have symptoms, but not in women in general. It does appear, however, that the longer an implant is in, the higher the chance for rupture. Some reports suggest that the rate of rupture is as high as 55 percent 10 to 15 years after surgery.[7] As a result, some plastic surgeons recommend that implants be replaced every 10 years.

Rupture is usually diagnosed by seeing a change in the size, shape, or consistency of the implant. It can also be detected through mammography coupled with ultrasound. The most sensitive tool, however, is MRI, which can show very accurately whether there has been a rupture and where.

The idea of a "rupture" sounds ominous, but what does it really mean? For one thing, it can defeat the purpose of the implant by creating a cosmetically unappealing effect. But the more serious question is whether it is dangerous. What does the body do when exposed to silicone? As it does to any foreign body, the immune system will respond to the silicone by trying to clean it up with an inflammatory reaction. This response is what ultimately leads to fibrosis, or capsule formation. This capsule, or scar, varies in degree, and it is what causes hardness around the implant. In some cases, it can be accompanied by local symptoms of pressure sensation and even pain. There have been cases in which the leaked silicone has migrated to the vicinity of the brachial plexus and nerves to the arm, causing chronic irritation and pain. But we don't know if that leakage is dangerous or not. There has never been a randomized study done on the long-term health of women who had silicone injections before they were banned: such a study might tell us if silicone in the breast and other parts of the body causes harm. Dr. Shaw has had a number of patients who had silicone injections years ago, and has seen cases in which hard lumps have formed in the breast, making early cancer detection more difficult, and other cases in which there was infection and dead tissue in the breast itself. This does suggest that similar problems can occur with leakage from implants.

The mystery is why capsules occur in some women and not in all. It may be that some women are more sensitive to silicone than others.

But the biggest concern of the activists is one that remains unproven. They believe that the gel might cause an *autoimmune* disorder (a condition in which the immune system, once turned on, gets carried away and starts attacking the body and connective tissue). The most common of these are scleroderma, lupus, rheumatoid arthritis, dermatomyositis, and Sjorgen's syndrome. Many of the women testifying at the FDA hearings had such disorders, or conditions whose symptoms seemed to be related to them. However, we don't have any way of knowing yet what, if any, relationship there is between the disorder and the implants. It's perfectly possible that there is no relation—that the percentage of women with silicone implants who have these conditions is the same as that of women with no implants who have these conditions. No studies have made any connections between the incidence of such diseases and silicone implants. A comprehensive review of over 15 epidemiological studies covering 4,000 women demonstrated no increased risk of connective tissue diseases among women with breast implants.[8] This does not mean that women reporting symptoms are wrong. They undoubtedly have them. But we simply have no evidence to suggest that this is anything but coincidence. In one case, we can be certain that there was no connection: one of the plaintiff's own doctors testified that her condition had existed before she got the implants. (She won her case against Dow Corning Wright, the implants' manufacturer, anyway, getting $7.3 million.)

One hypothesis is that some women are allergic to silicone, and that for those women a leak causes autoimmune disorders or other health problems, while the women who aren't allergic to silicone have no negative reactions to it. In any case, we certainly can't rule out the possibility that the implants cause health problems until the proper studies have been done.

Another issue is whether silicone implants increase the risk of breast cancer. The best study was in Los Angeles county, where over 3,000 women who had silicone implants were studied for a number of years, and their breast cancer rates compared to the expected incidence of breast cancer in LA.[9] Not only was there no increase in breast cancer in women with implants, but there actually appeared to be a possibility of a decrease. This was substantiated by a second study in Alberta, Canada, in which 13,577 women with breast cancer were studied and only 41 of them had implants.[10] The researchers concluded that there was a lower risk of breast cancer in these women. This may be because plastic surgeons are less likely to put implants into women who are high risk for breast cancer. Women with implants also tend to be thinner and thus at lower risk. Interestingly, however, there are data in animals showing that silicone may protect against breast cancer. We have no idea at this point why this may be so. It does not, of course, suggest that women should run out and get implants as a way to protect themselves from breast cancer. But it certainly does suggest that silicone implants aren't a demonic force, as many opponents have portrayed them.

So there are some proven problems with silicone implants. But they aren't severe enough to justify the FDA's ban—and even if the worst suspicions about their connections with other diseases turn out to be accurate, I'm still not sure I'd support a ban. I'm also a little suspicious about the paternalism in permitting implants in certain categories of women while keeping it from others. I distrust the whole concept that an operation the FDA perceives as too dangerous for "normal" women is somehow all right for women it sees as suffering so much they're permitted to take the risk. It's insulting from both perspectives. It assumes that someone outside can judge subjective suffering. There are women with asymmetry, injured breasts, or even mastectomies who aren't traumatized by their condition and prefer not to use surgical procedures to change it. And there are women who are terribly traumatized by small breasts. It's not up to the government, the plastic surgeons, or even the feminist movement to judge an individual woman's pain.

I'm not convinced women should be deprived of an option that's very important to them. It might be a lot better to make certain that plastic surgeons give prospective patients full information about all the possible dangers they may be subjecting themselves to, and then let the women decide for themselves. Even if it turns out that the implants do cause health problems in a certain number of women, there's no reason to deprive a woman who, fully informed, chooses to take the risk. People take risks every day that others find foolish or dangerous. As my coauthor, Karen Lindsey, who had silicone injections in the mid-1960s, wrote in the feminist newspaper *Sojourner,* "I can, if I choose, drink a quart of whiskey a day and smoke a pack of cigarettes a day. I can eat fats and sugar by the pound. I can fly in airplanes and ride motorcycles and walk alone down dangerous dark streets. I can do all kinds of dangerous things if I choose to do them—and I should be able to." Implants, adds Dr. Shaw, aren't all bad or all good, and he too believes the ban goes too far. "The ban implies it's all bad. It limits what we can do, and it creates tremendous fear. It's too simplistic."

Luckily for women who want implants, there are now a number of studies about implants being done. First, each implant (silicone gel or saline) put in the body is documented in a prospective manner. Surgeons are required to keep information about implants in a prospective study and to report problems periodically. Over many years, this will give us much better information about the magnitude and nature of the potential implant-related problems. Second, plastic surgeons and manufacturers are now studying different alternative materials to be used as fillers in breast implants, in place of silicone material. While we might anticipate certain improvements, particularly in terms of mammogram, it is unlikely that future implants will be totally trouble-free. We don't know if they could cause infection. Further, they would still be in a silicone pouch; in addition to the possible problems with the pouch itself, we still don't know if there would be reactions caused by the silicone rubber interacting with the oil on the one side and the patient's body on the other. "In the best possibility, it's still a foreign implant," Dr. Shaw warns. "Not every patient will have a good result." Unfortunately there are no studies on possible substitutes for the silicone pouch, because no solid substance is less inert than silicone.

According to Dr. Shaw, after a patient spends many years with implants there may be reason to remove them surgically because of local problems with capsular contracture, poor results, or ruptures, or because of systemic conditions that may or may not have a direct link to the implants. Also, some patients, after many years, may not wish to have such large breasts anymore and do not want to live with possible future problems with implants. In all of these patients silicone breast implants may be removed surgically to improve the patient's sense of comfort and security. The problem is that the removal of silicone breast implants requires surgery that is often tedious. Another issue is that the reduction of the volume of the breasts may be a shock to a woman after so many years of having larger breasts. Finally, many breasts would become more saggy and relatively deformed after implant removal. Dr. Shaw says he gets better results by doing an immediate *mastopexy,* or reshaping of the breasts, similar to breast reduction or *ptosis* (sagging breasts) correction. Many women are pleased with their resulting smaller but more shapely breasts. In most cases, immediate mastopexy can be performed at the same time as implant removal surgery.

THE PROCEDURE

It's been my experience that, when considering surgery, some patients want to know all the details of the operation, while others just want to know what it will do for them and leave the details up to the doctor. For this reason I've begun each discussion of cosmetic surgery procedures with a brief mention of what the procedure sets out to accomplish. Those of my readers who are content with that can skip the rest. But for those of you who want the "gory details," read on!

BREAST AUGMENTATION

Before considering augmentation surgery, women over 35 should have a mammogram to make sure there's no cancer there. In addition, the surgeon should check for cysts that will require needle aspirations (see Chapter 8). As Robert Goldwyn, a plastic surgeon colleague in my Boston days, puts it, "You don't want to be sticking needles into the patient's breast when there's a silicone gel bag inside it." The plastic surgeon will also take a careful history.

The surgeon should show you pictures of breasts that have been augmented, including those that have left very visible scars, so you know both the best and the worst possible results of your operation. You and the surgeon should also discuss what size you want your new breasts to be, and you need to be realistic about that—you won't have enough breast tissue to turn tiny breasts into huge ones. Dr. Goldwyn tells of a petite woman who wanted to go from a size 34A to a size 34D. "Not only did she lack sufficient soft tissue to harbor such implants," he says, "but the results would have been poor, even bizarre." Dr. Shaw emphasizes that the augmentation should be appropriate for the size and build of the patient.

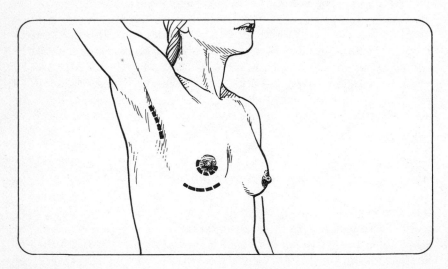

FIGURE 5-2

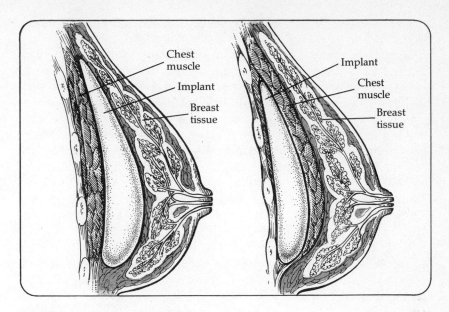

Chest muscle

Implant

Breast tissue

Implant

Chest muscle

Breast tissue

FIGURE 5-3

If you're married, some surgeons will want to make sure your husband feels okay about your having augmentation, since an angry husband might later try to sue the doctor. Dr Shaw points out that it is not so important for medical or legal reasons, but may be important for the marital relationship. If you feel that it is your decision alone, let the surgeon know, and try to work it out. If you can't, find a surgeon willing to do what you want.

The operation can be done under either local or general anesthetic. Some patients, says Dr. Shaw, prefer to use general anesthetic because they fear pain, and some surgeons also prefer it.

The incision is made either through the armpit, underneath the breast, or around the areola (Fig. 5-2). All of these have their proponents. The implant can be placed under the breast tissue between the breast and the muscles or under the muscle itself (Fig. 5-3). According to Dr Shaw, putting the implant under the muscles has two disadvantages: a tendency for a flatter breast and the possibility of movement of the breast with the muscle. But it has two advantages: it seems to carry less risk of contracture and, even more important, it's less likely to hide a cancer if one develops in the future.

The operation is usually done on an outpatient basis; it takes about two hours or more, depending on whether or not the surgeon puts the implant under the muscle, which takes more time. You go home after the operation. The stitches will be removed about 10 days later. You'll be out of work for about two to five days, and shouldn't drive a car for a week. In three weeks you'll be able to jog or play tennis.

Side effects can include infection, which occurs in less than 1 percent of cases, and bleeding, which is equally rare. There may be permanent altering of sensation in the nipple or areola, which occurs in less than 2 percent of cases, and there is also a slight possibility of reduced sensation in the breast itself. There's also the possibility of visible scarring and of contracture, both of which we mentioned earlier. And there is some possibility that lactation will be interfered with, unless the surgeon makes sure the scar is not next to the areola and no ducts are severed.

Implant rupture, as we discussed earlier, is a possible serious complication, though not a common one. It can occur through strenuous physical force or just spontaneously. The implant needs to be removed immediately and the surgeon must try to take out all the silicone in a procedure known as *explantation.* This is difficult surgery because it involves trying to remove all of the silicone, so it requires a surgeon experienced in the procedure.

Unfortunately, for now at least, some form of implant is the best we can do for women wanting to have their breasts enlarged. There are operations using the body's own tissue that are done for breast reconstruction after mastectomy (see Chapter 26), but they really don't make much sense for less drastic cosmetic purposes, says Dr. Shaw. "It's a big operation, and you'd have large scars on the area the tissue is taken from, so you'd create an aesthetic problem as great as the one you're trying to fix. Particularly for a very young woman, it wouldn't be worth it. For a middle-aged woman with very, very small breasts, whose tummy is probably pushing out a bit and whose cosmetic expectations may not be as great, it's a possibility, especially if she's had implants and now needs to have them removed." He warns also that insurance rarely pays for this kind of operation.

SURGERY FOR ASYMMETRY

To correct asymmetry, the doctor can use one of three procedures, and it's important for you as the patient to know which of the three you want. You can have an implant put in one, or you can have the other made smaller, or you can have a combination of both. Your doctor may assume you want the smaller breast augmented; if you don't, make that clear. (Silicone, as I noted earlier, is still legal for this kind of surgery, provided you're followed up in the NCI's study.)

The procedures used to reconstruct a breast are also possible, but they're far more drastic since they involve using flaps of skin, muscle, and fat from your back or abdomen. Particularly if you're young and healthy, it might be worth putting your body through the discomfort one time, knowing that with an implant you're likely to have it removed and replaced at a later date. If your asymmetry results from Poland's syndrome or an injury such as we discussed in Chapter 4, appropriate breast reconstruction utilizing expanders, implants, or one's own tissues will achieve a reasonable result. Unlike the situation of the woman with small but symmetrical breasts, the scars created in the area the tissue is taken from are likely to disturb you less than the cosmetic problems themselves.

If you're thinking of implants for asymmetry, keep in mind that exact matching is unlikely. If there's a difference in nipple and areola size, the implant operation will stretch the nipple and areola on the smaller breast. And, since silicone has now been added under tight skin, the augmented breast will tend not to sag like a normal breast does as you age. Still, these differences are minor compared to the original asymmetry, and it's likely that you yourself will be the only one to notice. Remember, you may need to have your implant replaced at some point, so be sure you know what size it is.

BREAST REDUCTION

Most women come for this operation because they're embarrassed by their large breasts or because they have discomfort from neck and back pain. As with the other operations described in this chapter, if a woman is over 35 she should have a mammogram to make sure there's no cancer.

On the patient's first visit, says my colleague Dr. Goldwyn, "I show them photos of breasts that have had reduction surgery to make sure they know there will be scars." The doctor will explain what sizes are possible; most of Dr. Goldwyn's patients want to be a B, and some want to be a C. Dr. Shaw points out that it is difficult to be sure that the patient and the surgeon both have the same idea of what a "B" or "C" cup is. He often has patients bring in pictures from magazines to be sure he knows what their expectations are. It's not always possible to get exactly the size you want, but a good surgeon can approximate it well. Then the operation is scheduled. There are a number of variations of the breast reduction operation, but all start with the same basic procedure.

The operation is usually done under general anesthesia and takes place the day you're admitted to the hospital. It may last up to four hours. Your nipples can be either removed and grafted back, or left on breast tissue and transposed. Most doctors today prefer not to graft the nipples except in extremely large reductions, since they lose sensitivity if all the nerves are severed.

Most procedures involve some variation of the "keyhole" technique. The amount of tissue to be removed is determined and a pattern drawn on the breast (Fig. 5-4). The nipple is preserved on a small flap of tissue while the tissue to be removed is taken from below and from the sides. This allows the surgeon to elevate the nipple and bring the flaps of tissue together, giving both uplift and reduction. The resulting scars are below the breast in the inframammary fold and come right up the center to the nipple. In recent years, says Dr. Shaw, there is a preference for shorter incisions under the breast. In some cases only a circular scar around the nipple is used—the so-called doughnut, or concentric, reduction pattern.

Patients experience pain the first day after the operation, but there's not much pain after that. You can go home the next morning, wearing a bra or some form of support. The stitches are out in one to two weeks, and you can go back to work; in three to four weeks you can be playing tennis.

Side effects include infection, which can occur with any operation. There's a slight risk that you'll need blood transfusions, but it's very rare. If you're worried, however, give your own blood to the hospital two or three months in advance, and it will be there in case you need it. There's some danger of the operation interfering with the blood supply of the nipple and areola; if this happens the nipple and areola die and need to be artificially reconstructed. It's not a very great danger— it happens in less than 4 percent of operations. The larger your breasts are, the greater the danger. Reduction does not affect a woman's risk of cancer. Your ability to breast-feed will be decreased; studies show that about half of women who have had reductions can still nurse their babies.

Some of the erotic sensation in your nipples may be reduced, though for many women the increased relaxation actually makes sex more pleasurable after reduction surgery. Also, because the nerves in the nipple of the overlarge breast are so stretched out, the nipple is unlikely to have much sensitivity to begin with, and the loss of sensation—in terms of both sexual activity and breast feeding—will probably go unnoticed. There's also a possibility of some reduction of sensitivity in the breast itself, although again this is minimal. There's no way to know in advance whether or not you'll experience reduced sensation, so you have to decide for yourself how important full sensation is, compared to whatever physical or emotional discomfort your large

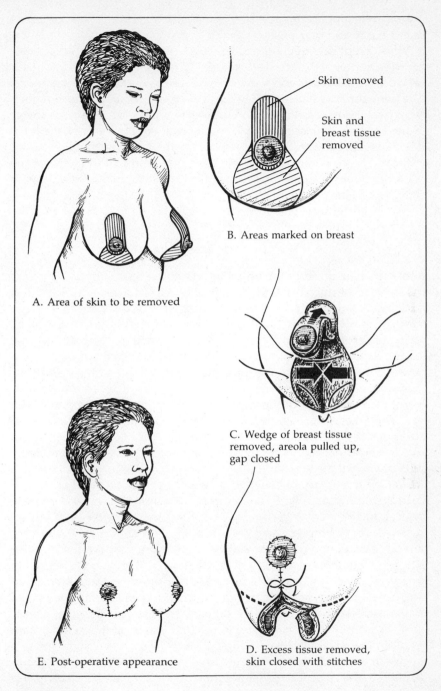

A. Area of skin to be removed

B. Areas marked on breast

Skin removed

Skin and
breast tissue
removed

C. Wedge of breast tissue
removed, areola pulled up,
gap closed

D. Excess tissue removed,
skin closed with stitches

E. Post-operative appearance

FIGURE 5-4

breasts create for you. In any case, you'll still retain most of your breast sensation.

If you do decide to get reduction surgery, be aware that if you later gain weight, your breasts will probably also gain weight, just as they would without the surgery. This happened to a number of my patients. One woman had her size 36EE breasts reduced to a 36B, but they ended up a 36D. According to Dr. Goldwyn and Dr. Shaw, the more the patient sees the operation as reconstructive, the happier she'll be, while the more she sees it as cosmetic, the more critical she'll be about the result. When it's only cosmetic, she's more likely to focus on the scars; if it relieves pain and discomfort, she'll focus on how much better she feels.

THE BREAST LIFT

As mentioned earlier, sagging breasts (known medically as "ptosis") can be made firmer through an operation called a mastopexy, which Dr. Goldwyn describes as "a face-lift of the breasts." A mastopexy can give your breasts uplift, but Dr. Goldwyn warns that it will not make your breasts look like a 20-year-old's. And it will leave scars—sometimes bad ones, depending on how your body usually scars. Like a face-lift, it won't last forever: remember, you've got gravity and time working against you.

Your first step is to set up a meeting with your plastic surgeon, who will take a very thorough medical history. You should get a mammogram before proceeding further, if you haven't had one recently. Be sure to get a full description of both the best and the worst possible results of a mastopexy.

This operation usually involves removing excess skin and fat and elevating the nipple (Fig. 5-5). If you're very large-breasted, you may want reduction surgery as well, especially since a mastopexy is less effective on very large breasts: gravity pulls them down. If you're very small-breasted, you may want an augmentation. (Both of these procedures were described earlier in this chapter.)

If your operation doesn't involve reduction or augmentation, it's a simpler procedure, and can be done either in the hospital under general anesthetic or in the doctor's office with local anesthesia. Since insurance won't pay for it, most women prefer the latter. The operation lasts about two and a half hours; the stitches are removed in two weeks. By three weeks, you'll be able to participate in sports. You should wear a bra constantly for many weeks after surgery. Follow-up is minimal—three or four visits during the year after surgery.

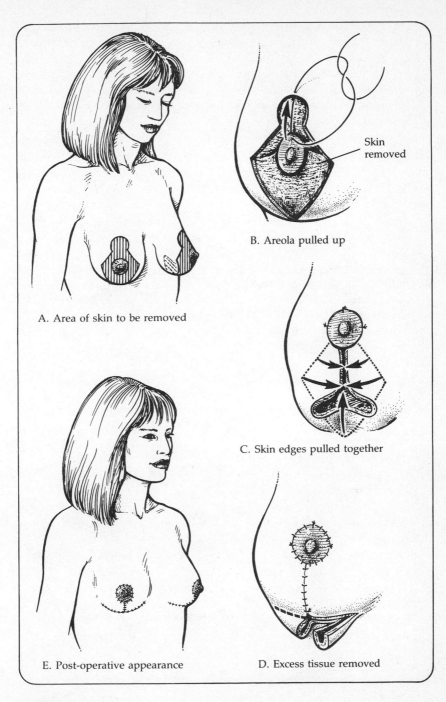

A. Area of skin to be removed

B. Areola pulled up

Skin removed

C. Skin edges pulled together

D. Excess tissue removed

E. Post-operative appearance

FIGURE 5-5

You may experience some very slight loss of sensation in the nipple or areola. Other than that, there are no particular side effects to mastopexy.

INVERTED NIPPLES

There is an operation that can reverse inversion of nipples, but it doesn't always work, and the inversion may recur. It's a very simple procedure, usually done under local anesthetic with no intravenous medication, and you can go back to work the next day. The stitches will come out in about two weeks.

Nipples are usually inverted because they are tethered down by scar or other tissue from birth. To reverse it, the surgeon will reach down and pull the nipple, stretch it, and make an incision, releasing the constricting tissue (Fig. 5-6). There are a number of procedures, and each one has its advocates. If the inversion recurs, the operation can be redone.

This operation can make a psychological difference for teenagers, who often feel extremely self-conscious about their inverted nipples. It

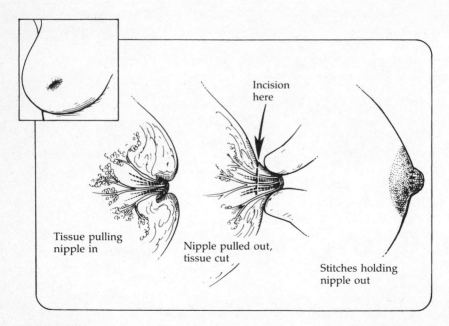

FIGURE 5-6

definitely interferes with breast feeding, but women with inverted nipples usually already have difficulty with breast feeding.

THINKING ABOUT PLASTIC SURGERY

None of these operations is medically necessary. Still, we're lucky to live in an age when they're available. For a woman deeply unhappy with the way her breasts look, plastic surgery offers a solution that can make a major psychological difference in her life. No operation will make you look "perfect" (whatever that is), but all of these procedures will help you look more normal and feel more comfortable in your body.

If you're thinking about plastic surgery, you should ask yourself a few questions. The first and probably most important is, who wants the surgery? If you're contented with your breasts, but your mother or boyfriend or someone else is pressuring you into surgery, you probably shouldn't do it. It's your body, not theirs.

The second question is, how realistic are your expectations, and how clear an idea do you have about the kind of breasts you want? Dr. John T. Heuston, a noted plastic surgeon, has written some wise words about reduction surgery that can equally well apply to all forms of cosmetic surgery for the breasts.[11] "The concept of an ideal operation," he writes, "carries with it the concept of an ideal breast. The surgeon seeks the best means to construct the breast form—but for whom? For him or her, or for the patient, or both?" As Heuston notes, there is no objectively ideal breast; each of us has her or his own ideal. So you should have a clear sense of what size and shape breast you want, and what your own goals are. The surgeon can't make your breasts absolutely perfect, but if your goals are fairly reasonable, they can come pretty close to being met. If you do decide on plastic surgery make sure you know the range of possible results. Some plastic surgeons like to "sell" their operation—a practice Dr. Goldwyn abhors. "Too often doctors use pictures to seduce patients into surgery," he says. "I think it's a form of hucksterism. If you're shown pictures of a surgeon's best results, insist upon seeing pictures of the average and worst results as well." Dr. Shaw concurs. "Communication between plastic surgeon and patient can be very tricky," he says. "It requires a tremendous amount of honesty and self-restraint. Both the patient and the surgeon constantly need to separate wishes for perfection from the reality of what can be reasonably expected."

Once you know what you want, don't hesitate to shop around for the right plastic surgeon. You should choose someone you feel abso-

lutely comfortable with and confident in. Above all, it should be someone who respects your ideal and doesn't seek to impose her or his ideal
on you. The surgeon's "beautiful breast" and yours may be very dis-
similar. Make sure you find someone who will construct *your* breast.
And make sure you find someone who respects who you are, and why
you're making your decision. One woman I know went to a plastic surgeon when she was 20, hoping to have her painfully large breasts reduced. The surgeon wanted her to wait until she had children and
had breast-fed them. She told him she was a lesbian and didn't plan
to have children. "In that case," he told her, "you won't need your
breasts—why don't we just cut them both off?" The experience so em-
bittered and intimidated the woman that she still, more than 30 years
later, hasn't had her breasts reduced. Remember that you don't have to
submit yourself to the surgeon's prejudices. If the surgeon you've approached acts insulting or condescending, go out and find someone
with a more professional, more humane approach.

Of course, there's no guarantee that you'll be happy with your operation after it's done, even if you have taken every precaution possible.
But the odds are on your side. I've had very few patients who regretted
having their breasts cosmetically altered, but I've had several who regretted not having it done. One of my Boston patients was an 80-year-
old woman with huge, uncomfortable breasts. When she was younger,
she went to a surgeon to try and get her breasts reduced. He told her
she shouldn't have the operation. She took his advice—those were the
days when doctors were gods; you didn't question them—and since
then had been uncomfortable and unhappy with her breasts. After we
talked she decided to have the surgery done. She was very happy with
her small breasts—and very sad about all the years she could have
been this comfortable.

Another of my patients was a sophisticated career woman in her
early 30s. During our first visit I noticed that her breasts were extremely asymmetrical, and after a few visits I asked her if she'd ever
thought about plastic surgery. Her face lit up. "Can I really do that?"
she asked me. I assured her that she could, and gave her a list of plastic
surgeons. She didn't even wait till she got out of the building to call
them; she found a phone booth downstairs, made an appointment, and
had her implant within the month. She's absolutely delighted with it—
but she needed me to suggest it and to give her "permission" to seek
help for her asymmetry. My coauthor, who had silicone injections for
her asymmetry, has found that her breasts are no longer perfectly
matched, and, as she grows older, the augmented breast sags much
more than the natural one. But she is very happy about her decision and says she would make the same choice again today. She keeps
in her closet an old V-necked sweater her mother gave her after she

finished her injections—a symbol of a freedom she hadn't known before.

We have seen so much news in the past few years about women who are unhappy with their silicone implants that it's easy to forget that the vast majority of patients—those that don't get in the news—are happy with their decision to alter their breasts. Psychologist Sanford Gifford writes about a patient feeling she had "gained something lost in early puberty."[12] He observes that the degree of satisfaction is much greater among women who have had plastic surgery for their breasts than among those who have had face-lifts or nose jobs—they don't have the same unrealistic expectations. Often they're happier with their still-imperfect breasts than the surgeon thinks they should be. For some reason people don't go into this kind of plastic surgery with the same dreams of impossible perfection they bring to facial surgery.

If you want plastic surgery for your breasts, make sure you have all the information you need about risks, dangers, and reasonable expectations—and then do what you want. And don't let age deter you from the cosmetic surgery you want. My 80-year-old patient was delighted with her belated operation, and I've had many women in their 50s, 60s, and 70s who have had their breasts reduced or augmented. If your health is good enough to sustain surgery, it doesn't matter how old you are.

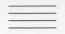

PART TWO

COMMON PROBLEMS
OF THE BREAST

6

"Fibrocystic Disease" and Breast Pain

You're concerned about your breasts: they get swollen and hard just before your period. Or they're painful, so painful you can't get any work done. Or there's discharge when you squeeze your nipple.

So you talk to a friend who says, "Oh, I know what that is! I had it a few years ago, and my doctor told me it was fibrocystic disease!"

You decide, quite sensibly, to talk to *your* doctor. After all, if you've got a disease you want to know about it. Probably nowadays your doctor will tell you not to worry about "fibrocystic disease" and will then go on to look at your specific symptom. But if your doctor is a bit more old-school, you may hear that you do indeed have fibrocystic disease.

Well, you *don't* have fibrocystic disease—any more than you have a werewolf bite. In both cases, there's no such animal. "Fibrocystic disease" is a meaningless umbrella term—a wastebasket into which doctors throw every breast problem that isn't cancerous. The symptoms it encompasses are so varied and so unrelated to each other that the term is wholly without meaning. To an examining doctor, "fibrocystic disease" can be swelling, pain, tenderness, lumpy breasts (a condition not to be confused with breast lumps—see Chapter 8), nipple discharge—any noncancerous thing that can happen in or on the breast. That's the clinical version of our mythical disease.

To a pathologist, fibrocystic disease is any one of about 15 microscopic findings that exist in virtually every woman's breasts, and that never reveal themselves except through a microscope. They cause no trouble, and they have no relation to cancer—or to anything else, except the body's natural aging process. They were found in the particular breast tissue that was biopsied only because it *was* biopsied, not because they had any relation to whatever symptom the examining doctor was concerned with. Only one of these microscopic findings is a danger sign: it's called *atypical hyperplasia,* and, combined with a family history of breast cancer, it can suggest an increased breast cancer risk (see Chapter 16).

The radiologists who read mammograms have another version of fibrocystic disease altogether—dense breasts. Dense breasts are normal in young women, as we discussed in Chapter 1. Breast tissue that is unusually dense for one's age is, however, related to hormonal stimulation of the breast which has been implicated in the increased risk of breast cancer.[1]

So whatever problem you have with your breasts, it isn't fibrocystic disease. But the invention of this mythical disease has caused a number of problems. Insurance companies have refused to cover women diagnosed with the "disease"—or have covered them, but excluded coverage of breast problems. If such women do develop breast diseases, their medical bills can be devastating.

Women have also been subjected to a number of "treatments"— ranging from eliminating caffeine from their diets to getting prophy-

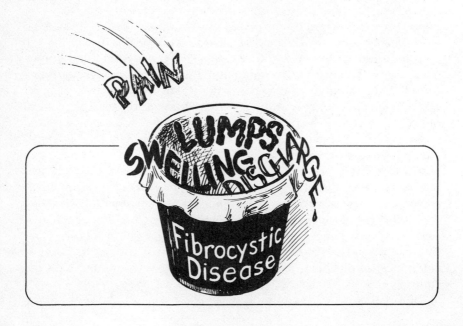

lactic mastectomies. Finally, for a long time researchers didn't bother to study any of the conditions defined as fibrocystic disease, since they believed a diagnosis already existed. As a result, we haven't had the studies necessary to help us learn what does cause some of the real problems, such as breast pain, that women actually do experience.

I'm proud to have been a pioneer in debunking the myth of fibrocystic disease. After doing a lot of research into the studies claiming to define the "disease," I wrote about my findings in the *New England Journal of Medicine* in 1982. Interestingly, no doctors wrote to the journal to argue against my findings. But it took four years for the College of American Pathologists to come out with a statement that fibrocystic disease doesn't increase the risk of cancer.[2]

Nevertheless, many doctors still insist that such a condition exists. Some of them now call it "fibrocystic changes" instead of disease. But that's ridiculous—what has changed, and what has it changed into? Frequently, they prescribe abstinence from caffeine to help clear up the dangers of this nonexistent condition. When challenged they argue that patients are reassured when they're offered treatments, and that coffee is bad for people anyway.

I have a lot of problems with this. If someone decides to give up caffeine because it's bad for her nerves or keeps her awake or any other reason, that's fine. But if she's depriving herself of something she enjoys in order to prevent a nonexistent disease from escalating into breast cancer, that's not fine at all. It may make sense to lie to children for their own good (though I doubt that very much), but it's patronizing and unethical to do it to adults.

Fortunately, fewer and fewer doctors are perpetuating the concept of fibrocystic disease. In Europe it's still used, but always only for one specific symptom—lumpy breasts. I'm still not happy about that, since lumpy breasts are no more a disease than curly hair or large feet—but at least it's reduced to only one situation. Europeans call breast pain "mastalgia," a sensible enough term since *mast* is Latin for breast and *algia* is Latin for pain. By separating out the different symptoms they allow each symptom to be studied on its own—a vast improvement.

Our own history provides an even better model. In the late 19th and early 20th centuries there was no "fibrocystic disease"; there were simply symptoms: you had breast pain, or lumpiness, or nipple discharge. It was only later that the silly term came into existence and became the wastebasket into which everything that wasn't cancer got thrown. Fortunately, we're coming back to that. Fibrocystic disease, that wastebasket term, is finally finding *itself* in the wastebasket.

In this chapter, and the two following, we'll discuss the various kinds of benign breast conditions. One common breast symptom is pain—frequently called either "mastalgia" or "mastodynia" (one's

Latin, the other's Greek, and they both translate to "breast pain"). It can run the gamut of discomfort—from a minor irritation a couple of days a month through permanent, nearly disabling agony, and everything in between.

A clinic in Cardiff, Wales, documented three main categories of breast pain: cyclical (pain related to the menstrual cycle), noncyclical ("trigger zone" pain), and pain that is non-breast in origin. Of these the most common by far is cyclical.[3]

The best way to determine which kind of pain you have is to keep a breast pain chart.[4] This is no more than a calendar where you mark every day whether your pain is severe, mild, or gone. In addition, you mark the days of your period. Looking at this you can easily determine whether your pain is premenstrual or everyday (that is, cyclical or noncyclical) or non-breast in origin.

CYCLICAL PAIN

We know that cyclical mastalgia is related to hormonal variations. The breasts are sensitive right before menstruation, then less sensitive once the period begins. For some women, tenderness begins at the time of ovulation and continues until their period, leaving only a couple of pain-free weeks during their cycles. Sometimes it's barely noticeable, but some women are in such pain they can't wear a T-shirt, lie on their stomachs, or tolerate hugs. Sometimes it's only in one breast, and other times it radiates into the armpit, and even down to the elbows, causing its poor victim to think she's got cancer spreading to her lymph nodes.

Understanding precisely the part hormones play in cyclical mastalgia is clouded by the fact that women's hormonal cycles haven't themselves been all that well researched. Although we know roughly how the levels of estrogen and progesterone go up and down during each cycle and that FSH and LH are the main pituitary hormones, we don't yet understand the "fine tuning" of these hormones, and how the hormones regulate and affect the different parts of the body. Just as we don't understand menstrual cramps and bloating and PMS, we don't understand breast pain.

Some studies in Europe have given us preliminary clues to the role of hormones in breast pain. Dr. P. Mauvais-Jarvis in France has shown that the amount of progesterone put out by the ovary in the second half of the menstrual cycle seems to vary in patients with breast pain: he found a decreased ratio of progesterone to estrogen in patients with mastalgia.[5] Other investigators have found that an abnormality in the regulation of prolactin seems to affect breast pain.[6] [7] Although prolactin blood levels in the subjects of these studies appear to be normal, these women are much more sensitive to stimulation with thyroid-stimulating hormone: they are "hyperreactive." In a study comparing women with pain to women with no pain Dr. J. Ayres found that patients with mastalgia had a lower progesterone to estrogen ratio as well as a hyperreactiveness in the regulation of prolactin, while the women in the control group did not.[8] Predictably, lumpiness demonstrated on ultrasound did not relate to the hormonal aberrations—only pain did.

Hormones may also affect cyclical breast pain in a more subtle way—for example, as a result of stress. We know that stress can affect the menstrual cycle: you can miss your period, or have a particularly heavy period, or an early or late period, when you're under a great deal of stress, positive or negative. Similarly, your breast pain can increase or change in its pattern with the hormone changes of stress. We also know that hormones vary at different points in your life and that the incidence of breast pain often follows these shifts. It's usually most intense in the teens and then again in the 40s—at both ends of the fertile years. It almost always ends with menopause, though in some rare cases it lasts beyond menopause—perhaps because of the continuing estrogen production of the ovaries and breast tissue (see Chapter 1). And of course, if a postmenopausal woman is taking hormones, her body thinks she's still premenopausal and she's as likely to get breast pain as she was before.[9] We also know it's common in pregnant women; indeed, unusual breast pain can be an early sign of pregnancy.

The relation to hormones doesn't appear to be absolute—there must be other factors, since most often the pain is more severe in one breast than in the other, and a purely hormonal symptom would have to affect both equally. It appears to be caused by a combination of the hormonal activity and something in the breast tissue that responds to that activity. More research clearly needs to be done.

Breast pain is annoying, but it usually isn't unbearable—what *can* be unbearable is the fear that it's cancer. The best "treatment," therefore, is reassurance. The study in Cardiff suggests that 85 percent of women with breast pain are worried much more about the possibility of cancer than about the pain itself. Most of them, when reassured that their problem has no relation to cancer, are relieved, and feel they can live with their pain. This study was repeated in Brazil just to see if it was only Welsh women who responded to reassurance. Sure enough, Brazilian women also responded to reassurance with a success rate of 70.2 percent.[10] Only 10–15 percent of the women have pain that's incapacitating and needs treatment.

The treatments of cyclical breast pain that have been proposed are many and varied. Some work and some don't. Many clinicians suggest stopping caffeine or taking vitamin E, despite studies showing that this approach does not work. Some physicians who believe the pain comes from water retention recommend diuretics ("water pills"). These give little relief. Others have tried everything from ginseng tea, vitamin A, vitamin B complex, and antibiotics, to just a firm support bra.

If you have breast pain, the first step is to get a good examination from a breast specialist, or someone knowledgeable in the field who will take your symptoms and concerns seriously (this may take some searching). If you're over 35, have a mammogram. Once you know you don't have cancer you can decide whether you are able to live with your discomfort or want to further explore treatment. You might also want to look into Chinese herbs and acupuncture, both of which have been used for centuries in China. In some cases, herbs and acupuncture are used together; in others, the patient and/or practitioner prefer to use one or the other. They can also be used for noncylical pain (see below.)

Another possibility is the use of meditation and visualization techniques, such as those discussed in Chapter 29. A number of studies have shown that these techniques can be effective in reducing pain, and they may well help relieve both cyclical and noncyclical breast pain.

If you are in your 20s, you may want to try the pill. Analgesics like aspirin, Tylenol, and ibuprofen can offer some relief, and wearing a firm bra will at least prevent bouncing breasts from increasing your discomfort.

A reasonable treatment plan for moderate to severe mastalgia has been proposed by the breast pain group in Wales. Although different women will respond better to different drugs, they assure relief of pain in 70–80 percent of women when their regimen has been followed.[11] They recommend evening primrose oil (a natural form of gamolenic acid) as the first step for women with moderate pain and those who are taking oral contraceptives. It can be obtained in health food stores as tablets containing 500 mg of gamolenic acid. Six capsules should be taken twice a day. It has minor side effects, but the reaction to therapy can take a while so a trial of treatment should last at least four months and be monitored by keeping your pain chart. This treatment has been shown to benefit 44–58 percent of women. If pain has decreased, evening primrose oil is continued for one to two months more and then discontinued. Many women will have long-lasting effects even after discontinuing therapy.[12] But don't take it if you're pregnant or trying to get pregnant as it can cause a miscarriage.

The next step for treatment in those women for whom evening primrose oil doesn't work is hormonal. Danazol and bromocriptine have been shown to have some benefit. Both drugs should be used only in women who are not taking oral contraceptives and who are using adequate mechanical contraception. Danazol is given at 200–300 mg per day and slowly reduced to 100 mg a day after relief of symptoms. Danazol will relieve pain in 70–80 percent of women.[13] Side effects are common, including menstrual irregularities, leg cramps, weight gain, and decreased libido. The symptoms are related to the dose and so the recommendation is to start with 200 mg a day for a month and, if the pain is diminished, to reduce it to 100 mg a day for the second month and then to stop. Women rarely need a longer course of therapy.

Bromocriptine inhibits the release of prolactin and has been shown to be effective in up to 65 percent of women treated for cyclical breast pain at doses of 5 mg a day. These results were demonstrated in a European multicenter randomized controlled trial.[14] Mild side effects such as nausea, dizziness, headaches, and irritability have been reported in 30 percent of women and 10 percent complained of severe side effects. Most of these effects can be avoided by gradually increasing the dose, taking the drug with meals, and using the smallest amount necessary to get an effect. (See Fig. 6-1 for an explanation of where the treatments described have their effects.) If bromocriptine is tried first and does not work, about 30 percent of women will respond to danazol, and vice versa if danazol is tried first. These two drugs are the only ones approved for the treatment of breast pain at this time. Other drugs have been shown to be effective but are not as yet approved for that purpose.

Tamoxifen is an estrogen blocker (see Chapter 28). According to an English study, it's very good at relieving mastalgia (80–90%).[15] Side effects include hot flashes and menstrual irregularities. Luckily, it was shown to be just as effective at 10 mg per day as at 20, and three months of treatment were just as good as six. A group in Minnesota reports using 10 mg for two months with good results and only a 30 percent recurrence rate.[16] LH-RH analogues are drugs that put you into a reversible menopause. In one study they achieved an 81 percent response rate when given by injection.[17] Side effects include hot flashes, headaches, nausea, and irritability. Because these drugs decrease bone density (see Chapter 23) they should only be used for a short period of time.

A more benign remedy, a low-fat diet, has been studied and shown to have some effect on cyclical mastalgia and hormone levels.[18] W. R. Ghent and colleagues have theorized that the absence of dietary iodine may render duct lining cells more sensitive to estrogen stimulation.[19] As a result, they have been studying the use of molecular iodine as a treatment for breast pain with some success.

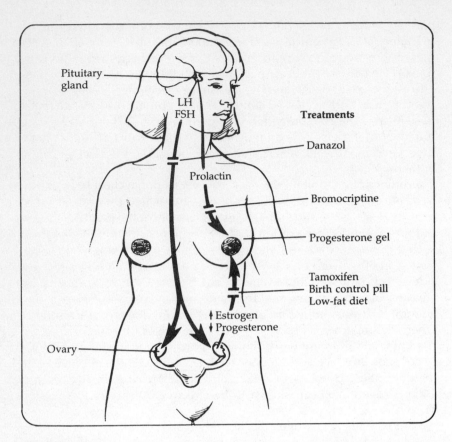

FIGURE 6-1

Eventually we will be able to invent something specifically for breast pain like the prostaglandin inhibitors (ibuprofen) that work so well with menstrual cramps, and women will no longer have to suffer from it.

NONCYCLICAL PAIN

Noncyclical pain is far less common than cyclical pain. It also feels a lot different. To begin with, it doesn't vary with your menstrual cycle—it's there, and it stays there. It's also known as "trigger zone" breast pain because it's almost always in one specific area: you can point exactly to where it hurts. It's anatomical rather than hormonal—something in the breast tissue is causing it (although we usually don't know what).

Rarely, it can be a sign of cancer, so it's always worth checking out with your doctor, especially if you are over 30.

One cause of noncyclical breast pain is trauma—a blow to the breast will obviously cause it to hurt, and a breast biopsy is likely to leave some pain (see Chapter 11). Many women get slight shooting or stabbing pains up to two years or more after a biopsy. And you're never quite perfect after any surgery—just as after breaking a leg you can always tell when it will rain. This kind of pain is usually pretty obvious: it's on the spot where your scar is. It's unpleasant, but it's nothing to worry about.

Often, we simply don't know what causes noncyclical breast pain; we'll operate and remove the area, have the tissue studied, and find nothing abnormal. Unfortunately we don't relieve the pain.

Treatment for this kind of breast pain is more difficult than for cyclical breast pain. Again, start with a good exam, and, if you're over 35, a mammogram. If there's an obvious abnormality it can then be taken care of. For example, sometimes a gross cyst (see Chapter 8) causing localized breast pain or tenderness can be cured by needle aspiration.

Since noncyclical pain is rarely caused by hormones, hormonal treatments are less likely to work. Some women, however, find relief with the other kinds of treatments mentioned under cyclical breast pain.[20] You may want to try them. Sometimes, though not invariably, having a biopsy relieves the pain—though, of course, you will have the pain of the biopsy itself. A good test is for your doctor to inject some local anesthesia into the spot. If it gives relief then surgery may work well; if not, then it probably isn't worth it.

The best treatment is most likely a good exam and a negative mammogram with the reassurance that goes with it. This, of course, does nothing to relieve your pain, but it does relieve what's usually much worse than the pain—the fear that you have cancer.

NON-BREAST-ORIGIN PAIN

This third category isn't really a form of breast pain, though that's what it feels like to the patient. It's usually in the middle of the chest, and doesn't change with your period. Most frequently, it's arthritic pain, in the place where the ribs and breastbone connect—an arthritis called *costochondritis*[21] (Fig. 6-2). When men get costochondritis they think it's a heart attack; when women get it, they think it's breast cancer. You can tell it's arthritis by pushing down on your breastbone where your ribs are—if it hurts a lot more, that's probably what you've got. Similarly, if you take a deep breath and the middle part of your

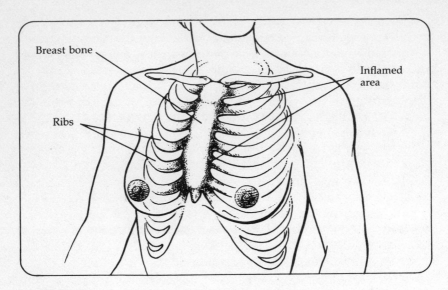

FIGURE 6-2

breast hurts, it's probably arthritis. If you take aspirin or Motrin and it relieves the pain, it's probably arthritis, since they're anti-inflammatory agents and thus work especially effectively on conditions like arthritis. Having your doctor inject the spot with local anesthetic and 40 mg of methylprednisolone (steriods) will relieve 90 percent of chest wall pain.[22]

You can also get non-breast-origin pain from arthritis in the neck (a pinched nerve).[23] This pain can radiate down into the breast the way lower back arthritis goes into the legs. There's also a special kind of phlebitis (inflamed vein) that can occur in the breast, called Mondor's syndrome. It gives you a drawing sensation around the outer edge of your breast that extends down into your abdomen. Sometimes you can even feel a cord where it is most tender. None of these problems is serious. When a non-breast condition appears in the breast area it's treated as it would be in any other part of the body. That usually means, for the conditions just mentioned, aspirin or another anti-inflammatory agent. These pains are usually self-limited and will go away in time.

CANCER CONCERNS

How likely are any of these forms of breast pain to be cancer? Cyclical pain has no relation to cancer at all, so don't worry. Noncyclical pain is rarely a sign of cancer, but it can be, so it's worth checking out. One of my patients discovered while she was traveling in Europe that her breast hurt when she lay on her stomach; though she couldn't feel any lump she had it checked when she came home and discovered she did indeed have a very tiny cancer on the spot. About 10 percent of all "target zone" breast pain is cancer. Non-breast-origin pain, as I said before, is probably arthritis, and you can confirm this by the methods I suggested. If you're still in doubt, have it checked by your doctor.

7

Breast Infections and Nipple Problems

Breast infections and nipple discharge are fairly uncommon, usually not much more than a nuisance, but can cause much anxiety to the woman who experiences them. There are two major categories of breast infection: intrinsic and extrinsic. Intrinsic breast infections—those occurring only to the breast itself—break down into three categories: lactational mastitis, nonlactational mastitis, and chronic subareolar abscess.

BREAST INFECTIONS: INTRINSIC

Lactational Mastitis

Lactational mastitis is the most common of these infections.[1] It occurs, as its name suggests, when the woman is breast-feeding. The breast is filled with milk, a medium that encourages the growth of bacteria. You've got a baby biting and sucking on your breast on a regular basis, causing cracks in the skin and introducing bacteria—it's really amazing that more nursing mothers don't get infections.

Probably it happens as seldom as it does because milk is always flowing through and flushing the bacteria out. However, sometimes when you're breast-feeding a duct will get blocked up with thick milk that doesn't flow very well. Then it's a setup for infection: the bacteria is trapped in the breast, the milk helps it grow, and suddenly you've got a reddened, hot, and very painful breast (Fig. 7-1).

Your doctor will probably initially suggest that you try to unblock the duct with massage and warm soaks; sometimes a doctor suggests heat (which liquifies the milk for better flow, but unfortunately increases the metabolic rate of breast tissue and thus accelerates the bacteria's growth) or ice packs (which slow the bacteria's growth rate but unfortunately harden the milk). If the infection persists, antibiotics are the next step. Usually that will take care of it. Don't worry about the antibiotics affecting your nursing child. Your obstetrician will know which antibiotics are safe for children to ingest, and will be careful about which are given to you. Nor will the bacteria hurt the child; since it's going into the gastrointestinal system, the bacteria will be killed by the baby's stomach acid. It's actually good for you if the child goes on nursing. The sucking helps keep the duct unblocked.

Antibiotics almost always get rid of infection, but in about 10 percent of cases an abscess forms, and antibiotics are useless in eliminating abscesses. An abscess, like a boil, is basically a collection of pus, and the doctor has to drain the pus. If it's an extremely small ab-

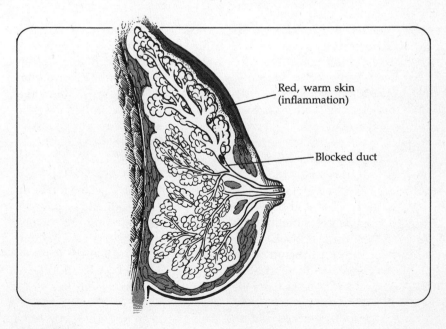

Red, warm skin (inflammation)

Blocked duct

FIGURE 7-1

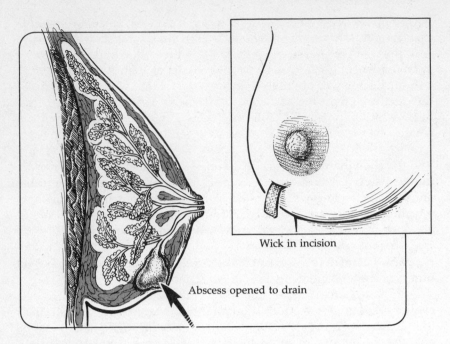

Wick in incision

Abscess opened to drain

FIGURE 7-2

scess, the pus can be aspirated with a needle. If it's fairly big, the doctor will have to make an incision large enough to allow the pus to drain (Fig. 7-2). This can be done under local anesthetic, but it's difficult because the inflamed tissue is highly sensitive and it's hard to inject an anesthetic that will really numb the area well. If my patient had an extremely small infected area, I'd tell her to bite the bullet, the pain would soon be over, and go with the local. But if it was a large area, I found it far more effective to put the patient to sleep. (See Chapter 25 for a discussion of general anesthetic.)

Once the cut is made, the pus drains out and the pain abates quickly. Surgeons never sew up a drained abscess; that would lock bacteria into the cavity and almost ensure the infection's return. I'd tell my patients to go home and rest, then, after 24 hours, begin taking daily showers; let the water run over the breast and wash away the bacteria. Then put a dressing over it to absorb oozing fluids from the incision. Some surgeons will put a wick, or drain, in the corner of the incision to keep it open; that way it heals from the inside out and closes within a week or two.

Some surgeons will tell you that if you need an operation you have to stop breast-feeding. Many women really want to breast-feed, and there's no reason they should give it up. It's messy, since not only are you oozing fluids, you're also oozing milk. But if you're willing to put up with the mess there's no reason not to breast-feed. It's usually just one breast, and just a segment of the breast at that; there's plenty of room for your baby to suckle.

Nonlactational Mastitis

Though the kind of mastitis described above is usually found only in lactating women, it can sometimes occur in nonlactating women, especially in particular circumstances. For example, it may occur in women who've had lumpectomies followed by radiation (see Chapter 27), in diabetics, or in women whose immune system is otherwise depressed: such women are prone to infections either because some of the lymph nodes, which help fight infection, have been removed, or because their immune systems are generally less strong than those of most people. This type of infection will usually be a *cellulitis*—an infection of the skin—red, hot, and swollen all over rather than just on one spot. It's generally accompanied by high fever and headache, both characteristics of a strep infection (staph infections, by contrast, are usually local). It will be treated by your doctor with antibiotics, usually penicillin, and you may be briefly hospitalized.

Skin boils (or staph infections) can form on the breast, as they can on other parts of the body. If you're a carrier of staph and prone to infection as well—as in the case of diabetics—this is more likely to occur than in noncarriers or people less infection prone. It's also possible to get an abscess in the breast when you're not lactating and don't have any of the other risk factors, although this is unusual. Both cellulitis and these abscesses can mask cancer (as we'll discuss below), so, though such cancer is rare, if you've got one of these conditions it's important to have it checked out by a doctor.

I had several patients with what has been called "chronic mastitis." In each case the patient had an infection, which her doctor had drained. Unlike lactational mastitis, discussed earlier, these infections are abscesses, and so the first treatment should be to drain them. If the abscess recurs or fails to heal completely the patients are sent to an infectious disease specialist who starts them on antibiotics. Some of the women I saw had been on these antibiotics for years, often given intravenously at home through a Hickman catheter (see Chapter 28). Most of the time I found that the problem could have been easily treated with a minor operation, a solution the infectious disease specialist, lacking experience in breast surgery, had overlooked. If you have a so-called chronic infection, make sure you see a breast surgeon early on.

You may save yourself a lot of suffering and expense. Diseased tissue, like the chronic subareolar abscess which I discuss next, has to be removed surgically.

Chronic Subareolar Abscess

The second most common breast infection—and it's pretty infrequent—is the chronic subareolar abscess, which we don't understand very well, though there is some evidence that it is more common in smokers. Two theories about its cause demonstrate the fact that we also don't really understand the anatomy of the breast ducts and the nipples (see Chapter 1). One theory states that this infection is caused by ducts that become blocked with keratin and then get infected.[2] But Dr. Bruce Derrick at Temple University and Dr. Otto Sartorius put forth a different view which I find more compelling.[3,4] As you'll recall from Chapter 1, there are little glands on the nipple, as well as ducts. These small, dead-ended glands can get infections, whether you're nursing or not. Bacteria from the skin or mouth of your child or lover gets into the gland; thickened secretions block it so it can't drain well, and it gets infected. This kind of infection is most common in women with inverted nipples, because their glands have narrower openings.

Whether the culprit in this condition is the ducts or the glands doesn't matter much to the patient. Either way, an abscess forms that can't drain through the usual exit and therefore tries to drain through the weakest part of the skin in the area—the border of the areola and the regular skin (Fig. 7-3). The abscess is a red, hot, sore area on part of the border of the nipple—like a boil. It looks and feels fairly awful, and the frightened woman often thinks she's got breast cancer. She doesn't, and the infection doesn't affect her vulnerability to breast cancer.

If the infection is caught very early, before an abscess forms, it can be helped by antibiotics, but often it can't be; it needs an incision and draining. I think it's best to do the incision on the border of the areola, so that it doesn't show later. Once the pus is drained, it's okay—for the time being. The trouble is that this type of infection is apt to recur. The gland is a little blind passage, with no internal opening, so it can reinfect itself and drain again at the same point. Eventually this leaves a permanent open tract.

We've had some luck reducing these recurrences by removing the entire gland or tract. To get the whole tract, the surgeon must excise a wedge of nipple. The method isn't perfect, but its success rate is a lot better than that of other methods.

Since the gland is small and the surgery relatively minor, I used to do it under local anesthetic. But it's hard to get a chronically infected

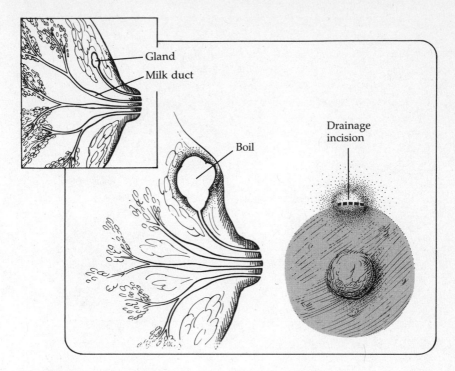

Gland

Milk duct

Boil

Drainage incision

FIGURE 7-3

area thoroughly numb, especially one as sensitive as the nipple—the same problem as in lactational mastitis, only more severe. So I found that, in my anxiousness to end my patient's discomfort, I sometimes didn't get the whole gland out, and the infection would often recur. Later I gave women short-acting drugs to complement the local. I passed a probe through the tract and then took out the wedge of nipple that contained the tract, including both openings (Fig. 7-4). I then closed the nipple and sewed it up.

There's some controversy about whether or not to close the incision: some doctors are afraid that if there are lots of bacteria to begin with there's a greater chance that the gland will reinfect itself if it's closed off; others are more concerned about the cosmetics of a nipple with a hole in it. I prefer to close it, but I always tell my patient the pros and cons, then do what she wants.

Unfortunately, even in the best-done operations, the problem often recurs.[5] Perhaps the infection spreads from one gland to another, or perhaps there's still lining left from the old gland that the surgeon isn't aware of. So if you have a chronic subareolar abscess, it's well worth trying to have it taken care of. But understand that you might have to

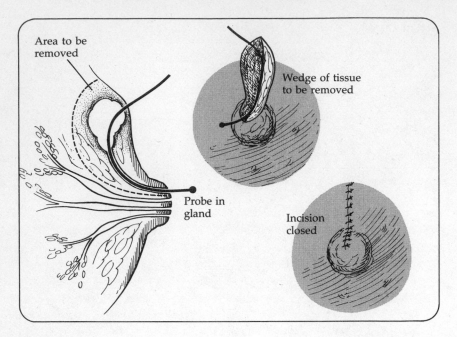

FIGURE 7-4

keep dealing with it. About 40 percent of these infections do recur, sometimes as often as every few months.

As so often happens, many doctors think disfiguring surgery on women's bodies is called for. One patient came to me after her doctor said he was fed up with these recurrences and wanted to remove both breasts. Fortunately, she had the sense not to listen to him. A well-planned, nonmutilating operation solved her problem—but even if it hadn't, the most drastic procedure that would have made any sense at all would have been to remove the nipple and leave the breast—then at least a plastic surgeon could reconstruct a new nipple, leaving the breast intact (see Chapter 5).

But if you have this condition it's unlikely you'd want even that done. It's unpleasant and a nuisance, but not life-threatening. It doesn't interfere with breast feeding, nor should it restrict your sexual life, except insofar as you're obviously not likely to want your nipple touched while it's hurting from the infection.

BREAST INFECTIONS: EXTRINSIC

Extrinsic breast infections are those that involve the whole body but show first on the breast. These are extremely rare, especially in this country, so I'll mention them only briefly. TB and syphilis have both been known to emerge first on the breast; such infections are treated the same way the diseases would be treated if they showed first anywhere else.

INFECTION AND CANCER

As I said earlier, breast infections never lead to breast cancer. However, some breast cancers lead to infections, or can look like infections (see Chapter 20): as the cancer cells grow, noncancer cells die off for lack of blood supply, and the necrotic (dead) tissue can get infected. So it's possible, though extremely unusual, for a breast cancer to show up first as a breast abscess.

There is a form of breast cancer called *inflammatory breast cancer* that can be mistaken for infection (see Chapter 20). This starts with redness of the skin, warmth, and swelling. There usually is no lump. What distinguishes it from infection is that it doesn't get better with antibiotics. Anyone with a breast infection that persists after 10 days to two weeks of antibiotics should see a breast surgeon, who will probably want to do a biopsy.

If you get an infection, don't worry about it—but do see your doctor right away. The infection won't give you cancer, but it should be treated and gotten rid of, and you do want to make sure it *is* an infection.

NIPPLE PROBLEMS

Discharge

The nipple is an especially sensitive area and subject to a number of problems, such as the subareolar abscess discussed earlier. The most common nipple problem—or rather concern, since it's not always a problem—is discharge. As we discussed at length in Chapter 2, most women do have some amount of discharge or fluid when their breasts are squeezed, and it's perfectly normal (Fig. 7-5). In a study at Boston's Lying-in Hospital breast clinic women had little suction cups, like breast pumps, put on their nipples and gentle suction applied.[6] Eighty-three percent of these women—old, young, mothers, nonmothers, previously pregnant, never pregnant—had some amount of fluid. As we will discuss in Chapter 17, this fluid can be analyzed for precancerous cells.

The ducts of the nipple are pipelines; they're made to carry milk to the nipple, so a little fluid in the pipes shouldn't be surprising. (It

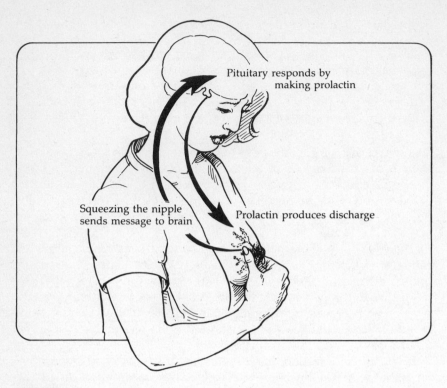

Pituitary responds by
making prolactin

Squeezing the nipple
sends message to brain

Prolactin produces discharge

FIGURE 7-5

can come in a number of colors—gray, green, and brown, as well as white.)

Sometimes people confuse nipple discharge with other problems— weepy sores, infections, abscesses (see above). Inverted nipples (see Chapter 2) can sometimes get dirt and dried-up sweat trapped in them, and this can be confused with discharge.

Some women are more prone to lots of discharge than others: women on birth control pills, antihypertensives such as Aldomet, or major tranquilizers such as thorazine tend to notice more discharge, because these medications increase prolactin levels. It may seem aesthetically displeasing, but beyond that there's nothing to worry about.

There are also different life periods when you're more likely to get discharge than others: there's more discharge at puberty and at meno-pause than in the years between. And there's the "witch's milk" that newborn babies get (see Chapter 1). This makes sense, since the dis-charge is a result of hormonal processes.

When Should You Worry?

The time to worry about nipple discharge is when it's spontaneous, persistent, and unilateral (only on one side). It comes out by itself without squeezing; it keeps on happening; and it's only from one nipple and usually one duct. It's either clear and sticky, like an egg white, or bloody. You should go to the doctor right away. There are several possible causes:

1. Intraductal papilloma. This is a little wartlike growth on the lining of the duct. It gets eroded and bleeds, creating a bloody discharge. It's benign; the surgeon removes it to make sure that's what it is.
2. Intraductal papillomatosis. Instead of one wart, you've got a lot of little warts.
3. Intraductal carcinoma *in situ*. This is a precancer that clogs up the duct like rust: it's discussed in detail in Chapter 16.
4. Cancer. Cancers are rarely the cause of discharge. Only about 4 percent of all spontaneous unilateral bloody discharges are cancerous. (See Chapter 20 for further discussion of discharge with cancer.)

Your clinician should first test for blood by taking a sample, putting it on a card, and adding a chemical (hemacult test). If it turns blue, there's blood (which may not be visible to the eye alone, because of the color of the discharge itself). The doctor may do a Pap smear, very like the Pap smear you get to test for cervical cancer. Discharge is put on a glass slide and sent to the lab for the cells to be examined. This is not as accurate as testing for blood in the discharge, but occasionally it can demonstrate the presence of abnormal cells.

Next the doctor will try and figure out the "trigger zone" by going around the breast to find out which duct the discharge is coming from, though often the woman herself can give the doctor this information. If you're over 30 you'll be sent for a mammogram to see if there's a tumor underneath the duct.

You can then have your duct lavaged (see Chapter 17). If the cells are abnormal you can then be given a ductogram—a tool I find vital. The radiologist takes a very fine plastic catheter and, with a magnifying glass, threads it into the duct, squirts dye into it, and takes a picture (Fig. 7-6). The procedure sounds uncomfortable, but it really isn't that bad—the duct is an open tube already, and the discharge has dilated it. The ductogram provides a "map" for the surgeon who may do a biopsy and may also show the source of the discharge. Not every surgeon will order a ductogram or lavage, but I find them extremely worthwhile.

A biopsy itself is fairly simple; it's a specialized form of the regular

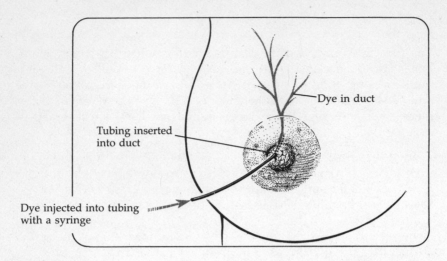

FIGURE 7-6

breast biopsy (see Chapter 11). It can be done under local anesthetic, and on an outpatient basis. A tiny incision is made at the edge of the areola; the areola is flipped up, and the blood-filled duct located and removed (Fig. 7-7). Sometimes the radiologist will cut a fine suture and pass it into the duct to the point to be removed, or blue dye can be injected into the duct to help identify it. Both of these techniques will help to pinpoint the right area. Sometimes if the ductogram has shown the lesion to be far from the nipple, the surgeon will localize the area with a wire, as described in Chapter 11. That way the duct won't get blocked, which interferes with breast feeding, or numbed, which interferes with sexual pleasure.

Because the lesion can be far from the nipple itself, the old standard surgical practice of removing all of the ductal system to make sure that the discharge has stopped has largely been abandoned. Though this procedure stops the discharge (by disconnecting the ducts from the nipple), it may or may not remove the pathology causing the discharge.

Some centers are using duct endoscopy to figure out what's causing the discharge. An endoscope is a thin tube put directly into the nipple duct, by which the surgeon can view the inside of the ducts on a video screen. They have reported success in seeing intraductal papillomas and other pathology.

Another form of problematic discharge is one that is spontaneous, bilateral (on both sides), and milky. If you're not breast-feeding, and

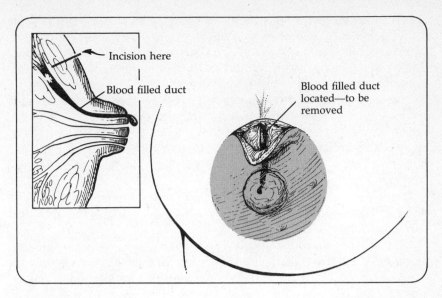

Incision here

Blood filled duct

Blood filled duct located—to be removed

FIGURE 7-7

haven't been in the past year, this is probably a condition called *galactorrhea*—excessive or spontaneous milk flow. It occurs because something is increasing the prolactin levels—sometimes a small tumor in the brain. This may not be as alarming as it sounds: often it's a tiny tumor which may not require surgery. A neurosurgeon and an endocrinologist together need to check this out. You may be given bromocriptine to block the prolactin. Galactorrhea is often associated with amenorrhea—failure to get your period. It can also be caused by major tranquilizers, marijuana consumption, or high estrogen doses.

Galactorrhea is diagnosed only when the discharge is bilateral. Many doctors don't understand this, and send patients with any discharge for prolactin level tests. They shouldn't; the unilateral discharges are not associated with hormonal problems. Unilateral spontaneous discharge is anatomical, not hormonal, and the money spent on prolactin tests is wasted.

Other Nipple Problems

There are a few other problems women can have with their nipples. Some patients complain of itchy nipples. Usually this doesn't indicate anything dangerous, especially if both nipples itch. You can get dry skin on your nipples as elsewhere. You may be allergic to your bra, or to the detergent it's washed in. Pubescent girls with growing breasts often experience itching as the skin stretches itself. Otherwise, we don't know what causes itchy nipples. If they bother you, you can use calamine lotion or other anti-itch medication.

There is a form of cancer known as Paget's disease that doctors and patients often confuse with eczema of the nipple. It looks like an open sore area, and it itches. If it's only on one nipple, and it doesn't go away with standard eczema treatments, check it out. A biopsy can be performed on a small section of the nipple. (Paget's disease is discussed at length in Chapter 24.)

If the rash is on both nipples and you tend to get eczema anyway, don't worry. Anything that can happen to other parts of the skin can happen to the nipple.

Most of these various infections and irritations are benign—they're more of a nuisance than anything else. If they appear, get them checked out, just to make sure they're what they appear to be, and to get the relief available.

8

Lumps and Lumpiness

To begin with, you need to remember that lumpiness, as I discussed in Chapter 2, isn't the same as having one dominant lump. It's a general pattern of many little lumps, in both breasts, and it's perfectly normal. The distinction between "lumps" and "lumpiness" is an important one; the confusion of the two can cause a woman days and weeks of needless mental anguish. Lumpiness is not a disease—"fibrocystic" or otherwise. It's simply normal breast tissue.

Patients aren't the only ones who get lumpiness and lumps confused: doctors who don't usually work with breast cancer—family practitioners and gynecologists—often get nervous about lumpy breasts and are afraid they're malignant. So your doctor may send you to a specialist—a surgeon or a breast specialist—to make sure you don't have a cancerous lump. If you or your doctor are uncertain about whether you've got a lump or just lumpy breasts, it's probably not a bad idea to check it out further. But understanding more about what a lump really is might make the trip to the specialist unnecessary.

Ellen Mahoney, a fellow breast surgeon, tells her patients to visualize what their breasts might be like inside—from butter to gravel to bubble wrap—and if it's the same all over, it's just the way they're made. The only area to be concerned about is the one that is different from all the rest. The most important thing to know about dominant lumps—benign or malignant—is that they're almost never subtle. They're not like little beebee gun pellets: they're usually at least a centimeter or two, almost an inch, or the size of a grape. The lump will stick out prominently in the midst of the smaller lumps that constitute normal lumpiness. You'll know it's something different. In fact, that's why most breast cancers are found by the woman herself—the lumps are so clearly distinct from the rest of her breast tissue.

The obvious question here is, how do I know the beebee-sized thing isn't an early cancer? The answer is that you usually don't feel a malignant lump when it's small. The cancer has to grow to a large enough size for the body to begin to create a reaction to it—a fibrous, scarlike tissue forms around the cancer, and this, combined with the cancer itself, makes up the palpable lump. The body won't create that reaction when the cancer is tiny, and you won't feel the cancerous lump until the reaction is formed.

At the same time, if it's much bigger than a walnut—if it feels like a quarter of the breast itself—you're probably still okay. You'll know by checking it through a couple of menstrual cycles, when you'll see that it changes through different parts of your cycle. A cancer lump that large would probably have been noticed earlier by even the most absentminded person. But if it doesn't go away or change significantly after two menstrual cycles, have it checked out; it's not likely that it's a cancer, but it could be, and you don't want to take the chance. It will be easier for you to notice changes if you've become acquainted with your breasts, as we discussed in Chapter 2.

There are four types of dominant lumps, three of which—cysts, fibroadenomas, and pseudolumps—are virtually harmless. It's the fourth type, of course—the malignant lump—that you're worrying about when you have your lump examined by a doctor. (I'll discuss cancerous lumps at length in Chapter 20.) Only one in 12 dominant lumps in premenopausal women is malignant. We don't know the cause of any of the noncancerous lumps, though we do know they're somehow related to hormonal variations (see Chapter 1). Two kinds of lumps—cysts and fibroadenomas—form only during a woman's menstruating years, but can show up years later, when breast tissue has shifted. Pseudolumps can occur in women of any age. It's interesting that two of the three kinds occur most often at opposite ends of a woman's fertile years: fibroadenomas occur when the woman is just starting to menstruate, and cysts when she's heading toward menopause.

CYSTS

Usually when you think of nonmalignant lumps you think of cysts, because doctors have a tendency to describe all nonmalignant lumps as cysts. They're not. A cyst is a particular, distinct kind of lump. Typically it occurs in women in their 30s, 40s, and early 50s, and is most common in women approaching menopause. It rarely occurs in a younger woman, or in a woman who's past menopause. However, I've had patients in both categories—including a teenager and a woman who'd finished with her menopause long ago and wasn't on artificial hormones. (As I said earlier, a woman taking estrogen to combat menopausal symptoms fools her body into thinking it's still premenopausal.)

A gross cyst—gross meaning "large," not, as in popular usage, "disgusting"—is a fluid-filled sac, very much like a large blister, which grows in the midst of the breast tissue. It's smooth on the outside and "ballotable"—squishy—on the inside, so that if you push on it, you can feel that it's got fluid inside.

This, however, can be deceptive. Cysts feel like cysts only when they're close to the surface (Fig. 8-1). Cysts that are deeply imbedded in breast tissue tend to distend that tissue and push it forward, so that what you're feeling is the hard breast tissue, not the soft cyst. In these cases the cyst feels like a hard lump.

The classical cyst story goes something like this. A woman in her 40s comes to a specialist and says, "I went to the gynecologist six weeks ago and everything was fine. I had a mammogram, and that was fine

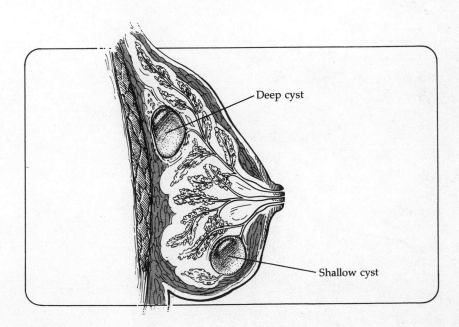

FIGURE 8-1

too. Then all of a sudden, in the shower last night, I found this lump in my breast, and I know it wasn't there before." So the doctor examines her and sure enough, there's a hard lump in her breast.

Because of its overnight appearance, the doctor is pretty sure it's a harmless cyst, but of course it's something the doctor—not to mention the patient—wants to be absolutely certain about: cancers sometimes do seem to appear overnight. So the doctor tries to aspirate it.

To aspirate a cyst, the doctor takes a tiny needle, like the kind used for insulin injections, and anesthetizes the sensitive skin over the breast lump (Fig. 8-2). Then a larger needle—like the kind used to draw blood—is attached to a syringe and stuck into the breast, where it draws out the fluid. The cyst collapses like a punctured blister, and that's that.

Aspirating cysts was one of the medical procedures I most enjoyed doing. It's very easy, and as soon as it was done, my patient and I both knew she was okay. We were both delighted that she didn't have cancer, and she thought I was the greatest doctor in the world, having simultaneously diagnosed and cured her condition. It did wonders for my ego.

An added pleasure is that it's usually almost painless for the patient. It sounds scary and grim—a little like descriptions of acupuncture—but in reality, most of the nerves in the breast are in the skin,

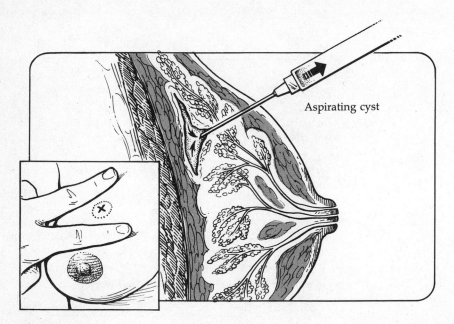

Aspirating cyst

FIGURE 8-2

and that's been anesthetized. Some women with greater sensitivity to pain or especially sensitive breasts do find it painful, but most don't. The only possible complications from aspirating a cyst are bruising or bleeding into the cyst, neither of which is more than slightly uncomfortable.

The fluid itself looks pretty disgusting, but it's harmless. It can be almost any color—usually it's green, brown, or yellow. Sometimes the fluid can even be milk—a breast-feeding woman can form a milk-filled cyst, called a galactocele, which is treated the way any other cyst is. There can be any amount of it—from a few drops to as much as a cup. One patient came to me with asymmetrical breasts; after I aspirated her cyst, her breasts were the same size.

Some doctors have the fluid analyzed in the lab, but frankly, I think it's pointless. The chances of getting a correct diagnosis from cyst fluid are very low, and false positives are common. The fluid's usually been around awhile and it's old, and its cells, though harmless, often seem weird when they're checked. The tests are virtually useless, and they're costly. Most specialists just throw the stuff down the sink.

In Sweden they think injecting air into the cyst after it's been aspirated prevents the cyst from recurring.[1] It's an interesting theory, but it hasn't been proved. Still, it's worth a try if the cyst has recurred many times.

Usually a woman will get only one or two cysts in her entire life. But some get many, and they get them often. If a patient had recurring multiple cysts, I would see her every three to six months, and aspirate as many as I could to keep the multiplication of cysts under control. If a malignant lump is forming, the cysts, harmless in themselves, can obscure it, and that, of course, is dangerous. When a woman has multiple cysts chances are she'll go on getting them until menopause—only rarely are they a one-time occurrence.

If cysts are harmless why do we bother to aspirate them? There are a number of reasons, but the most important one is that we need to be sure it *is* a cyst. You can't be sure a lump in the breast isn't cancer until you find out what it really is. Once we know it's a cyst, doctor and patient can both rest easy.

There are other ways of finding out you have a cyst—it may show up as an area of density on a routine mammogram, and then you can have an ultrasound test done to see whether it's a cyst or a solid lump. The ultrasound test works like radar. If you have a solid lump, the waves from the ultrasound will bounce back and there'll be a shadow behind it. If it is a cyst, however, the sound waves will go right through it and there won't be a shadow. (See Chapters 9 and 10 for discussions of mammograms and ultrasound techniques.)

If you've discovered a cyst through a mammogram and ultrasound

and it doesn't worry you, don't bother having it aspirated as well—
you already know it isn't cancer. Sometimes a cyst is painful, especially
if it developed very quickly. Aspirating the cyst will relieve the pain.

Cysts themselves are almost never malignant. There's a 1 percent incidence of cancer in cysts, and it's a seldom-dangerous cancer called
intracystic papillary carcinoma (Fig. 8-3). It usually doesn't spread beyond the lining of the cyst, and unless there are specific signs that it
might be present, it's not worth the risk of a biopsy. A biopsy is surgery, though minor surgery, and it's better to avoid it when you can.

If there are signs that cancer might be present in the cyst, I'd operate
on it—never otherwise, and only after I'd aspirated it. I'd operate if the
cyst had recurred after I'd aspirated it three times. I'd also operate if
the fluid came out bloody—that usually means something else is going
on, and I'd want to find out what it was. Finally, I'd do a biopsy if the
lump didn't go away after I'd aspirated the cyst.

Sometimes a doctor will aspirate a cyst and won't get any fluid. This
isn't a cause for panic. It can happen for a number of reasons. The
lump may not be a cyst after all, but a nonmalignant solid lump like
those discussed below. Or the doctor may have missed the middle
of the cyst. The doctor tries to get the cyst between her or his fingers
and then puncture it, but it's easy to miss the middle, especially in a
fairly small cyst. When this happened to me, I'd decide how sure I was
that it was a cyst and, if I had doubts, I'd send the patient for an ultrasound test rather than operate. Operating on a cyst should only be a
last resort.

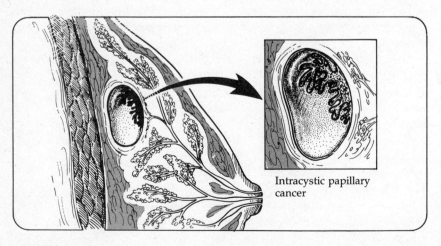

Intracystic papillary
cancer

FIGURE 8-3

It used to be believed that aspirating a cyst was dangerous if some-one unknowingly had breast cancer—that the process of aspiration would spread the cancer over the needle's track. We now know that's completely untrue.[2] Any dominant lump should be aspirated before it's biopsied. It might be a cyst, and surgery can be avoided.

Cysts don't increase the risk of cancer. Only one study—Dr. Cush-man Haagensen of Columbia's—suggests it does, and his evidence is sketchy.[3] Dr. David Page's research is a little better; he's found that there is a slight risk increase in women who have gross cysts and who have a first-degree relative with breast cancer—a mother or sister.[4] Most other research shows no relation between cysts and cancer.

The real risk is mental rather than physical. A woman with frequent cysts is likely to feel a lump and shrug it off as just another cyst—only to learn later that it was a malignant growth. Every lump should be checked out, to be sure it isn't dangerous.

FIBROADENOMAS

Another very common nonmalignant lump is the fibroadenoma. This is a smooth, round lump that feels the way most people think a cyst

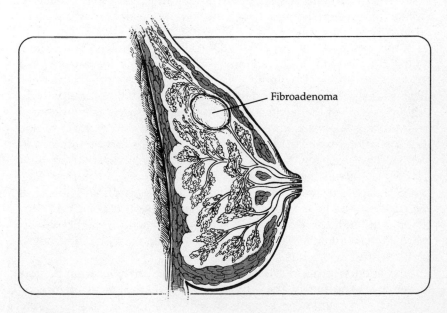

FIGURE 8-4

should feel—it's smooth and hard, like a marble dropped into the breast tissue (Fig. 8-4) where it can move around easily. It's often found near the nipple, but can grow anywhere in the breast. It's also very distinct from the rest of the breast tissue. It can vary from a tiny 5 mm to a lemon-sized 5 cm. The largest are called "giant fibroadenomas." A doctor can usually tell simply by feeling the lump that it's a fibroadenoma; if a needle aspiration is done and no fluid comes out, the doctor knows it isn't a cyst and is even more convinced it's a fibroadenoma. We can get a diagnosis by doing a core biopsy (see Chapter 11) and sending the tissue off to the lab just to make doubly sure. Fibroadenomas are usually distinct on a mammogram or ultrasound test (see Chapter 9 and 10). They are harmless in themselves, and don't have to be removed as long as we're sure they're fibroadenomas. Most investigators believe that fibroadenomas usually grow over a 12-month period to a size of approximately 2–3 cm, after which they remain unchanged for several years.[5] Studies in which women were followed for up to 29 years found that the fibroadenoma shrunk or disappeared in 16–59 percent of all cases. They concluded that a fibroadenoma would probably dissappear after five years in approximately 50 percent of cases and that in the others its lifetime is about 15 years.[6]

Since fibroadenomas develop at puberty, teenagers are both more prone to them and less likely to get breast cancer than are older women, so we might consider not removing fibroadenomas in teens. In women middle-aged or older, we tend to remove all fibroadenomas to be sure they're not cancer.

In the spring of 1993 a study by Dr. D. L. Page showed that women with a certain kind of fibroadenoma might have an increased risk of subsequent cancer.[7] This lump was called a "complex fibroadenoma" because not only were there glands and surrounding tissue as is usual in this lesion, but the women also had other microscopic entities such as sclerosing adenosis or apocrine metaplasia. It is important to note that the complex fibroadenomas studied had not turned into cancer. Rather, they were a marker for a future risk, like having a strong family history. About one third of all fibroadenomas are complex. Page found that, when associated with a family history in a first-degree relative, these fibroadenomas increased the subsequent risk of cancer three times. Although this does not change the treatment, it might make us more likely to remove a fibroadenoma in a woman with a first-degree family history to see if it is a complex one.

Fibroadenomas are easy to remove, and the procedure can be done under local anesthetic. The surgeon simply makes a small incision, finds the lump, and takes it right out (Fig. 8-5). (Some surgeons prefer to make a small incision around the nipple and then tunnel their way to the lump, since an incision at the nipple scars less noticeably. I don't

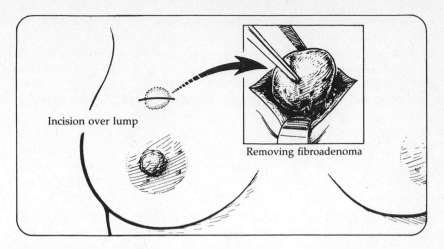

Incision over lump

Removing fibroadenoma

FIGURE 8-5

think this is a great idea, however; it's harder to find the lesion that way. If you cut over the fibroadenoma you're bound to get it, and the scarring doesn't usually remain all that noticeable in most patients.) If you feel nervous about your fibroadenomas, it's probably a good idea to get them removed for your own peace of mind; if there's no reason to get them removed and you don't want to, don't worry about it.

In most cases a woman has only one fibroadenoma; it's removed, and she never gets any more. But some women do get several during their lives—and a few women get many of them. One of my patients had a fibroadenoma in her left breast, and I removed it; she returned a couple of years later with another one on the exact same spot in her other breast—a kind of mirror image. Occasionally a woman will have multiple fibroadenomas at once. Once they are removed, more form. I had one woman with this problem and I must admit it is a difficult one. Obviously a surgeon can't keep removing them, but equally obviously a woman with this condition will be worried. One woman I talked to was told to have prophylactic mastectomies so the surgeon would not have to worry. This is pretty drastic for a benign condition that does not increase breast cancer risk. I'd generally recommend surgery only for the patient's needs, not for her doctor's peace of mind. A more sensible suggestion is to try danazol, a drug used for breast pain (see Chapter 6), which will put you into a reversible menopause. Stopping the hormonal stimulation of the breast should help to control the fibroadenomas.

Patients often call their fibroadenomas "fibroids"—and, while it's inaccurate, it makes sense in a way. Fibroids by definition exist only in the uterus, but there are similarities between the two conditions. In both cases, one section of glandular tissue becomes autonomous, growing as a ball in the midst of the rest of the tissue. But there's no correlation except for that—having one doesn't mean you're likely to get the other. In fact, they usually occur at different times in a woman's life: fibroids when you're heading toward menopause, fibroadenomas in your teens or early 20s.

They can, however, occur at any age, up until menopause. As with cysts, you can get them after menopause if you're taking hormones that trick your body into thinking it's premenopausal. It's true that, as we do more mammograms on "normal" women, we find more and more fibroadenomas in women in their 60s and 70s. Probably they've had them since their teens and simply, in those premammography days, didn't know about them. There are some very rare cancers that can look like fibroadenomas on a mammogram, so, in postmenopausal women, we usually do either a fine-needle aspiration, core biopsy, or, if those don't give us the information, an excisional biopsy (removal of the whole lump), just to make sure it is a fibroadenoma.

Ellen Mahoney, a breast surgeon friend of mine, says, "I tell people it has to come out if it bothers you, or if it grows—following this rule, I have never missed the occasional indolent cancer. One of my patients had three in the same quadrant. A baseline was done and repeated in six months—two had grown. All were removed and all were cancer. Following this rule, too, I have diagnosed some of the 2–3 mm tumors sitting next to fibroadenomas and stimulating them. I think there are two types of fibroadenomas: hamartomas, which rarely grow larger than 2.5 cm (like the sponge toys in the gelatin capsules), and neoplasms, which may grow in response to a number of factors. I make sure I have a good measurement by ultrasound or by my little cloth tape measure, whichever is appropriate to the location."

There's also a rare cancer called *cystosarcoma phylloides* (see Chapter 24) which can occur in a fibroadenoma. It occurs only in about 1 percent of fibroadenomas, and those are usually giant fibroadenomas—lemon-sized or larger. It's generally a relatively harmless cancer in that it doesn't tend to spread to other parts of the body. Some doctors will insist on removing all fibroadenomas on the theory that this cancer might be present. It's not a very sensible attitude, because of both the rarity and the lack of danger. Unless the lump is large, it's almost never going to be this cancer—and even if the cancer is present for a long time, it probably isn't going to kill you. When it's discovered, the surgeon simply has to remove the lump and it's gone.

Finally, fibroadenomas do not turn into cancer. They're a nuisance, and they can scare you into thinking you might have cancer—but that's the only bad thing about them. Cancer can rarely arise in fibro-adenomas, and it won't be missed as long as you check the size at diagnosis and at six months. If all is stable, then size doesn't have to be checked again until there is a suspicion of change.

PSEUDOLUMPS

Studies have shown that pseudolumps are the lumps that most confuse surgeons. If you line up patients with fibroadenomas, with cysts, and with breast cancers, and have surgeons who haven't been told which patient has which kind of lump examine them, usually the surgeons will agree in their diagnoses. Give them patients with pseudolumps, however, and you'll get all kinds of different diagnoses. These innocent lumps of breast tissue cause no physical problems, but all kinds of confusion.

"Pseudolump" is a descriptive term for an area of breast tissue that feels more prominent and persistent than usual. The surgeon checks it out and just can't be sure that it isn't another kind of lump.

If I thought a patient had a pseudolump, I'd usually see her at least twice, several months apart and at different parts of her cycle, just to make sure it wasn't normal lumpiness. Deciding what is or isn't a lump in these cases can be very subjective. If I'd recently done a lot of biopsies and they'd all turned out to be pseudolumps, I'd tend not to operate; but if I'd missed a cancer, I'd operate on a lot of them. Unfortunately, diagnosis is not an exact science. That's the other reason that before operating I liked to see the patient again, a few months after my first diagnosis, to balance out whatever effect my mood had had on my decision.

A pseudolump, then, is usually just exaggerated lumpiness. It's distinct and persistent enough, however, that we have to check to be certain that's all it is. It's usually what's meant when doctors say you have fibrocystic disease (see Chapter 6). Or a pseudolump can be caused by a rib pushing against breast tissue and causing it to feel hard and lumpy (Fig. 8-6). Sometimes women who had silicone injections years ago to enlarge one or both breasts (see Chapter 5) will get lumps that turn out to be hardened chunks of the silicone. If you've had injections and get a lump, check with either a breast surgeon or a plastic surgeon (preferably one who's old enough to have worked with silicone injections when they were legal). Surgery on the breast can cause pseudolumps through hardened scar tissue. A pseudolump can also be caused by "fat necrosis"—dead fat—resulting from trauma due to a lumpectomy and radiation in the removal of an earlier, cancerous lump (see

117

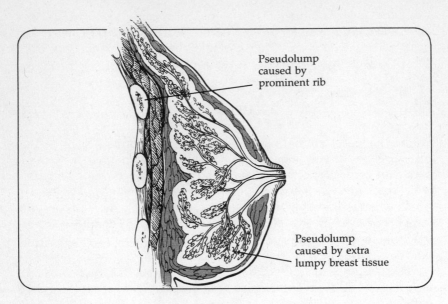

Pseudolump caused by prominent rib

Pseudolump caused by extra lumpy breast tissue

FIGURE 8-6

Chapter 27), or to breast reconstruction surgery (see Chapter 26). But in all these cases the best judge will be a breast surgeon who's done all the procedures.

CANCER

The fear of cancer is, of course, the main reason we worry about any of these lumps. You get a cyst aspirated, or a fibroadenoma or pseudolump biopsied, chiefly to make sure they aren't cancer.

It's reasonable to be afraid of getting breast cancer, and to check out any suspicious lump. But remember that a dominant lump doesn't mean you have cancer. In premenopausal women there are 12 benign lumps for every malignant one. The statistics change dramatically in postmenopausal women who aren't taking hormones, not because they get that much more cancer but because they no longer get the lumps that come with hormonal changes, cysts and fibroadenomas. Yet even for postmenopausal women it's only a 50–50 chance that a lump is cancer. We'll discuss malignant lumps in Chapter 20. The main thing to remember is to be cautious, but not frantic. If you've got a lump, it may be cancer, but it probably isn't. Get it checked out right away. Then if it's cancer, you can start working on it; if it isn't, you can stop worrying.

WHAT TO DO IF YOU THINK YOU HAVE A LUMP

If you have something that feels like it might be a lump, the first thing to do, obviously, is go to your doctor. Chances are that the doctor will check it out, tell you it's not a lump, and send you home. But a doctor who's a general practitioner or a gynecologist and hasn't spent years working on breasts might not be sure, and may send you to a breast surgeon for further examination. Often when you hear the word "surgeon" you get scared—sure that the doctor knows you've got something awful and that you will have to undergo major surgery.

Probably you won't. The doctor is simply, and sensibly, taking no chances, and sending you on to someone with more experience with breast lumps who is thus better able to determine whether or not it's a true dominant lump. But sometimes even the surgeon can't be sure. In this case, depending on your age, the surgeon will probably send you for a mammogram to get additional information. The mammogram might show evidence of a real lump, or a pseudolump. If it doesn't—if even the combination of an examination and a mammogram doesn't give the surgeon the necessary clarification—it's wise to do a biopsy to find out what it is. In the past we were afraid of unnecessary surgery and didn't want to biopsy these "gray-area" lumps. The problem is, you don't know until you have done the biopsy that it is a pseudolump, so it isn't unnecessary surgery at all. It's far wiser to risk a fairly safe operation than to take a chance on letting a cancer go.

One thing is important to stress. If you're certain that something is wrong with your breast, get it biopsied, whatever the doctor's diagnosis. Often a woman is sure she has a lump, the doctor is sure she doesn't, and a year or two later a lump shows up on her mammogram. She believes the doctor was careless. Usually that's not the case: a cancer that shows on a mammogram probably wasn't a lump two years earlier, or it would be a huge lump at that point. But I think it's very likely that the patient—who, after all, experiences her breast from both inside and outside, while the doctor can only experience the patient's breast from outside—has sensed something wrong, and interpreted that in terms of the concept most familiar to her, a lump. I'm convinced that this is the basis of many of the malpractice suits that arise when a doctor has "failed" to detect what later proves to be cancer. If you really feel something is wrong in your breast, insist on a biopsy. If you're wrong, you'll put your mind at rest—and if you're right, you may just save your own life. It's a minor procedure with low risks and potentially high gains.

PART THREE

DIAGNOSIS OF BREAST PROBLEMS

9

Mammography

Although mammography is most commonly thought of in relation to cancer, it's actually a diagnostic tool for a variety of breast problems. It shares this capacity with a number of other imaging techniques. ("Imaging" means ways of seeing body tissue; see Chapter 10.) For example, a woman with localized breast pain might have a mammogram to see if she has a cyst. A woman with an abscess might need an ultrasound to delineate its extent. A woman with nipple discharge might have a ductogram (type of mammogram; see Chapter 7) to find the lesion and plan surgery. Both magnetic resonance imaging (MRI) and ultrasound are being used to determine whether silicone implants have leaked.

In this chapter we'll look at diagnostic mammography, and in the next we'll discuss other commonly used diagnostic tools. Later, in Chapter 19, we will discuss the use of mammography as a method of screening for breast cancer. (The same equipment is used for screening and for diagnostic mammography, but different types of pictures may be taken.)

A mammogram is an x ray of the breast—"mammo" means breast and "gram" means picture. It isn't the same as a chest x ray, which looks through the breast and photographs the lungs. Mammograms look at the breast itself, and take pictures of the soft tissue within it, allowing the radiologist to see anything unusual or suspicious. Mammography can pick up very small lesions—about 0.5 cm (or 0.2 inch), whereas you usually can't feel a lump till it's at least a centimeter (0.4 inch). These lesions can be benign or malignant. In addition, mammograms can sometimes pick up precancers (see Chapter 16).

Mammography has its limits, though. The mammogram can take a picture of only the part of the breast that sticks out—the plates are put underneath the breast, or on the sides of the breast—so it's easier to get an accurate picture of a large breast than of a small one. The periphery of the breast will not get into the picture at all (Fig. 9-1). In addition, if your breasts are dense, the lump may not be visible through the tissue. So a mammogram isn't perfect. Physical exams and mammograms are complementary, not substitutions for each other. You can see some lumps on a mammogram that you can't feel, and you can feel some lumps (palpation) that you can't see on an x ray.

You get a diagnostic mammogram when you find a lump or have another breast complaint and your doctor wants to get a better sense of what the problem is. If, for example, you have lumpy breasts and there's one area that may be a dominant lump, your doctor may send you for a mammogram. If a lump looks jagged, not smooth, on the mammogram, it's a sign that further investigation may be called for. If you've got a lump your doctor thinks may be cancerous, a mam-

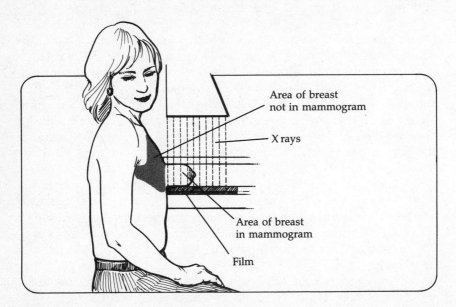

Area of breast
not in mammogram

X rays

Area of breast
in mammogram

Film

FIGURE 9-1

mogram can help determine if there are other lumps that should be biopsied at the same time; it can also document the location of the lump.

RADIATION RISKS

When mammography was first used, it was seen as the Great New Hope; in typical American fashion, it was hyped as the answer to all breast problems. All a woman had to do was get a mammogram every six months and she had nothing to worry about. Then, in 1976, Dr. John C. Bailar III calculated that if young women in their 20s started having mammograms every six months, we'd cause more cancer than we'd cure.[1] There were scary news stories, and mammograms were viewed as a major health hazard.

Predictably, the truth is somewhere in between. These days, mammography contains very little radiation risk, since we've reduced the amount of radiation significantly in recent years. As we note in Chapter 13, the risk of getting cancer from exposure to radiation is greater when you're young, and decreases as you grow older. This works out well, since mammography is less useful in most young women, who tend to have much more dense breast tissue than fat, and it's increasingly useful as women age and breast tissue gives way to fat. Most specialists now feel that the radiation risk of mammography after age 35 is negligible or nonexistent.

WHAT MAMMOGRAMS SHOW

A mammogram, like any other x ray, presents a two-dimensional view of a three-dimensional structure. Denser areas appear as shadows. Breast tissue, for example, is very dense, and shows up white on the mammogram. Fat, which is not very dense at all, shows up gray (see photographs on pages 126-127).

As you'll recall from our discussion in Chapter 1, when you're young—in your teens and early 20s—your breasts are usually made up mostly of breast tissue, and are very dense. As you grow older, the breast ages, much as your skin does, and as it ages there's less breast tissue and more fat. When you're in your 30s and 40s, it's about half and half. (This varies with your weight; if you're very heavy there'll be a lot more fat; if you're thinner, there'll be more breast tissue.) Once you're in menopause, the breast tissue goes away, and there are usually only a few strands of it left. However, women vary in the propor-

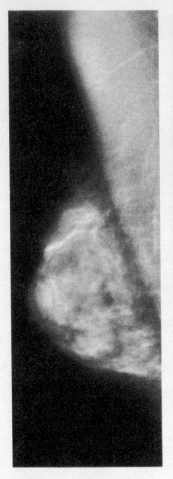 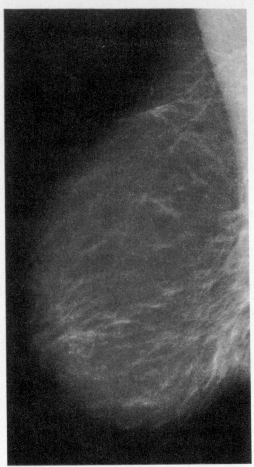

Dense breast in young woman   **Fatty breast in older woman**

tion of breast tissue remaining after menopause. And if they take hormone replacement therapy (see Chapter 13) their tissue may remain as dense as it was, or may even become more dense.

How does this affect the reading of a mammogram? Cancer and benign lumps are the same density as breast tissue. So if you've got a white lump in the middle of an area of dense tissue, it won't show up on the mammogram—the tissue will hide it. It's like looking for a polar bear in the snow. But if the same lump is sitting in the middle of fat, it'll be very obvious—a white spot in the midst of gray. So mammography is more accurate in older women, who have more fat, than in younger women, who have more breast tissue. Sometimes I'd get a pa-

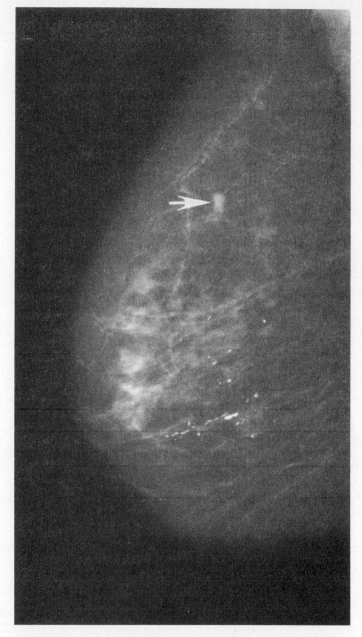

Small cancer in fatty breast (arrow) and benign calcifications

tient who'd been for a mammogram and had been told that her breasts were so dense that mammography wasn't useful to her. That's ridiculous—what it means is that mammography wasn't as useful to her now as it would have been if she had fatty breasts. Often the woman is around 30, when her breasts should be dense. What it really means is that there's a higher chance that something could be missed (9–20 percent; but there's also an 80–90 percent chance of picking up something. This isn't to say I'm recommending screening mammograms for women at 30, but that a diagnostic mammogram may have some value if there is a breast problem that needs to be explored.

When mammograms show something round and smooth, it's likely to be a cyst or a fibroadenoma (see Chapter 8). The mammogram can't distinguish between cysts and fibroadenomas; you'd follow up with an ultrasound (see next chapter) to see if it's a cyst. If a mammogram shows jagged, distinct, radiating strands, pulling inward, it's more likely to be cancer. But until it is biopsied, we can't tell for sure. Several benign conditions can mimic cancer on a mammogram. Scarring or fat necrosis (dead fat) will look very suspicious; as will a noncancerous entity called a *radial scar*. This lesion can be confusing even under the microscope and often requires an expert breast pathologist to be sure it is not cancer.

A mammogram may also show intramammary (in the breast) lymph nodes. In fact, until the invention of the mammogram, we didn't know there *were* lymph nodes in the breast. We now know that about 5.4 percent of women will have them. Sometimes you'll hear about a "normal" mammogram. But there's really no one pattern you can call normal, since there's no real "normal" breast.

In mammography reports, some radiologists use words loosely—as if they can see what the pathology is when they're looking at the shadows on the mammogram. So they'll tell you you've got "cystic changes," which is a variation of our old nemesis fibrocystic disease. All that means is that you've got dense breast tissue. Or they'll tell you you've got "mammary dysplasia," which sounds very serious and means you've got abnormal cells—cells en route to cancer. But the cells aren't visible on the mammogram—only a biopsy can show cells. What they really mean is, once again, you've got dense tissue in your breasts. All a radiologist can tell you is how much breast tissue there is and how much fat tissue, and whether there are abnormal areas of density.

Just as 20 percent of women have some degree of variation in the size of their breasts, variation exists on the inside as well. It will appear on the report as "asymmetry," and it probably doesn't mean anything at all—though sometimes, rarely, an asymmetry can be caused by cancer, so you might want to get a second mammogram several months later, just to make sure. If it's cancer, it's likely to have changed somewhat during that time. One of the most absurd cases I've come across is that of a patient who'd had a mastectomy on one side, with a reconstruction. She came to me because the report on the mammogram said it showed "marked asymmetry." Of course it did! The breasts were completely different in their composition; they were meant to look the same on the outside, not the inside.

TYPES OF MAMMOGRAMS

Mammography has changed over the years. In the beginning, in the 1950s, they used big x-ray machines—the same ones they used for chest or bone x rays. These produced a fair amount of radiation, and the pictures weren't very clear. So they began refining the process, and designed an x-ray machine specifically geared to do mammograms, one that could be aimed more precisely at the breast and could rotate to get most of the breast tissue. Over the years they've also refined the x-ray techniques, so that now very little radiation is actually used. It's commonly said that a mammogram exposes you to the same amount of radiation you'd get in a plane flying over Denver. One radiologist I used to work with in Boston explained it in more colorful terms: the amount of radiation of one mammogram is equal to the amount of radiation you would get by walking on the beach nude for 10 minutes or until you got caught.[2]

Film-screen mammography, the technique used now, gives a precise definition of what the tissue looks like. It can be a bit uncomfortable because the breasts have to be squeezed between the plates to get an accurate picture. The slight discomfort is well worth the increased accuracy and low radiation. A 1993 study tried letting women control the compression themselves. Not surprisingly, they ended up with the same amount of compression, equally good quality films, and fewer complaints.[3]

A new technique, called digital mammography, has been developed. Like a digital camera, digital mammography is a way of computerizing the image and then printing it back out again. Because it's a computerized rather than a photographic technique, the radiologist can magnify different areas to see what she or he wants to see. Just as you can play with digital photos on your computer and remove Uncle Jack, on a digital mammogram all the fat could be blocked out so only breast tissue would show up, or it could erase the breast tissue so that only fat would show up. Our hope is that this technique will solve some of the limitations of film-screen mammograms. It may be more accurate in women with dense breasts, for example, since it could erase some of the breast tissue and make a lump more evident. (It still involves radiation, so will continue to have limited application in very young women.) In addition, digital mammography will facilitate computerized reading of mammograms. Don't panic; we won't leave all of the reading up to a computer. What the computer will do is pre-screen mammograms and point out the worrisome areas so that the mammographers can examine them more carefully. We hope this will make reading more accurate as computers don't get easily distracted or blink at the wrong moment.

I think we've gotten almost as far as we can with mammography. Each advance is incremental. Other imaging techniques are being developed as well (see Chapter 10).

CALCIFICATIONS

One of the more important discoveries from the study of mammograms is that cancer is often associated with some very fine specks of calcium that appear on the picture—they look a bit like tiny pieces of dust on a film.

We discovered that these microcalcifications, as we called them, were sometimes an indication of cancer or precancer (see Chapter 16). So the radiologist will always mention in a report any microcalcifications that show up. But it's nothing to panic about—80 percent of microcalcifications have nothing to do with cancer; they're probably just the result of normal wear and tear on your breast.[4] Ironically, when you age, calcium leaves your bones, where it's needed, and shows up in other places, where it's not. It can show up in arteries, causing them to harden, and in joints, causing arthritis. The microcalcifications in your breast won't cause any problems if they're not indications of cancer or precancer. (The appearance of this calcium in your body has no relation to how much calcium you eat or drink, by the way.)

How can we tell which are the bad and which are the harmless kinds of calcifications? We look at the shape, the size, and how many there are. If they're very tiny and tightly clustered, and there aren't a whole lot of them, they're more likely to be precancer. If they're all over the place they're more likely to be benign.

Precancer occurs in the duct, which is very small. For the calcifications to fit in a duct, they have to be very tightly clustered and very small. The big chunks of calcium we see on the mammogram couldn't possibly fit in the ductal system, so we know they're benign. They're usually old fibroadenomas that you had as a teenager, which have faded and become soft and less dense and now are calcifying. Or they can be calcifications in a blood vessel as it gets older and harder.

There's a middle group of calcifications that are less easy to characterize. They may be new, but there are just one or two of them. In that situation, we'll usually repeat the mammogram in six months.[5] If it's precancer, we might see more calcifications, or a change in the shape or size, whereas if there's no change, it's more likely to be benign. Patients get nervous about that; if it's cancer and we wait six months, won't it grow and kill you? But in fact, if we wait six months it's probably because we don't think it's cancer. And even in the worst-case scenario, it's precancer, not cancer, and precancer takes 10 years to develop into cancer. So six months won't make any difference, and you don't want to have needless biopsies.

It's true that some precancerous calcifications don't grow or change, so they don't get picked up on the second mammogram. But that's because they aren't growing and thus aren't becoming cancer.

Any time that doctors are worried about calcifications they can of course proceed to a biopsy. This can be a core biopsy or an open biopsy depending on the available facilities (see Chapter 11).

MAMMOGRAPHIC WORKUP

Screening is for asymptomatic women. In contrast, diagnostic mammography involves the workup of a lump felt by a woman or her doctor or the workup of an abnormal finding on a screening mammogram.

One way to do this workup is to do a compression spot view. We do this when there is a dense area on the original mammogram that we're unsure of. It's an extra view on the mammogram; the radiologic technologist uses a small plate to press right over the abnormal area and takes a picture of that area. Since a mammogram is a two-dimensional picture of a three-dimensional structure, we see overlapping shadows. (It's as if you had a transparent balloon with different pictures on each side. If you took a photo from the front, it would look like one complex image. If you looked at each picture on the balloon from a different direction you'd see them as separate.) Another thing the technologist can do is press on your breast at an angle and change it so that things aren't perfectly juxtaposed.

If there is an abnormal density on mammogram, or a lump that you can feel but isn't visible on a mammogram, you may be sent to get an ultrasound (see Chapter 10).

If you have a palpable lump, the mammographer should put a marker on your breast to be sure that the lump is on the film. If it is at the periphery of the breast it may be necessary to take special mammographic views to get it in the picture—like changing the angle of your camera to make sure Aunt Mabel's head doesn't get cut off in the photo. This is especially important for lumps that are near the armpit or in the lower fold of the breast.

If you have calcifications, we very often do a magnification view, which is a mammogram that magnifies the area of the breast with the calcifications, so we can see them and characterize them better. So, for the most part, if you're told that the calcifications on your mammogram are worrisome, you should make sure they do a magnified view to see if the calcifications still look bad and how many there are. Sometimes mammographers will want to skip this step and send you for a biopsy. Don't let them. Why subject yourself to surgery if it may not be necessary?

Some problems arise because some radiologists don't have enough experience reading mammograms (see Quality of Mammograms below). How familiar your radiologist is with the procedure may well reflect how well the x ray is read. A more experienced mammographer may be willing to state his or her opinion that something is almost certainly benign. A radiologist anxious about missing something will be more likely to say, "I don't think it's cancer, but it could be, and a biopsy is recommended to be absolutely sure." As a result of these kinds of readings, we're doing more biopsies than ever on benign lumps.

For this reason it's very important, if you're told you need a biopsy for an abnormal mammogram, that you get a second opinion. Take your mammogram to another center—preferably a place that specializes in mammography—and have them review it. Studies show that 60 to 70 percent of biopsies done for abnormal mammograms could be avoided if the mammogram were reviewed by an expert.

A mammogram can't tell for certain what you have. To do that we need to have tissue we can look at under a microscope. But there are some situations in which the view from the mammogram shows signs that clearly suggest a diagnosis. It's a bit like seeing someone from the back. You don't know for sure that it's your friend Mary until she turns around and faces you, but if it's Mary's shade of red hair, in the kind of pony tail Mary always wears, and she walks like Mary does and carries the kind of large briefcase Mary likes to carry, you can make a pretty good guess that it's Mary. How often you are right will of course depend on how well you know Mary. An experienced mammographer is better able to diagnose breast problems than an inexperienced one.

A typical story in my practice was that of a patient who in her early 60s came to my office after her first mammogram and told me they found something strange. I looked at the x rays and saw a little asymmetry, so I sent her back for a compression spot mammogram—and the asymmetry completely disappeared. Because the radiologist didn't take it the next step, the patient had been scared needlessly.

In another frequent scenario a woman would tell me they found something strange on her mammogram. I would look at the x rays and see a small and smooth lump, like a fibroadenoma, but it would be new. The radiologist had written, "possible fibroadenoma; cancer can't be ruled out." I could have done one of two things. I could have had her wait six months and check it out again; if it was cancer, it probably would have grown. If she was really anxious, I could have done a stereotactic core biopsy, under x-ray control. If it wasn't cancer, that was fine; if it was, we could plan for the cancer surgery. If a diagnosis couldn't be made this way, we could do a wire localization biopsy. (We'll discuss these forms of biopsy further in Chapter 11.)

QUALITY OF MAMMOGRAMS

Today, all mammography units must be accredited by an FDA-approved accreditation body (certified by the FDA as meeting the standards) and prominently display the certificate issued by the agency. The initial quality standards for mammography facilities to meet FDA certification went into effect in December 1994. They include the following: radiologic technologists who perform mammography, physicians who interpret mammograms, and medical physicists who survey equipment must all have adequate training and experience; each facility must have a system for following up on mammograms that reveal problems and for obtaining biopsy results. In 1996 the FDA along with the National Mammography Quality Assurance Advisory Committee developed additional and more comprehensive final standards, which include: (1) a consumer complaint mechanism to provide women with a process for addressing their concerns about mammography facilities; (2) special techniques and personnel qualifications related to mammography of women with breast implants; (3) communication of mammography results to referring physicians and *all examinees (that means you)* in writing; and (4) additional clinical image review and examinee notification requirements when a facility's images are determined to be substandard. In addition, there is standardized reading of mammograms (called the BIRADS system) whereby all mammograms are classified according to five categories (see Table 9-1).

Mammography now is the one place where we really do have quality control—something we have little of in the rest of breast care, and indeed in much of medicine.

PROCEDURE

How do you actually experience the process of getting a mammogram? It starts before you leave the house. Don't wear talcum powder or deodorant the day you're scheduled for a mammogram—flecks of

Table 9-1. Breast Imaging-Reporting and Data System (BI-RADS)

Category	Assessment	Description, Recommendation
1	Negative	There is nothing to comment on. Routine screening.
2	Benign finding	A definitely benign finding. Routine screening.
3	Probably benign finding	Very high probability of benignity. Short-term follow-up recommended to establish stability.
4	Suspicious looking abnormality	Not characteristic but has reasonable probability of malignancy. Biopsy should be considered.
5	Highly suggestive of malignancy	Very high probability of maignancy. Appropriate action should be taken.

talcum can show up as calcifications on the mammogram. You should also avoid lotions that can make the breast slippery. Some places will tell you not to take in caffeine for two weeks before the x ray; unless you have experienced some problem with caffeine, ignore them.

The atmosphere you face when you get there will vary from hospital to hospital. Some are cold and clinical; others provide a warm ambience and reassuring, friendly personnel. But the actual procedure is pretty standard. You have to undress from the waist up, and you're usually given some kind of hospital gown. You'll probably be x-rayed standing up. The technologist—usually, but not always, a woman—will have you lean over a metal plate, and help you place your breast on the plate. It can be cold and a bit uncomfortable, and when the plates press your breast together, it can be somewhat unpleasant. Two pictures of each breast are usually taken, one in a lateral position, the other vertical. But 20 percent of the time it will be necessary to take additional views, or do special magnification or spot pictures. This isn't a sign that you have cancer—it just means that the mammography technologists and radiologists are being painstakingly careful to get accurate pictures. In addition, the way the technologist takes the x rays is important. The tighter they can squeeze your breasts, the more accurate a picture they can get.

The process really isn't all that painful. Paul Stomper did a multicenter study interviewing people right after their mammograms, asking how painful the process was, and what point they were at in their menstrual cycle.[6] He was pleased that 88 percent of the women reported no pain or discomfort at all, and was surprised to learn that their cycle didn't seem to have any effect on their comfort level.

There's a small percentage of women whose breasts are unusually sensitive, and for them a mammogram can be painful. In Stomper's study none of the women who reported that the procedure was painful felt that it would stop them from having another mammogram exam. It's unfortunate that it's not painless, but I think it's well worth the slight—and brief—pain. At UCLA we actually timed the technologists, and we found that compression lasted at most 10 seconds. It's only uncomfortable for a few seconds, and it doesn't leave bruises or tender spots when it's over.

Women with disabilities may have difficulty getting a clear mammogram, particularly if they're unable to stand up. Fortunately there is a new setup called the Bennett Contour Mammography System that allows women to sit for the procedure.

The whole process lasts only a few minutes; when it's done, you have to wait for a while till the pictures are developed, so you might want to bring along a good book or a Walkman. The radiologist (an M.D., not the technologist) who looks at the pictures will sometimes see something on the periphery that isn't completely clear, and will want to take another picture, focusing on that area. Or she or he will want a magnification view, which can magnify the breast in a certain area to show it more clearly. This latter is usually done when there are microcalcifications.

In some places, the radiologist will come out and tell you what the mammogram shows. If you have your x ray at a high-volume, low-cost center, the x rays aren't read right away, and you have to wait several days to a week to find out the results.

Don't ask your technologist to interpret the mammogram for you. Technologists aren't M.D.s: their job is taking the pictures, not reading them.

Although, as I have often been quoted as saying, diagnostic mammography must have been invented by a man (and there should be an equally fun test for men), it is the best tool we currently have. We have to be careful when we discuss the risks and benefits of screening (see Chapter 19) not to throw the baby out with the bath water. It's an imperfect tool but, particularly for women with confusing breast problems, it's an important one.

10

Other Imaging Techniques

Frustration with some of the limitations of mammography has led to the exploration of other ways of looking at the breast. The reasons we're looking for other tests are that mammography uses radiation, which is potentially dangerous, and that it is limited in its ability to see through dense breast tissue and to determine clearly whether a lump is benign or malignant. These issues are especially important for young, high-risk women. Some of the techniques we've looked at are old techniques, and some are new. The amount of promise varies significantly with each technique. So far none of these techniques promises to do away with mammography. Most are being proposed as an adjunct to mammography either to help figure out which suspicious lesions on mammogram are really worrisome or to image dense breasts where mammograms may miss something.

ULTRASOUND

In the ultrasound method, high-frequency sound waves are sent off in little pulses, like radar, toward the breast. A gel is put on the breast to make it slippery, and a small transducer (a device which picks up sound waves) is slid along the skin, sending waves through it. If something gets in the way of the waves, they bounce back again, and if nothing gets in the way, they pass through the breast. It never picks out the small details, as an x ray can, but it can show other characteristics of a lump. Ultrasound is appealing because it doesn't use radiation.

This technique is used mostly for looking at a specific area; if we know a lump is there, we can use ultrasound to get more information about it. It can help determine whether a lump is fluid-filled or solid— if it's fluid-filled, like a cyst, the sound waves go through it, and if it's solid, like a fibroadenoma, pseudolump, or cancerous lump, the sound waves will bounce back. So if a lump shows up on a mammogram that we can't feel in a physical examination, and we want to determine whether it's a cyst or a solid lump, ultrasound can give us the answer.

Ultrasound can also be quite useful in helping us interpret a mammogram. If the doctor feels a lump and the mammogram shows just dense breast tissue, the ultrasound can sometimes see if there's a lump within the dense breast tissue. Mammography will only show overlapping shadows, but ultrasound can sometimes distinguish differences in the density of the tissues causing the shadows. Remember the image of the transparent balloon in Chapter 9? Now imagine that the balloon has a few colored balls inside it. An ultrasound can distinguish the balls inside, which are different from the balloon itself. Ultrasound isn't perfect, but it adds another dimension to the imaging possible with mammography. Many cancer centers, therefore, if there is a lesion on a mammogram, will also do an ultrasound.

Because there is no radiation involved, and, as far as we know, sound waves are harmless, ultrasound is also often the best tool for studying benign problems at length, particularly in women under 35. So if a doctor has a younger patient who has a lump, and wants to determine if it's likely to be a fibroadenoma or just dense breast tissue, ultrasound in that area can differentiate between a distinct lesion with edges or a mixed area without any definite lumps.

A limitation of ultrasound is that it is more dependent than mammography on the experience of the person operating the equipment. Unlike mammography, which shows the whole breast on each picture, each ultrasound picture shows only a small section of the breast. Therefore, the technologist or physician who operates the ultrasound equipment must be able to first find the abnormality and then demonstrate it well on the pictures he or she takes. The technologist or physician holds the transducer directly over the lesion, and the angle at which it is held changes the image. Looking at the photograph of the image at another time can be difficult. The technologist or physician needs to be standing at the patient's side looking at the screen while performing the examination and taking the pictures. It may be hard for the physician to pick up an ultrasound picture after the fact and be able to interpret it accurately.

Ultrasound might appear like the ideal test, with no radiation and the capacity to tell cyst from solid tissue. Why then don't we just use ultrasound and not mammography? One problem is that it is not easy to accurately ultrasound the whole breast. There are a few ultrasonographers who are doing it, but it takes a lot of time, patience, and experience. It shows so many changes in contour and density that it becomes very difficult to differentiate normal breast tissue from a lesion. Also, microcalcifications or other lesions visible on a mammogram may not be identifiable on an ultrasound. It may be worth it for women who have dense breasts and are high risk, but other imaging techniques such as MRI may be just as good and less operator dependent. The best use of ultrasound is in investigating one lump or area that has already been detected by physical exam or mammography.

We can also use ultrasound in much the same way we use mammograms to guide needle biopsies (see Chapter 11).[1] Sometimes ultrasound is a more effective tool for guiding us into the lesion than mammography. Physicians experienced in breast ultrasound can approach the lesion from different directions, which can make it easier to biopsy hard-to-reach areas in the breast, and many find the ultrasound method faster and more comfortable for the patient.

Ultrasound has also been used to look at women with silicone implants to decide whether the implant has ruptured or leaked. With a highly skilled technologist and radiologist, it's very accurate for that purpose.[2]

Just as digital mammography is attempting to make mammography clearer, there are many scientists working on improving the resolution of ultrasound. Three-dimensional ultrasound with even better resolution will be more useful in the diagnosis of breast problems, especially in young women with dense breasts. Color Doppler ultrasound and power Doppler ultrasound are used to show whether there are increased blood vessels associated with a mass. Cancers often have an increase in blood supply (see angiogenesis in Chapter 13), but so do some benign lesions. One study compared the color Doppler images with later examinations of the tumors under the microscope. They found that increased blood flow shown on the color Doppler ultrasound correlated with the size of the tumor and the number of involved lymph nodes but did not correlate with the tiny new blood vessels in the tumor (micro vessel density). In other words, color Doppler ultrasound is better at picking up bigger blood vessels than at showing the very new ones that we think are important at predicting the behavior of tumors.[3]

Whether these new and improved ultrasound technologies will finally prove to be useful for detecting more abnormalities or in making diagnostic decisions will depend on clinical research studies. Meanwhile, ultrasound continues to be an important diagnostic tool for breast cancer diagnosis.

MRI

Magnetic resonance imaging (MRI) takes advantage of the electromagnetic qualities of the hydrogen nucleus. Hydrogen is part of water, and water is part of our bodies. MRI is a huge magnet. You are put in the middle of the magnet, and the hydrogen nucleus lines up with the magnetic field. Then the technician turns on a radiofrequency wave to tip the hydrogen nucleus off the new magnetic axis. When the radiofrequency wave is turned off, the hydrogen realigns with the strong magnetic field. The way the hydrogen realigns with the field allows the MRI machine to make an image of the tissues.

This test was initially used in the brain, and has been very accurate in diagnosing brain tumors. It's finally finding its place in breast diagnosis. It is now recognized as the most sensitive and specific way to evaluate whether a silicone breast implant has leaked. It is also gaining acceptance as a technique that can identify breast cancer and further define abnormalities identified on mammography or ultrasound.

A silicone-specific technique has been developed to differentiate rupture of the capsule from other benign breast problems. This has been accurate in experienced hands. Detection of invasive breast cancer is not quite as good.

Most of the studies on MRI and breast cancer are done with contrast material (a dye) that is injected into the woman's veins. This material is picked up rapidly by lesions with lots of blood vessels and therefore by cancers. Unfortunately, a few cancers are slow growing and do not have increased blood vessels, and a large number of benign lesions also have an increased number of blood vessels. MRI also does not pick up many precancers that show up on mammograms as calcifications. The lesions that look like cancers but aren't are called false positives, while the cancers that are missed are false negatives. Their preponderance limits MRI's value for screening. Its best potential application appears to be preoperative planning for possible breast-conserving therapy. It can tell you if there are other lesions in the breast that should be removed, and it can show the true extent of the lesion that has been diagnosed.

The MRI exam is done with the patient lying face down on a table with her breasts hanging into the machine. To get good results, the woman should have an injection of contrast material that is picked up by lesions and not by normal tissue. We do this by injecting a dye called gadolinium intravenously before the procedure. The dye is absorbed better and faster by cancers than by benign lesions. Though this improves the accuracy of the MRI, it is not foolproof; it often lights up with a fibroadenoma, and it still misses some cancers.

MRI is not going to replace mammography, at least at this stage. It's not as good a screening test—it's too expensive; it's too hard to do; and it is not yet accurate enough. Nonetheless much research is going on to determine the exact role MRI can have in the detection and diagnosis of breast cancer. I predict we will see more of it in the future.

PET SCANNING

Positron emission tomography (PET) is another technique that's gotten a lot of press. Other techniques create pictures, but PET is a completely different way of imaging breast tissue. We look not at the structure itself, but at the activity going on in it. All tissues need glucose as fuel to survive. Cancers are rapidly growing and turning over, so they use more glucose than normal tissue. PET scanning looks at how much and how fast glucose is being used by a tissue. Like MRI, PET was first developed to study the brain, and has been very useful for that.

To do this scan we give the patient a radioactively labeled glucose molecule, which is taken up and metabolized by the tissue. The scanner can demonstrate how much and how fast glucose is taken up by the tissues. When imaging the brain with the PET scan, we can have the patient do a number of things that use different parts of the brain. If the patient talks, the scan lights up in the area of the brain that connects for talking; if the patient reads, it lights up another area. So it's very useful in mapping the brain and seeing where different problems lie.

Potentially PET scanning could be the answer to detecting virtually any cancer, since it can examine the whole body. Cancers are faster growing and use more glucose than normal tissues, so they should light up better. PET scans have been able to demonstrate areas of metastatic disease that cannot be seen by other imaging techniques. The major question is how small a lesion it can pick up—how sensitive it really is. If it can pick up micrometastatic disease, it could be very helpful. At this stage in its development, it does not show the area involved very clearly and therefore is not good for finding a cancer and helping us know where to biopsy. As with MRI, we are still in the process of determining its usefulness. It may have a role in distinguishing benign lesions from malignant ones based on how much glucose they use.

Another thing we're looking at with PET scanning is whether it can be used to monitor how well a tumor is responding to chemotherapy. If we give a person chemotherapy and then follow up with a scan to see if there's less glucose utilization than there was before the treatment, we might be able to tell if the chemotherapy is slowing the tumor growth. Newer scans are using radioactive estrogen to try to delineate tumors that are estrogen sensitive.

One of the biggests drawbacks to the PET scan is that it is very expensive and can only be found in selected centers. Researchers are trying to develop a PET scanner that would work only on the breast and therefore would be both easier to buy and operate and less expensive.

MIBI SCAN

MIBI scan (Sesta MIBI scan) is a nuclear medicine scan. MIBI stands for 2-Methoxy IsoButyl Isonitral. It can be useful in determining the difference between benign lumps and cancer. The radioactive particle Tc-99m Sestamibi is injected intravenously (through the foot), and a scanner, much like a bone scan machine, takes a picture and shows whether the radioactive particle is taken up by the breast lump more than by the rest of the tissue. Since cancer is likely to pick up more Sestamibi, it will often light up. It was hoped that the MIBI scan would prove useful in determining the difference between benign lumps and cancer. Review of several studies suggests that this technique in women with palpable lesions has a high sensitivity (84–94%) and specificity (72–94%).[4] *Sensitivity* is the ability to find cancers; that is, it has a 6–16 percent chance of missing them. *Specificity* is the ability to correctly diagnose them as cancer; that is, it has a 6–28 percent chance of being wrong. It is not as good in nonpalpable or mammographically negative lesions, with a reported sensitivity as low as 50 percent. It is therefore best for palpable lesions that are hard to interpret on mammogram. This might be especially helpful for a young woman with dense breasts who feels a lump that her doctor can't find. A negative MIBI scan is not 100 percent accurate but should certainly put her mind at rest. It's not particularly good for screening, because you need an injection of radioactive material, and also because it doesn't localize things very well. It's very fuzzy and far less distinct than a mammogram.

CT SCANNING

Another type of test, CT scanning (the CAT scan), also uses radiation—far more than mammography does. It works by visually cutting a part of the body into cross-sectional slices. It's very good for detecting brain tumors and cancer in the belly and the lungs, because of the composition of those organs. But the amount of radiation needed to make a slice close enough to pick up a 5-millimeter lump in the breast is simply too high for safety, and you're wiser to stick with mammograms.

One recent study used contrast to enhance the CAT scan in women who had been diagnosed with cancer.[5] The contrast-enhanced CT was good at detecting the extent of disease and therefore in planning surgery. On the other hand, MRI, which does not involve radiation, is also good at this.

THERMOGRAPHY

Thermography is based on the concept that cancer gives off more heat than normal tissue. It was originally a much-heralded technique, since it doesn't involve radiation, or putting anything else into the body. A sensor is put on the breast, and heat coming from different parts of the breast is measured. From this a map is constructed, making beautiful colored pictures in which blue shows cold areas and red shows hot areas. The hot areas are supposed to be the cancerous ones. Unfortunately, this technique hasn't proved accurate—there are too many false positives and false negatives. Not all cancers give off heat, and of those that do, some are too deep, or located under wedges of fat, and the heat doesn't register on the device. More recently an Australian company has developed what is said to be a more accurate thermography machine. It has yet to be tested in the U.S. A Scottish group has developed an interesting device called the Chronobra[6]—a bra fitted with heat sensors and an electronic memory chip that can record the level of heat in the breast. According to its developer, Dr. Hugh Simpson, women who are high risk tend to reach their peak breast temperature a day or two earlier in the menstrual cycle than their low-risk counterparts. As this book was being written, thermography was getting press again for a device that uses computers to calculate results. How this will be used is difficult to predict.

Though thermography doesn't detect cancer, some doctors in Europe believe it can define the aggressiveness of a cancer that they know already exists: the more aggressive a cancer is, the more heat it gives off. This hasn't been substantiated, and thermography hasn't been used in the United States for this purpose.

TRANSILLUMINATION AND DIAPHANOGRAPHY

Transillumination is a very old technique that was used long before mammography appeared on the scene. Its purpose was to help determine whether a lump was a cyst or solid. It functioned like a flashlight; if the light shone through the lump, it was assumed to be a cyst, and if it didn't, the lump was solid and potentially dangerous.

That technique became more sophisticated, and equipment was developed that could monitor the exact amount of light in transmission. This advanced form of transillumination is called *diaphanography*. Since it doesn't use radiation, there was great hope that diaphanography would replace mammography, but it hasn't proved to be a great screening test. I have known some practitioners who have found it useful in conjunction with mammography.

THE FUTURE

All of these are attempts to find ways other than mammography to diagnose breast lesions, because what we really need is some kind of diagnostic test that does not involve radiation and that can determine the difference between dense breast tissue and benign lumps and cancer.

A new device was introduced in early 1998 that claimed to measure differences in electrical impulses coming from breast cells. It was found to be particularly useful in women with palpable lumps.

One possibility is combining biology and imaging. New techniques are exploiting the fact that cancers need a new blood supply if they are going to grow and spread. The process called angiogenesis is discussed further in Chapter 13. New MRI techniques are trying to use this to make the imaging more sensitive. Other work in animals combines antibodies to certain tumor genes with tags which can be seen on imaging. The future of breast cancer imaging will certainly be a long way from the rather crude tools that are available today.

Researchers are also exploring whether there are diagnostic tests that are different from imaging, like a blood test that could determine whether or not a lesion is malignant. As you'll see in Chapter 17, we now have a way to analyze nipple duct fluid that may point the way to the future of screening.

11

Biopsy

When the doctor tells you you need a biopsy, you'll want to find out what kind. There are four different kinds of biopsies—two done with needles, and two "open" biopsies that require surgical cutting (Fig. 11-1). A fine-needle (like the kind used to draw blood) biopsy takes only a few cells out of the lump; a larger-needle biopsy, called a core, cuts a small piece out of the lump. An incisional biopsy takes a much larger piece of the lump out, while in an excisional biopsy the entire lump is removed (Fig. 11–2).

If you aren't clear about what kind of biopsy the surgeon or radiologist is planning, you might discover that you are assuming only a little piece will be removed whereas the surgeon really means to remove the whole thing. Then you'll end up angry because you've had an operation, and the surgeon will end up defensive, because you were told you were getting a biopsy done.

The term *biopsy*, by the way, refers to the operation itself, not to the process of studying the lump in the laboratory, which the pathologist does later. Anything that we cut out of the body is always sent to the pathologist for analysis, and the connection between the two procedures causes people to confuse them with each other. If you're having a biopsy performed, it's useful for you to know the precise meaning of the term.

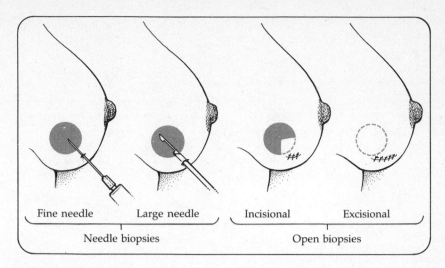

FIGURE 11-1

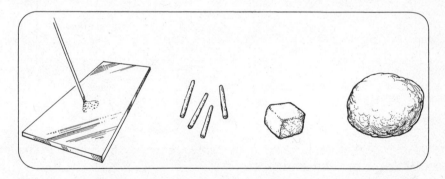

FIGURE 11-2

FINE-NEEDLE BIOPSY

If the patient has a palpable lump, the surgeon will anesthetize the breast with a small amount of lidocaine and then use a needle and syringe to try to get a few cells (Fig. 11-3). Then the material is squirted onto a slide, which is examined under a microscope. This can often show whether something is benign or cancerous.[1] However, since there's no tissue to look at, just the individual cells, the procedure requires a good cytologist—a specialist in the field of looking at cells rather than tissue—who can look at cells out of context.

Fine-needle biopsies can also be done on lesions that can only be

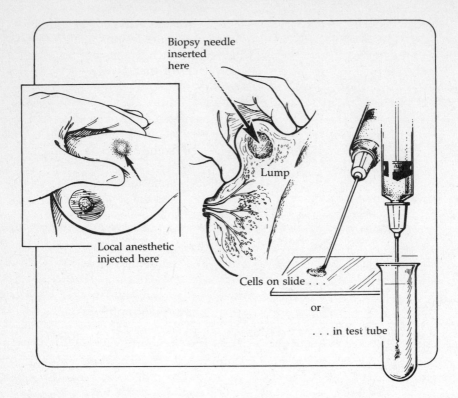

Biopsy needle inserted here

Lump

Local anesthetic injected here

Cells on slide . . .

or

. . . in test tube

FIGURE 11-3

seen on mammogram, although usually we use a core biopsy in that setting.

The rule of thumb with needle aspiration is that three elements should be consistent to determine that the lesion is benign.[2] So if I think on examination that it's a fibroadenoma, and it looks like one on the mammogram, and it also looks like one under the microscope after a needle aspiration, then I feel certain that's what it is. But if one of those elements is different—if it seems like it's not a fibroadenoma to me, even though the mammogram and needle aspiration suggest it is; or if I think it is but either the mammogram or needle aspiration biopsy suggests something different—then we go on to a larger biopsy.

CORE BIOPSY

A core biopsy is done in much the same way as a fine-needle biopsy. The major difference is that we use a larger needle. We've always done needle biopsies on palpable lumps. But with the increased use of mammography, doctors were finding more and more lesions that couldn't be felt. There's always a good chance that such lesions are harmless, but of course there's no way to be certain of that. So we were faced with the question of what to do about them.

One way we tried was with wire localization, a form of biopsy described later in this chapter. But it always made some of us uncomfortable. Here was a lesion we couldn't even feel, and yet we were doing surgery—always invasive and always with some risk. So a procedure was developed called *stereotactic core biopsy*.

When stereotactic core biopsies are done on lesions that can be seen only on mammogram, we use a machine called the stereotactic biopsy machine (Fig. 11-4). This procedure is now widely used. Sometimes it's done by a radiologist, sometimes by a surgeon; it doesn't matter which, as long as they know what they're doing. The American College of Surgeons has established voluntary guidelines for who should do the procedure. The radiologist or surgeon should have performed at least 12 stereotactic core biopsies, or at least three under the supervision of a physician qualified to interpret mammography who has performed at least 24 of the procedures. A radiologist must get some training in pathology, and a surgeon must get some training in how to read mammograms, so that whoever does the procedure is able to give the patient accurate information about the results.

There are some cases in which stereotactic core biopsies shouldn't be done. Large, diffuse areas of calcification are better surgically removed with a wide excision because a core only biopsies part of the lesion and may not be representative. Radial scars (see Chapter 9), which can be confused with cancer, are better taken out entirely, because the doctor may have difficulty diagnosing a small piece. In addition, there are other reasons that stereotactic biopsies may not work. People who weigh over 300 pounds won't fit on the machine. The patient has to be able to remain immobile in a prone position for as long as 45 minutes. This eliminates anyone with significant anxiety (unless the anxiety is being controlled successfully with medication), with arthritis in the neck or back, with chronic cough, with severe kyphosis (a condition that causes the person to hunch over), or anything else that prevents absolute immobility for 45 minutes. It's also a problem if the lesion is very superficial because the needle will poke through the skin. The needle is less than 3 centimeters thick, so if the breast, when compressed, is less than 3 cm, it won't work. Often this happens in very elderly women: although their breasts may appear fairly large when they hang down, there actually isn't much breast tissue there for the machine to grasp.

Luckily, core biopsies can also be done with ultrasound, using a handheld device which can accomodate these situations. It will also work better if a lesion that's palpable can't be seen on a mammogram. Even if the lesion is not palpable but can be visualized on ultrasound, a core biopsy can be done this way.

This approach is becoming more popular because it does not require equipment such as x-ray machines and does not expose the woman to radiation. Surgeons may have an ultrasound machine in their offices but will rarely have the x-ray equipment necessary for a stereotactic core. Why don't we do all core biopsies that way? Because not all lesions are visible on ultrasound. Microcalcifications, for example, are too small for an ultrasound machine to detect and so will require a stereotactic core.

No doctor should ever do a core biopsy in place of doing follow-up; it should be done in place of surgical biopsy. So the question, when a doctor is first examining a lesion, is always, "Should we do a biopsy?" If the answer is no, we should repeat the mammogram.

When, then, should biopsies be done? Different surgeons have different ideas on this. Many feel as I do, that when a biopsy is needed, it should be a core rather than a surgical biopsy whenever possible. This gives the surgeon the information, and after that the surgeon and patient can sit down and talk about what comes next. If the core biopsy shows cancer, you can then have the surgery you need, and you've had only one surgical procedure, rather than the two that you might have with a regular biopsy.

Some surgeons, on the other hand, feel that if the lesion appears likely to be malignant, they'd rather just do a wire localization biopsy (see below), diagnosing the lesion and removing it once and for all. Core biopsy is ideal if it seems likely that you'll want a mastectomy, since it entails only one surgery. People with multiple lesions do better with core biopsies, because multiple surgical biopsies are likely to leave your breast looking like Swiss cheese, and multiple core biopsies are far less disfiguring. If it's very likely that the lesion is a fibroadenoma (see Chapter 8), a core is also ideal, because it will assure you and your surgeon that it is indeed a harmless lump. But if you know it's going to worry you and you want the lump removed whatever it is, then you may as well just have that done right away and not bother with the core.

There are some new techniques coming out. Medical device manufacturers have been mobilized by the success of core biopsies and are trying to come up with machines that will allow a surgeon to do an entire lumpectomy this way. Their theory is that surgery could be altogether avoided if there were a needle bigger than that used for core—enlarged a centimeter or two—that could take out an entire lesion. One such device already out is the ABBI (advanced breast biopsy instrument). At first it seemed perfect, but it hasn't lived up to its promise. With malignant lesions it can seem that the machine is getting everything out, but when the pathologist looks at the edges of the removed tissue and they show cancer, more tissue will need to be taken out anyway. In addition, since the larger core takes a bigger piece out, there's more chance for bleeding and other complications. Theoretically, if a doctor is doing a large lumpectomy, which is essentially what ABBI does, there's less likelihood of part of the lesion being missed; but on the other hand, more tissue may be taken out than needs to be.

Another variation on this theme is a device called the *mammotome*. Instead of cutting out a core of tissue, this suctions it out. It gets out more tissue than the core method, and it's becoming more popular among doctors. Because of the amount of tissue it pulls out, it's better at finding microcalcifications than the other core procedures.

The problem with doing a lumpectomy with a device rather than doing an open, surgical one is always the difficulty of assuring that the doctor gets clean margins. There are some situations where this is more important than others; for example, when there's a small lesion that the doctor realizes is probably benign but which the patient wants removed, margins won't matter. In the rare case where the lesion turns out to be cancerous, a surgical re-excision can be done. This kind of lumpectomy also works well if the patient is in her 60s or older, with fairly fatty breasts, and has a small, well-circumscribed cancerous lesion. In this case the doctor should be able to remove the lesion and still get good margins.

The Procedure

Core biopsy differs mainly in whether it is being done under x-ray guidance or ultrasound. When x ray is used (stereotactic) the patient lies down on the table with her breast suspended below her between two x-ray plates (Fig. 11-4). The patient is given local anesthesia. A small incision is made over the site where the biopsy needle will go in. After exactly localizing the area with mammograms and a computer, the biopsy device enters the breast at 72 mph and drills a core of tissue. Often several passes are taken to make sure the lesion is well-sampled. The size of the incision depends on how big the core biopsy needle is. With the ABBI, it's big enough that it will have to be sutured closed when the procedure is finished. With others, if they're taking out only a small core, they can put a small, bandagelike covering called a steri-strip on it. Usually they take out five cores for lumps; for microcalci-

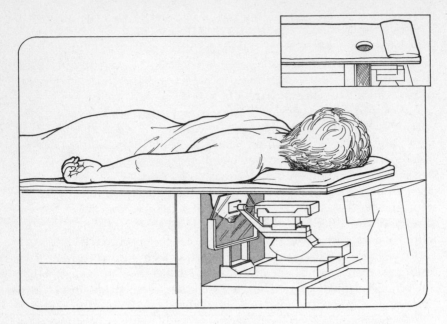

FIGURE 11-4

fications it may be 10 or more. After the biopsy they can take an x ray of the breast, see the line of air in the middle of the lump, and know that they've taken out what they were going after. (The inventor of these things was clearly a man: they were first called "biopsy guns." Only a man would think of aiming a gun at women's breasts! In the UCLA breast center, I got them to use the less militaristic term "biopsy device.") Afterward they use a metal clip to permanently mark the site of the biopsy, then hold pressure on the breast for a few minutes, until it's stopped bleeding. If the swelling seems bad, they may put an ice pack on it.

When the procedure is done by ultrasound the woman will lie on her back on a table and the radiologist or surgeon will identify the lesion using a handheld ultrasound device. Once the lesion is identified, the doctor will proceed with the biopsy, watching the core needle enter the lesion on the ultrasound monitor. The core biopsy is done by the physician with a handheld device.

There are few complications, whether done under x ray or ultrasound. The doctor might miss the lesion, but this very rarely happens. There may be infection or hematoma (blood blister), but these occur in only about 1 percent of patients. You may have some minor bruising.

SURGICAL BIOPSY

What is the process of an incisional or excisional biopsy like? Well, to begin with, there's the setting. You may have your biopsy performed in your doctor's office or, more frequently, in the hospital's "minor" operating room. If you had a biopsy several years ago, you might find this confusing—especially the minor operating room. In the past, most surgery was performed in what we now call the main operating room, and the surgical rituals may be very different from those you recall.

Most hospitals have two or three kinds of operating rooms. I like to think of them as similar to restaurant types, in which the food is basically the same, but there are different varieties served in different places and the rituals accompanying them are different.

In the hospital where I worked in Boston, there were three kinds of rooms. The minor operating room is like the snack bar—you can go in barefoot and wearing your bathing suit, and order your hamburger, and it's cheap and it tastes good. The ambulatory surgery room is more like the coffee shop; you have to wear shoes and be fully dressed, but it's okay to wear jeans, and you sit at a table and are waited on. There's a larger menu, which still includes your hamburger. And finally there's the main operating room, which is like the formal dining

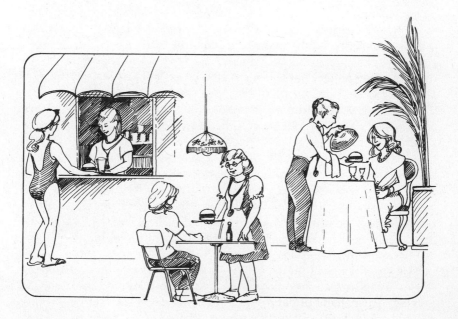

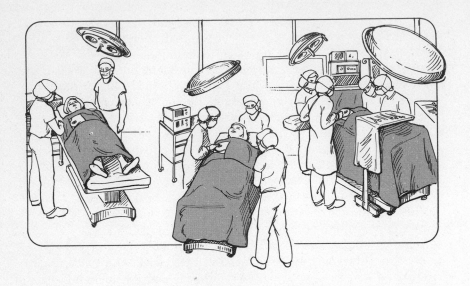

room—you've got to be a bit dressed up, there's a fancier menu, and the waiter grinds pepper onto your salad. Again, you can still get your hamburger, though it will cost you more. In each place, the hamburger's the same, but the rituals around it are different.

Similarly, you can have your biopsy in any of the three operating rooms, though the ambulatory and main rooms are equipped with a larger "menu" that includes more complex operations as well. The difference is in the ritual. And the rituals are always defined by the room they're performed in, not by the particular operation.

There's nothing wrong with the rituals—every profession has its rituals, and they're very useful to us. But if you don't know what the rituals are, or even that they *are* rituals, they can be intimidating.

Most of the surgical rituals are holdovers from the turn of the century, when they served a very practical purpose. Earlier, little was known about germs and the danger of spreading them through unsanitary practices. The majority of the rituals began then—the frequent hand-washing, the surgical gowns and masks, and so on—but nowadays, when people shower every day and wash their hands a lot and we have antibiotics to combat infections, the extreme degree of attention to totally sterile cleanliness is less necessary and, as I said, partially ritualistic. Predictably, the fancier the operating room, the fancier its attendant ritual.

Much of the breast surgery done today is done in either outpatient, freestanding ambulatory clinics or in the minor operating room. It's much cheaper than the same surgery performed in the main operating room. In the latter, you're paying for all that specialized equipment used for complicated procedures like open-heart surgery. Neither patients nor their insurance companies want that, so more and more the "snack bar" facilities are being used. (The ambulatory room is a bit more sophisticated than the minor operating room, but far less so than the main.) Often the ambulatory and minor operating rooms are used interchangeably. Keep in mind, however, that all this varies from hospital to hospital, and region to region.

So, if you had a biopsy 20 years ago in the "formal dining room," you may be expecting all the formal ritual, and be disturbed by its absence. Don't be. The operation and the care you're receiving are the same, and they are what matter.

If a patient has other medical problems—a heart or a respiratory condition, for example—then it's probably wiser to perform the operation in the main operating room, in case any complications arise that need more sophisticated equipment. If you're concerned about possible complications and how they'll be handled, talk with your doctor beforehand about which room will be used and what you're likely to need.

So much for the setting—now let's get to the procedure itself.

Wire Localization Biopsies

One form of surgery we might use, if your lesion cannot be felt and a needle biopsy is not possible, is a wire localization biopsy. As you might imagine, it's difficult to biopsy something you can see only on an x ray. In this procedure we use a thin wire to show the surgeon where the lesion is. It's usually done in the x-ray department. The radiologist will give you a local anesthetic, put a small needle into your breast under x-ray guidance, pointing toward the lesion (Fig. 11-5). She or he will then pass a wire and a hook on the end through the needle, and then position the hook so the end of the wire is on the site of the calcifications or density. The wire is left in the breast and you're taken to the operating room. The biopsy procedure is very similar to the procedure used to take a lump out, except that we use the wire to direct where we'll remove the tissue from. The surgeon gives you more local anesthetic, makes an incision, follows the wire, and then takes out the area of tissue around it, hoping it's the right place. The tissue is then sent to the radiology department. There they x-ray it to make sure it's from the area with the calcifications or lesion and then send it to the pathology department where they make slides and look at it under the microscope. Meanwhile the surgeon sews you up.

The x ray of the specimen will tell you if the surgeon got the calcifications or area that was seen on the mammogram. Since the surgeon

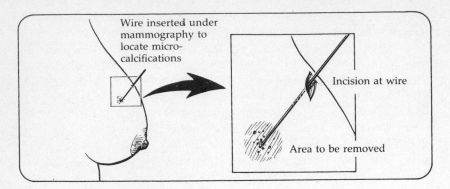

Wire inserted under mammography to locate micro-calcifications

Incision at wire

Area to be removed

FIGURE 11-5

can't see or feel calcifications, it is also possible to miss them with the surgery. In this case the x ray of the specimen will not show calcifications and you may need to get another biopsy.

The specimen won't, however, tell you if the surgeon got all the calcifications in your entire breast. If the area is benign this won't matter, but you will want to know whether there are still some benign calcifications inside. So it's important that you get another mammogram three to six months later to show how you look after the surgery.

Biopsy Procedures

Whether a wire local or a regular biopsy, the procedure can be done under either local or general anesthetic, but most doctors and patients prefer local. Some doctors like to give their patients a tranquilizer, but I prefer to help them stay calm through reassuring conversation. It is important to use a device called a pulse oximeter. This fits over your finger (like the pulse monitors often used by fitness enthusiasts) and monitors both your pulse and the amount of oxygen in your blood. It is an important safeguard whenever sedation is used. In some cases "local/standby" is used. This means the operation is done under local anesthesia, but an anesthesiologist or nurse-anesthetist is standing by in case you need some mild drugs that will make you indifferent to the procedure. The anesthesiologist can also put you to sleep if general anesthesia becomes necessary. There are now drugs that are very fast acting and don't last long. They put you into a kind of twilight sleep, in which you don't care about what happens and won't remember it, but you're not totally unconscious. These are often used in conjunction with a local anesthetic. This is known as monitored anesthesia, or MAC. If MAC is used, we need to do all the preoperative preparation in the same way we do for general anesthesia. When local anesthesia alone is used, you arrive, have your procedure, and go home. So it's a trade-off between being relatively more comfortable with a longer procedure and having more discomfort but getting in and out more quickly. MAC is definitely a coffee shop, not a snack bar, procedure. Which anesthetic people choose depends very much on their own personalities. Some people just don't want to know what's going on, and they're willing to put up with the extra inconvenience. Others hate being out of control and want to know what's happening. You should discuss with your doctor which way makes more sense for you. It is important to note that some of the drugs we use allow the patient to be awake and conversing but to have no memory of the experience afterward. If a woman wants to remember what happens during surgery, she needs to tell the anesthesiologist or anesthetist so that a drug such as Versed, for example, is not given to her.

If the biopsy takes place in the minor operating room or the doctor's office, the patient usually just has to change from the waist up; in the main operating room, where the dress code is more formal, the patient has to change into a hospital johnny and the surgeon wears a scrub suit. Depending on whether you are being operated on under local anesthesia or MAC, you may be more or less aware of what happens next.

Often in a biopsy, the surgeon will use a machine called an electric cautery to seal off the small blood vessels and prevent bleeding. Since there's a small risk of a short circuit, which would give the patient an electric shock, a grounding pad will be put on your leg, back, or abdomen to ground the current and prevent electric shock. It's a plastic pad with a cool gel inside which will initially feel freezing cold.

Next, the surgeon washes her or his hands, puts on surgical gloves, and then paints you with an antiseptic solution. Usually this is done two or three times—no particular reason, but three is a nice ritualistic number, so why not? Then sterilized towels (paper or cloth, depending on which room you're in) are framed around the area that's going to be operated on (Fig. 11-6).

With a sterile felt-tipped pen, the surgeon marks the spot over the lump, and then injects, through a small needle, the local anesthetic. (We usually use lidocaine, not novocaine, these days, but "novocaine" is still the popular term—like calling any facial tissues "kleenex.") When the needle first goes in, there can be a little pain and a little burning.

Don't be misled by the "novocaine"—it's not exactly like the anes-

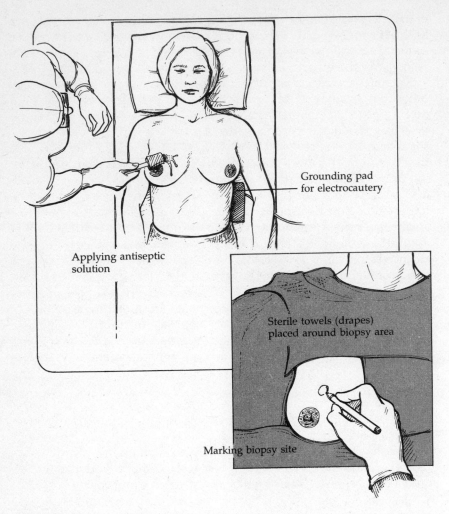

Grounding pad for electrocautery

Applying antiseptic solution

Sterile towels (drapes) placed around biopsy area

Marking biopsy site

FIGURE 11-6

thetic you get at the dentist's. For one thing, it hurts a lot less. The dentist has to poke around your mouth looking for a nerve, and then deaden it, and you have to wait till the novocaine takes effect, and then your whole mouth goes out and you end up chewing the inside of your cheek. It's not the dentist's fault: dental work requires a nerve block, since drilling into a tooth is felt all through the jaw.

But the process in the biopsy is different. Since we're cutting only into soft tissue, we can use "local infiltration," which numbs only the area where it's put, not the whole breast. And it works immediately. (This confuses some alert patients, who get scared when the surgeon starts to work right after injecting the anesthetic.) It's possible that you will feel some pain, even with the local anesthetic we give you for the biopsy. Some people are especially pain sensitive. This is not bad, nor are you being weak. Everyone's pain sensitivity is different and can change, depending on a number of factors, including medications you may be taking, stress, and prior experience. You can always ask for more anesthetic or sedation. Don't try to be "polite," or a "good girl"—there's no reason for you to suffer.

Now the surgeon makes the incision, going through skin, fat, and tissue to get to the lump. Most of the process isn't actually cutting; it's just spreading tissue apart till the lump is reached. There's little bleeding, because there aren't many blood vessels here, and the cautery takes care of the few there are. The lump is cut away from the surrounding tissue and removed (Fig. 11-7).

The incision is then sewn up, usually in layers—tissue, then fat, then skin. This prevents a dent from forming in the breast when it heals. Most surgeons use dissolvable stitches that tend to leave less scarring.

After the operation, the surgeon, who has bandaged the incision, will probably tell you when you can take the bandage off and when you can shower. I usually had the patient remove the bandage the next day and shower as soon as she wanted to. We used to think that you shouldn't shower until the stitches came out, but we've found that water doesn't hurt stitches at all.

The more you bounce, the sorer you'll be, so whether or not you usually wear a bra, it's a good idea to wear one for a couple of days after the surgery—a good firm, sensible bra, not a pretty, lacy, flimsy one. You'll probably want to keep it on all night as well. Some women, though, find the bra so uncomfortable in bed that they prefer the soreness. If the incision is near the bra line, the bra may cause more discomfort than it's worth. Use your own judgment; the point is to make you as comfortable as possible.

The anesthetic wears off much more quickly than the dentist's does: just as it goes to work right away, it wears off right away, generally within an hour after the biopsy is finished. You're usually not in much pain after the operation—many patients find that Tylenol is all they need. Do not, however, take aspirin or any nonsteroidal pain medication such as Motrin, Nuprin, or Aleve: they increase the chance of bleeding or bruising postoperatively. By the next day you can usually go back to work and resume your normal activities. (Be sensible, of course: if your normal activities include weight lifting, give it another couple of days.)

There will be some scarring, though usually very little. You should talk with your surgeon about it before you have the procedure done.

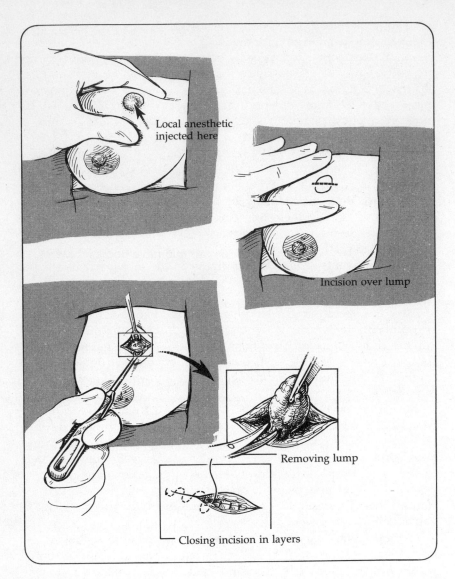

Local anesthetic injected here

Incision over lump

Removing lump

Closing incision in layers

FIGURE 11-7

You and your surgeon may have different ideas about what makes an acceptable scar. For example, surgeons have often learned in training that the most cosmetic scar results if they make the incision right around the areola and then tunnel up to the lesion, so that the scar is camouflaged by the color change between the areola and the rest of the breast. If that's done well, it can indeed give you a very unobtrusive scar. Sometimes, however, depending on the length of the scar or the amount of tissue that's removed, it can decrease the sexual sensation in your nipple, or create other changes in your nipple and areola such as numbness or puckering. Also, the scarring might cause difficulties in breast feeding. Further, the tunneling increases the chance that you'll have bleeding complications and a hematoma (see below).

An alternative, and one I personally favor, is to make the incision directly over the lesion and just take out the lump. It's usually a smaller incision that way, and there's less chance of damaging the nipple.

You really have to discuss your preferences with your surgeon, who will otherwise make assumptions about your wishes that may or may not be accurate. Most surgeons are sensitive to their patient's concerns and will try to give you the incision you want. If you feel the surgeon is being flippant or not taking your concerns seriously, find another one. At the same time, be aware that some people have bodies that make big keloid (thick) scars, and the best surgeon in the world can't prevent that. You probably know if you're one of these people from your own experience, although there's always the chance that, if you've never had a major cut before, you won't know till after the surgery.

With wire localization biopsies, it's important to know how much tissue the surgeon plans to remove. Some surgeons make their incision where the wire enters the skin, and will take out the tissue surrounding the whole length of the wire. This usually creates more deformity than making the incision over the place where the end of the wire is—going in directly and taking out only the lesion. With the increasing use of the core biopsy and the stereotactic needle aspiration, doctors can diagnose these things before the surgery, and don't have to remove as much tissue. So find out exactly how much tissue the surgeon plans to remove, and ask questions if it seems to you that it will be too much.

While you're resting up from the operation and getting on with your life, the lump is being analyzed by the pathologist, to whom the surgeon has immediately sent it. Sometimes the pathologist will do a "frozen section," which is a quick but crude method of testing the lump. The lump is cut in half; a piece is quick-frozen to make it solid, then thinly sliced, placed on a slide, and stained right away. Sometimes this will give you the answer, but it's not 100 percent accurate. In the old days, when we were doing immediate mastectomies if the lump was found to be malignant, this method was always used to allow the surgeon to proceed with the operation immediately. Nowadays, however, we usually do it in two steps—the biopsy is performed, the results are discussed with the patient, and, if further surgery is called for it's done later (see Chapter 25). So we don't often do a frozen section anymore.

Far more reliable is the regular procedure, the "permanent section." Here the tissue is removed and cut into small pieces. It goes through several stages. First it's dehydrated by putting it in different strengths of alcohol, then imbedded in a block of paraffin wax. This is then put on a microtome, a knife that cuts it into very thin slices. Each slice is then put on a slide, the wax melted away, and the tissue stained with different colors. This whole process takes between 24 and 36 hours.

When the slides are ready, the pathologist looks at them and makes a diagnosis; this takes a few hours. The pathologist then dictates a report, which is sent to the doctor, who will probably have it in a week. Some doctors wait till the report comes in, but others prefer to call the pathologist the day after the operation. This is what I used to do, because I liked to let my patients know what was happening as soon as possible, and because for all patients the waiting and uncertainty can be terrifying. Whatever your doctor's practice, you'll know in a week or so what the biopsy has shown.

As with any surgical procedure, in a breast biopsy there are sometimes complications. The two most common are hematoma and infection. If a hematoma occurs it will usually be within a day or two of the procedure. It's caused by bleeding inside the area where the surgery was done, causing a blood blister to form (Fig. 11-8). It turns blue and forms a lump right under the skin. The body usually simply absorbs and recycles it, as it does with any bruise. But sometimes, before the body can do that, you'll bump into something or someone will bump into you, and it will burst open, causing dark blood to come out. It looks gross and disgusting and you'll think you're dying, but don't

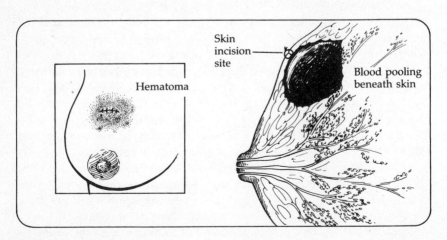

Skin incision site

Hematoma

Blood pooling beneath skin

FIGURE 11-8

worry—you're not. It's old blood; you're not bleeding now. What you need to do is go home, clean up the mess, and take a shower. If you're worried about it, call your doctor.

If an infection occurs, it will show up a week or two after surgery—there'll be redness and swelling and fever, and the doctor will treat it as infections are usually treated, with antibiotics. Again, it's more of a nuisance than anything else.

Sometimes, you'll get a combination of infection and hematoma—the blood mixes with pus, like an abscess or a boil, and needs to be drained by the doctor. Sometimes when stitches are removed after breast surgery—either biopsies or cosmetic procedures—a small non-dissolvable stitch is overlooked and remains in the breast, which will then get infected, as was the case with one of my patients (no, I wasn't the surgeon who removed the stitches!). It's easy to treat with antibiotics and removal of the stitch.

And, yes, the worst patient nightmares do occasionally occur—I had one patient who had a persistent infection following a biopsy, and when they finally operated on her they discovered that her surgeon had left a sponge inside her. I'm not quite sure how a surgeon could manage to do that, but this one did. Fortunately, it's very, very rare—and my patient is fine now.

These complications are pretty infrequent—they only occur in about 10 percent of breast biopsies, and, while they're unpleasant and inconvenient, they're not life threatening and they don't have any long-term effects.

HOW TO READ YOUR BIOPSY REPORT

There are three possible findings when the biopsy is done and the tissue studied—benign, cancer, or not certain. The latter happens because, by nature of the procedure, the doctor has gotten only a piece of the lesion. It's possible that the pathologist will find atypical hyperplasia, which often exists with cancer (see Chapter 19). If that's the case, the doctor is obligated to go back in and take more tissue out, to be certain that there are no cancer cells as well. According to a research article by H. A. Pass, about 50 percent of atypical hyperplasia diagnosed from a core biopsy on a mammographic lesion turn out to be accompanied by cancer.[3] Three elements should be consistent to determine that it's benign.[4] The physical exam, mammogram, and biopsy have to match. But if one of those elements is different—if it seems to the doctor that it's not a fibroadenoma, even though the mammogram and needle aspiration suggest it is; or if the doctor thinks it is but either the

mammogram or needle aspiration biopsy suggests something different—then it's important to go on to a larger biopsy.

Even when the doctor tells you that the lump was benign, it's very
important to find out exactly what it was. "Benign" isn't enough. So
you should ask to see a copy of your pathology report.

The report will have two parts. The first is the "gross description." It
describes what the surgeon gave the pathologist and the pathologist
could see just by looking at it—a slide with some cells on it, or a core,
or a piece of tissue measuring 3 by 5 centimeters. Then it will often describe cutting the tissue and what it looked like. It will say whether the
surgeon saw a distinct mass, or whether the lump just looked like
breast tissue. If what was removed was a fibroadenoma, it will often be
described as a distinct mass that's round and smooth and measures
such and such number of centimeters. If it's a psuedolump and it's just
breast tissue, it may be described as a piece of fibro-fatty tissue that
contains no obvious lesions. If it's microcalcifications, the pathologist
won't see these with the naked eye, so it won't be described.

The second part describes what the lump looks like under the microscope. Some reports will give you a detailed description—what the
cells look like, what the surrounding tissue is like, and so on. Others
cut to the chase and give just the final diagnosis. So it might read,
"1. fibroadenoma." It almost always adds, "2. fibrocystic disease"
or "fibrocystic change." That's because, as we said in Chapter 6, the
"fibrocystic change" is the background that we see normally in breast
tissue, so it's always there. The report may say "fibrocystic change"
alone if it's just breast tissue. That's not an adequate diagnosis. If your
report says that, you should ask for a more specific diagnosis, even if it
means making the pathologist go back, look at the slides again, and describe exactly what's there. Under the rubric of "fibrocystic disease"
there is one entity that does increase your risk of subsequent breast
cancer: atypical hyperplasia, which we describe in Chapter 16. You
want to know if that's what you have. Usually if it says fibrocystic disease (or change) alone, you don't have atypical hyperplasia, because
today most pathologists are aware of its importance, and are likely to
mention it if it's there. But they might not: I wouldn't risk assuming
they would have mentioned it and doing nothing. Often you'll have
hyperplasia that isn't atypical—extra cells in the lining of the duct that
are normal. So if it says "hyperplasia of the usual kind," that's fine.

In addition, if you had a biopsy that was done for calcifications, you
want to be sure that the pathologist saw calcifications under the microscope, so you can be sure that they're looking at the right tissue. Sometimes, if you have a very small area of calcifications and a big piece of
tissue taken out, when they make the slides they don't get the area

where the calcifications are. Then they can look at the tissue and say "totally benign." That's happened to me: I took out calcifications and the report came back benign. I asked if they'd seen the calcifications and they said no, but they'd put all the tissue through. I said, "You need to see the calcifications." So they took the blocks of paraffin, x-rayed them, found which ones had the calcifications, and made additional slides. Then they found the calcifications, and indeed there was precancer, which they would have missed. So it's important to make sure the pathologists have seen what they were supposed to see. You may think it's your doctor's job to take care of all that, and you're right. But you can't assume that's happening, and you need to double-check.

Then you should get a copy of the report and save it. It may become relevant at some later time and it's important for you to have it in your records. One of the things we're starting to realize is that some of the changes in the basic molecular biology of the breast tissue (see Chapter 15) can be identified in earlier biopsy tissue. For example, suppose you have a family history of breast cancer and you have a biopsy for what turns out to be a fibroadenoma. In the past we thought that was all you needed to know. But, as we discussed in Chapter 8, we've recently discovered that one kind of fibroadenoma can, when you have a family history of breast cancer, markedly increase your risk. It is important for you to be able to have the pathologist go back and look at the slides and determine what kind of fibroadenoma you actually had. Probably they won't keep the tissue, but if you at least keep a record of your biopsy, with the date and the hospital, you can go back and find the slides. That can be very important.

In fact, however, you may be able to have them keep some of the tissue itself. You can ask your doctor if there's any possibility of saving extra tissue from the biopsy in a tissue bank. As we do more and more research on benign and malignant breast problems, there's an enormous need to have tissue to test. Some of that needs to be saved fresh, and some can be saved in paraffin blocks. It's to your advantage to have the tissue saved because as new discoveries come along we can go back and test them out on this tissue. One of the things we're trying to do on a political level is create a regional network of tissue banks, so that everybody will be able to have some tissue saved when they have surgery.

It's really important, if you've had your biopsy because of a lesion seen on mammogram, to have a new baseline mammogram a month or two after the procedure. If the doctor doesn't suggest it, you should. Sometimes even when we take out calcifications we may not get all of them. If it's benign, that doesn't matter. But it's good to have it documented so that a year from now if you have a mammogram, it won't seem like there are new calcifications.

Similarly, if you have something taken out, your breast is going to look different: there will be scarring. A year later that might look like something new and alarming, unless there's a baseline fairly soon after the surgery for comparison.

PART FOUR

PREDICTION AND PREVENTION OF CANCER

12

*Understanding Studies
and Clinical Trials*

Nearly every day you turn on the television or read the newspaper and see that "a new study" has shown that this procedure cures this disease, or that medication prevents that condition. The next week you discover that another new study shows that the procedure doesn't work after all or the medication causes a new and unforeseen problem. And you're confused—as well you may be.

The problem is that the media don't distinguish between kinds of studies. Different studies have different values, and to understand what a particular study means, you need information about the process of the study itself.

There are many ways to conduct studies of various conditions and of possible ways to control, treat, or prevent them. Unfortunately, doing a completely accurate, comprehensive study is virtually impossible. There are too many elements in even the simplest area of study. But some studies are better than others. To understand how accurate a study is, you need to be able to look at all of its elements. It may be weak in one area, stronger in another, and excellent in a third. Different aspects of a study will make it more or less believable.

Few people actually understand study design. Doctors are as predisposed to self-deception as anyone else: we all tend to believe the studies that feed our biases rather than the ones that don't. This same tendency is reflected by the media. Reporters often don't understand the nuances of a study, and their quick-story reports usually fail to address limitations in the study's design. In addition, they often exaggerate the study's implications. Data that are only one brick in a complexly designed wall are presented as if they were the cornerstone. It's no wonder the layperson is confused about what a study's results might mean in real life.

KINDS OF STUDIES

There are two basic categories of study, each with several subcategories. Each has its own values and limitations. One category is the *observational study*, which observes, without intervention, people doing what they would normally do. The other category is the *clinical trial*, or *intervention study*, in which a certain treatment is tested on a group of people who are assigned to use the treatment in certain ways over a certain period of time.

Observational Studies

Observational studies are great for generating a hypothesis. They observe a phenomenon and then try to think of an explanation. They do not, however, prove cause and effect. For example, a study done in Boston and reported as I was writing this section observed that women with breast cancer were more likely to use dry cleaners, have exterminators come to their homes, and use lawn treatments. The hypothesis was that these poisons might lead to breast cancer. This is an interesting possibility, but it's far from proven. The next step might be to do an animal study and see if dry cleaning fluid increased cancers. We could also study women who work at dry cleaners to see if they have more cancer. If these studies still seemed to show a relationship, we could then go on to a controlled study in which women are randomized to use dry cleaners or not and then see how many developed breast cancer. This last study, of course, would be difficult to do, but it would be the one to give us the final proof. Many of the studies we read about in the news are observational, but they are presented as if they demonstrate cause and effect. This does not mean they are useless. They are great at telling us what to study. They may even function as a warning sign for possible temporary actions: you might decide to use one of the new "wet cleaners" who don't use chemicals, in case the original study turns out to be true. On the other hand, you might decide that your local dry cleaner does a great job, and you'll wait to decide about making a change until the definitive study is done.

Observational studies take the form of cross-sectional studies, case control studies, and cohort studies. In a *cross-sectional study* a large number of people are asked about symptoms at a specific time. It might study all 50-year-old women who have breast cancer and ask whether they were taking "hormone replacement therapy" (HRT) at the time their cancer was diagnosed. This might find what percent of women diagnosed with breast cancer at age 50 were taking postmenopausal hormone therapy at the time of diagnosis. But it wouldn't prove that HRT caused breast cancer. It would just tell us how often the two factors are found together. There could be other reasons for the relationship: maybe women on HRT are also more likely to go to the doctor and to get mammograms, so their breast cancer would be found while they were on the hormones.

Another example, this one not hypothetical, is the association of fibrocystic change with breast cancer. In examinations of breasts with cancer, we almost always find fibrocystic change as well. For years this was interpreted as showing that fibrocystic change caused breast cancer. But it turned out that when the breasts of women *without* breast cancer were studied, the same amount of fibrocystic change was found. All it proved is that most women have some degree of fibrocystic changes. The key is that the study is done at one point in time, and needs further studies to explain what the finding means.

The next step is often a *case control study* because it is easy and cheap to do. A case control study looks at a group of people with a certain condition, comparing them to another group without that condition but with other similarities to the first group. For example, we could take 100 women who had taken HRT for 10 years and match them as carefully as possible with 100 women who had not. Then we could see how many breast cancers occurred in each group. This is a cheap and relatively easy way to test the hypothesis generated by an observational study. If the difference between the two groups is statistically significant (couldn't happen by chance alone) we conclude that there is an association between HRT and breast cancer. This does not prove, however, that one caused the other, a fact often missed by the media.

If many case control studies support the hypothesis and findings then it may be worth doing a *cohort* (or *follow-up*) *study*. In a cohort study a particular group of people are followed over time. Cohort studies have subcategories of their own. *Retrospective* cohort studies, using information gathered years before, examine subjects at a defined time, usually years later, to see the relationship between the factor being studied and the outcome of interest. For example, they might look at women with breast cancer and find out how many of them had a high-fat diet as children. This is not as expensive and time-consuming as a *prospective* cohort study, which starts at the opposite end. These are done only if many case control studies are positive and the question is of considerable clinical or social importance. A group of subjects is followed forward over a period of years. Let's say we look at 100 45-year-old women with lobular carcinoma *in situ* who were examined every year for 10 years. This might give us a better idea of how many cases of lobular carcinoma lead to breast cancer. The Nurse's Health Study conducted by investigators in Boston is a prospective cohort study that has carefully followed a group of 121,700 nurses since 1976. Information on various potential risk factors for breast and other cancers and other conditions is collected in a mailed questionnaire every two years. Since there is a large number of subjects, the data are compelling. But there is no control over the behavior of the women in the study. The researchers can't, for example, assign one group to get yearly mammograms and another to use only doctors' examinations. So it is conceivable that women at risk for breast cancer are getting mammograms more frequently than women who are not at risk, and this will skew the results of the study. This cohort is also examined retrospectively as new questions arise. Because they don't count on the vagaries of the participants' memories, prospective studies are generally thought to be more accurate than retrospective studies. But prospective studies are more difficult and time-consuming to conduct.

Both case control and cohort studies have their limitations. We could take a group of recent lung cancer patients and compare them with nonsmokers chosen randomly out of the phone book to see how many from each group carried cigarette lighters. We might learn that more people who carried cigarette lighters got lung cancer. But there's always the possibility of other factors entering into the equation. So we might conclude that the lighter fluid in cigarette lighters causes lung cancer, completely missing the fact that the people were using them to light cigarettes, and it's the cigarettes, not the lighters, that cause the cancer.

It sounds silly, but only because we already know the cigarette and lung cancer connection. There are many actual cases of similar things happening. It may well be what has happened in the studies connecting estrogen therapy and heart disease prevention, which now are turning out to be questionable. To finally prove cause and effect, a randomized clinical trial is necessary.

Clinical Trials

Clinical trials (also known as *interventional studies*) are prospective trials that study a new treatment by having one group of subjects get the treatment while another group, known as the *control group,* doesn't get the treatment. This is where we actually test the hypothesis. The people are followed closely for a given amount of time, after which researchers compare the two groups. If, for example, a new drug, like tamoxifen, is believed to prevent cancer in women at risk, the study group will be given the treatment and the control group will be given a *placebo* (an inert pill) with no one knowing which group got which. If 20 percent of the women who got the drug got breast cancer, and 40 percent of those who got the placebo did, we'd know that the treatment did some good. Not all clinical studies use placebos. If there is a standard therapy, the new treatment will be compared to it. In the bone marrow transplant studies, high-dose chemotherapy with stem cell rescue (bone marrow transplant) was given to one group and standard chemotherapy was given to the other. (The studies showed no difference in survival between the two groups.)

These studies are usually *randomized.* This means that each subject's treatment is picked at random, usually by a computer, so there is no possibility that subjects will be chosen based on situations they're already in. If, for example, all of the women with atypical hyperplasia are put on one treatment regimen to prevent breast cancer and all the women without it are put on another, the second treatment will end up looking an awful lot better than it really was.

It's important that neither the researchers nor the subjects know who's getting the treatment and who's getting the placebo. That way the subjects won't be tempted to alter their behaviors based on the treatment they're getting or to unconsciously misreport symptoms, and the researchers won't be tempted to treat one group differently, or interpret the results differently. Because neither researcher nor subject knows who's getting the treatment, these studies are called *double-blind.*

The controlled study that is prospective, randomized, and double-blind has the fewest potential flaws, and so it's the most reliable. It's still not perfect, because people who decide to participate in a study like that may not be like most of us—usually people prefer to know what treatment they're getting and don't want to risk being given nothing or a placebo. But it's the closest we can get to good data.

A good example of a randomized controlled study is The Women's Health Initiative, which was started several years ago to investigate the use of Premarin and Provera, calcium, vitamin D, and low-fat diet on breast cancer, as well as on heart disease and osteoporosis. The HRT part is double-blind and obviously the diet part is not. Its completion in 2008 should give us important data about the risks and benefits of these treatments.

EVALUATING STUDIES

What Is the Study Studying?

Sometimes statistics from studies can be confusing because researchers are looking for one thing while people who hear about the studies are looking for another. An example is the study of raloxifene (Evista) in women with osteoporosis.[1] Postmenopausal women with a diagnosis of osteoporosis were randomized to get either raloxifene or placebo. At the end of two years there was a 2–3 percent improvement in bone density. In addition, there was a decrease in breast cancer in the women on raloxifene. On the surface this sounds terrific. But its impressiveness diminishes when you look at who was in the study. Women with osteoporosis are known to be at lower risk for breast cancer in the first place, and postmenopausal women are more likely to get estrogen-sensitive tumors. So raloxifene is good for preventing cancer in that group. This does not necessarily mean that it will work in women at risk of breast cancer, in premenopausal women, or in women with breast cancer. But this data is enough to initiate a randomized controlled study of raloxifene and tamoxifen (STAR trial) in high-risk women. Another example is the fact that since women who are on hormones are more likely to go to the doctor, they are also more likely to get mammograms and other screening for cancer. It's possible, therefore, that when these women get breast cancer they're more likely to be diagnosed early and do better. So they might have an increased incidence of breast cancer, but not an increased death rate. These are two different things. One study may be looking at how many breast cancers occur, while another looks at how many deaths from breast cancer there are. So it's very important to know what a study has been set up to determine. This is known as its *endpoint*.

We also need to look at the size of the study. If there is a big difference in the effect of a treatment, it will show up in a relatively small study. If, for example, a treatment decreases the death rate from breast cancer by 300 percent, it might become obvious after studying 100 women, half of whom get the treatment and half a placebo, that three times as many women in the first group are alive after 10 years. But if the effect is smaller it will emerge only if there are more subjects in the study. For example, the Nurses' Health Study, looking at 121,700 women, reported in the summer of 1995 that estrogen and progesterone therapy increased the incidence of breast cancer by 70 percent—that is, 70 percent more women on hormone therapy got breast cancer than women not on hormones.[2] Within a week another study came out in which no increased risk of breast cancer in women taking estrogen and progesterone was found. The second study had only 1,029 subjects, so it was too small to show a 70 percent effect.[3]

What Numbers Mean

In order to evaluate the information we have from available studies and to understand the figures your doctor may quote you, we need to spend a moment looking at what the numbers mean. Research studies about cancer therapy can be very confusing. Some studies will talk about the "percentage reduction in mortality." This refers to the percentage of patients who died compared to the number of deaths that were expected. For example, if a study showed that eight patients died in the control group and only six in the study group, there were two fewer deaths than expected. This is then reported out as a 25 percent reduction in mortality, or two divided by eight. A similar study with more patients might show that 40 patients died in the control group compared to 30 in the study group. The reduction of 10 deaths over a possible 40 is still 25 percent. In the second study, 10 patients' lives were saved, while in the first it was only two. So these percentages are only helpful if you know the expected mortality.

There are still other complications. One is the time frame. Since breast cancer is a slow disease, even the women who are going to die of it often don't do so for many years. Therefore any study has to follow patients for ten or even twenty years to be able to determine with confidence the effect of a treatment on the death rate (or, conversely, the cure rate). Many investigators, and indeed many patients, don't want to wait that long to look at the results of studies so they look instead at the "time to recurrence"—the time between the diagnosis of the disease and the first recurrence (if there is one).

This still has much value. Although lengthening the time to recurrence isn't the same as a cure, it is very important. For example, let's say you were diagnosed with breast cancer that, with the old treatment, would have killed you in one year. A new treatment increases your time to recurrence, or disease-free survival time, by three years and so you die four years after your diagnosis. Your cure rate at five years would be zero either way, but you have had three extra years of quality time.

Some studies will report on the *median* time to recurrence. The reason that the median, or middle, is used is actually a good one. An *average* adds up all the times to recurrence and divides by two. Since many cancers will never recur, it is impossible to do that. The median is the middle of the times to recurrence at the time that the study was completed. Some women will have a longer time to recurrence and some shorter. And, of course, some will never recur at all. It is a helpful way to look at early data in a study.

STUDY BIASES

Sometimes I'll hear someone say, "How can you say that you don't believe that hormone therapy does a lot to protect the heart, but you *do* believe it increases breast cancer risk? You're using the same studies!" But there's a reason. It's not only the information in the studies, but factors in how to interpret them.

For the relationships between cardiac disease and hormone therapy, we have only three randomized control studies, but many observational studies. Something that has come up in these observational studies is that most of the biases in these studies would lead to overestimating the effects on heart disease. The women who use hormone therapy are more likely to eat well, be thin, exercise—in other words, have lifestyles that would lead to better heart health. So it seems likely that the benefits of hormone therapy to the heart are being overestimated.

But with breast cancer, it's the reverse. Almost all the biases are such that they should *under*estimate the risk. There are two reasons. The first is that among women on hormone therapy, a higher percentage have had hysterectomies, including ovary removal, and this has usually happened premenopausally, because the chief reasons for non-cancer-related hysterectomies are to get rid of fibroids or end heavy bleeding. And having her ovaries removed before natural menopause, like having an early menopause, decreases a woman's risk of getting breast cancer.

The second reason is that women who are thin or who have low estrogen levels—and these tend to go together—tend to have more perimenopausal symptoms. Remember that these are also women who should be at low breast cancer risk. Add to this that most doctors are leery of putting women with known breast cancer risk on hormone therapy, and you see that the women taking hormones are a population that should have a lower risk than the average population. If there were no danger from hormones, we'd see the incidence of breast cancer going down among these women. So the 30 to 40 percent increase probably represents a lower estimation of the actual risk. Doctors must prove that a drug isn't harmful and not use it because it hasn't been proved absolutely to be harmful. "Innocent until proven guilty" is a good policy when someone is suspected of a crime, but it's a bad policy in medicine.

Luckily there are randomized studies that will help answer this. A European study called WISDOM—Women's International Study of long-Duration Oestrogen after Menopause—is ongoing.

The biggest U.S. study, the Women's Health Initiative, is looking at primary prevention. Healthy women are randomized to take estrogen alone, estrogen plus Provera, or a placebo. They're being monitored for heart disease, breast cancer, osteoporosis, colon cancer, and Alzheimer's disease. The data will be out in 2008. Though this wait is frustrating for women wanting to know what to do now, it's important that the study be allowed to go on long enough to give us really good results.

Preliminary results from the WHI reported out in early 2000 surprised everyone when they showed a small increase in heart disease and stroke in women on either estrogen and Provera or estrogen alone.[4] This confirmed the HERS trial of Premarin and Provera in women with heart disease, which showed an initial increase in deaths from heart disease in women on HRT. A third randomized controlled study, the Estrogen Replacement and Atherosclerosis Regression Trial (ERA) which used an estrogen patch and placebo in women with heart disease, reported no benefit to taking hormones in women with heart disease.[5] More studies are to come including the Women's Angiographic Vitamin and Estrogen Trial.

WAVE is studying between 400 and 450 women, all taking vitamins C and E, with hormone therapy in one group and without it in the other. Using angiography (x rays of the coronary blood vessels), they are looking at the progression of atherosclerosis, a blockage of the arteries that can lead to severe pain (angina) and ultimately heart attack. The Women's Estrogen, Progesterone, and Lipid Lowering Atherosclerosis Regression Trial (WELL-HART) is looking at estrogen with progestin and placebo in 226 women with high cholesterol.

There's also the RUTH Trial—Raloxifene Use for the Heart Trial. This is a big study—10,000 women over 55 from 26 countries who are at risk for coronary artery disease. They have been taking either raloxifene or a placebo, and the trial is set to last for seven years.

So results of studies are never simple. Any reporter who sums one up in a brief article or a "sound bite" is doing a great disservice. If you really want to know what a given study means, you'll have to do a little research of your own, and find out what kind of a study it is.

BECOMING PART OF A STUDY

So learning what studies mean is vital for every woman who is considering using a study as part of a basis for any decision she makes. But you can also take a further step. You can become part of a study—helping others, and very possibly helping yourself. The work that I discuss in Chapter 17 could never have been done if volunteers, both with and without breast disease, hadn't been subjects in my studies.

As a woman and a physician, I've always been frustrated by the lack of information about women's health. Virtually all of the research in the past was done on men. Even the rat research was done on male rats. In the course of reading this book you've probably noticed how often I have said, "We don't know whether . . ." or "More research is needed before we know. . . ." You're probably tired of reading it. I know I'm tired of writing it. But the answers aren't there.

As women, we can't complain that there are no data on diseases relevant to us and then remain aloof from studies when they exist. Our demands for research are slowly getting met, and there is some very important research going on now that offers women the opportunity to participate. There are several studies on adjuvant treatment for breast cancer. As we have mentioned, the STAR trial will help us to learn whether raloxifene is as good as tamoxifen in helping women at high risk for breast cancer (see Chapter 18). And the Women's Health Initiative will inform us about the health issues faced by postmenopausal women, including the safety of taking estrogen and Provera, and the efficacy of calcium and vitamin D supplements. I think women should seek out these studies—especially women who have been underrepresented in research in the past: lesbians, older women, women of color. I realize this may be hard for some people, since I'm asking women who have already suffered from the insensitivity of the health establishment to involve themselves deeply with that establishment. But the only way to learn about women's health is to have women in studies, and the way to be in studies is to sign up for them.

The high-dose chemotherapy with stem cell rescue (bone marrow transplant) controversy has dramatically demonstrated the problem with adopting a new treatment before there is proof that it works. Over 30,000 women had undergone stem cell rescue when the first randomized studies came out showing no benefit over standard chemotherapy (see Chapter 33).

All these studies are what we call *research protocols* (sometimes also known as clinical trials). Although "protocol" sounds like we're talking about who goes into the operating room first, a medical protocol is actually a program designed to answer some specific questions about the effectiveness of a particular approach. The questions can be about methods of diagnosis, types of treatment, dosage of drugs, timing of administration of drugs, or type of drugs used. So a protocol for breast cancer treatment, for example, will study node-negative breast cancers in premenopausal women to see whether they would benefit from chemotherapy. A large-enough group of patients who fit the criteria is recruited, and they're randomized (picked at random either to receive the treatment or not). Those selected to receive the drugs will be given them on a very strict regimen: for instance, they will be given x amount, on day 1 and 3, and a particular blood test will be given on day 5. This precision is important for the question to be answered—no variation is permitted, or our understanding of how well the treatment works will be impaired. The other women, or control group, will not receive the new drugs but will be followed just as rigorously, and will be given the standard treatment. What makes it a protocol is the fact that it is asking a question: will the women receiving the chemotherapy do better than the women who are not? Other protocols might compare two different treatments to see which is the best. By participating in such studies these women will get reasonable treatments and at the same time help us to figure out the answer.

New treatments used in protocols are tried out in three phases. Phase-one treatments are aimed at determining the safety of a technique or the toxicity and most effective dose. For example, each woman may get a dose higher than the one before until the toxic dose is identified. One of my Boston patients flew to Los Angeles to participate in the phase-one Herceptin study. She had an excellent response.

In the case of chemotherapy drugs, phase-one studies usually involve people who have advanced disease and are informed and willing to try unproven therapies, on the long shot that this may be the miracle that saves them. In addition, the researchers are giving patients the drugs in various doses to see which drugs do work. These are usually new drugs, and there is always the chance that one of them will be effective. If phase one shows the drug to be tolerated by patients, the study moves on to phase two, with the best and safest dose found in phase one. Here we are testing to see if the drug has any effect on the disease. A phase-two drug study looking at breast cancer is often done on women whose cancer has spread but who are not in an immediately life-threatening situation—women who have metastatic disease but are still asymptomatic, and are willing to gamble on the long shot that some experimental new treatment will be the breakthrough that they've been hoping for. Taxol, a new chemotherapy drug, is a good example of that—it turned out to be a very effective drug for metastatic disease.

Once we've determined the effectiveness and safety of the technique or drugs (and, with drugs, the best dosages), we're at phase three. With drugs, phase-three studies might take a new drug that seems to show some effectiveness without undue toxicity, and compare it to the standard treatment.

People often have an inaccurate perception of phase-three trials. They think it's all or nothing: the experimental group gets the new treatment and the control group gets nothing. But that's never the case. The trials compare new treatment against the standard treatment. So, for example, if you're part of a study comparing very high-dose chemotherapy with the standard dose, and you end up in the control group, you'll still get the doses of chemotherapy that you would have gotten if you weren't in the study. The new treatment group would get the higher doses to see if more is better. We don't know if the new treatment will be better or less effective. It's a good gamble: phase three can be thought of as a comparison of between what we hope will be the next step and the best we currently have.

This is an ethical way to experiment with drugs and new techniques, but it does create some limitations. Since in phase one we use only patients who have not responded well to standard therapy, we can't be sure that, if our new treatment fails also, it would not have worked with a patient whose disease was less widespread. In fact, there are now efforts to try some new drugs earlier, at the first sign of recurrence, which may indeed be a more revealing way to test them. Even with the current limitation, however, we've made amazing advances in treatments and techniques in the past decade.

If you're considering being part of a study, you have a right to know everything about it. Ask the researchers what exactly they're giving you; find out the possible side effects; find out what they know and don't know. You have to sign an informed consent form, which is often many pages long. (The form for the study of high-dosage chemotherapy was 27 pages long.) Read it, thoroughly; it's worth the effort. Write your questions down. Sit down with the doctor, go over questions about anything that's unclear. Also ask to speak to another woman with breast cancer who has gone through the same program ahead of you.

There are safeguards in most trials. In addition, there is a Human Subjects Protection Committee in every hospital that reviews each protocol to make sure it is safe and well designed. They oversee all clinical trials and are responsible for making sure that the informed consent is readable and the potential benefits of the study outweigh its risks for the subjects being studied. Of course, you'll always be given the choice. It's both unethical and illegal for a doctor to put you on a protocol treatment or clinical trial without your full and informed consent, and you have every right to refuse. If you're in an experiment and become convinced that it's harming you, you can leave it. You and your doctor both have the right to take you off the study at any time.

There are very good reasons for participating in a protocol. Aside from its usefulness to women in the future, studies assure the patient herself that she will get the most up-to-date care. For these reasons many women are eager to be part of studies. Susan McKenney, a nurse practitioner and oncology nurse who works extensively with breast cancer patients, has talked with many patients at the Dana Farber Institute and finds that, once they understand they're not just guinea pigs and the treatments can be helpful both to them and to other women, they are often anxious to participate. "Breast cancer treatment has changed over the last 20 years because women have participated in protocols," she says.

Patients I've spoken with back this up. One woman who was diagnosed in 1990 with a stage 3 cancer became involved in a study using far higher doses of chemotherapy than the standard—the dose was adjusted upward as far as the patient's tolerance allowed. Aside from the treatments in the hospital, which occurred every three weeks, she gave herself nightly injections of a material that stimulated the growth of the bone marrow that had been destroyed by the chemotherapy.

She had a difficult time with the treatment, throwing up so often that she slept on the bathroom floor for weeks. "They called me the nausea queen," she recalls ruefully. But her experiment paid off. Although in this study the patients went straight into chemotherapy without having had surgery or radiation beforehand, they had been warned that they would probably require both when the chemotherapy course was over. But her tumor shrunk so dramatically and so completely that she did not need either. "I feel that the only reason I'm alive is because I did that trial," she says. One of the other women in the trial, with whom she became close friends, survived in spite of the fact that she had a very aggressive inflammatory cancer.

Some studies are actually begun by patients themselves. You can get a group in the community together and initiate a study on your own terms. For example, if you want to research lesbians and breast cancer, you can go to the local medical school or a researcher and say, "This is a study we want to see done. We'll supply the participants—do you have anyone who can work with us?" A number of recent studies have begun that way. For example, a group of women in Long Island were very disturbed at the high level of breast cancer in their community. They lobbied the National Cancer Institute and got a study that investigated the possible relationship between environmental pollutants in Long Island and breast cancer. Other women on Cape Cod set up a similar study for Massachusetts.

Women need to be encouraged to participate in studies. So far, we haven't done so to a large enough extent. Only about 3 percent of breast cancer patients in the U.S. participate in protocols. This is much lower than in Europe, and not something for us to be proud of. But we can't wholly blame the patients for this. Many hospitals or doctors here simply don't offer protocols. If you're being treated at a research hospital or major cancer center you'll usually be offered protocols if you qualify, and large numbers of patients there do participate. Women who choose such hospitals for treatment tend to be those who seek out the most advanced, sophisticated treatments; that's why they go to a big research hospital. They feel safer in an environment where the major purpose is to study and fight cancer. But the ability to offer protocols isn't limited to these hospitals. There is now a mechanism allowing community hospitals to offer participation in protocols through a program called CCOP (Cancer Center Outreach Program) that links community hospitals with large medical centers and allows you to participate in the same studies in your local area. That participation assures that your doctor is keeping up to date, and that you're getting the best medicine has to offer.

If you're a patient, I think it's important that you seriously think about being in a study. If you ask about trials and your doctor doesn't know of any and doesn't want to bother finding out, you can call 1–800 4 CANCER at the National Cancer Institute or check their website at www.cancernet.nci.nih.gov. They'll hook you into their Physician Data Query (PDQ) computer program and give you a list of every clinical trial you're eligible for. They'll also tell you what area the trials are in so you'll know whether or not a given study is being conducted near you. Then you can go with that information to your doctor and work with it from there.

We should also mention the financial aspects of studies, since they vary greatly depending on the nature of the study. For a study that offers no benefit and some inconvenience to the subject, payment may be offered as an incentive—those are the studies college kids often get into to earn a couple of hundred dollars. In fact, I participated in a study of DES as a contraceptive to pay my tuition when I was in medical school. Some studies that might benefit the subject, or that cause the subject no inconvenience, involve no financial exchange at all. Occasionally a study of a treatment that can benefit the patient will offer a reduced fee for the treatment, like an asthma and visualization study my coauthor participated in. Finally, as is the case with the chemotherapy studies comparing drugs already approved by the FDA, the patient (or the insurance company) pays the full price for the procedure. When new drugs are being tested, the drug company generally pays for the treatment. Many hospitals will not allow studies involving an experimental drug or device in which the patient must pay. Political action has led some states to mandate insurance coverage for care as part of a clinical trial.

Unfortunately, even when they're offered protocols, only a small percentage of women accept the offer. Here too there are a number of reasons. Some women are afraid of being randomized. They want to get the best treatment and they find it hard to believe that the medical profession doesn't know what that is. Or they have strong feelings about getting a particular treatment and they don't want to experiment with anything else.

Often women don't want to be in studies because they can't decide which group they'll be in. "I'll be in a study comparing chemotherapy and tamoxifen," a woman will tell me, "if I can choose which one I'll get." That can't be done in a study since the treatments need to be chosen randomly for the study to be valid.

Another reason some women don't participate in clinical trials is that they think we already have the answers. For example, they assume that the standard treatments will save their lives, and they don't want to rock the boat with something new. But it's precisely because the standard treatments *don't* always work that we do experiments. The courageous women who participated in the phase-one and -two trials of Adriamycin and Taxol have benefited not only themselves but the many women who have followed.

Some women fail to understand the whole idea of a study. They want to choose their own treatment, rather than participate in a protocol. After the treatment is finished, they want that treatment and its effects on them to be studied. But of course, that isn't the way it works. For a study of a treatment to give us clear information, it must be done under controlled circumstances, defined by the researchers and strictly followed. After-the-fact statistics have their use, but that's not the same as following a particular subject on a particular treatment, and we can never get the same level of information with this kind of observational study that we can with randomized control studies. You can't have your cake and eat it too. If you want the information that comes with being part of a controlled study, you have to be part of that study from the beginning.

Ironically, some women swing to the other extreme, and I find that equally frustrating. Once in a while a highly publicized experimental procedure comes along that people think is the miracle we've been searching for. Then the attitude toward being in a study turns around. You don't fear being part of an experiment; you demand what you think will be your share of the miracle.

Of course, after learning what protocols are available you may decide that none of them offers the treatment you want. But you owe it to yourself, and to other women, to find out what protocols you are eligible for and what they involve, before you decide. My patient who took part in the high-dose chemotherapy experiment says that if she had a friend newly diagnosed with breast cancer she would strongly urge her to look into protocols. "I'd tell her not to jump into anything," she says, "but to explore everything. Find out what's there; weigh it in your mind. 'Latest' isn't always best, and it may be that what you find isn't right for you. But there's a very good chance that you'll find that what's best for you is in a clinical trial."

Whether or not you decide to become part of a clinical trial in terms of your treatment, there's another way you can contribute to the research on breast cancer—and do yourself a favor as well. If you have any surgical procedure—whether a biopsy, a wide excision, a mastectomy, or even breast reduction—make sure tissue removed from your breast is kept in a tissue bank (see Chapter 11). This is becoming more and more possible because one of the things we're pushing for politically is regional and national tissue banks. You can have this done in any hospital you're in. Both benign and cancerous tissue are useful in medical studies.

We have no guaranteed cures—if we did there'd be no need for trials. But with trials, the guarantee we do have is that whatever can be done to help women in the future is being done. Already we see some of the results of trials. Not too long ago a woman with breast cancer had no choice but to lose her breast. But a number of women participated in the first breast conservation studies and were randomized to get either mastectomy, lumpectomy, or radiation. They were very courageous women, going against the standard thinking to see if there was an alternative. Thanks to them, thousands of women today have been able to save their breasts. As you make the complex, difficult decisions about your own treatment, keep those women in mind—the brave experimenters, and all of us who have benefited from their courage.

13

The Molecular Biology
of Breast Cancer

Some of you are going to be like my coauthor: you got Ds in college biology and you still hate it. So the title of this chapter may put you off. And it *is* pretty complicated stuff. I'm including it because, in order to understand both the causes of cancer and the workings of all the new drugs and treatments that are becoming available, it helps to know how your body works at the most basic, molecular level. It's truly fascinating. But if the thought of reading about biology makes you unhappy, feel free to skip on to the next chapter. Those of you who like to know how things work—read on!

DNA, RNA, AND PROTEINS

The way life works is through a magnificently elegant system. Every bacteria, every tree, every dog, every human being has its vital information coded in its DNA (deoxyribonucleic acid) in the nucleus of cells. This is responsible for transferring genetic characteristics. With a single system of four bases (like four letters), everything that's alive is programmed. It's like realizing that with a single alphabet of 26 letters we have Shakespeare and Agatha Christie and the *National Inquirer*.

DNA codes all the information in your body. It determines the color of your eyes and your hair; it tells your lungs how to exchange oxygen. It's been called a blueprint, but I prefer the metaphor used by Mahlon Hoagland and Bert Dodson in *The Way Life Works*.[1] They call it a recipe. This recipe uses a definite code—four different *base pairs*, to which we have assigned letters (Fig. 13-1). Each letter represents a *nucleotide*—the smallest unit of information, which in itself doesn't convey a message but contributes to the creation of the message. The four nucleotides are adenosine (represented by the letter A), thymine (T), cytosine (C), and guanine (G). Each nucleotide is a specific arrangement of carbon, nitrogen, oxygen, and hydrogen atoms called a *base*. Each nucleotide is also bonded to a sugar called *deoxyribose*, as well as to a *phosphate*. The nucleotides combine in pairs, and these pairs become the basis of what-

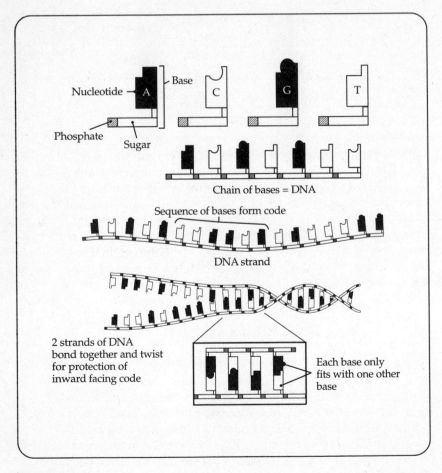

FIGURE 13-1

ever comes next; hence they are known as *base pairs*. This pairing is very precise, like a tiny jigsaw puzzle. A and T fit together, as do G and C, and that can never vary.

Hoagland and Dodson use the analogy of the letters of the alphabet and the paragraphs the letters make, which I'm adapting here and changing slightly for my own use. These letters and paragraphs will all combine to create our "cookbook." The base pairs can be seen as letters, and they come together in a chain to form a gene, which can thus be seen as a recipe made with those letters. The genes are arranged in a long row, side by side, to form a chromosome (a volume of the book). All the chromosomes together form the *genome* (or a set of volumes that contains all the recipes needed to make a full-scale banquet—a human being) (Fig. 13-2). Here's a multivolumed creation indeed!

There are hundreds of millions of bases. There are many genes as well—about 5,000 per chromosome, which equals over 100,000 per person. Each of us has 23 pairs of chromosomes, or two copies of every gene. Each gene (or recipe) codes for one protein.

Not all base pairs on a chromosome represent a gene. There are punctuation and spaces in between genes that affect how the gene is expressed. Thus, some series of these bases are important, telling you something crucial, while others represent a dash or a semicolon. The punctuation and spaces in between genes are just as important in one's chromosomal makeup as the actual genes that are expressed.

Why do the bases have to come in pairs? Each message is encoded only in one chromosome strand. But genes need to be able to replicate themselves, or no growth takes place. So the bases come in pairs that are actually mirror images of one another. This is the famous *double helix*. When a cell needs to divide—as it will for any number of reasons, from healing a scratch on the body to creating a pregnancy—it can do so because there is a mirror image attached to the original strand. In order to replicate, the helix separates, and mirror images are made of each strand from other bases that are floating around in the cell (see Fig. 13-1). The two mirror images then reconnect as a new double helix—a nifty way to make sure the code is unaltered.

The Cell Cycle

This process of *mitosis*, or cell division, is carefully orchestrated in what is called the *cell cycle*. This cycle has different phases (Fig. 13-3). The quiescent phase, G0, is the phase most cells are usually in. They're just sitting around, doing nothing. Then something wakes them up and says, "Time to divide!" sending them into the first *active* phase, the G1 phase. This lasts approximately nine hours, during which time the

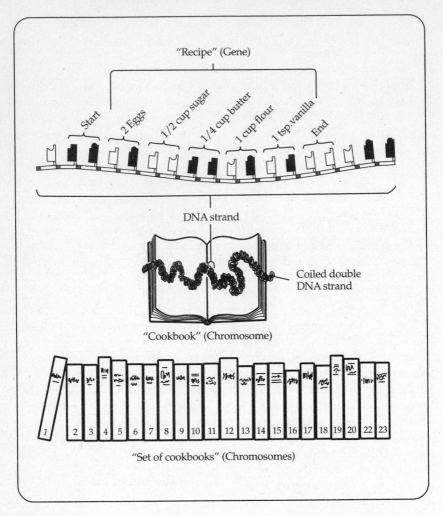

"Recipe" (Gene)

Start
2 Eggs
1/2 cup sugar
1/4 cup butter
1 cup flour
1 tsp. vanilla
End

DNA strand

Coiled double
DNA strand

"Cookbook" (Chromosome)

"Set of cookbooks" (Chromosomes)

FIGURE 13-2

cells get ready. At the end they must pass inspection at the G1 check-point and be found free of serious mutations before they can pass into the next phase and begin duplicating their DNA. There is a repair shop at the checkpoint as well, so that minor mutations can be fixed before they are passed on. P53 is a tumor suppressor gene that works at this checkpoint. But problems can occur with p53. It can become mutated. If that happens, it lets other mutations through, and defective genes will be allowed to pass.

Having passed the checkpoint, the gene then goes into the next

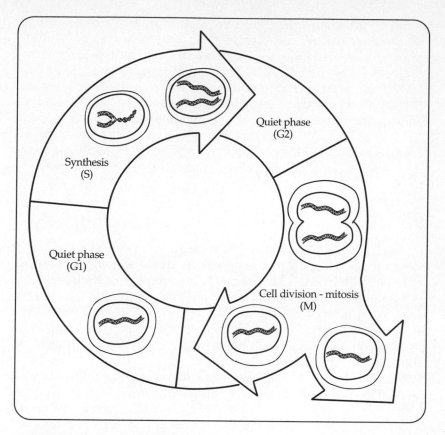

FIGURE 13-3   The Cell Cycle

phase, the S phase. This lasts six hours. At the end of the S phase the cell has replicated its entire genetic material and has two sets of paired chromosomes.

Then comes the G2 phase, another gap, which takes another four hours and involves another inspection and, if necessary, repair. It is the final checkpoint, or quality control, before the cell enters mitosis M phase, where it will divide and become two cells.

During G1, S phase, and G2, all the parts of the cell are duplicating so that there will be enough material to make two cells when the DNA is duplicated and ready to be passed on. The most variable period of the cell cycle is G1, the first gap, which essentially determines the length of the cycle by responding to signals within or outside of the cell that might trigger cell division and the entry into S phase. Its duration can be almost instantaneous (e.g., when an embryo is dividing every second) to indefinite (when your body doesn't need any more cells in this area). When cells are going to be quiescent and nonpro-liferating, they are shunted off to a special G1 phase, which, since it's quiescent, is also called G0. During each cell cycle some cells are also shunted into what's called terminal differentiation, which sounds terri-ble but only means that, like a postmenopausal woman, they can't re-produce. Though no longer capable of dividing, they remain fully func-tional. There are a lot of controls and redundancy in the cell cycle and scientists are still working out all the components. Nonetheless, we do know that it is the basis of all of life—including the life of cancer cells.

RNA

In case DNA hasn't confused you enough, you need to know that it doesn't work alone. It's got a temporary partner, called RNA. DNA, re-member, is just a code—a code for creating proteins. By itself, it doesn't do anything. Let's use our recipe image here. You've got a wonderful recipe book in your kitchen, but it's a very rare, expensive old book and you don't want to splatter stuff on it while you're cooking. What you'd like to do is have a copy of one page, which you can bring to the table and use to make your pie.

Well, the RNA provides that copy. It duplicates the gene that it needs at the moment. Then it takes the coding message to another part of the cell and translates that piece of code into a protein. When the copy is no longer used, it disappears (you throw it into the trashbin).

The RNA copy can be produced frequently for certain genes (like your daily breakfast cereal) or it can be produced less frequently (like a special dinner). The production of RNA determines how much protein will be produced and therefore the levels of expression of a particular protein.

So the gene is like one recipe: it will make one thing. The DNA is the information that has gone into writing that recipe. The chromosome is one volume of the cookbook. And the RNA is the disposable copy of the recipe that prevents the whole chromosome from being carted around.

Proteins

Proteins are the body's building blocks, which are needed throughout our lives—making this recipe system of vital importance. As Hoagland and Dodson write, proteins "do the daily business of living, giving cells their shapes and unique abilities."[2] There are many kinds of proteins (just as there are many dishes)—enzymes, transporters, movers, etc. There are 21 amino acids (ingredients) that are hooked together as proteins, and the RNA is what directs how they're strung together. Proteins are the end-product of a recipe—your delicious soufflé (Fig. 13-4).

Of course, you don't want to make all the recipes in the book at the same time. The whole point of a recipe book is to have a collection of recipes available for when you want them. There are pancake recipes that are great for Sunday brunch, and cranberry sauce recipes for Thanksgiving, and plain old mashed potato recipes for weekday din-

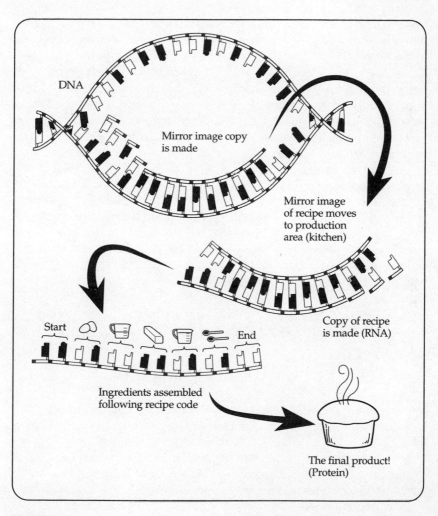

FIGURE 13-4

ners. Let's say you're rich enough to have several cooks: you need mechanisms for making sure they make only the right foods at the right time.

DNA too needs a control mechanism—it needs to be told which information to include for which "recipe" to be made at which time. So, for example, there are certain processes that DNA needs to do when a girl hits puberty: hair starts to grow under her arms; she starts growing breasts. But when she reaches adulthood she no longer needs some of those mechanisms. Her breasts don't need to keep growing once they've fully matured. Similarly, she doesn't want those breasts and hairy armpits too soon—at two or three, she's not ready for them. So there are many methods of regulation that are mechanisms for helping your body decide when you need one protein rather than another. The whole system is finely organized to have the right elements available just when you need them.

Needless to say, one of the major times you need them is when you are still in the uterus, when your body is beginning to make all its organs. But those organs get made just once. So their genes are turned off—recipes that remain in the book but that you never use again. Since the organs do need to grow, all the regulators are at work in the first few years of your life, making that happen.

Puberty and pregnancy are times that call for different "recipes." So at pregnancy, for example, your genes decide it's time to turn your breasts into milk machines, and make the proteins that are necessary to get things going. The correct gene is identified and told to make the milk. It then makes the proteins that tell the breast to develop into its next phase. It's all finely regulated so genes will make proteins that will turn on other genes. It's as though you wake up on Sunday morning and that triggers you to think, "Sunday—it's pancake day!" and you make your pancakes. And then at night there's another trigger that tells you it's time for your spaghetti dinner. Puberty and pregnancy are among the body's triggers.

GENES AND BREAST CANCER

When you understand DNA, RNA, and protein, you can begin to understand what can happen with cancer. The process can break down at any of these levels. The first level is at DNA. When your eggs are made, the cells divide and put only one DNA strand into each egg. So you give your child half of your DNA, the child's father gives half of his, and the combination makes a unique whole.

A mutation occurs when the wrong nucleotide gets inserted into the new strand as it's being made. Going back to our alphabet analogy,

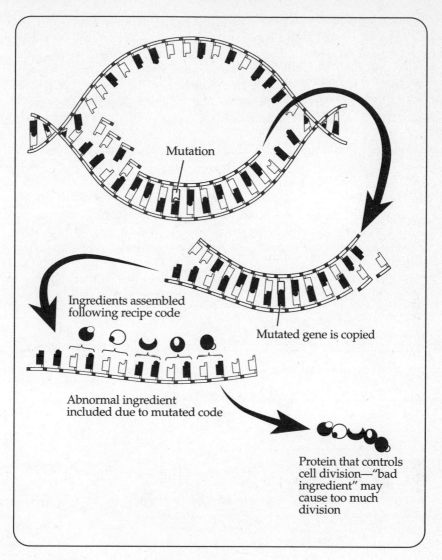

Mutation

Ingredients assembled
following recipe code

Mutated gene is copied

Abnormal ingredient
included due to mutated code

Protein that controls
cell division—"bad
ingredient" may
cause too much
division

FIGURE 13-5

there's a typo in the recipe (Fig. 13.5). Mutations can occur in somatic (cells that form the tissues of the body) or in germ cells (sperm and egg) which are passed on to our offspring. Both types of mutations are important: the first to the given individual and the second to the next generation.

Mutations happen with frequency over a person's lifetime: exposure to radiation, electricity, infrared light, and dozens of other things can create a mutation. But most are no problem. If you have a typo in a recipe no one ever uses, and it never gets retyped, it doesn't matter. This is especially true for adults: though infants and young children have constantly changing cells, as we grow older a lot of cell division stops. We don't, for example, make many more liver cells, and our brain cells, alas, are dying off more often than they are reproducing. So even if there are mutations, they don't much matter; they won't reproduce and be passed on to other cells.

There are other mutations that don't matter either, because "the typo" doesn't obscure meaning (Fig. 13-6). If your recipe says, "Add one cup of sigar," you may smile at it, but you know you need to add a cup of sugar. Once in a great while a mutation even creates an improvement. (If the recipe says to add a half cup of sugar, it may end up tasting just as good and being healthier.) In fact, there's an argument that civilization itself depends on mutations—the mutations involved in evolution.

But sometimes a mutation can be completely destructive, adding a lethal ingredient to the recipe. Birth deformities are caused by muta-

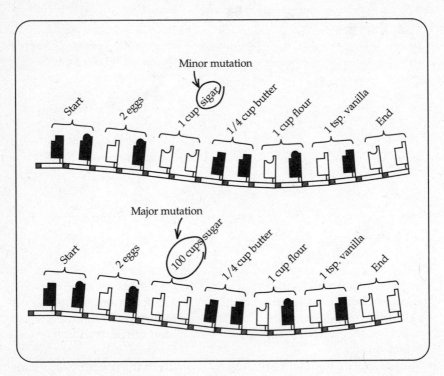

FIGURE 13-6

tions. The most severe are those in which the fetus miscarries, or is born dead. This occurs when the mutations are so bad that the body can't create a person. There are the less severe ones, in which a person can be created but is born with serious deformities such as the absence of limbs, or with serious genetic diseases, like the neurological condition AT in which the child seems healthy at birth but sickens and then dies because a protein necessary for brain growth is missing. These problems tend to be a result of DNA development rather than repair failures. Of course, there are minor and harmless variants of this kind of mutation. A child can be born with an oddly shaped toe, for example. It will never cause a medical illness, nor is it likely to limit the child's life through the years: it's simply there. Freckles are another example of a harmless mutation.

Some mutations can be either good or bad, depending on your situation. If you have a mutation that makes you exceptionally tall, it will be helpful if you plan to become a basketball player, or a hindrance if you want to be a jockey.

Then there are the cancer genes. These are genes that normally function in cell growth but which, if altered by mutation or loss, can lead to cancer. Mutations in these cancer genes can be caused by outside forces such as radiation, toxins in food, or environmental pollutants. If you're not exposed to these factors then the cancer-related genes won't be activated. Even if one of these genes is activated or altered, unless other cancer genes are also altered, cancer won't occur. In other words, cancers are due to multiple alterations in a number of genes, not just one.

It's as though the recipe gets typed by a number of different typists at different stages. The first typist makes the mistake, which then gets built into the manuscript, and it's always typed that way from then on. Then somewhere down the line another typist makes another error, and it too gets replicated. So now there are two mutations. And so on down the line. At some point the errors become such that the document's original meaning is destroyed.

Luckily the body has a technique for DNA repair—its own internal proofreader, enzymes called the *repair endonucleases* (Fig. 13-7). The proofreader reads through the recipe periodically, searching for mistakes, and then fixes them. These enzymes are responsible for quality control: they check every cell before allowing it to divide. So if, for example, you've been out too long in the sun and the ultraviolet rays cause a mutation, repair nucleases will catch it. It then has to decide what to do. How badly damaged is this cell? If it's in decent enough shape, then it's fixed. If the damage is too great, and the repair nuclease can't repair the damage in time, the cell senses this and self-destructs. It is estimated that our normal cells in the course of cell division contain thousands of DNA errors, which are fortunately detected

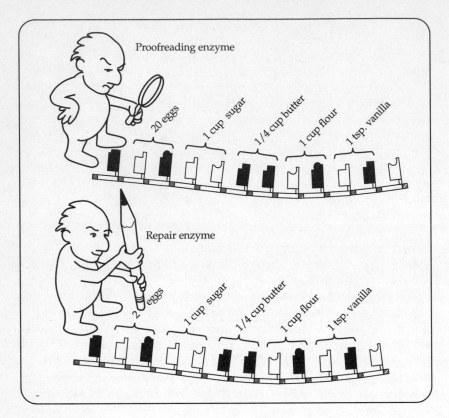

FIGURE 13-7

and repaired. This self-destruction is a form of cell suicide called *apoptosis* (Fig. 13-8). It occurs when there is something wrong with the cell itself or when the cell receives an abnormal signal from the environment. There may be too many mistakes in the DNA or a very central mistake.

The repair nucleases are usually pretty good workers, but once in a great while they fall asleep on the job, and the cell doesn't self-destruct. Like the proofreader who's daydreaming and misses a serious error in the text, the repair nuclease can sometimes let a mutated cell remain, and then divide. Now there are two mutated cells. Whether or not this will cause major problems depends on how important the mutation is.

The fact that this doesn't happen much more often than it does is testimony to the body's complex network of protection. There's a lot of redundancy built into the system. There's not just one pathway for repair; there are two or three (we've got several proofreaders and a copy editor at work here).

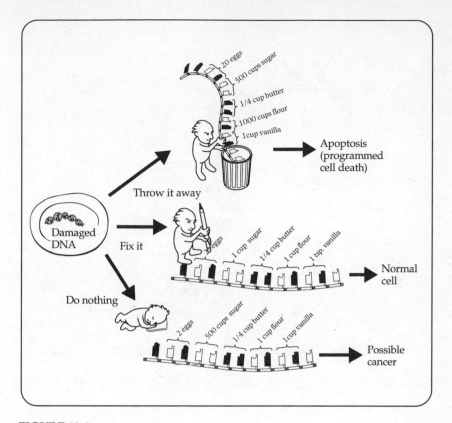

FIGURE 13-8

Apoptosis

The repair nucleases order the cell to kill itself, and the cell then releases a few enzymes that dissolve it (Fig. 13-9). The process doesn't cause inflammation or bruises, and you never know it's happening. There may be a little cleanup involved. It happens frequently, with a lot of minor mutations. So apoptosis is a good thing, a control system in your body. Apoptosis is also called "programmed cell death" because the cell controls its own fate. Chemotherapy can stimulate apoptosis.

Cells can also die through necrosis—getting attacked from both the outside and within and being injured during the process. In the case of necrosis, cells are damaged by external processes; like when you fall down the stairs and kill a few cells in the process. You know you have necrosis when you get a bruise or an inflammation. Then the macrophages (scavenger cells) clean the dead cells out and you heal. This

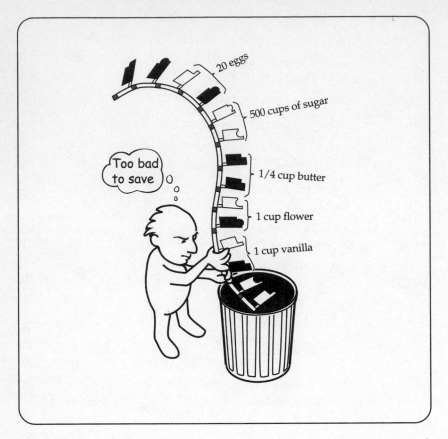

FIGURE 13-9

is completely different from apoptosis. It's usually apparent under a microscope which dead cells are necrotic and which apoptotic. The apoptotic cells have no reaction around them. Because apoptosis is an internal programmed event it has important implications for cancer, for two reasons: first, some cancer-related genes inhibit apoptosis. For example, a gene called bcl-2 is often rearranged in cancer and over-expressed. This gene blocks apoptosis and prevents cancer cells from dying. Second, chemotherapy is thought to induce apoptosis and certain genes like bcl-2 block the effects of chemotherapy.

Telomerase

Cells don't keep going round and round the cell cycle and dividing forever. This is fortunate, because every time the same DNA divides,

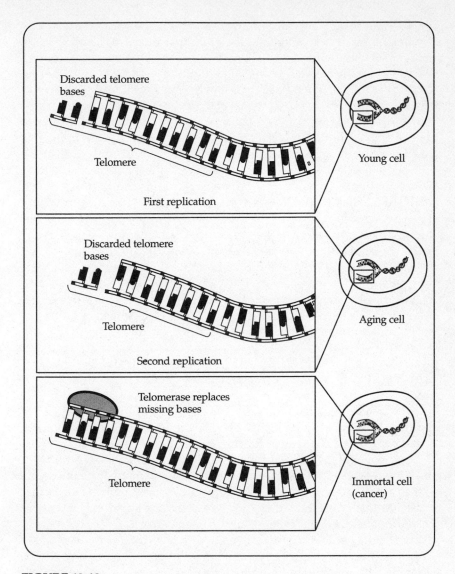

FIGURE 13-10

there are more opportunities for mutation. Knowing this, the body has a system to take care of it—a natural version of planned obsolescence. At the very end of the chromosome is a section called the *telomere*. Each time the cell makes new DNA, it snips off a little bit of the telomere. So the cell isn't actually completely copied; the very tip is gone from the duplicate. Thus each time the cell is copied it becomes a tiny bit shorter, until it gets to a point where it can't be copied anymore. This ensures that your body will copy this particular "recipe" only so many times. It can make new cells, but no one cell will be divided all that often. Telomerase is an enzyme in the body that reverses the process, by pasting the end of the DNA back on (Fig. 13-10). This enzyme is particularly important in cancer cells. It's another one of the things that allow cancer cells to keep dividing when they really should stop. In August 1999 scientists reported that they had done experiments trying to cause a cell in a petri dish to become cancerous by introducing two specific mutations. But it wasn't until they added telomerase to the mix that the cell became "immortal," as the scientists wistfully call it. So on both sides of the coin, normal regulatory mechanisms are getting blocked. Telomerase is of great interest to scientists, and it's getting a lot of study. They're looking for ways to block it so the cancer cells will die. They're also testing to see whether its presence in the blood or duct fluid can indicate whether or not a person has cancer. If someone had high levels of telomerase, they speculate, it could be a sign that cells that should be dying aren't. Although only a hypothesis, it's very intriguing.

As far as breast cancer is concerned, there are several types of genetic alterations involving key genes. Among these genes are oncogenes and tumor suppressor genes.

Oncogenes

There is a set of genes involved in making cells divide. When they're normal, these are called *proto-oncogenes;* when they're mutated they're called *oncogenes.* (The reason for the normal gene's name is that when we find something that's wrong, we try to track back and find out what it would do if it were normal. We found and named the oncogene first.) Proto-oncogenes involved in breast cancer are mostly ones that cause more cell division—they make the cell cycle go faster. They're involved in pushing cell division harder, faster, stronger.

One of the proto-oncogenes is related to the *epidermal growth factor receptor.* EGFR is necessary at certain times of your life, such as puberty, when big changes are going on in your growth, and you need growth factors egging on the cells, yelling "Grow! Grow! Grow!" The epidermal growth factor finds an epidermal growth factor receptor and signals the cell to grow. When the proto-oncogene for the receptor is overexpressed, it doesn't wait for EGFR to tell it to grow. Instead, it begins to grow independently, getting stuck in the "on" position (Fig. 13-11).

Another type of epidermal growth factor receptor is epidermal growth factor receptor 2. In the U.S. this is commonly known as Her-2 neu and in Europe as erbB2.

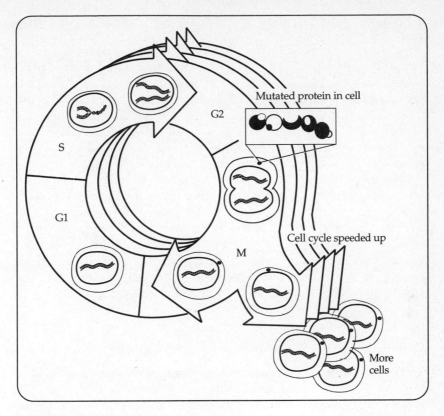

Mutated protein in cell

Cell cycle speeded up

More cells

G2

S

G1

M

FIGURE 13-11

The type of genetic alteration that Her-2 neu has is called *amplification*. Instead of having only one copy, the cell makes many (10–60) copies of this gene. When this happens, the cell has too many Her-2 neu receptors. Either the gene overexpression or the extra protein can be measured in a woman's tumor by studying the tissue that has been removed.

Since Her-2 neu is a growth factor receptor, it's involved in telling the cells to grow faster and faster. (It isn't involved in invasion, the other part of cancer, which we'll discuss a little later on in this chapter.)

About 70 to 80 percent of comedo DCIS (a form of precancer I discuss in Chapter 16) has overexpression of Her-2 neu. The cancer cells are still contained within the duct, but they have this "grow, grow, grow" receptor. Oddly, with invasive cancers, it's only about 30 percent. Although Her-2 neu was first identified in breast cancer, researchers are now studying other cancers (such as lung, pancreas, ovary, and prostate) to see if it is also present.

In order to have an invasive cancer you need more than one genetic alteration. As long as there's only overexpression of Her-2 neu and nothing else, the cancer (or precancer) will remain confined within the duct. If it acquires other alterations, one that tells it to move out of the ductal area or to make new blood vessels, then it can spread. If you have these invasive cancer alterations and one of the "grow-grow-grow" alterations, it's bad. People with both of these have a worse prognosis than those with the invasive alteration alone. Cancer not only requires too much proliferation, it also has to invade, grow new blood vessels, and get out of the breast territory.

One of the exciting things that's happened in recent years, which we'll discuss more in Chapter 23, is that there is now an antibody to the Her-2 neu receptor, which is given intravenously. It attaches only to cells with too much Her-2 neu receptor, not normal ones, so while it knocks out the Her-2 neu cells, it leaves the others alone. Unlike chemotherapy, which kills most dividing cells in your body, it's a targeted therapy. So far, this treatment has been tested only in metastatic disease, but it has implications for disease that hasn't yet spread.

Tumor Suppressor Genes

Tempering the oncogenes and proto-oncogenes are the *tumor suppressor genes*. These are the brakes in the cell system—so that while you have some genes that push the cells to grow and divide, you have others there to say, "Well, no, growing and dividing really isn't such a good idea." Sometimes they say this because the cell is defective; in which case the tumor suppressor genes tell the cell to stop dividing or, in some instances, they tell the cell to commit suicide. As you remember, the tumor suppressor genes hang out at the checkpoints of the cell cycle.

The suppressor gene p53 keeps cells with mutated DNA from dividing. It's believed that BRCA1 and 2 (Breast Cancer Genes) are actually tumor suppressor genes which may normally function as DNA repair enzymes such as the endonucleases mentioned previously. Since these genes are the quality control keepers, loss or mutations could be catastrophic for the cell.

For example, if you're missing p53 you have a rare condition called Li-Fraumeni syndrome. People in families with this syndrome have a very high incidence of all kinds of cancers—sarcomas, childhood cancers, breast cancers. Fortunately only about 100 families in the world have this. The absence of p53 creates a vulnerability to all kinds of cancers. Which cancer people get depends on which carcinogens they're exposed to. The brake isn't working, so none of the mutations caused by carcinogens will be stopped.

As we've seen, in most cancers, there are not just one but several mutations. One of the questions is whether the mutations come in specific orders. Will you get cancer only if you have the Her-2 neu mutation first and then the p53 one, in that sequence, but not if you get the p53 mutation first? Or will you get cancer if you have any of six mutations, in any order? Or if you get any 6 out of 12? We don't have these answers yet, but we're on the verge of finding them.

Gene Environment Interaction

Reading this chapter thus far you would think that all of cancer was genetic. In a way, it is. It's all based on altered genes. However, we're still not wholly certain what causes these genetic alterations. What is it in the woman's environment or in her life that does the damage? Is it hormones? If so, is it her own, or the ones she takes? Or is it pesticides or a virus or radiation or some completely unknown element that causes the genetic alterations? If we could identify the factors and block or eliminate them, it wouldn't matter quite as much which genes were being altered (Fig. 13-12). A good example is lung cancer. We know that smoking triggers the disease, so it must cause the alterations. Thus, it's less crucial to find out what the alterations are, because we don't have to try to neutralize these genetic alterations; we can just tell people to stay away from cigarette smoke and, if they do so, that will dramatically reduce their risk of lung cancer. So in terms of

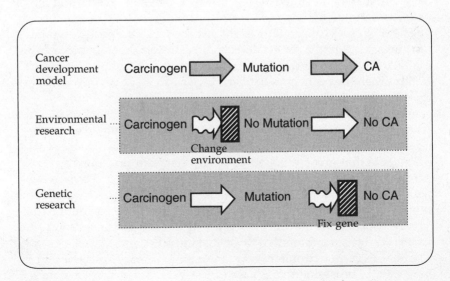

FIGURE 13-12

breast cancer we're studying things like diet, alcohol consumption, hormone medications, pesticides in the environment, and electromagnetic waves to find the carcinogens (see Chapter 15). But so far we're not finding anything equivalent to cigarette smoke.

Both the environmentalists and the basic scientists are correct, at least to an extent. You can't simply say, "Pesticides are the cause of cancer." Alone, they aren't. Many people are exposed to pesticides and never get cancer. But on the other hand, you can't simply say, "All cancers are genetic, so pesticides are irrelevant." It is the interaction between genes and the environment that will finally explain cancer.

INVASION

Oncogenes, tumor suppressor genes, and mutations are involved chiefly in the cell cycle—in division and proliferation. But they're not involved in the next step in cancer: invasion.

To become cancer, a cell needs more than the ability to divide and grow out of control. Noncancerous, benign tumors can also do that. What is ultimately crucial is the capacity to invade outside of their own normal territory. The cells in any given area are tightly attached to each other, forming a natural guard against invasion. So for a cell to break outside of its own area and into another requires special qualities.

One of the things we're all studying now in terms of cancer is that tight cell connection. There is a kind of "glue" called the *extracellular matrix* holding cells together. If a cell has an enzyme that can dissolve or consume the glue, it will have a much better chance of getting out of its area and into another.

The ability of cancer cells to invade may be caused by a number of things. One is the ability to secrete a protein, metalloproteinases, that actually tells the whole cell combination not to hang together so tightly. Then the other cells behave in a way that allows the cancer cell to escape.

Another possibility is that the cancer cell may be able to push its way out on its own. We discuss ducts and noninvasive cancer in Chapter 16, where we talk a bit about how Dr. Sanford Barksy's lab at UCLA discovered that myoepithelial cells, cells that surround the ducts, may help hold DCIS inside the ducts and prevent invasion. Perhaps what happens is not that the DCIS develops the ability to get out, but that the myoepthelial cells *allow* it to get out. Or maybe it's a combination. Maybe what allows it to get out is estrogen that you take. Maybe the DCIS secretes something that says, "Let me out," and the cells obey.

There are a lot of different ways it might happen. That's good in the long run, because there are a lot of potential ways we can interfere with the process. But it's difficult in the short run because it makes these complicated to figure out.

With the discovery of these various cancer genes, a new paradigm for thinking about breast cancer and subsequently treating it has emerged. To illustrate this paradigm, we need to switch metaphors temporarily. We're leaving the cozy world of cookbooks and jumping into the world of crime. (We'll be switching metaphors a few times throughout this chapter; we haven't found one that works all the way through.) What's amazing is that all these years we've been studying cancer cells by looking at them in isolation. Scientists take cancer cells and grow them in petri dishes and then study their behavior. It's a little like putting criminals in isolation chambers and then studying their personalities. They're not interacting with anyone, so there's really no way to measure how they behave. We've finally begun to realize that if we study cancer cells in their own environment we can learn a lot more, because they interact with the surrounding cells (stroma) and the surrounding cells have an effect on them.

Let's look at a hypothetical murderer. To begin with, maybe she's born with a sociopathic character—like the girl in *The Bad Seed*. But how is she raised, and in what environment? Let's say her parents are too busy with their social lives to pay much attention to her and there are no strong, loving family members; kind, responsible neighbors; solid school, or good community activities, to offer positive behavioral guidance. There are drug dealers at her school and she's impressed with them. Nothing prevents her from hanging out with them, and soon she's in a world where she learns criminal skills. Each of these factors plays its part in her ultimate criminal behavior. Had the original sociopathic tendencies been absent, the environment might not have made such a difference: she wouldn't be predisposed toward criminal acts. But even with the sociopathic tendencies, early training might have worked against the predisposition, developing a strong conscience that would prevent her acting on her instincts. Finally, even with the sociopathic tendencies and the amoral background, she might not have learned the skills to become an efficient criminal. Of course, her basic predisposition might not be permanently countered by the wholesome influences in childhood. As an adult, away from those influences, she might find herself in circumstances that nourish her basic character—"fall in with a bad crowd." And so that good little girl becomes a middle-aged murderer.

This may be how it works with cancer. Mina Bissel, a researcher in Berkeley, California, has begun studying breast cancer cells in a breast tissue environment. She has taken breast cancer cells that have the mutations of breast cancer and grown them in a culture of normal breast extracellular matrix. In that environment the cancer cells behaved like normal cells—they made ducts and did the other things that healthy breast cells do.[3] The healthy influence of the surrounding cells caused the cancer cells, even though they were genetically altered, to conduct themselves properly—like the sociopath in the perfect environment. When Dr. Bissel and her associates put the same cells in an artificial environment, the cells went back to behaving like cancer (Fig. 13-13).

How does this work? As the cells grow, they make certain proteins—growth factors, cytokines, enzymes—that are messengers telling the surrounding cells what to do. The surrounding cells then respond to these messages with messages of their own. This cross-talk is called *epigenetic interaction* (Fig. 13-14). It results in a change in a gene expression rather than structural alterations in the genes themselves. Epigenetic interaction is probably an important determinant of cancer cell growth and metastases, and thus it is likely to respond to therapeutic intervention. For an analogy, let us say there is a certain plant that can be pollinated only if there is a particular kind of bee in the environment that will take some of the pollen on its body to another plant. The original flower secretes a message, in the form of a smell, that attracts the bee. The bee then responds by cross-pollinating the plant. If you could block the scent of the flower, that species might well die out. Or you could change the environment so that it was inhospitable for the bee but not the flower. This also would eliminate the species. We don't want to eliminate any species of flower, of course. But it would be wonderful to be able to eliminate any species of cancer cells by blocking this type of interaction.

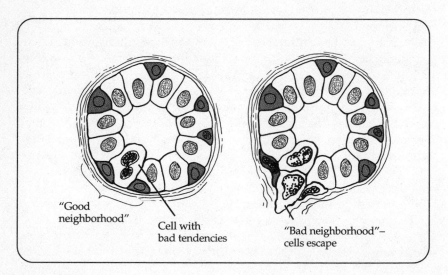

"Good neighborhood"

Cell with bad tendencies

"Bad neighborhood"– cells escape

FIGURE 13-13

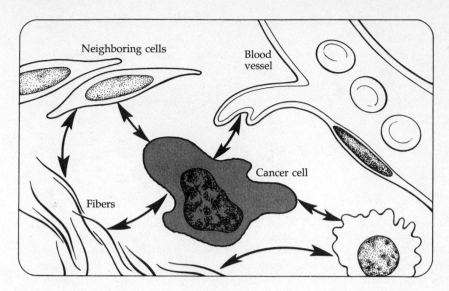

FIGURE 13-14

This means that, if we find the right tools, cancer may be reversible, or at least controllable, and we won't have to try to kill every last cancer cell. The ability to control or reverse cancer may also explain a phenomenon known as *tumor dormancy* (see Fig. 13-15). This is thought to happen in women who have had all of their treatment and appear to be cured, but then have a recurrence 10 years later. What were the cells doing for 10 years? They were asleep. What put them to sleep? What woke them up?

A cancer patient who came to one of my lectures found this notion very helpful. She had been trying to do visualization to help work with her therapy (see Chapter 29), but all the images suggested to her were aggressive ones: sharks inside her body attacking the cancer cells, bullets being shot at them. She had never been comfortable with the idea of these violent battles inside her. Now, she told me happily, she could change that. She could sing a lullaby to her tumor, sending all the cells peacefully off to sleep. It's an interesting idea.

ANGIOGENESIS

Once the cancer cells get out of the duct (or any other organ) and start to grow they need their own blood supply. Blood supply is the lifeline that gives them oxygen and nutrients so they can grow. It's as if you started a new colony or a commune out in the desert. You've found

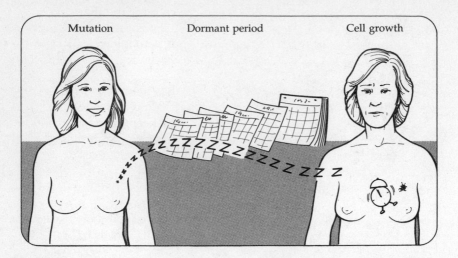

FIGURE 13-15

this nice place, but you need roads to bring in your supplies and to bring out your garbage. Without such roads, your community will die off quickly. In the same way, the cancer cells die off quickly if they don't have a blood supply. Tumors can grow only to about 2 millimeters, and then will stop growing unless they have more blood vessels. There are proteins that send the message saying, "Let's have new blood vessels growing."

These proteins are specific growth factors that are important. When you're an embryo, for example, you need new blood vessels that can go all the way down your arms and legs, so you'll have fingers and toes. Later, if you have an injury, you need new blood vessels to grow and heal it. That's part of the reason an injury turns red. One such protein which stimulates blood vessel growth called *veg-f—vascular endothelial cell growth factor*—is secreted by the cancer and then can fit into a specific receptor on the blood vessels and tell them to make more.

This is where the process of *angiogenesis* comes in—"angio" means vessels, and "genesis" means growth. If you look at tumors under a microscope you can see that some have more blood vessels than others. The more blood vessels you have, the more blood supply you have. Thus the more chances the cancer has of spreading, because there are more "roads" to spread out on (Fig. 13-16). Even in some DCIS, which is still trapped inside the duct, there is an increase in blood vessels around the outside of the duct. Those blood vessels can't do the DCIS cells any good, since they're too far away. But their presence means that the DCIS is secreting angiogenic factors such as veg-f to create new blood vessels even before the cells are out there and need them. This may be a clue that these are the cells that will eventually get out and invade. Some researchers think that perhaps we can measure veg-f in the bloodstream or duct fluid to see if there are new blood vessels growing.

Judah Folkman, a researcher in Boston, has made the startling discovery that cancer tumors actually secrete not only angiogenic factors, but also angiogenic inhibitors (a factor that keeps metastasis under control by not allowing new blood vessels to grow in), and that when the primary tumor is removed, the metastasis grows more because the angiogenic inhibitors have been removed.[4] It's interesting because there's always been a sort of folk belief that surgery to remove a tumor "lets the air get into it" and causes the cancer to spread. It's unlikely that the air has anything to do with it, but this may be some canny observers' way of interpreting something they realized was happening— that the cancer spread more quickly, the person got sicker, after the tumor was removed. Until we learned about this tumor-secreted angiogenesis inhibitor there was no way to account for these observations.

It seems odd that the cancer would do this—one would think it is in the nature of cancer to "want" to spread. It's fanciful, but I find myself thinking that the tumor doesn't like having rivals. It will grow in its

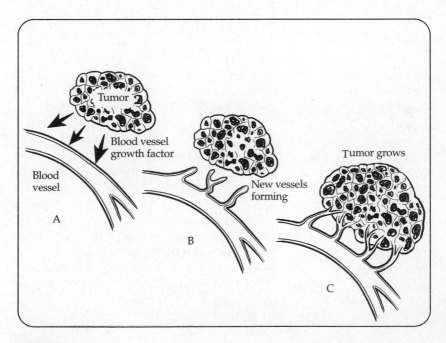

FIGURE 13-16

own area, but will keep any cells from growing in other organs. This isn't to suggest that if you have a tumor you should ignore it because it won't spread unless you encourage it by surgery. For one thing, it probably isn't true of all tumors. For another, the process is far from absolute. It doesn't stop the cancer from metastasizing; it only keeps the metastases already out there under control. The tumor wants to be king, and it sends some dukes out to oversee the provinces, but it doesn't want the dukes to become as strong as it is. Then when the king dies, the dukes all take advantage of his death and expand their own powers.

Anti-angiogenesis drugs are being tested now on humans. One of these, is thalidomide. Thalidomide blocks the growth of new blood vessels, which is why, when pregnant women took it for insomnia in the 1960s, their children were often born without arms and legs. But if you're not pregnant and you're an adult who doesn't need many more blood vessels, then it would be great if you could take it to block angiogenesis when you have a cancerous tumor. Certain anti-angiogenesis drugs being tested may not even have the drawbacks of thalidomide. Some new drugs that were developed for arthritis (Cox2 inhibitors) are also antiangiogenic, and are being tested in cancer prevention.

METASTATIC DISEASE

In order to metastasize, cancer cells have to grow too much, survive the immune system, make new blood vessels, crawl through the extracellular matrix, and break into the bloodstream. Having managed to survive all that, they must survive as they travel around the body, figure out what organ they get attracted to, break back out of the blood vessels and into the new organ, swim through *its* extracellular matrix, and set up shop there (Fig. 13-17). And maybe, after all that, the new organ isn't supportive of the cells. We don't yet know why some cancers end up in certain organs and not others. Is it that the cells don't grow well in some organs, and they know it, so they don't even bother to travel there? Or do they travel there and then get rejected by the organ, or die when they try to infiltrate? There's some evidence that there may be some kind of difference between blood vessels in certain organs—so that, for example, a breast cancer doesn't travel to the pancreas because the blood vessels there warn it away, whereas it travels with some confidence to the welcoming lungs or brain.

In any case, let us say that the cell has successfully made the journey to the lung. Now it has to make new blood vessels of its own in the lung, and the lung's environment may or may not be conducive to that. The question at this stage may be, do the lungs have the where-

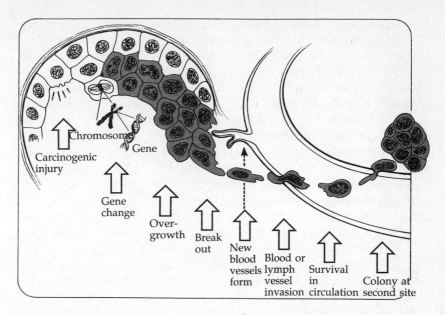

FIGURE 13-17

withal to keep the cells under control? Remember the cells that mutated like cancer but behaved normally in the normal breast? It's possible that even once they've metastasized, they'll behave normally, until something else happens—a change in the lung's environment, or a new genetic alteration that allows the cancer cells to grow in the lung.

We used to think that most cancer cells got knocked off in the bloodstream, that during the perilous journey from the breast to the lung they got killed by the immune system. But recently some elegant experiments were done in which researchers actually were able to follow the cells, found that the cells were very efficient and got to their target organs easily—the journey wasn't so perilous after all. So the question becomes, what happens once they've arrived?

An article in the *Journal of the National Cancer Institute* explores how tumors become dormant at the new site and how they wake up.[5] We're just beginning to understand this. How do they sneak through the immune system's surveillance? Where do they hide? When they hide, are they in the G0 phase, or are they dividing and just dying off as fast as they divide? We don't know. We do know that one hiding place is bone marrow; we found tumor cells in the bone marrow of people who never got metastasis. One possible model explains the process in stages. In stage 1, single cells or small groups lie dormant at a metastatic site until some genetic or intrinsic factor causes them to proliferate. In stage 2, clusters of about 2,000 to 150,000 cells have formed but they're unable to grow further because they don't have a blood supply. Finally, in stage 3, unrestrained growth occurs and the new blood supply necessary for further growth develops. What turns on this angiogenesis? It could be a mutation or the removal of some block in some antiangiogenic factor. Even when early metastasis has occurred, it doesn't necessarily spell doom. Some of these steps may well be reversible. If the cancer cells are sitting in the lung but the lung tissue cannot supply their needed growth factors, they may become dormant for a while (maybe years), waiting for just the right circumstances to arise in order to resume their growth (Fig. 13-18). This would explain why some women will have a recurrence of breast cancer many years after the first diagnosis. Those cells were there from the beginning but were dormant until the right conditions induced them to grow again.

This leads to a crucial question: should we reconsider our treatment of cancer? Instead of doing surgery and chemotherapy to eradicate every tumor, it might be wiser to treat the cancer the way we treat herpes: keep it under control, keep it dormant, instead of attempting to eradicate it.

As you see, metastasis isn't as simple a process as we once thought it was. It isn't simply that the cells spread, then grow, then kill you. If we can figure out the process in all its complexity, we may well reach a point where we can intervene and control metastasis at various points,

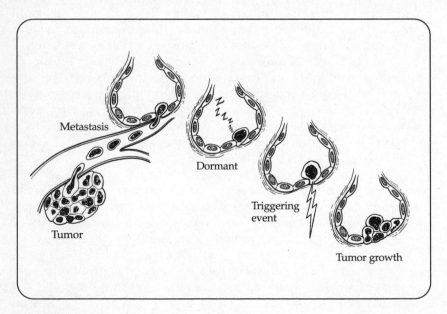

FIGURE 13-18

and keep people alive indefinitely, even with the metastasis present, virtually turning remission into cure.

To a certain extent, tamoxifen and the estrogen receptors are the model for this in breast cancer treatment. If a patient has metastatic cancer and is estrogen receptor positive, often the first thing we do is give her tamoxifen or toremifene, a similar hormone. The tumor shrinks and stays under control for a couple of years. Sometimes, this check can even last for 5 or 10 years. It doesn't kill cells the way chemotherapy does: none of the hormone manipulations we use kills cells. What they do is change the environment in the body—just as removing the ovaries does. They put the cells into a state of dormancy.

At this point, we're not certain why the cells eventually wake up and proliferate again. Possibly, with breast cancer, a subgroup of cells gets a mutation that makes it estrogen receptor negative. All the estrogen receptor positive cells remain under control, but this group that has escaped the control of the receptors multiplies and breaks free. The longer your cancer is around, the more chance there is for an alteration to affect these dormant cells, but in some women they stay dormant forever.

HORMONE RECEPTORS

The whole estrogen-progesterone story, like the others we've been talking about, is still a work-in-progress as far as science is concerned. And the story keeps changing. We realized a long time ago that estrogen had something to do with the breast, and we've learned a lot along the way, but we still don't know exactly how it works, how it interacts with breast cells, or what effect it has and how it has that effect.

When I wrote the first edition of this book, which came out in 1990, the medical community thought that there was a receptor in the nucleus of the cell and that the estrogen molecule was floating along, secreted by the ovary, and then got hooked into the receptor, causing the message to be sent. We thought that what tamoxifen did was to block the receptor so the estrogen couldn't get in. It was easy—like a key and a lock.

But it soon became clear that it wasn't that simple. There were several inconsistencies. How, for example, could tamoxifen act like estrogen in some organs and not in others? If it's just a key in a lock, the key either opens the lock or it doesn't.

Further, some organs that seemed to benefit from estrogen, like the bones and the bladder and the parts of the brain having to do with memory, had no estrogen receptors at all—no lock for the estrogen key to turn. Clearly our lock-and-key idea wasn't enough.

In 1995 researchers at the Karolinska Institute made an important discovery. It turns out there isn't just one estrogen receptor; there's also a second one. So now we have estrogen receptor alpha and estrogen receptor beta. Alpha is the one we've been looking at all along, the one we thought was *the* receptor. The beta receptor exists in some of the same organs as the alpha, and also in some others.[6] They can bind both estrogen and the antiestrogens tamoxifen and raloxifene. Some organs that didn't have the alpha receptor had the beta receptor. We wondered why these organs didn't have receptors yet still responded to estrogen. Now we know that they have another receptor which we didn't know existed. Estrogen beta receptor has been found in the central nervous system, blood vessels, breasts, uterus, bones, lungs, kidneys, intestines, ovaries, and bladder. Men, too, have estrogen: they have fewer and different estrogen receptors. And beta receptors have been found in the prostate.

That means that there are at least three ways estrogen can have an effect. It can act on the alpha receptor, the beta receptor, or both. So estrogen can function with a much greater subtlety—it has three locks, not one. This begins to explain why estrogen works in some organs and not others—why it causes cells to grow in some organs and stops their growth in others.

There are also some data suggesting that breast tissue itself can make estrogen. This might explain something that has puzzled me for some time: how can it happen, as it does, that sometimes women who have had total hysterectomies have estrogen receptor positive breast cancer? The little estrogen they get from their adrenal glands isn't enough to stimulate estrogen receptor positive breast cancer. Unfortunately this breast-created estrogen does not appear to have any of the good effects of estrogen: it can't help reduce osteoporosis, for example. All it seems able to do is stimulate breast cancer.

The story is not as simple as different keys and different locks; there may be different locking and unlocking mechanisms. For example, there's a three-dimensional quality to the estrogen receptor that we didn't realize until recently. When the estrogen (the key) fits into the receptor, it changes the shape of the receptor (the lock), uncovering a previously hidden connection point. This additional point may change the message that the particular hormone gives to the cell. So there's a shape change, as well as a chemical change, when the key goes into the lock. The whole lock changes. Depending on the hormone that fits in it, the receptor changes in different ways. Estrogen causes one kind of change. Tamoxifen causes a different one. In some organs, the tamoxifen changes the shape so it's unable to do its job any more and it becomes an estrogen blocker. But in other organs it changes its shape in ways that make it *able* to do its job. It can be both agonist and antagonist—it can block estrogen or mimic it, depending on the receptor. It may be that it changes differently in the beta receptor than in the alpha receptor. Now that we have observed this phenomenon we have named it. Tamoxifen is called a selective estrogen receptor modulator, or SERM. (We'll discuss SERMs in Chapters 18 and 23.)

Tamoxifen Resistance

Women who take tamoxifen for breast cancer for five years have a reduction in second cancers, but those who take it for 10 years get an increase in breast cancer (see Chapter 23). In mouse models, they found that getting rid of estrogen causes the tumor to shrink for four to six months, but then it starts growing again. It seems that the mouse's body resets its "thermostat" so that it becomes sensitive to a lower level of estrogen.

Complicating things still more are *co-activators* and *co-repressors*. They're like chaperones who travel with the receptor and influence the action that results. For example, tamoxifen, which, as we've noted, can both stimulate and block estrogen in the breast, is wishy-washy, and it can go either way. The protein chaperones can push it into being a blocker or an activator. In the past six years at least 10 different co-repressors and co-activators have been found—all of which modulate how hormones act. They interpose between receptor and transcription, and can affect how much protein your body makes.

Progesterone

Progesterone is less discussed than estrogen, but it's just as important. One of the big confusions comes with the conflation of progesterone with progestins. Progesterone is a hormone made by the ovaries; progestin is artificial. One might argue that there are also selective *progesterone* receptor modulators (though that would end up as SPERMs, so we'd have to find a new acronym), and that progesterone is the standard and progestins like Provera are the variants. Just like the SERMs, these might act differently on different organs. Unfortunately, in spite of the data proving there's a difference between progesterone and Provera, many doctors assume they're the same.

There are also A and B progesterone receptors, similar to the alpha and beta estrogen receptors. And there may turn out to be yet more receptors in either the estrogen or progesterone category which will be discovered.

Estrogen actually induces the growth of progesterone receptors.

They work as a team in the breast. Katherine Horwitz has shown that progesterone has a different effect on the breast cell when given alone than when given with estrogen. Alone it rushes the cell through the cell cycle and stops it at G1 all ready to go. And there it stays unless estrogen or another epithelial growth factor prompts the cell to divide and proliferate.[7] This may explain why studies show that postmenopausal women who take both estrogen and progestin have an increased risk of breast cancer over those who take estrogen alone. On the other hand, it also suggests that postmenopausal women or those who have had total hysterectomies who take progesterone alone may not be increasing their risk.

TRANSLATIONAL RESEARCH

Both tamoxifen and Herceptin are examples of how this biological research actually works in practice. In the case of tamoxifen, we started out with a drug we were using and then tried to figure out the mechanism by which it worked. With Herceptin we started out with biological observations and made a drug to fit them.

Although tamoxifen and Herceptin are good examples of this kind of research, which we call *translational research,* they also point out how hard it is. Let's say we want to block telomerase. If we give a blocker intravenously, will it survive or will it get eaten up by the immune system? Can it be swallowed? Injected into the tumor? Does it have to be specifically designed to block only the kind of telomerase the tumor makes, so that no other kind will work? The concept is good, but getting it to work takes a lot of steps. It's like saying, "Let's put on a production of *The Wizard of Oz.* We'll do it next Saturday night." But you need to hold auditions for the cast, find a crew, find a theater, do rehearsals . . . you need months to put it all together. And you'll have a lot of frustrations—30 women will audition for Dorothy, and none will be right. Similarly, a lot of work—a lot of trial and error—goes with any medical discovery. Unfortunately, while the media are good at announcing a supposedly great discovery, they're not so good at reporting that it turned out not to work, or to need a lot more honing. Most of the "breakthroughs" that get reported don't lead to changes in our therapies. One of the frustrating things with all this research is that while we're at the point of knowing how it works and realizing that it might be helpful, we're not at the point of knowing how to use most of it in patients. We're furthest along with Her-2 neu. But the good thing is that all of this is already in the pipeline. It's not fantasy; it's only a question of how soon we'll know what to do with our knowledge.

14

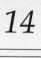

Risk Factors:
Genetic and Hormonal

Until about 1940, it was widely believed that cancer was an inevitable consequence of aging. Somehow the process of living included the inevitable creation of cancer cells at some significant frequency, and they were bound to get you eventually in one form or another, unless something else got you first, like an infectious disease (this was before the discovery of antibiotics). This theory wasn't completely crazy—as we saw in the previous chapter cells do mutate and cancer is created by lots of different kinds of genetic alterations (see Chapter 13). But there are diverse causes for cell mutations, some external and some internal—and many are not inevitable.

RISK

Every woman wants to know what her risk of getting breast cancer is and what she can do about it. Before discussing the figures, however, we need to be clear about their derivation, since they're often used in confusing and misleading ways. For example, an advertisement calling milk "99 percent fat-free" might suggest that it has 1 percent as much fat as whole milk. Actually, what it means is that 1 percent of the milk is made up of fat. Since only 3.6 percent of whole milk is made up of

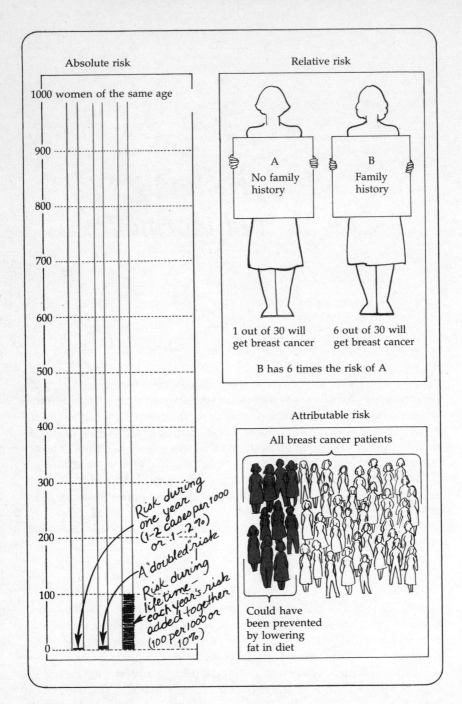

Absolute risk

1000 women of the same age

900

800

700

600

500

400

300

200

100

0

Risk during one year (1-2 cases per 1000 or .1-.2%)

A "doubled" risk

Risk during lifetime— each year's risk added together (100 per 1000 or 10%)

Relative risk

A
No family history

B
Family history

1 out of 30 will get breast cancer

6 out of 30 will get breast cancer

B has 6 times the risk of A

Attributable risk

All breast cancer patients

Could have been prevented by lowering fat in diet

FIGURE 14-1

216

Table 14-1. Probability of a Woman Developing Breast Cancer by Age 75 by Race/Ethnicity[a]

	%	No.
White	8.2	1 in 12
African-American	7.0	1 in 14
New-Mexican Hispanic	4.8	1 in 21
New-Mexican American Indian	2.5	1 in 40
Japanese-American	5.4	1 in 19
Chinese-American	6.1	1 in 16

[a] J.W. Berg, "Clinical Implications of Risk Factors for Breast Cancer," *Cancer* 53 (1984): 589. Reprinted with permission.

Note table calculates risk to age 75 (1 in 12) rather than the familiar 1 in 8 calculated to age 85.

fat, whole milk could be called "96.4 percent fat-free." Thus, a more helpful ad would say, "less than one third the fat of whole milk." Likewise, when the media headlines say that three drinks a week increase breast cancer risk by 50 percent they don't mean you have a 50-50 chance of getting breast cancer but rather that these drinks increase the relative risk by 50 percent and your lifetime risk is now about 5 percent rather than 3.3 percent. Thus, it is important that we examine the common statistics used about breast cancer and review exactly what they mean. There are three kinds of risk commonly referred to in discussing breast cancer: absolute risk, relative risk, and attributable risk (Fig. 14-1).

Absolute risk is the rate at which cancer or mortality from cancer occurs in a general population. It can be expressed either as the number of cases per a specified population (e.g., 50 cases per 100,000 annually) or as a cumulative risk up to a particular age. This cumulative risk is the source of the familiar 1 in 8 for non-Hispanic white women. (Other racial and ethnic groups actually have a lower risk—see Table 14-1.) It is important to recognize that this number can't be applied to any one individual woman. It describes the "average" risk of breast cancer in non-Hispanic white women and is calculated to take into consideration other causes of death over the life span. This figure will overestimate the number for the woman with no risk factors and underestimate for the one with risk factors.

Future risk at any one time depends to a great extent on your age. For the average white woman, it is something like 1/4000/year at age 30 to 34 (0.1%). This number increases with age, since breast cancer becomes more common as women get older: for example, by age 50 the average white woman has a 1/500/year (0.2%) risk of getting breast cancer (see Tables 14-2 and 14-3). For women of color, the risk is less (Table 14-1), although the mortality rate for African-American women is greater.

The second kind of risk we talk about determining is *relative risk*. This is the comparison of the incidence of breast cancer or deaths from breast cancer among people with a particular risk factor to that of people without that factor, or a "reference population." This type of measurement is more useful to an individual woman because she can determine her risk factors and thus calculate how they will affect her chances of getting the disease. Even here you have to be very care-

Table 14-2. The Average Risk of White Women Developing Breast Cancer in a Given Year By Age[a]

	Risk
30	1 in 5,900
35	1 in 2,300
40	1 in 1,200
50	1 in 590
60	1 in 420
70	1 in 330
80	1 in 290

[a]Adapted from P.C. Stomper, R.S. Gellman, J.E. Meyer, and G.S. Gross, "New England Mammography Survey 1988: Public Misconceptions of Breast Cancer Incidence," *Breast Disease*, May 1990.

Table 14-3. Probability of Breast Cancer for the Population of White Women[a]

Age Interval	Risk of Developing Breast Cancer	Risk of Dying of Breast Cancer
Birth to 110	10.2 %	3.60%
20–30	0.04	0.00
35–45	0.88	0.14
50–60	1.95	0.33
65–75	3.17	0.43

[a]H. Seidman et al., *CA: A Cancer Journal for Clinicians* 35 (1985): 36–56. Reprinted with permission.

Table 14-4. Family History and Risk of Breast Cancer[a]

	Relative Risk
First-degree relative with breast cancer (mother, sister, daughter)	2.3%
premenopausal	2.7
postmenopausal	2.5
mother	2.1
sister	2.1
mother and sister	13.6
Second degree relative (aunt or grandmother)	1.5
First and second degree relative	2.2

[a]Adapted from R.W. Sattin, G.L. Rubin, L.A. Webster, et al., "Family History and the Risk of Breast Cancer," *Journal of the American Medical Association* 253 (1985): 1908.

ful. For comparison, you can't use the 1 in 8, or 12 percent, generated in the absolute risk equation (see above) because that is based on all women regardless of risk factors. Rather, you need a number that will reflect the risk of a woman without the factors being considered. For a woman with no clear risk factors at all (no previous cancers, no family history, menarche after 11, menopause before 52, first pregnancy before 30) this is 1 in 30, or 3.3 percent, significantly lower than the "average" risk of 12 percent.[1]

If you call the risk of the woman without any particular risk factors 1.0, you can report the risk of those *with* a particular risk factor in relation to this. This is how relative risk is derived. A woman whose mother had breast cancer in both breasts before the age of 40, for example, has a relative risk of 2.7 over her lifetime—that is, 2.7 times that of the woman with no family history, not, as it might appear, 2.7 times the 12 percent we mentioned above (see Table 14-4).

How an increase in relative risk will affect your absolute risk also depends on your age at the time. For example, a threefold relative risk (compared to that of the general population) at a young age will increase your absolute risk by about 20 percent, while by age 50, the woman with the threefold increased relative risk has a lifetime risk of about 14 percent. One third of the breast cancers occur before age 50 and so her risk is only 2/3. She has about a 4.5 percent chance of developing breast cancer over the next 10 years and about 10.5 percent in the next 20 years, compared with the average risks of 1.5 and 3.5 percent, respectively.[2]

When you read a study or see one reported in the media it is impor-

Table 14-5. Reproductive Factors and Risk of Breast Cancer[a]

	Relative Risk
Menstrual History	
Age of first period < 12	1.3%
Age at menopause > 55 with > 40 menstruating years	2.0
Pregnancy	
First child before 20	0.8
First child 21–29	1.3
First child after age 30	1.4
Nulliparous (no pregnancies)	1.6

Adapted from W.D. Dupont and D.L. Page, "Breast Cancer Risk Associated with Proliferative Disease, Age at First Birth, and a Family History of Breast Cancer," *American Journal of Epidemiology* 125 (1987): 769.

tant to check the basis for the relative risk numbers. Most authors compare women with a specific risk factor to women without it. They assume that all the other risk factors are equal in both groups, so that only their risk in terms of the risk factor of interest is being compared. It's like the fat in the milk: the numbers can be very misleading if you don't take the time to put them in context.

Finally, we must consider the *attributable risk*. This concept relates more to public policy. It looks at the amount of disease in the population that could be prevented by alteration of risk factors. For example, a risk factor could convey a very large relative risk but be restricted to a few individuals, so changing it would only benefit a few individuals. Dr. Anthony B. Miller has hypothesized that if every woman in the world were to have a baby before 25, 17 percent of the world's breast cancer would be eliminated.[3] If you were looking at this from a public health policy perspective, you'd have to weigh the possible advantages of pushing early pregnancy against the problems of young and possibly immature parents, and possible increased population growth (Table 14-5).

But what do we mean by risk factors and how are they determined? "Risk factor" is a term referring to identifiable factors that make some people more susceptible than others to a particular disease; that is, smoking is a risk factor in lung cancer, and high cholesterol is a risk factor in heart disease. Medical researchers attempt to define risk factors in order to discover who is most likely to get a particular disease, and also to get clues as to the disease's cause and thus to the possible prevention and/or cure.

A risk factor is usually determined by taking a large population of people—say, 1,000–2,000 or more—and identifying a variety of features about them, determining who gets the disease under study, and then seeing what the relationship is between the disease and the features that commonly occur within the group. (Such a study is by definition observational, with all the limits of an observational study; see Chapter 12.)

You have to be careful how you use your findings. If you determine that out of your 2,000 people under study, 500 got the disease and all 500 drank milk as infants, you can't decide from this that milk-drinking causes cancer. If none of the other 1,500 drank milk as infants, you might be on the right track; if, as is more likely, all 1,500 did drink milk, you've learned nothing except that most people drink milk as children.

Sometimes, as in the case of lung cancer and smoking, risk factors are dramatic, and can make a clear difference in the individual's likelihood of getting the disease. Unfortunately, it usually doesn't work this way. In breast cancer, we have come up with some risk factors—such as family history—which we'll look at in this chapter. But so far, there is nothing comparable to the connections found between cholesterol and heart disease or between smoking and lung cancer. With breast cancer, the sad reality is that we can't say, as with lung cancer, "You're fairly safe because you're not in this particular population." In fact, 70 percent of breast cancer patients have none of the classical risk factors in their background.[4] It's important to understand this, for two reasons. Overestimating the importance of risk factors can cause needless mental anguish if you have one of them in your background. On the other hand, you may create a false sense of security if you don't have them. I can't count the number of times patients have come in to me with a suspicious lump that turns out to be malignant and, stunned, say, "I don't know how this happened! No one in my family ever had breast cancer!" I tell them they're in good company—most breast cancer patients don't have a family history of breast cancer. By virtue of being women, we are at risk for breast cancer.

Another thing to note is that risk factors don't necessarily increase in a simple arithmetical fashion: if one risk factor gives you a 20 percent risk of getting breast cancer, and another gives you a 10 percent chance, it doesn't always mean that now you're up to 30 percent. The interaction of risk factors is a tricky and complicated process. One interesting example is in the studies on alcohol and breast cancer (see Chapter 15) which show that women with other risk factors who also drank liquor didn't increase their risk very much, while women with no other risk factors who drank raised their risk dramatically.[5]

It would be much more convenient if we could say, "This causes breast cancer so don't do it." But breast cancer is what is known as a "multifactorial disease"—that is, it has many causes which interact with each other in ways we don't understand yet.

As I noted earlier, the older you are, the higher are your chances of getting breast cancer. The publicity about breast cancer, which has increased rapidly in recent years, gives the impression that the disease is hitting younger and younger women. That's partially true. The *percentage* of young women getting breast cancer is the same as it's always been. The number of younger women in the country has risen in recent years, because the baby boomers are in their 40s and 50s. If you take 10 percent of 40, you get 4; if you take 10 percent of 400, you get 40. There are more 40-something women with breast cancer because there are more 40-something women around. (There's no breast cancer rise among post-boomers, by the way. There are fewer of them than boomers, and breast cancer in really young women—teens and 20s—has always been unusual.)

Most breast cancer still occurs in women over 50—about 80 percent of cases. Your risk at age 30 (see Table 14-2) is one in 5,900 per year. By age 40, it's 1 in 1,200. So the risk of getting breast cancer before you're 50 is very small. The median age for breast cancer diagnosis is 64, which means that half of women who get breast cancer will get it before age 64 and half will get it after.

So whenever you look at risk factors, you need to correct for age. Other risk factors—family history, hormonal factors, etc.—will most likely cause breast cancer only in combination with rising age.

Another factor we need to look at is the variation among ethnic groups. Almost all the data you read are based on non-Hispanic Caucasian women. Table 14-1, although it is now dated, demonstrates that the risk for African-American and other women of color is less than for white women. This is a disease that is predominantly found in non-Hispanic Caucasian women. African-American women have rates similar to those of white women premenopausally, but lower than those of whites postmenopausally. That won't necessarily be comforting news to African-American women, however, since, though it's less common in that group, it's often more deadly. In one study five-year survival for African-American women diagnosed in 1986–1996 was 77 percent compared to 84 percent in white women diagnosed in the same time period.[6] That has to do in part with screening and being diagnosed early.

Interestingly, there's also a class variation—white women of higher socioeconomic status get more breast cancer than poorer white women.[7] Black women of higher socioeconomic status also have a higher risk than poorer black women. Breast cancer seems to "discriminate" opposite to the way our society discriminates.

The difference in vulnerability to breast cancer works on an international level as well. Third World countries have less breast cancer than highly industrialized countries.

The only likely possibility that we've come up with so far is one I'll discuss in a later chapter. These days many white middle- and upper-class women tend to have their first child later in life, and a small sub-set of these women choose to have no children at all. In addition, they are more likely to take hormones. This trend doesn't follow in women of color and women of lower socioeconomic groups in the U.S., nor in women of Third World countries. But that's not enough to explain the whole difference.

Risk in Lesbians

In 1993 there was a lot of publicity about the possibility that lesbians are at a higher risk of breast cancer—1 in 3 instead of 1 in 8. This was based on some research done by Suzanne Haynes from the National Cancer Institute.[8] She had looked at some studies that had been done on lesbians who frequented the gay bars in the 1950s and who had been asked to fill out questionnaires about their lifestyles. Then she took the characteristics that those studies had found and matched them with known breast cancer risk factors. She hypothesized that there should be a larger amount of breast cancer than in heterosexual women. The factors she was looking at were not directly related to their sexual preference, but to the lifestyle common to the lesbians who had been studied. Since they spent a lot of time at bars, they tended to drink a lot of alcohol, and were often obese. Most had not been pregnant. These are in themselves risk factors for breast cancer. Haynes did not necessarily believe lesbians had a greater risk of breast cancer than heterosexual women. But there hadn't been any studies on lesbians and breast cancer, and she was trying to show the research es-tablishment that it was a population that needed to be studied. As a re-sult of her work, studies are now being done. The Women's Health Ini-tiative (see Chapter 12), which is researching estrogen, diet, and other aspects of women's health, includes a question about sexual preference so that we can begin to get information that will tell us whether lesbi-ans are indeed at higher risk, or have particular risks.

In 1998, the *Journal of the Gay and Lesbian Medical Association* pub-lished a study by Stephanie Roberts, done for the Lyon Martins Women's Health Services. Roberts looked at a group of women 35 and older, half of whom were lesbians and half not. She asked them a num-ber of questions. Interestingly, though the lesbians didn't seem to have a greater incidence of breast cancer than the straight women, they did have more breast biopsies. This finding was a bit surprising and she is researching it further. They also had a higher body mass (possibly because they were less concerned with looking thin, which is perceived in our culture as necessary to "catch a man"). The heterosexual women had higher rates of smoking and—less confusingly—of birth control pill use, pregnancy, and miscarriages. So much for overall populations and their risks. Now let's look at the most complex category of risk—genetic.

GENETIC RISK FACTORS

Hereditary breast cancer first made its appearance in medical history in 1757. A French surgeon named LeGrand told of a nun with breast cancer who was treated by a surgeon in Avignon. The surgeon wanted to perform a mastectomy, but the nun, "fearing extirpation more than death," refused the operation. She was convinced, furthermore, that it would do no good, as her grandmother and maternal great grand uncle had died of the disease, and thus, she said, "her blood was corrupted by a cancerous vermin natural to her family." As the pain of her disease worsened, she gave in, had the mastectomy, and was, LeGrand tells us, restored to "perfect health." It would be nice to know how soon after the nun's surgery LeGrand wrote this, and how long her "perfect health" lasted.

Some things never change: the nun, just like many women today, tended to exaggerate her risk of breast cancer. While it's true that breast cancer in the family increases a woman's chance of getting breast cancer, the additional risk for most women may not be that great.

Genetically, we divide breast cancer occurrences into three groupings. The first, and most common, is sporadic—that's the 70 percent of women with breast cancer who have no known family history of the disease. The second is genetic—there's one dominant cancer gene, and it's passed on to every generation. Most people assume that these are the only two kinds of breast cancer: the kind that is inherited and the kind that isn't. In fact, there is a third group that is much more common than the genetic group. It's what we call "polygenic," and it occurs when there is a family history of breast cancer that isn't directly passed on through each generation in one dominant gene—some members of the family will get it and others won't. Women in this category are at greater risk for cancer than the general public, though less so than women with hereditary cancer.

Dr. Henry Lynch of Creighton Medical School's oncology clinic did a study estimating the percentages of these genetic groupings of breast cancer within a particular population.[9] He looked at 225 patients with breast cancer, and found that 82 percent had sporadic breast cancer (or no family history), while 13 percent had polygenic and only 5 percent had true genetic breast cancer. Other studies have put polygenic cancers at about 20 percent of breast cancers.

Most estimates are that pure hereditary breast cancer is rare, but it does occur—between 5 and 10 percent of all breast cancers fall into this category. In this case, the mother (or father) has a breast cancer gene, as mentioned in the previous chapter, and there's a 50-50 chance it will be passed on to the daughters (Fig. 14-2). If a daughter, or son, has inherited the gene, that gene again has a 50-50 chance of passing on to the next generation. I've had one family with a dramatic instance of genetic cancer. The grandmother had it, and the mother had it. The mother was fine the last time I saw her, years after her surgery, but two of her five daughters died of breast cancer, and two others have had the disease. (This is a very different situation from the more common one, when the family members with breast cancer are aunts or cousins rather than mother and sisters, and the risk is not so high.)

When we wrote the previous editions there was no test to pick out which women were at risk, and so doctors developed an elaborate system of guesswork based on what knowledge existed. It was sort of like searching for a criminal before the discovery of fingerprints or DNA, but with a fairly good description. If the suspect was a tall blond man with glasses, many tall blond bespectacled men might get rounded up, but only one would be the criminal.

So it was with determining cancer risk. If a woman's mother or sister had had bilateral breast cancer, or had gotten breast cancer at an early age, or if the woman had more than two relatives with breast cancer, we decided she was at risk. But, as we were to learn later, such a woman, though she had the risk factors, didn't necessarily have the one element that actually made her at genetic risk—the BRCA1 or 2 gene. Now that we have a way to test for the genes, the old rules are much less relevant.

Some women, we now know, have a family history of breast cancer without having an inherited gene. About 20 percent of breast cancers fall into this category. This doesn't mean the cancer is pure coincidence. These people may have inherited something that makes them more prone to breast cancer. What could make you more prone to breast cancer? Well, you may inherit a gene that causes you to begin menstruating at an early age, or a gene that makes you particularly susceptible to estrogen—which means other family members will be likely to get breast cancer.

Another possibility is exposure to similar external risk factors. I have a friend who is one of five sisters who got breast cancer. The sisters were all tested for BRCA1 and 2, and were shocked to discover they didn't have it. When all the cancer is in one generation, as in my friend's case, it's possible that they were all exposed to an environmental factor that caused the cancer. When this is the case, the gene won't be passed on to their children: it's not hereditary.

BRCA1 and 2

In 1990 the BRCA1 gene, which is a tumor suppressor gene linked to genetic breast cancer, was discovered; and in 1991 the gene was also shown to be linked with genetic ovarian cancer. The families who have this gene tend to have a high incidence of breast cancer, often at a young age, in both breasts, as well as ovarian cancer (see Table 14-4).

Amazingly soon after this discovery, in 1994, the gene was cloned. In that same year, a second gene was discovered, BRCA2. BRCA2 is less common than BRCA1. While BRCA1 affects only women, and also carries ovarian cancer, BRCA2 carries only breast cancer, and it can affect both women and men.

At first the researchers believed that anyone with the BRCA1 gene had an 80 percent lifetime risk of getting breast cancer based on their studies of families with a lot of breast and ovarian cancer.[10] Additional studies were then done, not just on women from families with an obvious high risk, but on women who had the gene but came from less clear situations—they had perhaps one or two relatives with breast cancer. They found, predictably, that the risk was commensurately lower in this group—more like a 30 to 50 percent chance.[11]

But why weren't *all* the carriers getting breast cancer? The word we have to describe this variability is *penetrance*. Whether or not the breast cancer gene develops depends on whether the mutation in the gene has an effect. We don't know what causes this difference in penetrance, but it probably relates to the fact that some of these people need an additional genetic alteration before the gene turns cancerous. As we noted in Chapter 13, several mutations in sequence are probably needed to get breast cancer (Fig. 14-2). For example, initially you'd be susceptible to a mutation caused by hormones; the second mutation would be caused by diet. The person with genetic breast cancer has passed the gene on to her daughter, so the girl is born with her first mutation and only needs the second to get breast cancer. If the second mutation were something that could be altered (e.g., diet, which we'll discuss in Chapter 15), it would be possible that changing the situation (e.g., switching to a different diet) really could prevent her from getting breast cancer. Unfortunately, at this stage we have no way of determining what the sequence is likely to be, or who is vulnerable to which risk factors, or if a different diet even works. But it's interesting

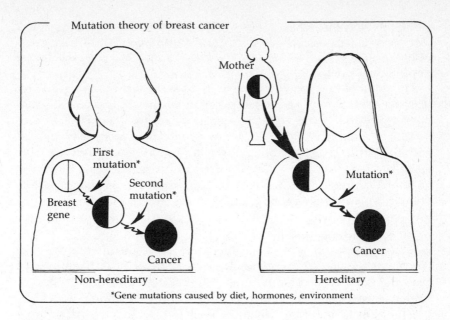

FIGURE 14-2

to think about, and if it turns out to be true it would tell us a lot about the link between environment and genetics.

There are over 100 mutations in each of the genes, just as the same word can be mistyped in a number of different ways. Shortly after the discovery of BRCA1 and 2, a researcher in Washington, D.C., studied a group of local residents who were Ashkenazi Jews (Jews whose ancestry is Eastern European).[12] He had about 800 vials of blood left over from testing that had been done years earlier for Tay-Sachs disease, a condition that Ashkenazi Jews are particularly prone to. These were both men and women, and they had no particular family histories of breast cancer. (Men can carry the genes for breast cancer, though they usually don't get the disease.) He ran the gene test and found that about 1 percent had mutations for BRCA1. Of these, the vast majority were one of two mutations, like a word always mistyped in one of the same two ways.

One of these BRCA1 mutations was 185delHG; the other, 617delIT. BRCA1 soon became known as "the Jewish gene." But this is a misnomer, in two ways. A more accurate phrase would be "the Ashkenazi mutation"—it isn't a gene itself but two of its mutations, and Sephardic Jews aren't particularly susceptible to either mutation.

Mutations of this sort are caused by what's known as the *founder effect,* because they're indications that there's been a lot of intermarriage within the population. The founder is the first person who got the gene, inadvertently "founding" it, and then passed it down to her or his descendents. Because of the intermarriage, the gene has lasted through many generations.

This kind of effect isn't exclusive to Ashkenazi Jews. When the researchers started looking at other populations they found similar situations. In Iceland[13] there's a lot of intermarriage, and there is also a predominant mutation of BRCA2. (Only 9 percent of people in Iceland with the BRCA gene have BRCA1, while 54 percent have BRCA2. This is the reverse of the case in most other countries, in which BRCA1 is far more common than BRCA2.) In Norway it's even more specific. Though Norwegians[14] get both BRCA genes, which mutation a person gets depends on which fjord she lives on. One fjord has one mutation, while another has one of the others.

Going back to our typo image, there are 300 to 400 different possible typos with the BRCA1 or 2 genes. It's as though all the Ashkenazi Jews used the same typewriter, with an "e" that didn't work. All the Icelanders used a different typewriter, on which the "t" didn't work.

All of this is important when it comes to testing. If you're from an Ashkenazi family and have breast or ovarian cancer, instead of trying to find any of the 300 to 400 possible mutations, the doctors look only for that one letter—that one typo—and it's much easier to test for. But if you're not, they have to study the whole paragraph to find the typo, and it's more time-consuming, and thus expensive, to test.

In some cases, there are mutations whose effects, if any, we haven't yet determined. Even within the known mutations of BRCA1, we can't be sure. Suppose the mutation is one that hasn't been well studied and might end up being a harmless mutation—you'd still test positive for BRCA1. Again, as research continues, we'll know more and more about this, but we don't have answers now.

Testing

The fact that we're still in the process of studying BRCA1 and 2, that it's still a work-in-progress, is important to know if you're considering getting tested. If you get tested and have the gene, we really don't know how to interpret it. We don't know whether to tell you you have a 30 percent or an 80 percent risk.

Thus, at the same time that we are researching the test, we're using it clinically. We aren't yet clear *who* should be tested, when they should be tested, or why they should be tested. If you test positive, we don't know how much of a risk that gives you. If you test negative, it doesn't mean you don't have *a* breast cancer gene, it just means you don't have BRCA1 or 2. You could have BRCA3 or 4, which we haven't discovered yet.

So all we can do is look for "typos" in these two different paragraphs. If you happen to have a typo in *another* paragraph, and that mutation causes breast cancer, we won't know it. Or if you have a typo that doesn't change the meaning of the sentence, you might test positive and not get breast cancer. With each new bit of discovery, the answers to those questions can change.

If you do want to be tested, it makes sense to find out if there is a breast cancer gene in your family by having a relative with breast cancer tested first. If your mother has breast cancer, is tested, and discovers that she doesn't have a genetic alteration, there's no need for you to get tested. If we find that she has a mutation in the BRCA1 gene and you don't, then we know you didn't inherit that gene. Again, that's no guarantee you won't get breast cancer. And again, she could pass on a gene we don't know about; we don't even have absolute assurance that *her* cancer came from her BRCA1 gene. It could be a complete fluke, like a flight attendant who gets killed in a plane crash when she's off duty and just a passenger.

An interesting article in the *Annals of Surgery* looked into the responses of women who were considering getting tested for BRCA genes and were counseled about it beforehand at the testing center.[15] Even after they had talked it over with the counselors, who had explained all the limitations of what testing could reveal, most women still retained the belief that if they were tested negative they wouldn't ever get breast cancer. When you desperately want something to be true, you often mentally edit what you hear to make it say what you want it to.

Whatever the limits of counseling, however, it's far more frightening when women go into testing without it. And for the most part, they do. Says J. D. Iglehart, "Physicians without genetic training are more likely to provide testing and least likely to provide counseling."[16] And in fact, few doctors have had genetic training.

In the Iglehart study, women who were likely to be positive were asked before testing to estimate their risk of having the gene. The patients far overestimated their risk. The doctors thought most patients had zero risk. They thought a few had a 10 percent risk, and a few had a 20 percent risk. The patients thought they all had a 100 percent risk. So while the doctors underrated the risk, the patients vastly overrated it.

Interestingly, women who go to those doctors who *do* have expertise—the ones who tend to work in clinics set up for such testing, where counseling is part of the process—are much less likely after the counseling to get tested. If they recognize the limits of what the test can do, they reconsider. Women who go to their local doctors and get no counseling are more likely to go ahead and have it done. Some people have asked why the test for the breast cancer gene is only being offered to women at high risk for the disease, and isn't being suggested for all women with breast cancer, or even all women in the country.

Part of the reason is that the chance of having the gene is so low for most people that it wouldn't be worth it. A study by Beth Newman, reported in the *Journal of the American Medical Association,* looked not at high risk women with BRCA1 but at a general group of women between 20 and 74 with breast cancer, to see how many had the mutation.[17] Only 3 percent had the BRCA1 gene.

J. Peto and his group did a study in the U.K. in the summer of 1999, looking at women with hereditary breast cancer[18]. They divided them into age groups and looked at the correlation between hereditary cancer and the BRCA genes. In the group most likely to have the gene, women who had gotten cancer before they were 36, only 3.5 percent had BRCA1 and 2.4 percent had BRCA2. In women between 36 and 45, 1.9 percent had BRCA1 and 2.2 percent had BRCA2. So it's a very small percentage, even among young women.

The Risks of Getting Tested

What precisely are the risks? Well, one is financial. The testing is expensive—and insurance companies don't pay for it. Typically, it costs $2,400 in the United States. If a particular mutation is identified, then other family members can get tested for around $400. That's because the really hard work is searching for the specific mutation. It's like proofreading the whole manuscript to find the typo: once you know where it is, finding it in other copies is fairly easy.

Initially there was great fear that there would be insurance discrimination against women who had been tested. So far this has not proved to be the case. Still, it would be smart to check out the laws in your state and to check out the policy of your insurance company before proceeding.

Further, it isn't only you who will need to deal with the consequences of your decision. It becomes a family issue. If I get tested and I'm positive, it will have implications for my sisters—who may or may not want to get tested. It has implications for my daughter.

If you choose to be tested, and know you have the gene, you will then need to decide what to do with the information. Should you start getting regular mammograms and physical exams? If your family has a history of breast cancer, you should be doing that anyway. If you do have the gene, you have a number of options. You can simply be frequently monitored to see whether or not you do get cancer: remember, even in that 80 percent category, 20 percent of women don't get the cancer. Should you have your breasts and/or ovaries removed? Preventive oophorectomy and/or mastectomy may help. You can take tamoxifen for five years. All these will be discussed at length in Chapter 18. Luckily there are many other options being studied so this should all be clearer by the next edition of this book.

If you feel strongly that you want to get tested, then you should be sure and do it at a research center. Don't go to your gynecologist or primary care doctor, or to the medical school in the next town. Even if it costs a lot to fly to wherever the closest research center is, do it. You'll only do this once, and it will affect the rest of your life, so do it well. A research center will have counseling, and they'll do the tests appropriately, giving you the most accurate information that's possible at this time. To find such a center, you can check with a nearby medical school. You can also call 1-800-FOR CANCER (see Appendix B, National Cancer Institute). There is a website that lists genetic counselors for cancer geographically throughout the U.S. (see Appendix B).

When you yourself have breast cancer, the emotional conflict becomes even more intense. You tend to think that you're unlucky and that you're bound to get it again, so you think that you must have the bad gene. Further, your own psychological issues get mixed into your perceptions. Were you mean to your mother when she had breast cancer, so now you're being punished by inheriting a killer gene? The most sophisticated of us are to some extent trapped by our own unconscious expectations.

There are, of course, more rational reasons for women with breast cancer to consider getting tested. They might want to know if others in their family are likely to get it. Or they might be considering having children, and the possibility of passing on a breast cancer gene could play a role in that decision. Women with cancer in one breast are more likely to get it in the other, and they might want to consider getting double mastectomies if they know they have the gene. In women without the gene, the risk of a second primary is between 0.5 and 1 percent a year, and 15 to 25 percent over their lifetime. For someone with the gene, it's probably between 1 and 2 percent a year, 30 to 50 percent over their lifetime. Similarly, a woman with BRCA1 might want to have her ovaries removed. People with the BRCA1 gene also have a slightly higher risk of getting colon cancer as well. So if you know you have the gene, you should also be getting regular colonoscopies. Some studies indicate that prostate cancer may also be more common among people with the gene.

It doesn't make sense for every woman with breast cancer to be tested since hereditary breast cancer is so rare. Still, there are some profiles showing your likelihood of carrying a genetic alteration. If you are a Jewish woman younger than 40 with breast cancer, there is about a 33 percent chance that you are a carrier. If you are not Jewish and have breast cancer before 30 you have a 12 percent chance of having a mutation. If you develop bilateral breast cancer between ages 40 and 50 and have a first- or second-degree relative with breast or ovarian cancer before 50 there is a 42 percent chance that you carry a mutation. If you got breast cancer after 50 there is a lower risk that it is hereditary; in fact, having more than two breast cancers in first- or second-degree relatives after 50 only gives you a risk of about 2 percent of having a mutation.[19][20]

And if you don't have breast cancer, who should get tested? I find this a difficult question to answer. The American Society of Clinical Oncology has recommended getting tested in several cases where there is a high probability that the test might be positive:

1. Women with more than two first-degree relatives with breast cancer and one or more with ovarian cancer, diagnosed at any age.
2. Those with more than three first-degree relatives with breast cancer diagnosed before age 50.
3. Those with two sisters who have been diagnosed with breast or ovarian cancer before age 50.
4. Women who have a first-degree relative who has had two breast cancers, two ovarian cancers, or breast and ovarian cancer.

If you decide to be tested, there are several possible results. Most satisfying are the true positives and true negatives. In a true positive the test is positive for a known mutation. In a true negative it is negative for a mutation that has been identified to be present in the woman's family. In this case she knows she did not inherit the family gene. More complex is the situation where no known mutation is found. Then you do not know whether there is a gene but it is not one of the ones we know how to look for, or if there isn't a genetic alteration. Also, genetic alterations of unknown clinical significance can be found that are abnormal but have not been linked to breast cancer before. In both of these situations the woman is left with as many questions as answers. This is a situation where ductal lavage (see Chapter 17) may be helpful. It can take you beyond the statistics of risk and tell you what your ductal lining cells look like and whether they appear to be en route to cancer.

And what should you do with the information? Luckily in the past year we have identified several prevention strategies from prophylactic oophorectomies to chemoprevention. These will be discussed further in Chapter 18.

The question of testing depends on you, your family, and your values. The answer will be different for each person. If you are considering it, by all means get counseling so that you can get up-to-date information on the risks and benefits for you and your family.

What Kind of Cancer?

One of the important questions still to be answered in our study of the BRCA genes is about prognosis. Does the woman with a cancer gene have a different *kind* of cancer than the one who doesn't have the gene? There is some evidence that BRCA2 cancers are more likely to be estrogen receptor positive, while BRCA1 cancers tend to be estrogen receptor negative. This is a concern, because tamoxifen doesn't usually work very well on estrogen receptor negative tumors. This goes back to the need for true early detection (see Chapter 17). All tumors start out estrogen receptor positive: it is only as they grow that they lose their receptivity. Normal tissue is always positive. Ninety percent of atypical hyperplasia is positive, as is 50 percent of DCIS. Only 30 percent of invasive cancer is positive. The genes get less and less receptive as the process progresses.

The strange thing is that even though these cancers *appear* to be more aggressive than most others, they don't tend to act that way. The mortality rates are about the same. As with so many other things here, we don't know why. Maybe it's because coming from a family with a breast cancer history causes women to have their breasts checked more often, to have more mammograms, and so on. Maybe not. There is some indication that medullary carcinomas (see Chapter 21), which tend to look very aggressive yet to not always act that badly, are more common in women with BRCA1. If that turns out to be true, it might at least partially explain the mortality rates.

HORMONAL RISK FACTORS

Aside from genetic risk factors, the other most obvious group of risk factors is hormonal. We know that hormones play a large part in breast cancer because it's a form of cancer common in women and rare in men, and, as we discussed in Chapter 1, women's breasts undergo a complex hormonal evolution that men's don't. We don't yet understand what the hormonal risk factors are, but we have some interesting clues. We know that it has something to do with age and menstrual cycle: the younger a woman is at her first period, and the older she is when she goes into menopause, the more likely she is to get breast cancer (Table 14-5). It seems that the longer a woman has reproductive levels of hormones, the more prone she is to breast cancer. If she menstruates for more than 40 years, she seems to have a particularly high risk. If your ovaries are removed early, and no hormone replacement are given, your risk of breast cancer is greatly reduced.[21] It's not exactly a cure-all, however, since it would also greatly increase your danger of osteoporosis. If you've had a hysterectomy, it may or may not influence your vulnerability to breast cancer, depending upon whether your ovaries, as well as your uterus, are removed. If you still have ovaries, your body is still going through hormonal cycles, even though you have no periods.

Pregnancy also appears to affect breast cancer risk. Women who have never been pregnant seem to be more at risk than women who have had a child before 30. And women who have their first pregnancies after 30 have a greater risk than women who have never been pregnant at all. The hormones of a pregnancy carried to term will mature the breast tissue in a young woman. The same hormones after 30 may actually stimulate breast tissue that has already been mutated. Some studies indicate that a pregnancy that ends in a miscarriage or abortion slightly increases your risk, while other studies have not been able to confirm this.[22,23]

The key seems to be the amount of time between the first period and the first pregnancy (Fig. 14-3). There are a lot of theories about why this is so. One possible explanation is that between menarche and the first pregnancy the breast tissue is especially sensitive to carcinogens. This seems to be true. As we'll discuss a little later, such factors as diet, alcohol consumption, and radiation exposure all seem to have a greater effect on a woman's breasts between her first period and her first pregnancy than they do later. So it may indeed be that the "developing breast" is more susceptible to carcinogens than the breast that has gone through its complete hormonal development. This increased sensitivity may relate to the breast cells' capability of mutating up until the first pregnancy. There may be something about the first pregnancy of a young woman that stops the cells from being able to sustain a mutation; thus, the more time cells have to sustain a mutation, the greater the chance that they'll mutate in response to a carcinogen and in a way that develops into cancer.

Dr. Malcolm Pike thinks the total number of ovulatory cycles a woman has gone through is a factor in her vulnerability to breast can-

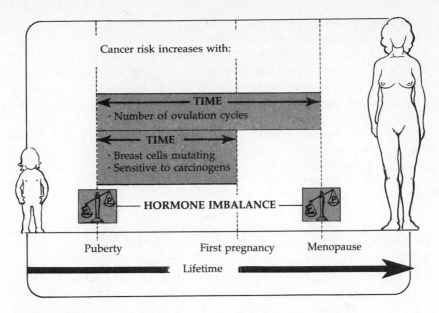

FIGURE 14-3

cer, since it's the length of time between menarche and menopause that seems to count.[24] In fact, a Swedish study found that the total number of regular menstrual cycles prior to the first full pregnancy was a better predictor of risk than age at first period or age at first pregnancy.[25] This may be because early menarche is associated with rapid onset of ovulatory menstrual cycles.[26] Within two years of early menarche (ages 8–11) all cycles become ovulatory; however, late menarche is associated with delayed onset of regular ovulatory cycles—that is, for young women who are 13 or older at menarche, no more than 50 percent of their cycles are ovulatory four years after their first period. Estrogen doesn't always become elevated if ovulation does not occur. Also, it is usually accompanied by a shortened *luteal* phase, which means less cumulative exposure to high levels of hormones. This has been shown by Leslie Bernstein at the University of Southern California. She suggests that this is another explanation for the difference in breast cancer rates in white and Japanese women in the United States. Asian women have a later age at menarche and menstrual cycles that are on average two days longer than those of white women in the U.S. (30 vs. 28 days). This increase in days is almost completely in the *follicular* phase, where estrogen levels are lower.[27]

Another factor relating to the number of menstrual cycles is breast feeding. Recent studies have shown that women who breast-feed for a long period of time (more than six consecutive years) have a decreased risk of breast cancer.[28] In addition, women who have had early pregnancies and have breast-fed have a decreased risk of subsequent breast cancer.[29] This is probably related to fewer ovulatory cycles at a crucial time in reproductive life.

As you see, we're still very much in the theorizing stage: as yet, we don't know why there is this vulnerable time in a woman's life and why or how internal hormones affect breast cancer. Theories are interesting, but more useful to scientists than to individual women, who can't control heredity, ethnicity, or menarche.

15

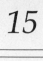

Risk Factors: External

There are two overall categories of risk factors, genetic and external. We discussed genetic factors in the previous chapter. Equally important are external, environmental factors which can create a breast-cancer-causing mutation or accelerate the growth of breast cancer—or, for that matter, prevent the growth of breast cancer. Diet, alcohol, and certain medications carry risks over which we have some control. The amount of fat and liquor you consume may play a role in increasing your susceptibility to breast cancer. Hormones taken by postmenopausal women, as well as birth control pills, are also a matter of choice and are being studied in relation to breast cancer. Radiation has always been known to increase cancer risk, and may or may not be something over which you have control.

DIET

The concept that dietary fat could cause breast cancer has been around for a long time. It began with the observation that breast cancer is lower in Japan than it is in the United States, and that the incidence increases when women move from Japan to the United States. As proponents of this theory note, one of the many cultural differences in the immigrant group has been diet. Charts of fat intake in different countries overlaid on charts of breast cancer incidence appear to confirm the association.

But, as I've mentioned a number of times here, this kind of parallel doesn't necessarily mean cause-and-effect. Northern Western European countries do tend to have both a high-fat diet and an increase in breast cancer. But they also have a high-calorie diet. Further, they tend to have the same genetic background, one that has been passed on to us in the New World. These, or other factors, might be equally or even solely significant.

The high-fat breast cancer hypothesis was put to the test in rats, and it was found that the total calorie count seems to be more important than the amount of fat. Further tests on human subjects suggest that this is true in women as well.

Some researchers feel that the *type* of fat may be important, but a recent analysis of the Nurses' Health Study failed to find an association between fat of any type and breast cancer.[1] Although the large numbers of women in this study increase its power to demonstrate a relationship, it is an observational study and thus not as conclusive as we'd like (see Chapter 12). The Women's Health Initiative, which is randomized and prospective, has the best chance of answering the fat and breast cancer question.

It won't, however, be the definitive study by any means. Postmenopausal women are more likely than younger ones to get breast cancer, but the factors that give them the cancer may, as we discussed earlier, begin during adolescence. So if it turns out that changing her diet at age 55 doesn't affect a woman's chance of getting breast cancer, that doesn't necessarily mean fat has no role in the disease. We need another study, one that starts in adolescence and monitors the young woman's diet throughout her life.

Getting such a study seems difficult at this point. My 12-year-old isn't fond of advice about what to eat. Still, we must figure out a way to create such a study. We desperately need research to tell us not only exactly what the culprits are in our Westernized high-fat diet, but also when they do their dirty work. If it's during adolescence, then it's pointless for us to encourage 50-year-old women to change their diets as a method of lessening breast cancer risk.

Of course, the fact that fat intake probably doesn't cause breast cancer doesn't mean you should scarf down a pound cake and a wheel of Brie every day. It still plays a large role in heart disease and other illnesses. And calorie count, as the rat study showed, does play a role in breast cancer. If you can find a way to eat high-fat foods and not get a lot of calories, you're a lot cleverer than I am!

Factors Other Than Fat

Some studies suggest that the amount of fat we eat may be a more indirect cause of breast cancer. Being high in calories, fat creates greater weight. Some data show that the taller and fatter a postmenopausal woman is, the more susceptible she is to breast cancer.

So it's quite possible that the problem isn't fat itself, but overall nutrition: people who eat more may be more vulnerable to breast cancer. Overnutrition might also have some connection with some of the other risk factors: girls with lower food consumption stay thinner and often begin menstruating later than more heavily nourished girls. People who eat more also tend to be those who can afford to—those with an overall higher standard of living, who appear to be at greater risk for breast cancer.

If fat intake does indeed increase the risk of breast cancer, what makes it happen? There are a number of theories. Some researchers think it changes the metabolism of estrogen. According to one study, people with a high-fat diet tend to have more estrogen in their blood and low urinary excretion of estrogen; vegetarians who eat dairy foods excrete more estrogen, leaving less in the blood, and people on macrobiotic diets, which include a very low amount of fat, have even lower levels of estrogen in their blood and secrete less in their urine.[2] As I noted in Chapter 1, your fat cells can make estrogen, so it is also possible that if you're obese you have an oversupply of estrogen, which could increase your vulnerability to cancer. Studies attempting to confirm this hypothesis have been inconsistent.

It's also possible that cancer cells grow better in an environment with a lot of overnourished cells, and the fatter you are the more such cells there are for the cancer cells to grow with. There's also some evidence that among women with breast cancer those on low-fat diets have a better prognosis than those on high-fat diets. The WINS study, which randomizes survivors to a low-fat diet or no change, will give us an important answer to this question.

It may be that fiber, rather than fat, is the important element. Usually diets very high in fiber are very low in fat. It may be that with a low-fat diet it's the fiber or the high-complex carbohydrates or the vegetables you're replacing the fat with that are helping you. Some evidence suggests that soy protein may be a protective element as well.[3] Maybe the problem is not that the Japanese start eating fat, but that they stop eating tofu. There's also growing evidence that certain vegetables, particularly antioxidants, which contain vitamins A, C, and E, may be protective against breast cancer.[4]

Vitamin A, particularly the vegetable form, betacarotene, seems to decrease the incidence of several cancers. People with lower betacarotene levels have been shown to get more lung cancer, for example. It's not clear that massive doses of vitamin A or beta carotene supplements will change anyone's risk of breast cancer. A recent study using 4HPR, which is a form of vitamin A, in women who had had breast cancer showed no decrease in second cancers, although there was a hint that there may be different, more beneficial effects in premenopausal women than in postmenopausal women. Vegetables with vitamin A include broccoli, kale, carrots, and lettuce. Vitamin C and folic acid both appear to be good against all cancers.

The National Cancer Institute has a major plan, the "five-a-day" plan, encouraging people to eat five servings of fruits and vegetables a day. That can sound pretty daunting, but when you find out what they call a serving, it's not all that bad—one carrot is a "serving."

The other possibility is that it isn't the food at all that contributes to breast cancer but the carcinogens and hormones that are in the food. Beef in this country, for example, still has artificial hormones. Unfortunately meat isn't the only problem. Fish are very much contaminated, since most of our fresh and coastal waters are contaminated. Among other things, there is a lot of mercury in the fish we eat. Even vegetables aren't that safe, since they're sprayed with pesticides.

Overall, it seems likely from the material in the various studies that weight and calorie intake do have some effect on your vulnerability to breast cancer. While there isn't nearly as solid proof as there is with smoking and lung cancer, the data are strong enough to make it worthwhile to seriously consider cutting back your calories and animal fat consumption—especially when you consider that animal fat has proved to be a factor in many other illnesses, and nothing good has

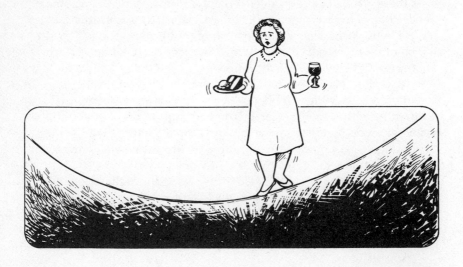

ever been shown about high animal fat consumption, except perhaps that it tastes nice. If you're the parent of a teen or preteen daughter, it may be particularly wise to consider encouraging her to eat a healthy diet, since the evidence suggests that much of the damage may be done early in life. You may do well to encourage your kids to spend a little less time at MacDonald's, and to eat a bit more low-fat, nutritional food. Don't, however, expect miracles. Even if changing your diet does have an effect, it is likely to be a small one.

ALCOHOL CONSUMPTION

Alcohol, the other major dietary substance that has been associated with breast cancer, has garnered much less attention—which is ironic, since the data are more solid. A number of studies suggest that drinking alcoholic beverages, even in moderate amounts, may increase your risk of breast cancer. Walt Willett of the Harvard School of Public Health conducted a study of the dietary habits of a group of nurses (cited earlier in this chapter).[5] He studied 89,538 nurses between 34 and 59 years old for four years after examining their nutritional habits. He found that consuming hard liquor, beer, and wine appeared to increase women's risk of breast cancer. Women who usually had between three and nine drinks a week had a 1.3 increase in relative risk of breast cancer (1 being the norm; see Chapter 14 for a description of relative risk). Those who had more than nine drinks a week had a 1.6 increase. It was interesting to note that in this study drinking had little effect on those women who were already at high risk—the effect was mainly on those women with no risk factors.

Also, women under 55 with no other risk factors who had more than nine drinks a week had a more dramatic increase than those over 55: they had a 2.5 increase—two and a half times the susceptibility to breast cancer of nondrinkers with no risk factors. (In all these cases, Dr. Willett looked to see if there were dietary differences as well: there weren't.)

Studies in France and Italy, where wine is consumed regularly by virtually everyone, have supported this connection. Women in these countries do have a higher incidence of breast cancer than do women in the U.S., though it's a fairly slight increase—only 1.2 to 1.9 times.

A recent analysis of six prospective studies found a consistent increase in the risk of breast cancer when larger amounts of alcohol are drunk.[6] This is regardless of the type of drink—beer, wine, and hard liquor all contribute to breast cancer risk, and as your consumption rises, so does your risk. It would be good to have a randomized controlled study, but I can't figure out how we'd do it. Consigning one group of subjects to be teetotalers and another to get drunk every day might create some legal and logistical problems. But the studies we do have are fairly good, and given the other problems alcohol consumption can cause, cutting back on drinking is probably a pretty good idea anyway.

As with fat consumption, the main effect of alcohol in increasing breast cancer risk may be during the vulnerable period of youth. More precise information as to when and how the effect manifests itself is needed before we can make concrete recommendations. Whether to stop drinking or not is unfortunately one of the many decisions we all must make on inadequate information. The risk increase isn't great, but it definitely exists. You alone know how much pleasure you get from your glass of wine or beer, and how alarmed you are at the thought of breast cancer. If it's not all that important to you to drink, you might want to reduce your alcohol consumption to a glass of champagne on New Year's Eve and major celebrations. Although it may be wise for any number of reasons to discourage your daughters from drinking, this is an area, like many in parenting, where you may not have a lot of control.

RADIATION

One of the known risk factors for breast cancer, as well as a variety of other cancers, is radiation. At least three major studies have confirmed that there is indeed a link between radiation and increased risk of breast cancer.

The first study came out of one of the major tragedies of the 20th century—the bombings of Hiroshima and Nagasaki at the end of World War II. The people in the immediate area of the bombings died instantly, or shortly after the bombs were dropped. But it has become evident that those within a 10-kilometer radius of the bomb sites developed far more cancer than others in comparable populations, and scientists began studying these survivors to learn more about the dangers of radiation. They measured the amount of radiation these people had been exposed to, and then followed them over the years to see what cancers they developed.[7]

The most recent analysis of this sample reports that women exposed to the bomb have a relative risk of developing breast cancer of 14.6 per unit of radiation if it happened before they were 20 and 3.0 if it happened when they were older.[8] The effects were greatest among women in their teens and early 20s, and nearly nonexistent in women in their 50s and 60s. Recent reports have indicated an increased risk in the women who were less than 10 years old at the time of the exposure.

The effect took longer to be revealed because it didn't appear until the women had reached the age at which breast cancer normally occurs. This supports other findings about the particular vulnerability of the developing breast to carcinogenic agents.

An interesting new finding among the A bomb survivors is that those who had early full-term pregnancies were at significantly lower risk than those who hadn't. Remarkably, this protection occurred among women who were exposed as children, as well as among those exposed as adults. Here is confirmation that the maturation of breast tissue that occurs during a full-term pregnancy drastically reduces the ability of a cell to progress to cancer, even if it has received earlier damage that would predispose it to breast cancer.[9] This provides us with yet more evidence that it often takes more than one factor to cause a breast cancer.

Other studies of radiation exposure support the atom bomb data. The first is a Canadian study that looked at women who had been treated for tuberculosis with fluoroscopy.[10] This was a common treatment in the 1930s and 1940s before we knew of the dangers of radiation and saw it as something of a magic cure-all. The typical treatment for TB was to collapse the infected lung to rest it, and then check it with x rays every day to see how it was doing. When the women were studied in the 1970s, they were found to have an increased incidence of breast cancer. I came across a similar case in my own practice. A 58-year-old patient I diagnosed with breast cancer had had TB in her early 20s. She lived in France and was treated with intensive radiation in the sanitarium. Her two best friends at the sanitarium, treated with the same radiation therapy she was given, also have developed breast cancer.

Another study examined a group of 606 women in Rochester, New York, who had suffered postpartum mastitis—painfully inflamed breasts (Chapter 6)—and had been given radiation averaging between 50 and 450 rads for both breasts to alleviate their pain.[11] They too had a rate of breast cancer higher than that of the general population. And the risk was dose related. This study is interesting for a second reason. The radiation was given after the first pregnancy, which should have been protective. But nonetheless it was during lactation, a time of high activity in the breast.

There are other studies confirming the existence of radiation-induced breast cancer. One showed an increase in the disease among women with scoliosis who had had a lot of x rays to monitor their backs during the crucial time of puberty.[12] Another showed an increase among a group of women who had had radiation therapy on their chests for acne—also during puberty.[13] Still another study looked at women who had their thymuses radiated in infancy or early childhood to shrink them. (The thymus, a normal gland in the middle of the chest, shrinks with age. At one time before we realized that it shrank normally, radiation therapy was used to shrink it.)[14]

All these studies show that the danger is from exposure to moderate doses of radiation (10–500 rads), and the last two show that the danger is only to the area of the body at which the radiation has been aimed. Thus people exposed to radiation for cancer of the cervix did not show an increased rate of breast cancer.[15] Obviously the survivors of Nagasaki and Hiroshima had their whole bodies exposed to the radiation, and, in fact, they have suffered increased vulnerability to virtually all kinds of cancer. Another interesting finding in all these studies is the long latency period. The excess risk does not appear until the age at which breast cancer commonly occurs. This suggests that radiation is only part of the early picture and that other moderating influences come later and affect the development of breast cancer. The duration of the increased risk from radiation is also not known, but in the atomic bomb survivors, fluoroscopy patients, and mastitis patients, it appears to have lasted at least 35 years from the time of exposure.

This kind of exposure is very different from the kind you get with occasional diagnostic x rays such as chest x rays and mammograms. Many people are legitimately concerned about getting such x rays, but it's a mistake to throw out a highly useful diagnostic tool. Remember that the danger comes with a total cumulative dose of radiation. If you had a chest x ray every week for two years you probably would increase your risk of getting breast cancer. But the danger of leaving pneumonia undetected, if you have reason to believe it may exist, is far greater than any danger from infrequent chest x rays. Similarly, the level of radiation in up-to-date mammograms (1/4 of a rad) won't increase your risk of breast cancer, except in very rare instances where you carry a gene that makes you more sensitive to radiation.

Radiation to treat cancer puts us at the other end of the spectrum: very high levels of radiation are used, on the order of 8,000 rads. In these cases, however, the risk of radiation is far outweighed by the risk of cancer. For example, radiation is used to treat Hodgkin's disease, a cancer of the lymph nodes. By itself and in conjunction with chemotherapy it has been responsible for many cures. However, some women who had this treatment many years ago are now showing up with breast cancer. We suspect that the radiation to their chests, which saved their lives, is responsible now for their second cancers.[16] In a study examining second cancers after treatment for childhood Hodgkin's disease, breast cancer was reported as the most common solid tumor detected. Women in the group studied had 75 times greater risk of developing breast cancer than did women in the general public, and the cancers almost all developed in the area in which the radiation had been done. The younger a woman had been when she was radiated, the higher her risk. A second study showed the relative risk of breast cancer after 15 years of follow-up was 11.4 for women who had been under 30 when they were treated and 41.9 for women who had been under 20 when they were treated. When you consider that most risk factors are 0.3, this increase is considerable.

Women who have received radiation exposure to their breasts, especially at a young age, might consider some of the current prevention practices such as taking tamoxifen for five years or even getting prophylactic mastectomy. If those approaches seem too drastic (as well they might), they should certainly make sure that they get regular breast exams and mammography beginning 10 years following their radiation.

The type of cancer that occurs after radiation therapy for Hodgkin's disease is similar to the type found in the general population, with 81 percent of lesions detectable by mammography. It usually occurs when the woman is about 40 (approximately 15 years after treatment). While it is for the most part unilateral, it occasionally will occur in both breasts. Treatment is usually a mastectomy because the woman has already had radiation to the chest and so cannot get radiation in that area again.

It won't be surprising if some of the children treated today for cancer with radiation in the chest region will also eventually have an increase in breast cancers.[17] This is unfortunate, but since radiation is probably responsible for their being around long enough to get a second cancer, few of those patients are likely to have regrets.

HORMONE MEDICATIONS

Birth Control Pills

We discussed earlier the effects of your body's hormonal system on breast cancer. Since your own hormones can affect breast cancer, it stands to reason that hormones taken externally as drugs will also have an effect—and studies have shown this to be the case.

The birth control pill, originally seen as the magic solution to unwanted pregnancy, quickly became vilified as its negative side effects became apparent. As is often the case, the reality of the pill falls somewhere between its panacea and demon images. The pill did indeed, especially in its early forms, seem to contribute to a number of illnesses, including stroke (especially in combination with cigarette smoking in women over 30). Later studies, however, have suggested that it may also be useful in protecting against certain diseases such as ovarian cancer. It stops ovulation, and the more you ovulate the more chance you have of getting ovarian cancer. So if you take the birth control pill and decrease the total number of ovulations, you can decrease your risk. It has consistently been shown to reduce endometrial cancer as well.[18][19]

Part of the problem in discussing "the pill" as though it were a single entity is that, like some other inventions, it has gone through many permutations. The earlier pills used much more estrogen and progestin than current pills do: we've changed both the amounts and the proportions of those hormones. So early findings aren't necessarily applicable to the pill used today. A study that says it's looking at women who have been on the pill for 10 or 20 years is actually likely to be looking at women who have been on a number of different pills at different times—which explains in part why we seem to get so many contradictory results with studies on the relationship between breast cancer and the pill. Dr. Leslie Bernstein, Professor of Preventive Medicine at the University of Southern California, along with Dr. Malcolm Pike, did a careful meta-analysis of birth control pill use and breast cancer risk and found that total months of use is the most important factor.[20] But even with that the increased risk is about 3.3 percent per year of use or 38 percent (relative risk of 1.38) for 10 years of use. This risk may be worth it for the benefit of a convenient, sure method of birth control. This is a decision only you can make, weighing any evidence of increased breast cancer against the risks of other contraceptives, of unwanted births, or of abortion.

DES

Another external hormone women have taken is the estrogen DES. It was used in the 1940s–1960s to increase fertility and to prevent miscarriage. A 1984 study showed a slight increase—1.4—in breast cancer among women who took DES while pregnant.[21] Since there's a lot of estrogen going through your body anyway when you're pregnant, it's not clear why an increased external dosage would be harmful, but it appears to have been, at least for some women. One theory is that exposure to estrogen during the period of rapid growth of breast tissue during pregnancy may increase risk.[22] We don't know yet what effects DES had on the breast cancer rate among daughters of women who'd taken it, since the daughters are only now approaching the age when breast cancer is most common. There has been an increase in vaginal cancer among this population, but it's not as aggressive as we once thought it was.

Postmenopausal Hormones

During the '40s and '50s it was popular to give estrogen to any woman going through menopause—gynecologists would routinely prescribe it whether the woman had any complaints or not. And since in those days most women did whatever their doctors told them to do, they took it. Then studies appeared linking long use of Premarin with uterine cancer: there was a big scandal, and everyone stopped taking it. Then, as the baby boomers began to hit middle age, it came back, with a vengeance.

Like birth control pills, estrogen therapy pills have been changed over the years. Provera, a progestin, has been added to balance the estrogen, and it seems to help protect against uterine cancer. Unfortunately there is no evidence that Provera acts the same way on the breast as it does on the endometrium (the uterine lining).

I have some problems with the idea that we're supposed to keep taking these hormones indefinitely—there is a reason that menopause exists in the first place. Our bodies need high levels of hormones to reproduce and they need the downshift to a more reasonable level postmenopausally (see Chapter 1). Those who favor hormone therapy argue that we're not "supposed" to live long enough to go into menopause in the first place: in the old days people died in their 30s and 40s. But in fact people *didn't* all die in their 30s and 40s. The "average life expectancy" was low—as low as 32 in 1640. But that average was drawn from all deaths, and did not represent a "typical age of death." Until modern medicine came along, there were large numbers of deaths at all ages, and especially in childhood. It was no more usual to die at 35 than it was to die at 65. Men were considered fit for military service until they were 60, and a fair number of people of both genders lived into their 90s.[23,24,25] So that argument makes no sense.

Originally, we believed that the ovaries stopped functioning at menopause. But recent studies have shown that also to be a biological fallacy. It turns out that, in most women, the ovaries *don't* stop functioning. It's simply that, until recently, there was no test available that could detect lower levels of estrogen, and so it was assumed that there weren't any such levels. But most women continue to produce hormones well into their 80s—testosterone, androstenedione (both "male" hormones), and even some estrogen.

And we are starting to understand the symptoms of menopause

better as well. The traditional belief is that the symptoms of perimenopause come from low levels of hormones, but recent studies have
shown that what's really at the core of symptoms is the *fluctuation* of
hormones as the body rebalances at a new level. The transition typically takes between three and six years, and then the body settles into
its new situation.

Although menopause is perfectly natural, it has been redefined as a
disease called "estrogen deficiency," no longer seen as a normal passage of life. And since it's a disease, the assumption is that it should be
treated. In reality if "estrogen deficiency" is a disease, then all men are
sick. Imagine how they could decrease their risk of heart disease, prostate cancer, and osteoporosis if they took the "miracle drug" menopausal women are so often prescribed! Notice we even call the treatment "hormone replacement therapy," which implies we are missing
something which needs to be replaced. A far better term is "hormone
therapy": that implies rightly that these are drugs being given to treat
or prevent disease—if and when they're needed.

Symptoms vs. Prevention

It's important, when discussing hormone therapy, to differentiate between the two very distinct reasons women might want to use it:
symptom control and disease prevention. For symptom relief, hormone therapy is used to help reduce hot flashes, vaginal dryness, insomnia, night sweats—the vast range of uncomfortable, usually short-
term symptoms many women experience during their perimenopausal
years. In natural menopause, these symptoms are usually transient—
they last about three to five years. After that, your body readjusts itself
and you're fine. The use of hormones short-term (three to five years)
for women who do not have breast cancer or clotting disorders is probably safe. At the end of the period they should taper off the hormones
over six to nine months in order to ensure that the abrupt change
doesn't bring back their symptoms. In women who have had breast
cancer it is better to explore alternative methods to decrease symptoms, which we discuss at length in Chapter 31 on menopause.

Disease prevention means taking hormones—whether or not you're
experiencing any symptoms—indefinitely. Ostensibly this is done to
prevent illnesses of old age—heart disease and/or osteoporosis.

The most important concern about osteoporosis is the incidence of
hip fractures, which occur at an average age of 79. A 50-year-old white
woman has a 15 percent lifetime probability of an eventual hip fracture. If she takes estrogen (we have no good evidence about progester-

one) therapy she can reduce this by 25% so that it now becomes 11.25 percent, according to observational data.[26] Although the initial data suggested that taking estrogen from age 50 on was the only way to prevent this problem, newer data have given us many alternatives. Non-hormonal drugs have been shown to prevent vertebral fractures as well as estrogen does. In addition, data have indicated that starting estrogen at a later age, such as 70, and at half the usual dose, will yield virtually the same increase in bone density as starting at 50.[27] As this field evolves and we begin to understand bone metabolism the treatments will become more specific and beneficial. Also, there are alternatives (such as Fosamax) which have been shown to work just as well.

Heart disease may be a more cogent problem. A 50-year-old white woman has a 46 percent lifetime probability of developing, and a 31 percent chance of dying of, heart disease. Death from coronary heart disease occurs at a median age of 74 years. Observational studies have shown a lower risk of coronary heart disease among estrogen users compared to nonusers. But most of this evidence is limited. The studies looking at this are all observational and therefore flawed (see Chapter 12). Women who take hormones tend to be white, educated, upper middle class, and usually thinner than women in lower socioeconomic groups and thus have a lower risk of heart disease than the women who don't take hormones. It may well be that healthy women take hormones, not that hormones make women healthy.

It was thought that the protective effect of estrogen would be highest in women who already had coronary heart disease. The HERS study (Heart and Estrogen-Progestin Replacement Study), designed to demonstrate this, randomized women with heart disease to take either estrogen and Provera or placebo. Much to everyone's surprise the results showed that there was no benefit from taking the hormones.[28] This was followed by the ERA study of women with coronary artery disease diagnosed by angiography. Again, women randomized to estrogen showed no decrease in heart attacks.[29] Finally, the preliminary results from the Women's Health Initiative, which randomized healthy women to Premarin and Provera versus placebo, showed an increase—albeit slight—in deaths from heart attack and stroke in the hormone group.[30]

All of these data certainly call into question the benfits of HRT for women trying to prevent heart disease. Meanwhile there are alternatives here as well, from lifestyle changes to statins, drugs developed specifically to lower cholesterol and proved in randomized controlled studies to prevent heart disease. What is more important for this book is whether taking postmenopausal hormones will increase breast cancer.

Hormone Therapy as a Risk Factor for Breast Cancer

This is a question for all women, given the fear that breast cancer engenders. It's even more charged for women who are at high risk, who have had DCIS, or who have actually had breast cancer.

The first thing to consider is the quality of the evidence for a connection between breast cancer and estrogen and progesterone. From an epidemiological, biological standpoint, there's fairly good evidence. We know that women who have their ovaries removed at an early age rarely get breast cancer. The younger a woman was at her first period and the older she is at menopause, the more likely she is to get the disease. In other words, the more years she is exposed to cycling estrogen and progesterone, the higher her risk. Those are biological implications.

We also know that women who have osteoporosis have a 60 percent lower risk of getting breast cancer. If you have inherently low levels of estrogen you tend to have bad bones and good breasts. Conversely, if you have inherently *high* levels of estrogen, you tend to have good bones and bad breasts. (A few lucky women have both strong bones and a low risk of breast cancer.) Obesity in postmenopausal women, which correlates with higher levels of estrogen, creates a higher risk of breast cancer. So we have lots of circumstantial evidence to suggest that higher levels of estrogen and progesterone create higher risk of breast cancer. There have also been test-tube studies showing that breast cancer cells in a petri dish don't grow very well unless hormones are added to them.

The fact that tamoxifen, which blocks estrogen, can successfully prevent and treat breast cancer is another strong clue. So is the fact that in the days before tamoxifen women with breast cancer were often treated by having their ovaries removed (see Chapter 18). This too helped cure or contain the cancer.

In addition, we have some observational data on the breast cancer risk of women who take hormone therapy comparing women who take hormone therapy with those who don't. These show that those who are on the hormones get more breast cancer than those who aren't.

The problem with observational studies is that we don't know whether the difference is actually caused by the hormones, or by something else. (Remember our invented cigarette-lighter study in Chapter 12?) For example, we know that breast cancer is most common among white women in high-socioeconomic categories. These are precisely the women most likely to take hormone therapy. We also know that women on hormone therapy see their gynecologists more often—they have to, if only to get their prescriptions refilled. So they're more likely to be reminded of the need to have yearly mammograms, and to follow through. Are they actually getting more breast cancer, or are we finding more breast cancer among them because we're looking for it more?

There is another reason that the connection between hormone therapy and breast cancer is biologically plausible. If you plot the rate of breast cancer against age, starting at age 20, there's a straight line. The rate of breast cancer remains the same—until menopause. After menopause the rate is less. Further, there's about a 1 percent increase per year of delayed menopause—that is, every year after 50 in which you're still menstruating, your risk goes up 1 percent more than it was the year before. The rate of increase you see with estrogen therapy use is exactly the same that you see with delayed menopause.

The studies, sadly, are not as strong as we'd like. Almost all of them look at short-term rather than long-term use, and they don't take into account how long the woman used them. So the woman who took hormones for one year is put in the same category as the woman who took them for 20 years. But if you *do* differentiate by duration, you find that women who are on hormones for 10 years or more are the ones who have the increased breast cancer risk. The general medical thought is that estrogen and progestins aren't so much a cause of cancer, but a promoter of cell division. As I discussed in Chapter 13, cells can acquire cancerous mutations, but if the cells don't divide it doesn't matter.

Women who take estrogen for between 5 and 10 years have a 35 to 50 percent increased risk of breast cancer. (That doesn't mean 50 percent of women who take estrogen for that long will get breast cancer. It means that the original risk is increased by half. So if your risk at 50 is 1 per 1,000 per year, it becomes 1.5 per 1,000. That's not a huge increase, but it's definitely an increase.) A study by Bruce Ettinger found that it doubled the risk in women who took it for 20 years.[31] Adding progestin doesn't help. A study reported in 2000 showed that women taking progestin plus estrogen increased their risk of breast cancer more than if they took estrogen alone.[32]

None of these studies is conclusive. The Women's Health Initiative, a randomized controlled double-blind study of healthy women assigned to take either hormone therapy or placebo (see Chapter 12), will have some data available in 2008. But there's enough evidence now to cause concern.

One reason it's been so difficult to establish with certainty the connection between breast cancer and hormone therapy is that it may affect some women more than others. One of the things current research such as the ductal lavage (described in Chapter 17) may help us do is distinguish between the women for whom hormone therapy is dangerous and those for whom it's not.

For example, one of the dangers of hormone therapy is that a third of women taking it have increased breast density on mammogram. As we said in Chapter 9, there are some epidemiological data showing that this is problematical for two reasons. One is that it makes it more difficult to see lumps on the mammogram. The other is that it shows us the stroma in the breast tissue is being stimulated. When I was first told this I thought it was foolish—the dense breast tissue that shows on the mammogram isn't what gets cancer; the cells within the ducts get cancer. But now we're learning that there is constant "cross-talk" between cells and their neighbors, and it isn't quite so easy to dismiss. And, as observational studies had suggested, progestin added to estrogen increases the density and resulting risk more than estrogen alone.[33] One appealing but not yet proven hypothesis is that if you begin hormone therapy and your mammograms start to get a lot denser, it *might* be a sign that you're one of the people who shouldn't be taking hormones. On the other hand, if your mammograms didn't show more density, *maybe* you could feel better about taking them.

There are more data to support this theory, though it's not yet conclusive. Malcolm Pike from the University of Southern California has developed a pill for breast cancer prevention that essentially puts a woman into a state of reversible menopause. It blocks all hormones (see Chapter 18). After six months in a small study, the volunteers' mammograms were much less dense. There are other factors that may be important. It appears, for example, that if you are a carrier of BRCA2 the cancers you develop are more sensitive to hormones, while those in women with BRCA1 may be less so.

Alcohol consumption may also play a role. A couple of studies have shown that the estrogen levels of a woman on hormone therapy are 300 percent higher after she's had a drink. This is particularly true when the medication used is Premarin, which is metabolized by the liver. The liver, as you know, is strongly affected by alcohol. This suggests that if you want to use hormone therapy, you should probably have fewer than three alcoholic drinks a week—maybe save your drinks for very special occasions. (Remember, as we discuss elsewhere in this chapter, drinking already increases your breast cancer risk.)

There is a recent, rather frightening, study showing that women who take both birth control pills and hormone therapy have a higher risk of getting breast cancer.[34] The baby boomers are the first group to do this: they were the young women on birth control pills, and now are the middle-aged women taking hormones. According to this study's findings, short-term use of either one doesn't seem to make a difference. But women who were on oral contraceptives for 10 years, and then took hormone therapy for three or more years, had a relative risk of 3.2—more than triple the risk of women who never used either. This was a small study of 25 women; it's too soon to be certain if its results will hold true in larger studies. But it's something to keep in mind: it points out one of the ways in which the baby boomers are different from past generations. If we base our estimates of risk on our mothers' experiences, it may not be realistic, because they weren't taking these hormones throughout their lives.[35]

Types of Cancer

Another concern is the survival of women who get breast cancer while they're on hormone therapy. This is fairly complicated. Studies show that women who take hormones get more breast cancer, but the mortality rate among these women is actually between 10 and 15 percent lower than that of other women with breast cancer. The Iowa Women's Health Study helped explain some of this finding. It showed that the cancers of the women on estrogen tended, not surprisingly, to be more sensitive to estrogen and to have a less aggressive pathology. The tumors were more likely to be colloid, tubular, or medullary than the standard infiltrating ductal (see Chapter 20). This has been used to justify hormone therapy: if it only causes the "good" kind of cancer, who cares if they get it? I have a number of problems with that. Though the mortality is lower, it's hardly nonexistent: more women are still dying.

Furthermore, breast cancer is no fun, even if you survive it. It's a bit disingenuous to say that it's no problem if it's not a killer cancer. You still need surgery, radiation, and possibly chemotherapy, because you can't be sure it isn't going to spread. And you still experience all the fear that goes with having had cancer: the worry that the itch on your breast might be a new cancer, or the gas pain might really be metastasis to the liver. No one who survives cancer ever takes it lightly.

All in all, although we do not as of yet know for certain whether estrogen and its companion progesterone increase breast cancer, there is a lot of circumstantial evidence.

If you're thinking of going onto hormone therapy, you need a full discussion with your doctor of all the pros and cons, and you should sign a consent form. If you decide against using hormone therapy, and are interested in alternatives for symptoms and/or prevention of other diseases, see the discussion in Chapter 31. For the woman with breast cancer or at high risk, the decision about long-term estrogen use is clearer, because the benefits, even to the extent that they're thought to exist, just aren't that great. And we have proven alternatives.

FERTILITY DRUGS

Fertility drugs are being used a lot these days as the baby boomers who postponed childbearing are now trying to get pregnant. We don't know how safe fertility drugs are or how they interact with breast cancer. There are data now that suggest that use of Clomid, which kicks your ovaries and makes them work harder, will increase ovarian cancer since the more you ovulate the stronger your chance is of getting ovarian cancer, and the drugs make you hyperovulate.[36] Then there are drugs like Perganol, which comes from the urine of pregnant mares, which also causes you to hyperovulate. These all stimulate the ovaries. There's also HCG, human chorionic gonadotropin—the hormone that actually goes up in pregnancy. By the time you're taking fertility drugs you're probably over 30 and haven't had a child yet—a combination that already increases your risk of breast cancer. The drugs and hormones might also add a promoter effect. It's very important for women to realize that we don't know the relationship of these drugs to breast cancer, but it's likely that they have some effect, since DES and the other hormones do.

I have mixed feelings about all this use of hormones. You have your first period, and a few years later you get on the pill. You stay on the pill, with a few interruptions to have your kids. Or maybe you're already in your 30s when you get off the pill, and you don't get pregnant for a while. So you use fertility drugs. Otherwise you have your kids and go back to the pill, and stay on it till you hit menopause. Then you take postmenopausal hormones the rest of your life. In this way, you're always on some kind of hormonal medication. That somehow says our bodies are wrong. It bothers me. It provides a great market for the pharmaceutical companies, but it may not do us any good in the long run. Rather than fixing our bodies we should be fixing the world we live in and fostering a healthy lifestyle from girlhood on. But that is harder and less lucrative.

PESTICIDES AND OTHER ENVIRONMENTAL HAZARDS

There are a number of other things we now believe may contribute to your vulnerability to breast cancer. Among them are DDT and PCBs, persistent environmental contaminants that have been identified throughout the global ecosystem, including in fish, wildlife, and human tissue, blood, and milk. There is some evidence to support this link. The most telling study has been done by Dr. Mary Wolff.[37] Wolff and her group looked at the levels of DDE (a breakdown product of DDT) in the breast fat of women with breast cancer, comparing them to

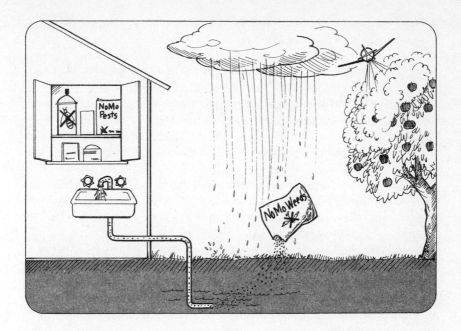

the fat of women without breast cancer.[38] The levels were significantly higher in the women with breast cancer. This doesn't mean that DDE is the cause of the breast cancer, but it certainly suggests a possibility.

Wolff's study has been criticized because it measured only DDT levels in the breast tissue at the time of diagnosis. A larger study by N. K. Krieger and others looked at levels prior to diagnosis and found no relationship between blood levels of organochlorides and subsequent breast cancer risk.[39]

One reason many people believe that DDT and PCBs are related to breast cancer is that a lot of them are broken down in the body to weak forms of estrogen, which, it's thought, can stimulate and cause breast cancer just as estrogen can.

But this isn't always the case with weak estrogens. Phytoestrogens like soy and the weak estrogen of tamoxifen have very different effects, as we'll discuss in Chapters 18 and 29. The fact that something is a weak estrogen is not enough to link it to the effects of estradiol. If we have learned anything since the last edition of this book, it's that the biology of estrogen, estrogen receptors, and the selective estrogen receptor modulators is very complex.

Several observational studies have been done and have failed to demonstrate a relationship between occupational exposure to pesticides and breast cancer. For example, the Nurses Health Study, a European study, and one from Mexico where levels are especially high have all shown no relationship between blood levels of DDE and PCBs and breast cancer.[40,41,42] At the same time, observational studies can miss connections.

Breast cancer activists on Cape Cod and Long Island (where there is very high risk of breast cancer) were responsible for some of the studies done in the early 1990s. They demanded that the Centers for Disease Control (CDC) investigate the high incidence of breast cancer in their areas. Though the studies[43] have not show a relation between breast cancer and pesticides, it opened the way to much breast cancer activism, and raised some questions that remain unanswered. Why were these populations getting more breast cancer?

Studies are being done with farm workers, who are exposed to high levels of pesticides, hormones, and other additives, to see if they have a higher risk of cancer than others. It may well be that people who live in smoggy Los Angeles are safer than people who live in farms in the San Joaquin Valley. So there are a variety of external factors that haven't been very well explored that we're just now starting to look at.

I think that the issue is complex and must take into consideration time of exposure and other associated risk factors. There still might be an environmental relationship, but it is probably small. Nonetheless, this lack of definitive answers is no excuse for not cleaning up the environment. There are enough known health problems from environmental pollution to convince us that it needs to be seriously curtailed. This is a fairly new area of scientific study. Who knows what we'll find in the next 5 or 10 years?

OCCUPATIONAL EXPOSURES

Many of the risks for breast cancer may be things you're unaware of. I used to ask all my patients if they had any environmental or occupational exposures to carcinogens. Almost to a woman, they'd say no. Then I'd ask what they did for a living. Very often it turned out that, in fact, they did have exposures. For example, one of my patients had been a manicurist for 15 years. She'd been inhaling all those fumes from the nail polish remover and nail polishes in a fairly close area for a long period of time. Could that be a carcinogen? Another woman was an artist who used oil paints. She was exposed to all the solvents used to clean the oil paint, as well as the cadmium in the paint, which some studies indicate is a very strong carcinogen.

There are probably a lot of environmental exposures that don't even occur to us because we're not used to thinking about life that way. In 1993 the National Cancer Institute held the first conference on occupational risks of cancer in women. (Until now, I think they assumed women didn't have occupations.) Women who work at home are ex-

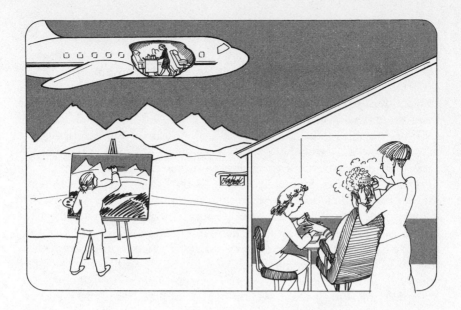

posed to many different cleaning solvents and insecticides. These may well be among the factors that lead to breast cancer.

Occupational exposure to radiation has been linked to an increased risk of breast cancer in a sample of medical diagnostic x-ray workers in China, in female employees at a nuclear plant, in female and male Finnish airline cabin attendants, and in radiologic technologists in the United States.[44,45,46,47]

As opposed to many of the carcinogenic exposures that simply promote cancer, radiation is known actually to cause mutations in the breast cells. In addition, there are certain other mutations that enhance the effects of radiation. At present at least 21 of these cancer-predisposing genes (see Chapter 14) have been isolated and cloned (9 tumor suppressor genes, 11 DNA repair genes, and 1 proto-oncogene). Also, at least eight other tumor suppressor genes and a gene involved in ataxia telangiectasia (AT), a neurological disease, have been found in a specific chromosome. These genes are involved in the control of cellular proliferation, programmed cell death (apoptosis), and DNA repair pathways. Several are examples of radiosensitizers.[48]

ELECTROMAGNETIC FIELD (EMF) EXPOSURE

Another issue that hasn't yet been well studied is that of electromagnetic fields. Electric and magnetic fields arise from the motion of electric charges. They are characterized as *non-ionizing radiation* when they lack sufficient energy to remove electrons from atoms, as opposed to *ionizing* radiation such as x rays and gamma rays. EMFs are emitted from devices that produce, transmit, or use electric power such as power lines, transmitters, and common household items like electric clocks, shavers, and blankets, computers, televisions, heated water-beds, and microwave ovens.

There has been concern that EMF exposure may increase the incidence of cancers, especially brain tumors and childhood leukemia, although studies have had inconsistent findings.

Artificial light is another source of EMFs. There's a very interesting study that was done in Seattle on *men* with breast cancer, and it showed that men who spent many hours using artificial light had a higher rate of breast cancer than men who didn't.[49] (Men were chosen because, since breast cancer is so rare in men, it's easier to find something in common than in the much larger female population. A similar study on women is now underway.) There are several possible theories to explain this. One is that the vitamin D in sunlight works as a form of breast cancer prevention, and artificial light, obviously, doesn't contain vitamin D.

The other argument, which the researchers in Seattle favor, is that the little gland under the brain called the pineal gland, which is involved in helping you distinguish day and night, produces a hormone, melatonin, which is excreted in a strong daily rhythm that peaks at night and decreases during the day. It appears that melatonin can be protective of the breast. Electric power produces light at night (electric lighting) and a range of non-ionizing electric and magnetic fields. According to a hypothesis developed by Richard Stevens, both light at night and low-level EMF may lower melatonin levels, which may in turn increase breast cancer risk.[50]

The effect of melatonin on breast cancer is based on studies in rats given a carcinogen.[51] The control group developed cancer, but the rats given melatonin didn't. The mechanism for this effect is unclear, but it may be through an increase in estrogen and prolactin, which stimulate breast tissue and/or prevent the growth and spread of cancer cells.

As appealing as this hypothesis is, it's only a hypothesis, accompanied by a lot of circumstantial evidence. One problem is the perennial limitation of animal studies: we are not rats. Further, there are vast differences between how light suppresses melatonin, nighttime melatonin levels, and patterns of melatonin release. And while there have been interesting laboratory studies, findings in the laboratory may not reproduce what happens in life. Charles Graham described his findings from double-blind studies in a human research laboratory, in which they found no effect of overnight exposure to EMF on levels of melatonin.[52] But real-world research on garment, utility, railway, and video display terminal workers indicated suppressed levels of melatonin. The different results may be due to differences between laboratory settings and the real world—laboratory research is over a short period of time, while chronic exposure may have more of an effect. Further, laboratory exposures are consistent, while real-world exposure may be relatively low over time with infrequent high exposures that occur in microseconds. These short-term high-energy peaks also occur in the home from utility operation and, unlike low-level EMF, may have enough power to alter cells. A study is going on to investigate this possibility.[53] We know that women who work on the telephone lines have a higher incidence of breast cancer.[54] There is another study of women who were completely blind (and therefore might have high melatonin levels): these women had less breast cancer than did the sighted women in the control group. Several other studies have been launched to investigate the potential association between EMFs and breast cancer. A study is in progress at Fred Hutchinson Cancer Center and another at the University Medical Center at Stony Brook in New York as part of the National Cancer Institute's Long Island Cancer Study. Both studies will measure in-home magnetic field exposures and proximity to power lines as possible risk factors. A project at the Brigham and Women's Hospital in Boston is evaluating whether electric blankets are associated with breast cancer in a group of 121,700 nurses who have been studied since 1976.

While we await these studies, you might want to consider some lifestyle modifications. Try to increase the space between yourself and devices that might emit magnetic fields. Avoid being too close to computers, microwave ovens, and televisions. Turn off electric devices when you aren't using them (this also saves on your electric bill and energy waste). Avoid electric blankets, and don't keep electric alarm clocks close to the bed. Discourage children from playing below power lines. Avoid prolonged use of cell phones. And sleep in a dark room.

How much you want to change your lifestyle to avoid a possible risk increase depends on you. My coauthor, for example, can't sleep in a completely dark room. Many people's livelihoods depend on frequent use of computers and cell phones. As with any risk question, there's always a compromise between your needs and your efforts to avoid risk.

The cause of breast cancer will probably not be just one thing. It will be a combination of the environment and the genetic components. Research needs to be done on both of these fronts if we are to find an answer.

16

<hr/>

Precancerous Conditions

As we discussed in Chapter 6, virtually none of the symptoms misnamed "fibrocystic disease" is related to breast cancer. There are, however, certain microscopic findings in breast tissue that may well lead to cancer.

You'll recall that I've described the breast as a milk factory, with two parts—lobules that make the milk, and ducts, like hollow branches, that carry it to the nipples (Fig. 16-1). Over the years, you can get a few extra cells lining the branch—sort of like a fungus. This is called *intraductal hyperplasia*, which simply translates to "too many cells in the duct." In itself, this is not a problem. Sometimes the cells can begin to get a bit strange looking, and this condition is called intraductal hyperplasia with atypia (also known as atypical hyperplasia, or ADH). If they keep on getting odd looking, and multiply within the duct, clogging it up, they're known as ductal carcinoma *in situ* (meaning "in place") or *intraductal carcinoma* or even DCIS (Fig. 16-2). These three steps are all reversible. We don't yet know how, but we suspect it has something to do with hormones. Finally, if cells break out of the ducts and into the surrounding fat, they are called invasive ductal cancer.

The first two conditions do not cause lumps (the third rarely does)—they take place inside the duct, so you can't feel them by examining your breast. Though they're often found during a biopsy, they

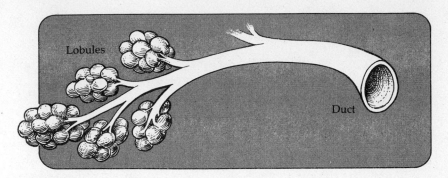

FIGURE 16-1

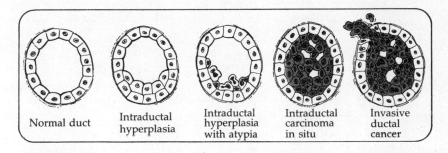

| Normal duct | Intraductal hyperplasia | Intraductal hyperplasia with atypia | Intraductal carcinoma in situ | Invasive ductal cancer |

FIGURE 16-2

aren't in the lump itself—they're next to the lump in the rim of apparently "normal" tissue and the pathologist comes across them by accident.

If you look at autopsy studies of women who've died of causes other than breast cancer, you'll see that 30 percent or so had some degree of either hyperplasia or atypical hyperplasia.[1] So probably a lot of us are walking around with these conditions, and we don't know it because we have no reason to have biopsies, and they don't show on mammograms.

David Page, of Vanderbilt University, studied 10,000 biopsies and found, not surprisingly, that there is a progression of increased risk with each of these entities.[2] The women with hyperplasia and no atypia had a slightly increased relative risk (barely significant), which was worse when compounded with family history (1.5 and 2.1, respectively). Interestingly, and not easily explained, he also found that women with gross cysts and family history had an increased relative risk of about 3, or 3 times the risk of a woman without gross cysts and a family history. Finally, and most significantly, the women with atypical hyperplasia had an increased relative risk of 3.5, and if they had a family history in a first-degree relative this rose to 8.9 over 15 years. Although this sounds high, I must point out that there were only 39 women who fulfilled these criteria. In fact, of the 10,000 benign biopsies Page reviewed, only 3 percent had atypical hyperplasia.

We're not quite sure whether atypical intraductal hyperplasia increases the risk of cancer because it's dangerous in itself, or because it's a response to something else that's dangerous and we don't yet know about—the way, for example, a bruise that doesn't heal isn't intrinsically harmful but may be failing to heal because it's over a cancer site. It is interesting to note that the risk of invasive cancer in the patients Dr. Page studied was equal in either breast, and some of the patients even had bilateral cancers. This makes it more likely that we are picking up women at high risk in this specific group rather than those with a condition that is dangerous in itself. It might be termed an intermediate marker.

There are obviously still many questions. The most vital, however, to the woman diagnosed with atypical hyperplasia is the question of what to do. At this time most surgeons would agree that the best program is close follow-up, to find an intraductal carcinoma or invasive cancer in its early stages. This would include physical exam by a doctor every six months and yearly mammograms. It might also be the perfect place for ductal lavage (see Chapter 17). You could have the duct with the atypical cells monitored every six months to find out whether the hyperplasia progressed, regressed, or stayed stable.

For those women who want a treatment, the recent studies using tamoxifen for prevention have given us another option. The women with ADH who took tamoxifen for five years had an 86 percent decrease in subsequent breast cancers.[3] It is certainly worth considering the risks and benefits of this approach (see Chapter 17). Some women may even consider a more drastic approach and have preventive mastectomies (see Chapter 18).

If we consider atypical hyperplasia as "pre-precancer," *in situ* cancer, the next step along the path, can be considered precancer. Some doctors prefer to call it "noninvasive cancer"—a term I find misleading, since in most people's minds cancer is by definition an invasive disease. I prefer the term "precancer" because the lack of invasion means that these lesions don't metastasize, and therefore can't kill you. I have had many battles over this nomenclature with some colleagues, doctors who say cancer is cancer whether it is invasive or not.

Precancers in the breast, like atypical hyperplasia, rarely cause lumps, pain, or any other symptoms. They are also usually found incidentally. Unlike atypical hyperplasia, however, they can sometimes show up on mammograms, and the increased use of mammography for screening has shown us that they're actually far more common than we'd thought. The process of learning about and treating breast precancers is similar to that of cervical precancers, which were rarely seen until the routine use of Pap smears showed them to be fairly frequent.

There are two kinds of precancer of the breast: *ductal carcinoma in situ*, which we have mentioned and will discuss more below, and *lobular carcinoma in situ* (LCIS). As its name suggests, lobular carcinoma *in situ* occurs in the lobules. The difference is not only in the lesions' locale: the two behave very differently.

LOBULAR CANCER IN SITU

Under the microscope, LCIS is seen as very small, round cells stuffing the lobules, which normally have no cells inside them (Fig. 16-3). If there are only a few cells and they're not too odd looking, you have lobular hyperplasia, while if they fill the whole lobule and look very atypical (odd), you have LCIS. Such lobules have been termed "multicentric" because they can be found scattered throughout both breasts. However, no one has tried to tie them to one ductal system the way they have with DCIS. Since the lobules are at the periphery of each ductal branch, they could appear scattered and really be part of the same branch of ducts.

The natural history of LCIS became better known when Cushman Haagensen, a leading breast specialist, did a study in which he care-

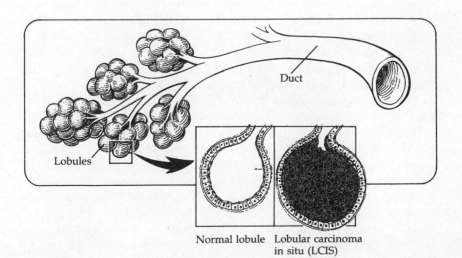

Normal lobule   Lobular carcinoma
in situ (LCIS)

FIGURE 16-3

fully monitored his patients who had LCIS, rather than perform mastectomies.[4] He saw them periodically for about 30 years, examining them every four months (this was in the early days of mammography, and Haagensen, who didn't much trust the procedure, used only physical examination). Out of 211 patients, only 36 (about 17%) developed invasive cancer over 30 years. This made their risk 7.2 times the normal risk. These cancers occurred in either breast, and any place within the breast: they weren't confined to the spot where the original LCIS was found, or even to the lobular system itself. This strongly suggests that LCIS doesn't grow into cancer, but simply is a sign that cancer is a possible danger—the way, for example, an overcast day warns you it might rain. Because of this, some experts believe that lobular carcinoma *in situ* isn't, in fact, a true precancer.

Having LCIS indicates a degree of risk similar to that faced by a woman whose mother and sister have breast cancer. It is cumulative risk, spread out over your entire life (see Chapter 14).

It's important to note that of the women in Haagensen's study who did develop breast cancer, only six died of it. And none of the six had come back for regular examinations. In Haagensen's opinion, they died because they ignored the warning sign of LCIS, and didn't monitor the condition of their breasts after the LCIS diagnosis.

Haagensen's was the benchmark study, but others that have followed have had similar results, showing that people with LCIS have a range of between 16 and 27 percent risk of breast cancer in either breast over 30 years.[5,6,7] This risk can be compounded by other risk factors for breast cancer (see Table 16-1).

What can you do if you have lobular carcinoma *in situ?* Removing the LCIS isn't enough, since the LCIS isn't what grows into cancer. Basically this is a prevention situation. You want to prevent yourself from ever getting breast cancer. There are a number of options; the most drastic is bilateral prophylactic mastectomy.

Some women choose this because they want to know they've done everything they could. They feel that if they get breast cancer, at least it isn't their fault, whereas if they hadn't done anything surgically and gotten the disease, they'd always wonder if they could have prevented it. One patient told me, "I knew instantly what my decision should be. I was astounded to see how greedy for life I was." This patient was already in a high-risk group because of her family history; she had seen members of her family go through breast cancer, and was determined to do all she could to avoid suffering with it herself. She was uncomfortable with the studies about monitoring, which she thought were too recent, while mastectomy had been around a long time. She had reconstruction through one of the flap procedures discussed in Chapter 26. Others have silicone implants.

Table 16-1. Benign Breast Disease and Risk of Breast Cancer[a]

	Relative Risk
Previous biopsy[b]	1.8%
Gross cysts	1.3
with first-degree family history	2.7
Atypical hyperplasia	4.4
with first-degree family history	8.9
with calcifications on mammogram	6.5
with first birth after 20	4.5
Lobular carcinoma *in situ*	7.2
Ductal carcinoma *in situ*	11.0

[a]Adapted from W.D. Dupont and D.L. Page, "Breast Cancer Risk with Proliferative Disease, Age at First Birth, and a Family History of Breast Cancer," *American Journal of Epidemiology* 125 (1987): 769.

[b]S.M. Love, R.S. Gelman, and W.S. Silen, "'Fibrocystic Disease': A Non-disease?," *New England Journal of Medicine* 307 (1982): 1010.

The alternative to surgery is to take the appearance of LCIS as a warning that you need to be closely watched. This means follow-up exams every six months, with a yearly mammogram. That way if a cancer does develop you're likely to catch it at an early stage and can decide then if you want to have a mastectomy, or a lumpectomy and radiation (see Chapter 23). If a cancer doesn't develop, you've been spared the ordeal of major and disfiguring surgery. This was Haagensen's recommendation, and for the most part I agree with him. Most of my patients have opted for this course. To monitor what the cells are doing in the breast, the new technique of ductal lavage may give an even earlier warning than mammogram that something is going awry (see Chapter 17).

The third possiblity is to take tamoxifen for less than five years. This has been shown to decrease the chance of getting breast cancer by 56 percent in women with LCIS. Although there is some question as to whether its effect will last beyond five years, we have reason to believe it might. Other drugs are being developed that might have a similar benefit. As of yet none of them, including raloxifene (or Evista), have been tried in women with LCIS. All of the drugs have side effects that must be taken into consideration. In addition, they are not safe to take if you are trying to get pregnant.

What's important is that you give yourself the time to figure out what you want to do. LCIS doesn't call for an immediate decision. A woman called me recently in a panic because she had been diagnosed with LCIS and told by her oncologist that she should start on tamoxifen immediately. She was uncomfortable with this choice and worried about what to do. It is important to remember that LCIS is a risk factor for subsequent cancer, not cancer itself. The risk of developing cancer is 1 percent per year, so there is no rush to begin a treatment. I suggested to this woman that she take the follow-up route initially, and see how she felt about it in six months or a year. If she was comfortable living with it, then she could continue this course for the rest of her life, or until a cancer occurred. You can always decide on tamoxifen or mastectomy later, but you can't undo a double mastectomy. However, if a woman finds herself living in a constant state of anxiety, waking up every morning thinking, "This is it—this is the day I'll find the lump," then maybe a bilateral mastectomy is best for her.

Radiation and chemotherapy are not necessary treatments for LCIS because it's not really cancer. Nor is there any reason to obtain clean margins surgically. Since it is only a marker for risk and does not become cancer itself, LCIS does not need to be excised. Some clinicians do not understand this. If your surgeon or oncologist starts talking about wide excision, radiation, or chemotherapy for LCIS make sure you get a second opinion from a doctor more familiar with this condition. A few years ago, I saw a woman from Southern California who had had a wide excision and radiation for LCIS. She was now being told to have chemotherapy "just in case." I reviewed her slides and indeed it was just LCIS. When I explained that she had been overtreated she said she had thought this was the case at the time: she had read the first edition of this book and had understood what she had. But she hadn't been able to convince her doctors, and had trusted their expertise. The moral is, when in doubt get a second opinion.

Sometimes when a patient has a lump that turns out to be cancer, the pathologist will find LCIS in the adjacent tissue. What does this mean? Well, it may just mean that the patient was at a higher risk for breast cancer, and sure enough she got it. But it may mean that the other breast is also at a higher risk for breast cancer than otherwise, so some surgeons like to do what we call a "blind biopsy" on that breast. It's called a blind biopsy because surgeons really have no way of knowing what they're looking for: sometimes they'll take out the upper outer quadrant because that's where most of the breast tissue is, or sometimes they'll take out the mirror image of the section they've removed from the breast with LCIS. It's pretty chancy since there's no evidence that cancer will occur in the mirror image, and they might find something that looks worrisome pathologically but is biologically insignificant. In addition, the biopsy might be negative but miss a cancer millimeters away. Most doctors have preferred simply to follow the woman closely, with breast examinations every three to four months and yearly mammograms. Now they might consider adding ductal lavage (see next chapter) as a way to monitor what may be going on in the other breast.

DUCTAL CARCINOMA IN SITU

DCIS is more complex than LCIS. It's also more than a marker that cancer may appear in the breast: it's a lesion that can in itself grow into a cancer. It rarely forms lumps, but may sometimes form a soft thickening (caused by the pliable ducts becoming less pliable because they're filled with cells; see Fig. 16-4).

DCIS is now found far more frequently because of mammograms, where it appears with microcalcifications. In fact, it's probably very common. Autopsies done on women who died from all kinds of causes show that between 6 and 16 percent had DCIS. [8,9] This would suggest that many of us have it and never know it—it is probably not, as we used to believe, a rare condition.

In the past, standard treatment was a mastectomy of the breast with the lesion. That worked most of the time. But it might not have been necessary—and since the breasts had all been removed, we had no way of studying what happened when a breast that had DCIS *wasn't* removed.

There have been a few small studies, however, that have given us a

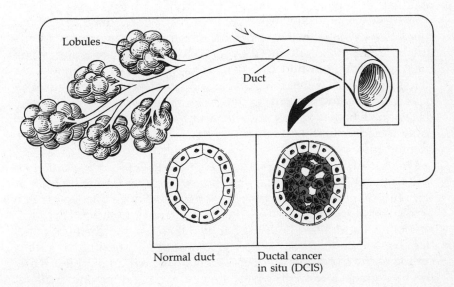

Lobules

Duct

Normal duct

Ductal cancer in situ (DCIS)

FIGURE 16-4

clue. Three studies followed people who were biopsied and thought to have something benign. W. L. Betsill at Sloan Kettering reviewed all the pathology the hospital had done on 10,000 breasts between 1940 and 1950 and, on reexamining the pathology reports, found 25 cases of people who had been misdiagnosed: the biopsied tissue had been described as benign but actually had had early intraductal lesions. (Such lesions are often small, and very easy to miss.) Obviously, no further treatment had been done. Of these 25, only 10 had been regularly followed for 22 years. They contacted these women and found out what their breast history had been since the biopsies had been performed. They found that 7 had developed invasive cancer in the 22 years after the original diagnosis.[10]

Other similar studies have led us to believe that about 20–25 percent of women with untreated low-grade DCIS will go on to get invasive cancer up to 25 years after the initial biopsy, and in the same area of the breast in which that biopsy was done. So the fact that low-grade lesions take a long time to turn into cancer is no guarantee that they won't do so eventually. This becomes important later in this discussion.[11]

Since all the studies together add up to only 78 patients, this is not enough to be sure they're representative. Furthermore, their lesions were on the border between atypical hyperplasia and DCIS, or they would have been diagnosed initially: the studies don't address the situation of women with obvious DCIS. What is clear from these studies, however, is that untreated DCIS can go on to invasive breast cancer and that in the majority of women it does not seem to do so.

A further complexity is that some of the lesions don't stay in the precancerous stage, but revert to either intraductal hyperplasia with atypia or just plain intraductal hyperplasia. Unfortunately, at the moment we don't know how to make this happen, nor do we know how to tell which ones will become cancer and which won't. There's a lot of research going on right now on the molecular biology level to try and determine whether there's some kind of a marker that would clearly show which lesions are on their way to cancer, and which won't ever become cancer.

One attempt to make this distinction is to look at the architecture of the DCIS. Researchers have discovered three general patterns (Fig. 16-5). One is called *micropapillary:* the cells fill the duct with a fingerlike mass sticking out into the duct's center. A second is called *cribriform:* it also fills in the duct but then there are punched-out holes like Swiss cheese. These are low-grade patterns. The third is called *comedo* for its resemblance to a comedon, or whitehead pimple. This is the high-grade pattern. The cells are stuffing the duct, and some of

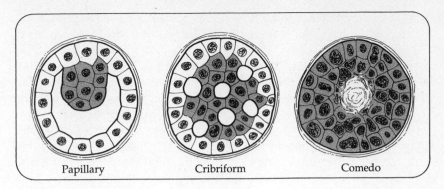

| Papillary | Cribriform | Comedo |

FIGURE 16-5

them are dead (necrotic). There is also a lot of apoptosis, and there are very aberrant cells. If the tissue around the duct is squeezed, white, cheesy material comes out, exactly as if you were squeezing a pimple.

More recently, a lot of different groups have come up with classification schemes they hope will help predict which DCIS is more aggressive. This is somewhat complicated by the fact that different doctors define "worse" and "less aggressive" differently. One criterion is the likelihood that it will recur locally after surgery and radiation; the other is its likelihood of turning invasive. However, of the groups that have been creating classification schemes, most have come up with fairly similar classifications. The two most important factors, they agree, are whether the cells are high grade or low grade, and whether or not there's necrosis.

We've found that these new categories are very helpful in predicting which DCIS is likely to become invasive, but not in predicting which will come back in the breast. Another factor determines that: whether or not the surgeon got all the DCIS out. This makes sense. By definition, DCIS is contained within part of the duct. If the surgeon gets it all out, there's none left to grow and cause a recurrence. If not, if some stays behind, it's likely to come back in the breast. We use margins (see Chapter 20) to help us guess whether there is any cancer left behind. This is true for both low- and high-grade DCIS: the difference is in the timing of the recurrence, not the recurrence itself. Recurrence of DCIS in the breast is never in itself life-threatening; it only means that you have to deal with DCIS again.

Ironically, high-grade DCIS—the kind that if it becomes cancer will be a very aggressive cancer—is the easiest to contain. It grows in a very concentrated area; it doesn't tend to spread itself out a lot. Further, it has calcifications (caused by the apoptosis and necrosis) that show up on mammogram, and serve as a guide for the surgeon. So it's easier to get it all out.

Low-grade DCIS, on the other hand, doesn't have necrosis and apoptosis. It sometimes has calcifications (caused by secretions), but they're nowhere near as definitive as the calcifications in high-grade DCIS. It also tends to be more widespread. While the high-grade version is tight and concentrated, the low-grade kind meanders all around the duct. So it's harder for the surgeon to get it all out. Our hope is that the intraductal approach (described in the next chapter) will help to outline the extent of the duct to aid the surgeon in this procedure. Even if it does, however, many ductal systems are quite extensive and removing them may mean removing a large portion of the breast.

This creates a paradoxical situation. The low-grade DCIS, which creates fewer and less aggressive cancers, may require a mastectomy. The high-grade DCIS, which is more likely to invade and to create aggressive cancers, may be treatable with wide excision and radiation.

Dr. Melvin Silverstein's group, previously in Van Nuys, California, but now at Norris Cancer Center at the University of Southern California, came out with a prognostic index in 1996,[12] in an attempt to figure out whether the DCIS was likely to come back in the breast and thus what treatment people should have. They looked for whether the lesion was high-grade or low-grade, necrosis or lack of it, size of tumor, and size of margin (how much normal tissue was between the DCIS and the edge of the tissue that had been removed). They found what we had already suspected: that the predictor that trumped the rest was the size of the margins—which translates to "Did we get it all out?" Even with a very high grade DCIS, if they get it out with a nice, clean margin, it doesn't come back in the breast.

The Van Nuys classification system was the first of the newer ones to come out, and it's the one used now. Once we find a test we can apply to the DCIS cells themselves that will predict the risk for recurrence in the breast (as well as the chance the tumor will become invasive), the Van Nuys system will have outlived its usefulness.

Here is the Van Nuys prognostic index. Each factor gets a score. Your DCIS will be based on a number between 3 and 9, with 9 as the worst. ("The worst" is defined by the likelihood of recurrence, not the likelihood of your ultimately dying from a cancer that grows from the DCIS.) A high score is bad; a low score much more hopeful.

Tumor size: 1 point for less than or equal to 15 mm; 2 points, 16–40 mm; 3 points, greater than or equal to 41 mm.
Margin width: 1 point for greater or equal to 10 mm; 2 points, 1–9 mm; 3 points, less than 1 mm.

Pathological classification: 1 point for low-grade and no necrosis; 2 points for low-grade with necrosis; 3 points for high-grade with or without necrosis.

The points are added up to see how likely your DCIS is to recur. This is an interesting index, but it's not foolproof.

DCIS and Invasion

We've always thought that invasive cancer cells were simply DCIS cells that have learned a new skill that allows them mobility, so they can break outside the ducts—sort of the way a tadpole grows into a frog. Perhaps a mutation gives them that ability, and from there they take off, make blood vessels, and become invasive cancer.

To determine this, researchers looked at DCIS cells and cancer cells, examining them for the molecular markers (such as p53, apoptosis, Her-2 neu; see Chapter 14) that are signs of cancer. They expected to find some of the markers in DCIS and many more in invasive cancers.

What they found, however, was that there were the same markers in both. We have yet to find anything that shows a difference between DCIS and invasive cells—something that would allow us to examine a lesion and say, "Okay, now it's not invasive, but if it develops X, we'll know it's crossed over that line." With such knowledge, we could probably catch invasive cancer at an extremely early stage, just by examining the DCIS.

We still may find it. But another hypothesis researchers are beginning to look at is the possibility that there may not really be any difference in the cells—that in both situations, they're the same cancer cells. In that case, what would cause DCIS to stay within the duct would be not its inability to get out, but the action of some other force keeping it inside. They're not acting, say the researchers; they're being acted on.

If the second theory is correct, something is holding the DCIS inside the duct. Dr. Sanford Barsky, the breast pathologist at UCLA, has done some very interesting work looking at the myoepithelial cells that form a rim around the outside of the duct.[13] The cells are just sitting there in the background and no one has paid much attention to them till now. Barsky's studies have found that they produce an enzyme that actively blocks invasion. In order for cancer cells to invade, they have to be able to eat away proteins and get through the cells, and the enzyme stops them from doing this.

Another component may be the local cellular neighborhood—the "cross-talk" between the cancer cells and the cells around them (see Chapter 13). Some of the tissues that these surrounding cells make up may also be involved in preventing invasion. Some hormones act differently on the myoepithelial cells. Think of these cells as a big line of prison guards standing there and not letting anyone through. Then someone gives the guards whiskey, and they get mellow and laid back and decide to let everyone pass. On the other hand, tell them the boss is watching them and they get even tougher. Estrogen is the whiskey; prednisone, another hormone, is the snoopy boss. Tamoxifen too tends to make them tougher—which may be one of the ways it works.

This is all preliminary—and probably is only one factor. It works in the lab, and that's a hopeful sign. But putting cells in a petri dish, dripping estrogen on them, and watching the myoepithelial cells get weaker doesn't tell us what happens in a human body. Still, it's promising. I'd love for it to work out, because if it does, we may discover that even invasive cancer could be reversible. If we knew the elements needed to confine the cells, we could give patients whatever those elements were, and confine the cells again.

Another significant change in the way we perceive DCIS is that we no longer necessarily see it as a simple progression from atypical hyperplasia to low-grade DCIS to high-grade DCIS and then to invasion. It looks like low-grade DCIS becomes low-grade cancer, and high-grade DCIS becomes high-grade cancer.[14] This lends credence to the idea that the cells aren't changing. Their "personality" will stay the same, whether they're high-grade or low-grade, and there's something external making them behave differently.

If the high-grade DCIS cells recur or become invasive, they do so more quickly—which makes sense: they're more aggressive to begin with. Low-grade tumors appear to grow or invade much more slowly: the recurrences that David Page found 15 to 20 years after the diagnosis were all low-grade DCIS. This is very important to realize when we're doing studies: if a DCIS study follows its subjects for only five years, it will look as though only high-grade DCIS recurs or becomes invasive. We need longer studies following subjects with DCIS, and we also need to address additional questions. What were those cells doing for 20 years?

There are other important things to consider. In women with breast cancer, DCIS cells are surrounded by microscopic extra blood vessels and also *stroma desmoplasia,* a hardening of the surrounding tissue. Both are reactions to something being secreted by the cancer cells. How can cancer cells trapped inside the duct get messages ordering the creation of new blood cells *outside* the duct? So far, we don't know. Maybe they're stimulating the myoepithelial cells to do it (the prison guards are getting messages to the gang outside). This ability to induce new blood vessels to grow and to increase the hardness of the surrounding tissue is shared with invasive cancer cells and may be an early indicator of which cells are likely to become invasive.

Without a thorough understanding of the natural history of DCIS, which we do not yet have, it's hard to devise a logical treatment. However, there is increasing interest in treatments for DCIS that are less drastic than mastectomy—chiefly, wide excision. This is the same principal as the lumpectomy in breast cancer (see Chapter 23), except that there's usually no lump involved, so the surgeon tries to remove the entire area that has the DCIS, along with a rim of normal breast tissue.

Some experts argue against this, claiming that DCIS, like LCIS, is multicentric.[15] Their idea is that these conditions mean that all the breast tissue is marching along toward cancer, and is precancerous to a greater or lesser degree, and this tissue has just gotten a little further on. So, says this theory, we really have to take off the whole breast or even both breasts, because just taking off part of one isn't going to solve the problem.

This unfortunate idea evolved from a number of studies in which breasts that had been removed for DCIS were analyzed. The breasts were cut into four quadrants, and then examined under the microscope. If they found DCIS in more than one quadrant, the researchers designated it as multicentric.[16]

The problem is this presupposes that breast tissue is arranged in quadrants. It isn't. It's not an orange with nicely defined sections. The ductal system isn't structured in quadrants at all. It's more like an arbor: it comes from the nipple, branches out, and fills up a certain amount of space. There are between five and nine separate ductal systems in each breast; they intertwine but they don't connect. So one system might take up the whole upper part of the breast. If the breast is cut into quadrants, we would find DCIS in both quadrants even though it's all part of one ductal system.

This was proved in a study done by Rolland Holland in Nijmegan in the Netherlands.[17] He took breasts that had been removed and cut them into four quadrants, and he too found that there was disease in several of the quadrants. But he went a step further. He very carefully mapped out the DCIS and found that in 80 of the 81 cases, even though it was in more than one quadrant, it was in the same duct, which branched into several parts of the breast.

The idea that DCIS is multicentric has been given less credence since the last edition of this book. One of the things that has caused this change in perspective is the discovery that DCIS is *monoclonal*.[18] A clone, remember, is an exact replica of the original cell. This means that all of the molecular markers would be exactly the same. If you could be cloned, for example, your clones would be far more like you than an identical twin would. Everything, down to the tiny mole on your left buttock, would be the same. The monoclonal model suggests that one cell keeps replicating and all the cells up and down the duct look exactly the same.

This is important not only in terms of our scientific understanding of DCIS but in an immediate way for patients diagnosed with the disease. If it were multicentric, it would lend itself to the argument that you may as well have mastectomies in both breasts, because it would only be a matter of time until the second breast got cancer. But if it's really unicentric and monoclonal, the wiser treatment would be to take the one section of the breast with DCIS out.

The problem with lumpectomy at this stage, however, is that the doctor probably can't tell where the ducts are. Since breast cancer originates in ducts, we've been working for several years to find a way to cut out an entire ductal system. I've mapped out the ducts and I know generally where they are (see Chapter 17), but so far this doesn't help with surgery. I can't tell exactly where a particular woman's breast ducts are. We need a way of marking the ductal system for excision. Now, when a surgeon tries to remove a duct, it's a hit or miss proposition. The ducts are suspended in fat and breast tissue, undetectable by any visual or tactile method. This is why we depend on evaluating the margins to help estimate how thorough the surgery has been.

Unfortunately, when pathologists look at DCIS on a slide, and see several duct profiles filled with cells, they also use the terms "multicentric" or "multifocal." The clinician interprets that as meaning there's DCIS all over the breast. But the pathologist just means that there are several different ducts (or sections of the same duct) seen in cross-section that have DCIS in them (Fig. 16-6). Pathologists don't have a whole breast under the microscope, just one little piece. All they can say is whether there is DCIS all over that piece. This means if a doctor says you have multicentric DCIS and need a mastectomy, you need to probe further what is meant. If necessary, see if you can talk directly to the pathologist and ask what exactly was under the microscope. This will give you a better perspective on the problem.

What we currently do is a wide excision based on our best guess of the extent of disease. We arrive at this guess by looking at the preoperative mammogram and then studying the tissue we remove from the breast. The pathologist examines the tissue and coats the outer surface with India ink. The tissue is then fixed and made into slides (see Chapter 20), which are examined. If there is DCIS near ink it is said to be a "dirty margin": if there is only normal breast tissue next to ink it is a "clean margin." But the pathologists can't look at every margin—it would be more than 2,000 slides. They are only sampling the mar-

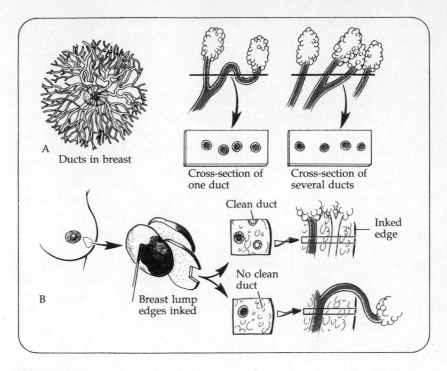

A
Ducts in breast

Cross-section of
one duct

Cross-section of
several ducts

Clean duct

Inked
edge

No clean
duct

B

Breast lump
edges inked

FIGURE 16-6

gins, so it's possible that even if all the margins they look at are negative there will be a DCIS-filled duct crossing into the breast that they
have missed. This is a different situation than when we remove a single lump; in which case, knowing precisely where the lesion is, we
know that we have gotten out the right surrounding tissue. So when
there's a "recurrence" of DCIS, it's probably not a recurrence at all; it's
DCIS that we left behind in the first place, in spite of what we thought
were clean margins. This doesn't happen frequently, but often enough
(about 10 to 20% of the time) to make it significant. That's why mastectomy, though imperfect, tends to give a lower recurrence rate—it's the
widest excision possible.

Unfortunately, they defined a "wide excision" as simply one in
which DCIS can't be seen in the ink around the lesion. But because
DCIS can go in and out of the plane of a section (see Fig. 16-6), a truly
clean margin should show normal breast tissue between the ink and
the DCIS. This is why most doctors now do measurements for margins: we say it has to be more than a centimeter. In reality, this isn't
true: it could be a millimeter, if we got all the DCIS within that millime-

ter out. But since we have no way of knowing when that is so, we give ourselves a big rim around the lesion to be certain.

It is also important to look at a post-biopsy mammogram. DCIS usually shows up on the mammogram as calcifications. Even if calcifications have been removed, there are often some left, and this picture can add information about residual disease.

Treatment for DCIS has been evolving since the last edition of this book, and we now have more data. The National Surgical Adjuvant Breast and Bowel Project (NSABP) has done a large study (B17) looking at whether radiation is an effective treatment for DCIS.[19] They took 818 women throughout the country with DCIS, randomly dividing them into one group that got wide excision alone and one that got wide excision plus radiation. After eight years of follow-up, the study found that DCIS recurrence was 26.7 percent when lumpectomy alone was done. Half of these recurrences—13.4 percent—were invasive. In the group receiving radiation, 12.1 percent had recurrences, and one third of those were invasive. This says two things: first, there are fewer recurrences in women who get radiation; and second, and more important, there were fewer *invasive* recurrences. Having DCIS recur is unpleasant, but it won't kill you. Having an invasive cancer show up puts your life at risk.

There are a number of possible reasons for this. Maybe some of the precancers were already on the road to being invasive and we just couldn't tell that under the microscope. Maybe radiation does what a surgeon cannot: picks out the DCIS destined to go on to invasion from DCIS that remains stable. This study established the value of using radiation for DCIS, but it has been recently challenged. Another randomized trial is being done in Europe by the European Organization for Research and Treatment of Cancer. The EORTC study looked at 1,010 cases of DCIS in 46 centers. They did lumpectomies on all the women, and then randomized them into one group getting radiation and the other getting just close follow-up. There are as yet no data showing that radiation makes a difference.

As usual the answer is probably somewhere in the middle. Mel Silverstein has been arguing for some time against treating all women with DCIS the same way. He says that if a woman has a tiny, 5-millimeter spot of DCIS that can be cut out with a centimeter of margin all around it, she may not need radiation. At the other extreme, if she has very aggressive and widespread DCIS, and the surgeon can't get a wide margin, she may need much more than radiation and lumpectomy: she may need a mastectomy.

In his Van Nuys study, Silverstein looked at his own data.[20] It wasn't a perfect group of women to study, since it was made up of the last 469 DCIS patients he saw, and the treatment they had had was based on what they wanted, not on participation in a controlled, randomized study. Still, it's a useful study. Silverstein found that if a woman had more than a centimeter margin, radiation made no difference in her recurrence rate. If her margin was between a millimeter and a centimeter, there was a 50 percent improvement with radiation. If her margin was less than a millimeter wide, whatever the size of the lesion, she had 2.5 times the chance of recurrence without radiation.

So we may be able to select out patients who need radiation. In order for the surgeon to get out a centimeter all around of margin, the lesion has to be small. With a bigger lesion, that large a margin would be a virtual mastectomy.

A 1999 study tested whether adding tamoxifen to lumpectomy and radiation had additional value.[21] To do this, researchers randomized 1,804 women who had been treated for DCIS to receive either tamoxifen or a placebo for five years (see Table 16-1). All had been treated by excision followed by radiation therapy. Forty women in the placebo group and 23 in the tamoxifen group developed subsequent invasive cancers in the treated breast. In other words, tamoxifen reduced the chance of developing invasive cancer from 4.2 percent to 2.1 percent. There were 47 noninvasive recurrences (more DCIS) in the placebo group and 40 in the tamoxifen group. Tamoxifen lowered the rate of noninvasive recurrences (new ones or DCIS left over from earlier treatment) from 5.1 to 3.9 percent.

Thirty-six cancers (noninvasive and invasive combined) developed in the placebo group and 18 in the tamoxifen group (3.45 to 2.0%). Most important, there were 10 recurrences—seven in the placebo group and three in the tamoxifen group—in the nodes, chest wall, or elsewhere in the body (metastases). Although the recurrence rate was less than half as great in the tamoxifen group, the numbers are too small to be statistically significant. There were six deaths from breast cancer (a very rare event for DCIS) in the placebo group, two from cancers in the same breast as the original DCIS. In comparison, there were four deaths in the tamoxifen group, including three that were attributed to cancers in the treated breast.

Overall, the risk of any breast-related event (recurrent invasive disease, noninvasive disease, second cancers in the opposite breast, and metastasis) went from 13.4 to 8.2 percent at five years. Side effects included two cases of phlebitis in the placebo group and nine in the tamoxifen group with one nonfatal pulmonary embolus in the placebo group and two in the tamoxifen group. There was about a 10-percent higher incidence of hot flashes, fluid retention, and vaginal discharge in the tamoxifen group than in the placebo group. There were about 3.5 times as many cases of uterine cancer in the tamoxifen group as in the placebo group, although there were no uterine cancer deaths.

This is obviously a complex issue. The advantages are small, but then so are the risks. It is important to remember that this study was in women who had been treated with lumpectomy and radiation. In women who underwent mastectomy the benefits are unknown, but are probably limited to a decrease of cancer in the other breast. In a woman who chooses bilateral mastectomy there would be little to no benefit. Each woman will probably evaluate these risks and benefits differently.

Treatment Options for DCIS

What does all this mean for you? How should you proceed? First, if your routine mammogram has shown a cluster of microcalcifications you'll need to have a core biopsy or a wire localization biopsy (see Chapter 11). This will determine whether you have DCIS. The next step should always be to have another mammogram to see if the biopsy has gotten rid of all the microcalcifications. However thorough your surgeon has been, there still may be a few remaining. Then you've got the four choices described above: wide excision alone, wide excision and radiation, a combination of those with tamoxifen, or mastectomy. Currently there is a lot of difference among doctors about the best ways to treat DCIS. Until more studies come out with definitive answers, the controversies will rage. A reasonable approach to treatment options is discussed in the following paragraphs.

You can have that breast removed, which is the ultimate wide excision. Most of the time this will be more than adequate, but even with this there have been reports of recurrence of DCIS in the remaining breast tissue.[22,23] It happens only in about 5 percent of cases. We do a mastectomy only if the DCIS is so extensive that it's the only choice, or if the patient strongly wants it.

The next option is a wide excision. This means taking out the area with a centimeter-wide rim of normal tissue around it. Sometimes this has been done on the first operation and other times it is necessary to go back and remove more tissue (a re-excision).

If your margins are less than a centimeter, you can have a wide excision combined with radiation. You can add five years of tamoxifen to any of the choices above (the biggest benefit of doing this may be not in treating the DCIS but in preventing an invasive cancer or one in the other breast).

There is no reason to remove lymph nodes for small areas of DCIS since precancer can't spread at this stage. But if the lesions are big (greater than 5 centimeters), some experts think they may hide microinvasion and recommend removing the lymph nodes as well. (Sentinel node biopsy is a good option here.) On the other hand, as we mention in Chapter 21, many surgeons will forego lymph node dissection in this group as well, since even with microinvasion the chance of having positive nodes is so low.[24]

Since DCIS is not capable of spreading there is no reason to use chemotherapy. The fact that DCIS doubles your risk of getting cancer in the other breast is another factor to consider. But remember that this "double" isn't as alarming as it sounds: it's about the same risk a woman without breast cancer has because of having had a late first pregnancy. (If your general risk at 50 is 1 in 500, it becomes 1 in 250.) Some doctors suggest that you really need double mastectomies. But it's an individual decision. Some women who have regular mastectomies feel that if they have to lose one breast they may as well lose both and get it over with. Others feel that losing one breast makes the remaining one even more precious and they really want to save it. For the latter group close follow-up alone is the standard, but tamoxifen might be an option.

For the reasons discussed in Chapter 12, I try to encourage every woman to participate in a study, unless she has a definite preference or unless there are reasons to pick a particular treatment. As new studies and information come in we will be able to refine our understanding of DCIS and have a better basis for determining treatment. Every patient should have the final say in what treatment she gets: some women don't want a mastectomy no matter how big the lesions are, while at the other extreme some patients don't want to gamble even on the smallest lesion. Remember, there's not one single treatment for precancer; there are a number of possible treatments. You don't have to rush into any one treatment because your doctor or your friend or anyone else says you should. It's your breast, and your life. Take the time to decide what's best for you.

17

The Intraductal Approach—A
Breast Pap Smear?

It would be wonderful if we had a way to find all problem cells before they grow into cancer. But unfortunately we don't. We can't find all DCIS on mammogram: only about half of all DCIS cases create calcifications that will show up on the x ray. We can rarely find atypical hyperplasia on mammogram: it usually gets discovered accidentally, when we do a biopsy on a fibroadenoma or pseudolump and happen to notice it. Mammography finds abnormal cells when they're already malignant, and have been for a while. What we need is to find cells before they become cancers: to predict, and then prevent. And especially we need an additional way to evaluate those women between 25 and 40 whom we know to be at high risk for breast cancer. Breast self-exam is not much help (see Chapter 2); mammography isn't all that useful for younger women. Manual examination by doctors can help, but again, it's very limited.

What we've needed is something like a Pap smear for breast cancer—something that would be able to find abnormal cells, cancerous or not, before they have developed the ability to spread outside the breast, when they can be treated and the progression reversed (Fig. 17-1). We've known for a while that all breast cancer starts in the milk ducts. Since milk comes out of these ducts, I've always felt that there should be a way that we could go *into* them. If we could do that, we

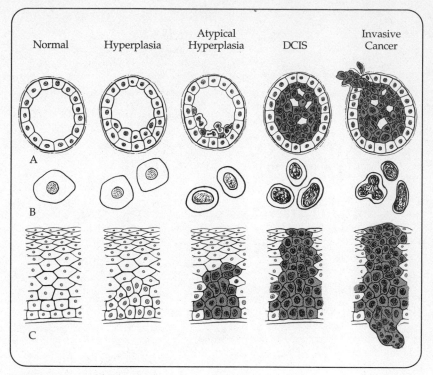

| Normal | Hyperplasia | Atypical Hyperplasia | DCIS | Invasive Cancer |

A. Breast Cancer Development
B. Cells from PAP Smear or Ductal Lavage
C. Cervical Cancer Development

FIGURE 17-1

could sample the lining of the duct and see what's happening to the cells inside it. In the mid-1980s I started a research project at the Faulkner Hospital on the intraductal approach to the breast that was to last almost 15 years and travel across country, finally developing into a company founded around the need to develop and make available a new technique.

Much as I'd like to be able to say that I came up with this idea on my own, I'm afraid it's just not true. The idea of studying the ducts and duct fluid was first mentioned back in 1946 when a Uruguayan doctor, LeBourgne, described a way to pass a small catheter into a breast duct and squirt saline in, take the catheter out, and collect the fluid as it dripped out.[1] He termed his procedure a "ductal rinse." Then in 1958 in the United States George Papanicolaou, the inventor of the cervical Pap smear, described applying suction to the nipple to obtain small drops of fluid from the milk ducts (Fig. 17-2). He termed it a "breast

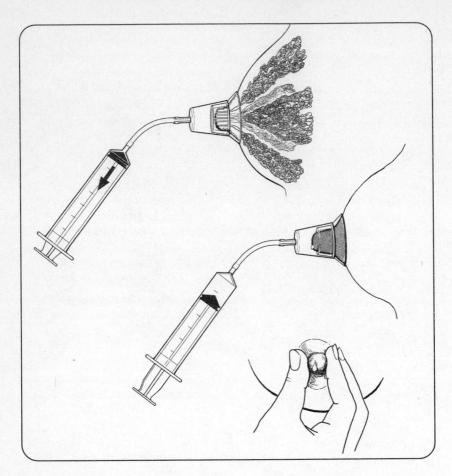

FIGURE 17-2

Pap smear."[2] (As I discussed in Chapter 7, it's not unusual to be able to get some fluid from a woman's breast.)

In spite of the fact that Papanicolaou had been able to diagnose one case of DCIS in nipple aspirate fluid (NAF), the technique languished for years. This was probably because no one knew in 1958 how the information could be used to help women. But curiosity remained, and in the 1970s, several researchers reevaluated Papanicolaou's approach. Three major series of studies took place, each advancing our understanding in a slightly different way: one by Gertrude Beuhring, another by Otto Sartorius, and the third by Eileen King and Nicholas Petrakis.[3,4,5] In all of them researchers were able to obtain fluid from about 80 percent of premenopausal women and 50 percent of postmenopausal women by using a suction cup on the nipple.

King and Petrakis took the long view. Between 1973 and 1980 they analyzed the fluid they obtained by aspirating the ducts on a series of 2,701 women. The researchers would try to get fluid from the woman's breast for five seconds. If no fluid appeared, the woman was classified as a "nonyielder." When they got fluid, it wasn't much—only a drop or so. They would collect this fluid on a slide. They then processed it, studied the cells, and classified these cells into normal, hyperplasia, atypical hyperplasia, and malignant. Margaret Wrensch joined them and they have been studying these women—all of whom were volunteers, and at no particular risk for breast cancer—for over 20 years. With a median of 21 years of follow-up, 285 of 3,633 women have developed breast cancer. The researchers compared the outcome with their initial evaluation of the fluid they'd taken 21 years earlier. Not surprisingly, they discovered that the women who had had no fluid also had the lowest incidence of breast cancer (4.7%). Those with fluid but with normal cells had a slightly higher incidence (8.2%) than those without fluid. Those with hyperplasia showed a bit higher (10.8%) incidence, and those with atypical cells the highest (13.8%). Account was taken of differences in the women's ages and the years they entered the study. The women with atypical cells had nearly three times the amount of breast cancer of the women with no fluid at all.

In a smaller group of 1,662 women from whom Petrakis, King, and colleagues attempted fluid collection between 1980 and 1985, 76 women have developed breast cancer in the intervening years. The women in this group who had either hyperplasia or atypical hyperplasia also had nearly three times the amount of breast cancer of the women with no fluid at all.

They also concluded from this study that women with atypical cells and a first-degree relative with breast cancer were nearly twice as likely to develop the disease as were women who had atypical cells but who did not have first-degree relatives with breast cancer. This certainly suggests that if you have both atypical cells and a family history of breast cancer you have a fairly high risk of getting the disease yourself. We are now arranging to do 20-year follow-up on the other two major studies, by Sartorius and Beuhring. So we should soon know how most of the 6,000 or so women who underwent the procedure more than 20 years ago have fared.

If you're very sharp-eyed (and have read every page of this book so far!) you'll notice that these numbers for increased risk due to abnormal cells are similar to those we find in biopsies that show atypical hyperplasia (see Chapter 11). Whether the cells are the same or not, the risk certainly appears to be.

Surprisingly, the early experiments with atypical cell detection didn't catch on, with either the public or the medical community.

There were two major reasons for this. For one thing, as in the 1950s we still did not know what to do with the information. If a woman had hyperplasia or even atypical hyperplasia, it was no guarantee that she would get breast cancer: in most cases, neither of those conditions grows into a cancer. What use, then, was the knowledge? Was the woman with hyperplasia going to get a mastectomy simply because she might one day have breast cancer? Or was she to spend years simply waiting nervously for the other shoe to drop?

At around the time all these studies were going on, mammography began to grow in popularity. It detected actual cancer or obvious pre-cancer (DCIS), not the processes leading to cancer—and the doctors knew what to do with that information. So the medical community greeted mammography with much more enthusiasm than it did the findings about ductal fluid.

But a few persistent researchers didn't give up. In Santa Barbara, Otto Sartorius didn't stop with NAF. He studied 2,000 women, using nipple aspiration. Of these women some produced either no fluid or too little fluid for him to analyze. Others were found to have atypical cells. He decided to literally probe this group of 400 women further. He threaded a tiny catheter into a duct opening at the nipple, squirted some contrast material through it into a duct, and did an x ray (ductogram). After this he instilled saline into the duct in an attempt to wash it out. He then removed the catheter and applied suction to the duct to retrieve the saline. He couldn't suction the fluid out through the catheter because the suction caused the flimsy duct to collapse (like sucking on a wet straw). He found that washing out the cells with saline usually provided enough cells to make a diagnosis.

Despite this improvement in cell yield, the procedure still was not adopted by the medical community. Doctors thought it was too hard to do and still didn't know what to do with the results.

But timing is everything. By the late 1990s as breast cancer rates continued to grow and the disease had become known as an "epidemic," researchers were desperately trying to find the means of detecting the earliest signs of breast cancer risk. They began to go back to the studies on breast duct fluid to see what possibilities these studies offered. They hoped that they could find a sign in the breast duct fluid of the early changes of cancer, something that could serve as a *marker* of what was going on biologically in the duct—a protein secreted by precancerous cells, for example. Ed Sauter, a surgeon from Fox Chase Hospital in Philadelphia, improved the suction technique (NAF) so that he was able to retrieve fluid from close to 100 percent of women.[6] He then looked for PSA, a protein marker which had proved valuable in the diagnosis of prostate cancer. Other researchers have looked for other markers, but as yet the perfect one that can predict who is at risk for breast cancer has not been identified.

In a different approach to the problem of identifying the woman with high-risk changes in the breast, Carol Fabian in Kansas explored the use of fine-needle aspirates (see Chapter 11)—sticking small needles into both breasts on both sides of the nipple and then suctioning out some cells.[7] Although this technique has demonstrated atypical changes in the tissue of high-risk women when compared to those of normal risk, it also has its limitations. The common thinking, as we discussed in Chapter 13, is that breast cancer starts in the lining of the milk ducts and that only one ductal system goes bad. If this is the case it would be important to identify a ductal system with abnormal cells and be able to recheck it after an intervention to see if the changes had disappeared. If atypical cells are identified by random needle sticks it is more difficult to be sure which duct they are in, and to get back to the very same spot in six months.

I was convinced that the answer to this problem was in accessing the ducts directly, not through suction of the whole nipple or randomly sampling the breast. My research team at Faulkner Hospital first tried using a ductoscope in the ducts to find abnormalities. This was not very successful because the ducts divide very early into many branches, like a bushy tree (see Fig. 1-4a). We tried the nipple aspirate fluid (NAF) collection with a suction device but were frustrated by the fact that the fluid had to be pooled for analysis, making it impossible for us to know which duct it came from. I also tried Otto Sartorius's technique with a catheter but was frustrated by the small amount of fluid I was able to recover. I decided that a double lumen catheter (catheter with two inner tubes) might fit the bill. We could thread it into the lactiferous sinus, squirt salt water into one lumen, and suck it out of the other. After much experimentation in women under anesthesia who were having mastectomies or on breasts that were freshly removed I was able to demonstrate that a double lumen catheter could retrieve cells from a duct. This success led me to found a company with an engineering friend, Julian Nikolchev. The company, known as Pro•Duct Health, set out to develop a catheter for washing out the duct (ductal lavage).

At the same time, with help from a grant from the Department of Defense, my research continued. I was often the guinea pig. We were initially stymied by the absence of a clear map of the ductal orifices. After studying breast-feeding women with the help of La Leche League, we determined that there were between five and nine openings in the nipple and that the pattern was fairly stable (See Fig. 1-6). We also reevaluated all of the ductograms done by Otto Sartorius and found that the ducts were distributed in the breasts in two concentric circles, with an inner group of three or four and a second, more peripheral, group of three or four (see Fig. 1-4C). These anatomical studies helped us find the openings of the ducts and we confirmed them by injecting blue dye into the nipples of breasts that had been removed by mastectomy and observing the holes the dye emerged from. I even tried it on myself a few times, much to my 11-year-old daughter's chagrin. I didn't find it particularly unpleasant—but Katie did. The dye turns the nipple blue for several days, and Katie walked into my room one day while I was getting dressed. She glared at me. "Mom!" she said angrily. "Do you know how *embarrassing* it is to have a mother with blue nipples?" I tried to explain to her that there was no need for her to be embarrassed; I had no intention of displaying my nipples,

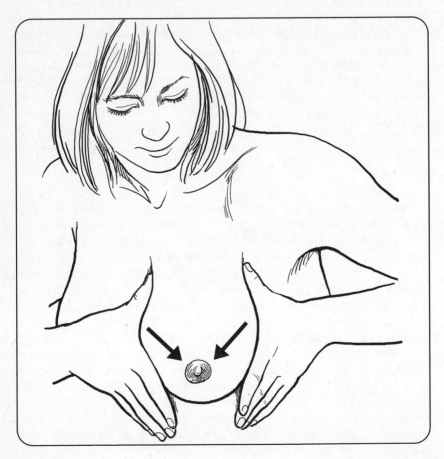

FIGURE 17-3

whatever their color, to any of her friends or their parents. It didn't matter. Mom was not to have blue nipples. Luckily we've moved on a bit, and are no longer using the blue dye—so no 11-year-old need ever again be embarrassed by the color of her mother's nipples.

Eventually it became clear that the ducts we wanted to study were the ones that yielded fluid on suction. These were the ones most likely to have pathology, according to the earlier studies of Petrakis and Sartorius. The company's first clinical trial designed to demonstrate the utility of this approach involved studying women at high risk for breast cancer. We first had the women massage their breasts (Fig. 17-3) and we applied suction to their nipples. Once a duct or ducts were identified a tiny ductal catheter was threaded into a milk duct for a distance of about 0.5 inch (1 cm) (Fig. 17-4). The duct was washed with salt water and then cells were retrieved from deep in each ductal tree. The fluid was sent to be examined by a cytologist (pathologist who studies cells) and we determined whether there were normal, atypical, or cancerous cells present. These cells were compared to those in the

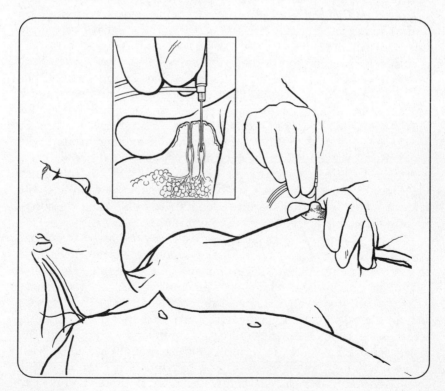

FIGURE 17-4

fluid obtained by suction alone (NAF). The preliminary results from this study were reported at the American Society of Clinical Oncology (ASCO) meeting in May 2000. In this study of 271 breasts which were subjected to both nipple aspiration and ductal lavage, the preliminary results demonstrated that lavage was better than NAF at finding atypical cells. Lavage identified 42 breasts with atypical or malignant cells while NAF found only 12. In addition, only 18 percent of the NAF cases yielded sufficient cells for diagnosis compared to 70 percent of the lavage cases. In this study of high-risk women who were normal by mammography and physical exam one year prior to enrolling in the study, researchers found one high-grade cancer.

Some of the first volunteers were moderately uncomfortable, depending on their sensitivity to pain and the ease with which their fluid came out. One woman, whose fluid came quite easily, describes the procedure as "less painful and invasive than a Pap smear," and compared it to going to the dentist. "It's more frightening to think about than to do," she laughs. "I'm pretty squeamish, so I didn't watch them do it, and that helped." In the earlier studies we used injections of lidocaine, and this patient found the anesthetic needle more uncomfortable than the process itself. When the anesthetic wore off, "I felt it—not quite pain, but tenderness: I was very aware that I had a nipple," she says. But she had no bruising or discomfort later.

Another volunteer found the process even less problematic. With both NAF and lavage, she found the sensations strange, rather than painful. "I nursed two kids when I was younger," she says, "and it seemed weird at first, having this pressure at my breast/nipple that wasn't connected to either sexual pleasure or suckling an infant. So you have to get used to the notion that they're messing around with your breast." She didn't like the anesthetic needles, but described them as "pinpricks." The discomfort, she says, was "so minor, it didn't matter." Since beginning the study we have improved our technique with a new catheter that doesn't require needle sticks or lidocaine injections, making the whole procedure more comfortable.

And what do you *do* with the information? By the year 2000 we had several options for managing high-risk women. For starters they could be followed more closely with exams and mammograms. Tamoxifen is another option. In the large NSABP tamoxifen prevention study, women with atypical hyperplasia who were treated with tamoxifen had an eighty-six percent reduction in their chances of developing breast cancer compared with similar women treated with placebo. This makes sense since nearly all atypical cells are thought to still be sensitive to estrogen. A more drastic approach, but one that women with a genetic risk and atypical cells might consider, is preventive mastectomy which Lynn Hartman from the Mayo Clinic showed would reduce the risk of breast cancer by 90 percent. Finally, women could participate in the STAR trial that randomizes women who are high-risk to take either tamoxifen or raloxifene, one of the new designer estrogens. If malignant cells are found in a woman with a normal mammogram and physical examination, a ductogram can be done (see Chapter 19) to delineate the area in question for surgery.

In 1999 the Santa Barbara Breast Cancer Institute, now known as the Susan Love, M.D., Breast Cancer Foundation, sponsored the first International Conference on nipple aspirate fluid in honor of its founder, Otto Sartorius, who died in 1995 after a lifetime of dedicated work on breast cancer. There were researchers from 10 or 15 breast centers from all over the U.S. as well as from the Czech Republic, England, and Japan. Essentially all the people researching NAF were there—Nicholas Petrakis, Gertrude Beuhring, Margaret Wrensch, and others. And the new generation was also there. We wanted all those doing work in the '90s to learn from those who had done the '70s work. We even managed to pull Dr. Petrakis's research nurse, Lynn Mason, out of retirement in Arizona, to help train those of us in the new wave. We wanted to jump-start this area of research by giving scientists all of the tools they might need.

One thing that came out of the conference was a consensus on which patients would not be good candidates for ductal lavage. Women who had the following conditions, we agreed, were poor candidates:

1. Anyone who had had radiation to her breast, since radiation dries up fluid.
2. Anyone who had had surgery around her nipple, since the ducts were likely to have been cut (in this case we could try; there would be only a slight chance it would work) (see Chapter 11).
3. Anyone who had had a subareolar abscess (see Chapter 11). Some ducts may still function after this, but there's no guarantee.
4. Anyone who has had breast reduction surgery: sometimes this involves the nipple being moved, and thus the ducts are cut (see Chapter 5).

If a woman has had a lumpectomy without accompanying radiation, the test wouldn't be useful in the ducts around the area that had been operated on, but the other ducts in that breast should remain unaffected.

The Susan Love, M.D. Breast Cancer Foundation has as one of its goals supporting research into these techniques. Apart from their immediate use in identifying women with normal, atypical, and malignant ductal cells, my hope is that the techniques of nipple aspirate fluid collection and ductal lavage will provide a new route for the study of the breast. It will help us answer questions about the concentration of pesticides in breast duct fluid as well as identify the early mutations that have to take place before a woman develops breast cancer. It will also allow us to proceed much more rapidly in identifying reliable ways to prevent breast cancer by allowing us to pick out the women truly at risk and monitor them as we try different treatment agents.

Ductal lavage will be available at some of the top breast centers around the country within the near future. When it initially becomes available, doctors will most likely use it in the population most likely to benefit from it: women at high risk for breast cancer and women with breast cancer. Ultimately, however, I think its usefulness will prove far greater than just to that population. As more data become available and use becomes more widespread, doctors may begin using it as routine testing. It's easy learn and fairly inexpensive. Back in 1958 Dr. Papanicolaou wrote, on the basis if his findings, that "examination of the breast in the presence of secretions in patients without symptoms" might help prevent breast cancers from occurring.[8] Those words may well prove to be prophetic.

18

===

Prevention

When we did the first edition of this book, we didn't have a separate chapter called "Prevention." That's because at the time there wasn't enough material for such a chapter. In the second edition we added a chapter, but it was more about hope for prevention than about reality. With this edition we go a step further. In the past two years we have established both chemoprevention and surgical prevention as means of reducing the risk of breast cancer. In addition, with gene testing and now nipple fluid analysis we have ways to determine who might benefit from such approaches. We have come a long way indeed.

LIFESTYLE CHANGES

According to Canadian epidemiologist Anthony Miller, the major factors that seem amenable to change and that therefore have potential for prevention are diet, reduction in obesity, reduction in the use of estrogens at menopause, and—more controversially—a shift back to women having their first babies at an earlier age.[1]

Table 18-1 lists Miller's attributable risks for some of these environmental and lifestyle risk factors. Remember, attributable risk is the amount of breast cancer that can be attributed to a certain risk factor

Table 18-1. Attributable Risks for Breast Cancer[a]
(percent of breast cancer cases that can be attributed to each factor)

	Attributable Risk
Age 25 or greater with first birth	17%
Estrogen replacement therapy	8
High-fat diet	26
Obesity	12

[a]A.B. Miller, "Epidemiology and Prevention," in J.R. Harris, S. Hellman, I.C. Henderson, and D.W. Kinne, eds., *Breast Diseases* (Philadelphia: J.B. Lippincott, 1987).

(or eliminated if that factor is changed). The degree of certainty varies for each risk factor. These are all very interesting from a public health standpoint, but may or may not be applicable to any one individual woman, and I don't advise using them as the sole influence in decision making. For example, I had my first child at 40 and do not regret it. The advantages to me far outweighed the slight potential increased risk for breast cancer that this may entail. Would I have been wiser to have had a child in my 20s, when I wasn't ready for it? Or, since having no children is actually less of a risk than having a first child later in life, should I have deprived myself of the joy Katie has brought me? For me, there was no question. On the other hand, I do eat a good diet high in fruits and vegetables and low in animal fat. The occasional twinge I feel at the sight of a juicy hamburger or wedge of Brie is a reasonable price to pay for the possibility that I may be decreasing my breast cancer risk and improving my overall health. These are very individual decisions.

Diet

As you'll recall from our discussion in Chapter 15, the possibilities that a low-fat diet may decrease breast cancer are looking less promising, but the final answer should come from the Women's Health Initiative. Whether you do it through a study or not, you can get onto a low-fat diet, and I still think it's wise for any woman to do so. I'm not sure that it prevents breast cancer, but it's certainly healthier in terms of preventing heart disease and stroke. Further, we do know that obesity is a risk factor for breast cancer in adult women, and a low-fat diet makes you less likely to be obese.

Your diet should also be high in fiber, in antioxidants, and in green leafy vegetables. I concur with the National Cancer Institute's recommendation of five servings of vegetables and/or fruits a day. Some interesting research is also suggesting benefits from soy protein, perhaps a factor in the low incidence of breast cancer in East Asia (see Chapter 15). It also makes sense to drink alcohol only in moderation, since, as we discussed in Chapter 15, regular consumption of liquor may affect your vulnerability to breast cancer, in addition to all of its other effects.

Exercise

Exercise is important for cardiovascular health and for preventing osteoporosis and heart disease—and, probably, breast cancer. A study by Leslie Bernstein at the University of Southern California came out in the fall of 1994 demonstrating that women who participated in four or more hours of exercise a week during their reproductive years have a 58 percent decrease in breast cancer risk.[2] This is very exciting because it is one of the first lifestyle changes that has been shown to decrease risk. The mechanism is hormonal. The study showed no association at all between body mass index, weight or height, and breast cancer risk. In fact, studies of body mass and breast cancer risk among premenopausal women are consistent in showing that obesity is not a risk factor for breast cancer at young ages. There is a correlation in young girls, however, with moderate exercise and alterations in menstrual cycle patterns and ovulatory frequency.[3] Since, as we discuss below, late onset of menstruation works against breast cancer, this is significant (Fig. 18-1). A prospective cohort study of Norwegian women aged 20–24 found that consistently active women had 37 percent less breast cancer than consistently sedentary women.[4]

A good, long-term prevention approach would be to increase adolescent athletics and thus get girls into the habit of exercising. Rose Frisch of Harvard Medical School and Harvard School of Public Health has also shown that women who were involved in athletics during high school and college have a decreased risk of breast cancer.[5]

As a result, a proposal has been very seriously put forth that I find delightful: put increased funding into high school athletics for girls. This would be likely to decrease breast cancer and also strengthen bones and prevent future osteoporosis and it would help to prevent heart disease. The next generation of women could probably dispense with the need for postmenopausal hormones for prevention if we could increase the exercise levels in girls and adolescents. (One caution in all this. There has been a near epidemic of eating disorders among teenage girls desperate to conform to our culture's "thin is beautiful" image. "Low-fat" doesn't translate to "no food," and to be beneficial,

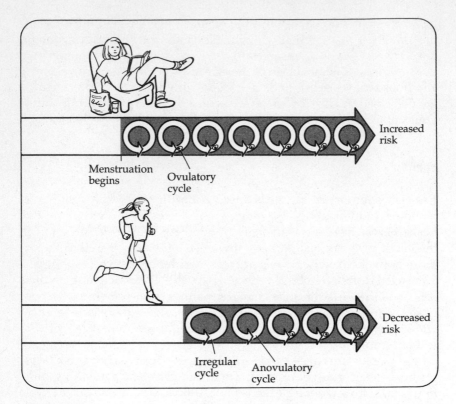

FIGURE 18-1

exercise requires a well-nourished body. Breast cancer will not be a big issue if a girl has so badly damaged her body with starvation that she doesn't live long enough to worry about it.)

Exercise in adult women is undoubtedly of value as well, in terms of a number of health concerns, although its effectiveness in terms of breast cancer is less clear. Besides, when you exercise every day you get to feel morally superior.

HORMONES

Another approach to preventing breast cancer has been through studying hormones. As we mentioned in Chapter 14, the earlier you have your first period and the later your menopause—the more menstruating years—the higher your risk of breast cancer. And the younger you are when you have your first child, the lower your risk. So there has been some thought that we might have an effect on breast cancer risk by coming up with a way to induce a hormonal "pregnancy," in which

294

a teenager would be given the hormones of pregnancy for nine months to mature the breast tissue. To my knowledge, this has only been tried in rats so far, but it's an interesting possibility.

A related idea, which is actually being tried at USC by Doctors Malcolm Pike and Darcy Spicer, is devising a type of contraceptive that might protect against breast cancer, based on the fact that reproductive hormone levels lead to an increased risk.[6] The women in the study are given GnRH inhibitors, which are drugs that inhibit the pituitary gland from stimulating the ovary (see Chapter 1). This puts the woman into a reversible menopause (Fig. 18-2). Staying indefinitely in this state would put young women at risk for osteoporosis, so they are put on a low dose of estrogen, just enough to help prevent hot flashes, but less than they'd have if they were regularly menstruating. Since if they received estrogen alone they would be at risk for endometrial cancer, every two or three months they receive a small amount of progesterone. The women have been carefully monitored (which includes regular mammograms), and it was found after the first six to nine months of the study that they had an increase in bone loss, so a bit of androgen has been added.

This particular "cocktail" will, in theory, reduce breast, ovarian, and uterine cancer, while acting as a contraceptive. An interesting effect in

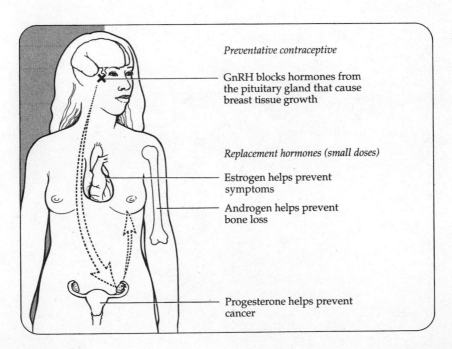

Preventative contraceptive

GnRH blocks hormones from the pituitary gland that cause breast tissue growth

Replacement hormones (small doses)

Estrogen helps prevent symptoms

Androgen helps prevent bone loss

Progesterone helps prevent cancer

FIGURE 18-2

the first 20 women to be studied on this new contraceptive was a change in their mammograms.[7] After a year on the study they were found to have reduced density of tissue. We don't as yet know whether this means that they are successfully preventing breast cancer or whether it will just make a cancer easier to detect. It is provocative, however, and lends credence to Pike and Spicer's approach. It's a fairly complicated contraceptive, and it wouldn't be used by everyone. But it might be good for a woman whose family has hereditary breast cancer and who has a gene that makes it more likely that she'll get the disease. Again, I'm not too crazy about using medicine to prevent disease, but this could be right for a certain population of young women.

TAMOXIFEN AND OTHER SERMS

The drugs used for prevention of breast cancer all have to do with the fact that the precancerous cell has four possible actions (Fig. 18-3). It

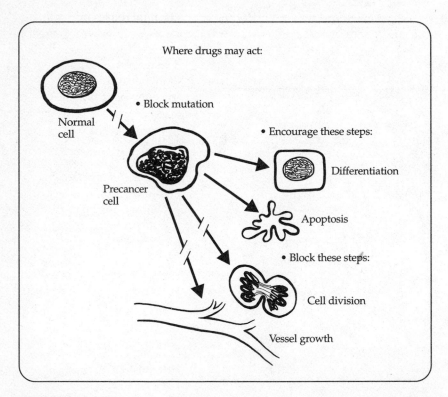

FIGURE 18-3

can terminally differentiate and become a functional, nondividing cell. It can commit suicide, which is called "apoptosis" (see Chapter 13). It can proliferate, grow and create more cells, and it can incite more blood vessels to grow in (see Chapter 13).

Estrogen increases proliferation and decreases apoptosis. Blocking estrogen, then, should be helpful in preventing breast cancer. This is the theory behind the efforts to prevent breast cancer by giving women tamoxifen.

Tamoxifen didn't begin its life as a cancer treatment. It was actually developed in 1967 as a fertility drug. But then the researchers realized it could block estrogen, so they decided to try it in treating breast cancer.

There was initially some concern about the possibility that its use would lead to more heart disease, since it blocked estrogen. I voiced that concern in the first edition of this book. As it turns out, however, not only does tamoxifen block estrogen in the breast but it also acts as a weak estrogen in the liver, resulting in a good effect on cholesterol rates, lowering the dangerous LDL. It doesn't, however, raise the helpful HDL. And its effect on LDL is only half as good as that of estrogen. It neither lessened nor increased osteoporosis: it increases bone density slightly, but doesn't affect the number of fractures.

The real surprise was that it seems to cause uterine cancer. Why, we wondered, would something that blocked estrogen increase uterine cancer, which is *caused* by estrogen? It soon became apparent that tamoxifen acted like estrogen in some organs even as it blocked estrogen in other organs.

With this discovery, a new term was coined—selected estrogen receptor modulator, or SERM. We all like to act now as if we set out to make the SERMs (also known as "designer estrogens") and, after much research, finally succeeded. But the reality is quite different: we stumbled on the phenomenon, and then gave it a name. Still, if we weren't clever enough to figure out how useful SERMs would be until we'd stumbled on them, we quickly learned, and many drug companies set out to capitalize on the discovery. Soon raloxifene was on the market, to be shortly followed by several others.

Even before the marvels of tamoxifen as a breast cancer prevention tool had given it its fancy new category, researchers who had been using it for treatment of already existing cancers had begun to realize that when women with breast cancer took tamoxifen, not only would they have decreased recurrences of the original cancer, but they also had 30 to 50 percent fewer cancers in the opposite breast. A woman who usually had a 10-percent risk of breast cancer now had a 5 to 7 percent risk. If the drug could prevent new cancers in women who already had the disease, thought the researchers, perhaps it could further reduce the susceptibility of women who were at high risk. A study, the National Surgical Adjuvant Breast and Bowel Project (NSABP), was devised to examine that possibility.[8] It was a huge study—13,388 women. First they used the Gail Model, a statistical combination of risk factors to calculate who was at increased risk.[9] These factors included a woman's age at her first period, age at her first pregnancy, whether or not she'd ever had a breast biopsy before, family history, and whether she had atypical hyperplasia or LCIS (see Chapter 14).

They decided that they would consider any woman 60 or over to be at high risk. If a woman under 60 had risk factors that added up to those of a 60-year-old, she could take part in the study. Thus, a woman over 60 in the study might have only one risk factor—for example, she had her first child at a late age. But a 30-year-old would have to have three family members with breast cancer. (There are limitations to the Gail model, which are discussed later in the chapter.)

Having picked the subjects for their study group, they then randomized them (see Chapter 12), giving half the group tamoxifen and half a placebo. Among these women, some had lobular carcinoma *in situ* and some had atypical ductal hyperplasia (see Chapter 16). Although the study included women with a risk of 1.6 percent or more, most women in the study had a higher risk—and half of them had more than a 3 percent risk.

Overall, the study showed that taking tamoxifen decreased by 49 percent the danger of getting invasive cancer. What this means is that there were fewer cases of breast cancer among the women who took tamoxifen than among those who didn't. But the numbers aren't huge: 89 women in the tamoxifen group got cancer, while 175 women in the placebo group did. In an overall group of more than 13,000 women, those aren't very large figures.

The benefit persisted in all age groups, though the numbers were small. In some groups the difference was more dramatic. For example, the women with previously diagnosed atypical hyperplasia had an 86 percent decreased risk. This was based on a small number of cases: 3 cases in the tamoxifen group and 23 in the placebo group. Perhaps the most important finding in the study is that intervening at an earlier point, when most cells are still sensitive to estrogen, is the key to real prevention. This gives more power to the likelihood of detecting atypical breast duct cells in breast duct fluid (see Chapter 17).

Another interesting thing about this tamoxifen study is that all the cancers the placebo group got and the tamoxifen group didn't were estrogen receptor positive. This makes sense, since tamoxifen is an estrogen blocker. But it also shows the limitations of tamoxifen. It will have its strongest effect if all tumors start out sensitive to hormones.

In addition, we know that women with estrogen receptor positive tumors have a better prognosis. This raises a big question: is it really worth taking tamoxifen? Is preventing breast cancer, in these conditions, better than curing it if it happens? If we prevent only cancers that we could cure if we caught them early on mammography, is it worthwhile? Prevention is certainly better than finding and not curing, but we can't be sure yet if it's better than finding and curing. Do we want long-term use, or short-term use?

This study lasted only four years, and that too is a serious limitation. It couldn't look at death from breast cancer, because cancer takes time to develop, be detected, and kill. So there's no way of knowing if the tamoxifen prevented cancer deaths, or only prevented the appearance of cancers that wouldn't have been fatal anyway.

Confusing the issue even more is the fact that the current study includes the prevention of DCIS. But only a third of DCIS becomes invasive cancer. So we can't say that preventing DCIS equates with preventing invasive cancer, let alone fatal cancer.

Another issue is that a lot of the prevention happened immediately, within the first year or two. So we need to question whether it's really preventing cancer, or treating a cancer that isn't yet detectable—remember that cancers are around for years before we're able to detect them.

It might be that tamoxifen prevention still saves lives, but we won't know that until we have a long enough study. Luckily two European studies are going on that will help us be able to look and see whether more of the women who took the placebo died of breast cancer over time.

Because of all these questions, the FDA did not grant the pharmaceutical company, Zeneca, permission to market tamoxifen as "cancer prevention." Breast cancer activists argued vociferously against this terminology, pointing out that the public is likely to interpret "prevention" as meaning those who take it will never get the disease. They pointed out too that, with only a few years of study, the most the company could claim is that they could "prevent" the disease for five years, no longer. So the FDA permitted them to use only the words "risk reduction."

Zeneca has been distributing a "risk disk" to help doctors determine who will benefit from taking tamoxifen. This "risk disk" has some limitations. It is based on the Gail model, one of many models developed to estimate a woman's risk of getting subsequent breast cancer. Although it comprises several factors, it leaves out others that may be equally important. For example, it doesn't ask if the woman is on hormones or whether she was exposed to radiation. The biggest problem though, is that of family history. The model deals only with breast cancer in a subject's mother, sister, or daughter, not with cousins, grandparents, or aunts. But hereditary breast cancer can be passed down through the father's or the mother's line. If your paternal grandmother and paternal aunts all had breast cancer, you would appear to be at low risk in the Gail model, but could have inherited BRCA1 or 2.

It's an interesting tool, but that is all it is. It can tell you only your statistical risk according to its criteria. It does not tell you if you actually will get breast cancer. It also doesn't tell you what would happen if you changed your diet, started exercising, and stopped taking hormones. So if you don't fit the model, don't feel confident that you're risk free. It's a good sign, but not conclusive in any way. By the same token, if you do fit the model, don't panic. There are many options for you to consider.

Risks and Benefits of Tamoxifen for Prevention

As with all drugs, there are risks in taking tamoxifen. In the study just mentioned some areas show more deaths among the placebo group (see Table 18-2). In others, though, there are more in the tamoxifen group. (Remember, there were the same number of women in both groups.)[10]

Most worrisome are the clotting problems leading to phlebitis, pulmonary emboli, and strokes, and the uterine cancers. These are probably risks worth taking to cure cancer. But prevention is a thornier question. You may well die from a pulmonary embolism you got trying to

Table 18-2. Risks and Benefits of Tamoxifen for Prevention

	Placebo	Tamoxifen
Breast cancer cases	175	89
Breast cancer deaths	6	3
Hip fracture	22	12
Endometrial cancer	15	36
Stroke	24	38
Pulmonary emboli	0	3
Deep vein thrombosis	22	35
Cataracts	507	574
Other fractures	54	37

M. Gail, J.P. Costantino, J. Bryant et al., "Weighing the Risks and Benefits of Tamoxifen Treatment for Preventing Breast Cancer," *Journal of the National Cancer Institute* 91 (1999): 1829–1846. Used by permission of M. Gail.

cure a cancer you may never have had. It is important to note that the absolute risks from tamoxifen of endometrial cancer, stroke, pulmonary embolism, and deep vein thrombosis increase with age. Most of the risk was in the women over 50. There were 75 percent more strokes and heart attacks among these women. Tamoxifen is also most beneficial for the women at highest risk of breast cancer. This leads to the conclusion that its greatest use should be in younger women with a high risk of breast cancer. In addition, the risks of heart attacks, strokes, and thrombosis are higher in black women, making the risk of tamoxifen higher in this group.

Dr. M. Gail, who created the Gail Index, has developed a complex model to determine the risks and benefits according to the age and race of the woman. For example, a 40-year-old white woman with a uterus and a risk of breast cancer of 2 percent who took tamoxifen for five years might look at a chart like Table 18-3.

The risks increase as the woman becomes older. The good news is that the greatest risk of uterine cancer appears to occur in women who have previously taken estrogen therapy (without Provera) for menopause. For a woman who has not been on ERT the risks may be lower

Table 18-3. Potential Risks and Benefits of Tamoxifen for Prevention

Type of Event	Expected Number of Cases per 10,000 Untreated Women	Expected Effect Among 10,000 Women Who Were Treated with Tamoxifen for Five Years
		Potential Benefit
Invasive breast cancer	200	97 cases may be prevented
In situ breast cancer	106	53 cases may be prevented
Hip fracture	2	1 case may be prevented
		Potential Risk
Endometrial cancer	10	16 more cases may be caused
Stroke	22	13 more cases may be caused
Pulmonary embolism	7	15 more cases may be caused
Deep vein thrombosis	24	15 more cases may be caused

Source: M. Gail, J.P. Costantino, J. Bryant, et al., "Weighing the Risks and Benefits of Tamoxifen Treatment for Preventing Breast Cancer," *Journal of the National Cancer Institute* 91 (1999): 1829–1846. Used by permission of M. Gail.

(see Chapter 15). There were also fewer severe problems—hot flashes and vaginal dryness.

In addition to the risks, women who want to take tamoxifen have a number of important questions to address. Since it will work only for four or five years, which four or five years are the most sensible for you? When you stop taking it, will your original risk return? Or will the tamoxifen have reversed the risk for a longer period of time? We have reason to think it may: in women who take it to cure breast cancer there is at least a 10-year benefit even after they stop. That may or may not apply to prevention: at this stage, we simply don't know.

There are two tamoxifen studies going on in Europe now. Both are continuing to study the long-term effects, and both are very good studies—randomized, double-blind, and so on. The one in England is a pilot study that has been looking at 2,471 women for 70 months, and to date has found virtually the same numbers of breast cancers in both groups—5 per 1,000 women in the placebo group; 4.7 per 1,000 in the tamoxifen group.[11] The study in Milan, looking at 5,400 women who weren't at especially high risk, also found no difference between the women who took tamoxifen and those on placebo after 46 months.[12] (All of these women had previously had total hysterectomies, since the researchers knew this would eliminate the problem of causing uterine cancer during the study.)

Why are there such conflicting studies? Unfortunately, we don't know. There are several possibilities. It may have to do with the fact that they're studying different populations. The NSABP P1 (Prevention 1) study used the Gail model to identify women at increased risk. This model focuses on hormonal risks such as age of first period and of menopause, and it can underestimate family and hereditary risk. The British study picked those who were at high risk because of family history—it was more skewed toward genetics. The Italian study didn't focus on high-risk women at all, but used only women who had had hysterectomies, which possibly created another slant, since women who have hysterectomies in their 40s or earlier are at lower risk than the general population, so it might take longer to see if there's any benefit in these groups than in the NSABP group.

In England, the International Breast Cancer Intervention Study (IBIS) is continuing to put women on tamoxifen, and it has 4,000 subjects so far. They will continue to follow them long-term. In continental Europe, there are two other studies going on comparing other SERMs against placebo. In the U.S., there's the STAR trial, comparing tamoxifen against raloxifene.

What I find truly exciting about tamoxifen is not so much its current uses in preventing breast cancer, but the fact that it opens up that possibility. It reminds me of the beginnings of antibiotics. The first antibiotic ever used was streptomycin, developed right after World War II. It was a miracle in its time, but was quite toxic. However, it paved the way for other antibiotics that were more specific for different bacteria and had fewer side effects. We never use streptomycin anymore.

So tamoxifen has opened up new vistas. It may or may not be one of the drugs we'll continue using indefinitely. But like streptomycin, it will always be remembered with gratitude.

Raloxifene

The accidental discovery of tamoxifen's potential effect on breast cancer was followed by furious research for drugs with similar capabilities. Raloxifene (Evista) is the first such drug—the first true designer SERM. It's been on the market since 1999. It was created to make a drug that has the positive effect of estrogen on the body with none of its negative effects—in particular, uterine cancer. The biggest study to date has been done by the pharmaceutical company Lilly. It's called the MORE study (Multiple Outcomes of Raloxifene Evaluations), and it's part of a study Lilly has been doing to see if raloxifene could affect the bones.[13]

The study has been done on women in their 60s who have low enough bone density to be diagnosed as having osteoporosis. This two-year study has shown that raloxifene does indeed improve bone density by about 3 to 4 percent—not as well as either alendronate (Fosamax) or estrogen (which improve bone density by 8 percent), but better than a placebo. This is important because it allowed Lilly to get FDA approval of the drug for osteoporosis prevention. Such approval takes only a year or two, because you can see the difference in bone density tests in two years. Once the FDA has approved a drug for one purpose, it can be prescribed for virtually any purpose.

As part of the overall study, Lilly also tried to discover whether raloxifene could prevent breast cancer. They found that in postmenopausal women with low breast cancer risk, risk of invasive breast cancer decreased by 76 percent during three years of treatment. (Remember that women with low bone density have less risk of breast cancer, and women with low risk of breast cancer have a higher risk of osteoporosis.) There were 13 cases of breast cancer in the 5,129 women given raloxifene vs. 27 in the 2,576 women given placebo. To prevent one case of breast cancer, 176 women had to take raloxifene. As with tamoxifen, raloxifene affected only estrogen receptor positive tumors (see Chapter 20). It also shared tamoxifen's effect on pulmonary emboli, increasing them by 300 percent. It did not, however, increase the incidence of uterine cancer. There was one case of pulmonary emboli per 155 women, and of the women who got pulmonary emboli, one died. It's also the same as tamoxifen in terms of causing hot flashes and vaginal dryness, so it's probably not good for women who have these symptoms already, since it intensifies them.

It might appear that a 76 percent reduction of breast cancer trumps tamoxifen's 49 percent decrease, but the data really aren't comparable. To begin with, while the tamoxifen study looked at women at high risk, the raloxifene study looked at women who, because they had low bone density and thus by definition had little estrogen in their bodies, were at *low* risk for breast cancer.

Unfortunately, a lot of doctors are jumping on the bandwagon and putting their high-risk patients on raloxifene. They may be doing good for these women; they may be doing harm. But they're not using a drug that's been studied long enough to use outside of a trial context. It hasn't been studied in high-risk women or women with breast cancer, and shouldn't at this point be used by women in those categories. And, according to ASCO (the American Society of Clinical Oncology), the data are insufficient to recommend it for breast cancer prevention. It should only be used for prevention of osteoporosis.[14]

The STAR Trial

Some of our questions about raloxifene will be answered in a new trial now under way, the STAR (study on tamoxifen and raloxifene). In this study high-risk postmenopausal women are randomized to take one of the two drugs for five years. Once the researchers know the safety in premenopausal women, they're planning to include such women in the STAR trial. I would encourage any eligible woman who wants to try raloxifene to do it by participating in this trial. It's quite extensive—there are 400 centers in the U.S. If women get on raloxifene without the necessary data, we may end up facing the same predicament that happened with bone marrow transplant and hormone therapy to prevent heart disease: they became the standard of care, and were later found not to work. Other studies going on looking at raloxifene, tamoxifen, and other SERMs will help us find the answers to some of these questions.

It's good that they're developing drugs like raloxifene that seem to cause fewer dangerous side effects in the process of offering possible cancer prevention. But it's equally important to come up with mechanisms for determining who should get such drugs. The drug that is without any side effects is rare indeed, and this means that any drug should be taken only when the benefits are worth risking the side effects.

Meanwhile, should you, the reader, take raloxifene or tamoxifen? It depends. Possibly if you're at extremely high risk for breast cancer, it would be worth it. In that case, however, you'd be better off doing it as part of a study such as STAR. And you need to be aware that this is very early in the development of SERMs. I think it's very likely that, just as raloxifene appears to be an improvement over tamoxifen, so there will be other SERMs in a few years that are even better. It's exciting that there are drugs that can be used for prevention. It's another step in moving forward, away from diagnosis and treatment of breast cancer and into prediction and prevention.

One SERM we know of actually occurs in nature—soy. It still needs further study (see Chapter 29), but it holds out promise for a dietary approach to breast cancer prevention.

RETINOIDS

Another study being done on a possible breast cancer preventive is the 4HPR study.[15] 4HPR is a relative of vitamin A, a type of retinoid. In many cancers, particularly lung cancer, it has been shown to be preventive. The National Cancer Institute funded a study in Milan looking at women who have had stage 1 breast cancer to see if 4HPR will reduce the incidence of cancer in the opposite breast. The initial data were reported in November 1999 and showed no reduction in risk. There was some suggestion, however, that the premenopausal women benefited while the postmenopausal women didn't.[16] We will need further studies to confirm this observation.

PREVENTIVE MASTECTOMY

Most people assume that the foolproof way to prevent breast cancer is to remove the breasts. If you don't have breasts, the reasoning goes, you won't get breast cancer. It's a pretty drastic solution: most women like their breasts for aesthetic and erotic reasons, even if they're not planning to use them for breast feeding. Yet there are some women who are so terrified of the possibility of breast cancer that preventive mastectomy still seems to be a good idea.

It's important to realize that this procedure doesn't completely eliminate the risk of breast cancer. No mastectomy can be guaranteed to get out all the breast tissue, which extends from the collarbone to below the rib cage, from the breastbone around to the back. Further, it doesn't separate itself out from the surrounding tissue in any obvious way (Fig. 18-4). The most brilliant surgeon in the world couldn't figure out

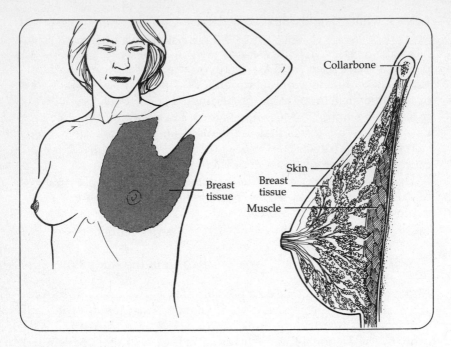

FIGURE 18-4

a way to be certain of digging all the breast tissue out of your body. When we do a mastectomy we do our best to get out as much as we possibly can.[17] The million-dollar question has been, does removing most of the tissue get rid of most of the risk?

In the 1950s a plastic surgeon in the Mayo Clinic did a large number of prophylactic mastectomies for a number of reasons, ranging from the reasonable to the appalling. If a patient had had multiple breast biopsies, family history of breast cancer, cancer phobia, "fibrocysitic disease," or lumpy breasts that were hard to examine, he recommended that she get her breasts removed, and a surprising number of women went along with him.

Excesses like this, and studies that showed the limits of prophylactic mastectomy, caused much of the medical community to frown on them for many years. But the zealous doctor has ended up doing some good after all. In 1999 researchers at the Mayo went back to look at the slides and records of those early operations—fortunately the Mayo Clinic keeps very thorough records.[18] They identified 639 women out of a group of 1,065 who had had the procedure done, and who also had a family history of breast cancer. They then divided them into high or moderate risk. If the relative with breast cancer had been a sister or aunt, the risk was deemed moderate; if it was the woman's mother, it was deemed high. (Their criteria for high risk were a little more liberal than most people would use. If the woman is young and has two or more first-degree relatives with breast cancer, or if she has one first-degree relative plus two or more second-degree relatives with the disease, she's usually considered at high risk.) The median length of follow-up was 14 years—one half of the women the clinic was looking at had been followed up for that time. The median age when the women had their surgery was 42. The women whose cancer is the result of the BRCA genes tend to be younger: 80 percent have breast cancer by 40. They recalculated the risk using the Gail model, figured out how many were in the moderate group, and compared that to how many they had expected to be in this group. They had expected to find 37.4 cancers, but there were only four. This was a risk reduction of 90 percent.

They then contacted sisters of the women in the study to see how many of them had gotten breast cancer. This would provide a good comparison, since the sisters presumably had the same risk as the original patients had. Of the sisters, 38.7 percent (156) had gotten breast cancer. Thirty-eight were diagnosed after their sisters' prophylactic mastectomies. Three of the 214 women who had had prophylactic mastectomies developed breast cancers in the remaining breast tissue. That's three cancers rather than the expected 38, or a 90 percent reduction. Adding together the two groups, seven women still got breast cancer after the prophylactic mastectomy, and two died of it. Overall, instead of 20 deaths from breast cancer, there were two. This is the first paper that really examines this issue. It gives us something to go on, in spite of the study's imperfections.

What we really want, though, is a prospective, randomized control study—to have identical twins living in the same places all their lives who have BRCA1 and give one a prophylactic mastectomy, and then see what happened to both. Since such a study is unlikely to happen, the Mayo Clinic one gives us a really good clue. It tells us that there's probably a significant reduction in breast cancer among women who have had prophylactic mastectomy. It may be 90 percent; it may be 80 percent.

An editorial discussing this study summarized it well: "In the end, what the study demonstrated most dramatically is the cost of prophylactic mastectomy. Even in the cases with an unprecedented 80 percent reduction of breast cancer and deaths from breast cancer, the fact remains that 639 women, because of the fear of breast cancer, underwent a disfiguring and potentially psychologically damaging operation. As a result, instead of the 20 deaths related to breast cancer that were expected during this period of observation, there were only two. The saving of those 18 lives was clearly important. But the 621 women who probably would have survived without prophylactic mastectomy paid a price that will probably be considered unacceptable in the future."[19]

It's ironic that the data supporting the efficacy of bilateral mastectomy for prevention should appear in an era in which the goal of surgical treatment of breast cancer is conservation. The good news, however, is that we are now much better able to pick out the women who are truly at high risk. This includes those who test positively for BRCA1 or 2. It is these women who are at very high risk that might benefit from chemo or surgical prevention.

BRCA1

What kind of prevention can you try if you have the BRCA1 gene? You need to monitor for breast and ovarian cancer. In many ways, as I noted earlier, ovarian cancer is more frightening than breast cancer, although it's also much less common. Breast cancer may or may not prove fatal; ovarian cancer almost always does. Unfortunately it is also a very sneaky cancer: there are no symptoms until it's very far developed. Pelvic exams rarely show signs of ovarian cancer. There's a blood test called CA125 that's good for monitoring metastatic ovarian cancer, but it works only about 50 percent of the time when the cancer is in an early stage. It's particularly tricky in premenopausal women—there are a lot of false positives, leaving the patient terrified that she has an incurable disease, and leading to unnecessary surgery. Transvaginal ultrasound is a more recent technique. An ultrasound tool is placed into the vagina and the technician can look around the ovarian area. The process has a very high resolution, but most of what it finds is benign. It might be a good idea for very high-risk women, but even then out of 1,000 women screened they'd find suspicious signs in 50 women, all of whom would undergo major surgery and only one of whom would turn out to have cancer.

Some data have shown that taking the birth control pill may prevent ovarian cancer. This makes sense, because ovarian cancer seems to be related to the frequency of ovulation, and the pill blocks ovulation. So if you have the BRCA1 gene and still want to have children, you can go onto the pill as a teenager, go off only at the specific times you want to get pregnant, go back on between children, and then have your ovaries removed after you're finished childbearing.

This also suggests that preventive oophorectomy may help. We know from old data that if your ovaries are removed when you're young, you have a much lower chance of getting breast cancer. In order to determine how much the risk of breast and ovarian cancer might be lowered by having both ovaries out preventatively, Barbara Weber's group at the University of Philadelphia collected all the cases that they could find in North America of women who had been diagnosed with the BRCA 1 gene and had had their ovaries, but not their breasts, prophylactically removed. They found 43 women, whom they then compared to 79 women with the gene who had not had any prophylactic surgery. After ten years, they discovered a 70% reduction in risk in the women who had had the surgery. Interestingly HRT did not seem to affect this lowered risk, probably because the hormones are given at a lower dose than that which one would expect premenopausal women to have naturally. It is not clear how much additional benefit bilateral mastectomies would contribute.[20]

Dr. D. Schrag from Boston's Dana Farber and others developed a statistical model to estimate the effect of oophorectomy and prophylactic mastectomy on life expectancy for high-risk women.[21] They found that on average a 40-year-old woman with the BRCA1 mutation would gain three years of life with bilateral mastectomy and one additional year for oophorectomy. Remember, however, that this is only an average. One woman could gain four years, another only one year. And remember also that not every woman with the gene gets the cancer at all. Further, it's very age related. If you're 60 with the BRCA1 gene, you don't gain anything by having your ovaries removed.

And of course you could take tamoxifen for four years and see what happens. It may be that the protection lasts for a significant time after you've stopped the tamoxifen; we don't know that yet. We also don't know whether tamoxifen works in women with BRCA1 since they often get estrogen receptor negative tumors. The tamoxifen prevention study has been examining the blood of the 13,000 women under study, and a percentage of these women had the BRC1 gene, so we may soon know the answer.

Remember, however, that you've only *reduced* the risk of breast and ovarian cancers. Both breast and ovarian tissue, as I've noted before, exist outside the actual organ involved. But it certainly does lessen the risk, so one possibility would be to have your ovaries removed after you've finished your childbearing—and possibly to plan your childbearing in such a way that you can do it at a fairly young age.

BRCA2

The options for BRCA2 are similar. Although you do not have the ovarian cancer risk, oophorectomy may still be an option to prevent the primarily estrogen receptor positive breast tumors. Tamoxifen is also likely to work in this group.

THE FUTURE

I think the next step in prevention will capitalize on the intraductal approach. Not only will we use it to identify which women are truly at risk, but we may be able to use it for prevention. Just as you can put Drano down the rusty pipe, so we can find forms of "Drano" for the ducts. Possibly we could do gene therapy, sending altering genes down the ductal system that's affected. Perhaps we could use the chemotherapy drugs that are now used systemically, sending them only into the relevant duct.

The true answer to prevention isn't systemic, it's local. We need to find ways to either block the carcinogens or do something that could reverse the damage to genes.

So once again—what can most women do? Not a whole lot—as I said in Chapters 14 and 15, there isn't one overriding factor in breast cancer, like cigarettes and lung cancer. But there are some things you can do to affect your own and your daughters' risk. Basically you should follow what your mother told you when you were a kid: eat your vegetables, exercise, and drink alcohol in moderation. You can get breast exams and mammograms when it becomes appropriate. In addition, you can participate in a high-risk program. At UCLA where I set up a breast program, there is a high-risk program to follow women with a strong family history. We have an integrated program including physical therapy, stress reduction, and nutritional counseling, as well as exams, mammograms, and participation in the latest research, such as the tamoxifen prevention trial. There are other high-risk programs around the country. It's a good option for someone at high risk who doesn't want a medical procedure but wants to be followed in the most thorough, up-to-date manner.

Finally, you can get involved in political action. It's vital that we continue with the pressure to fund research into prevention. We can't just do one study and then wait for it to be over, and then another and wait for that to be over. It will take too long. What we need to do is have several studies going on at once. And we have to demand that prevention become a priority.

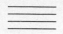

PART FIVE

DIAGNOSIS OF BREAST CANCER

19

Screening

Screening is the process of looking at healthy people with no symptoms in order to pick up early signs of disease. The PSA test for prostate cancer has allowed us to diagnose prostate cancers in men before they have any symptoms. In breast cancer we need something similar. We need a test that's easy to do, widely acceptable to patients (i.e., cheap and painless), sensitive enough to pick up the disease (avoid false negatives), and specific enough not to give false positives. Ductal lavage and nipple aspirate fluid collection may prove to fit the bill (see Chapter 17), but it is too soon to tell. Meanwhile, most breast cancer screening uses one of three tests which vary in their effectiveness— breast self-exam (BSE), breast exam by a doctor, and mammography. All these tests attempt to find cancers before they manifest themselves.

EVALUATING SCREENING TESTS

There have been several studies examining the value of screening for breast cancer. Accepting that not all cancers will be found early, what evidence is there that our current tools are making a difference? Before we get into the studies, it's useful to look at a few common biases that complicate the issue of early detection (Fig. 19-1).

The first is lead time bias—the assumption that catching a disease early in its existence will necessarily affect its rate of progress. This is sometimes true and sometimes not. Let's assume you have a disease that usually kills you eight years after it starts. If we diagnose the disease in the fifth year, you'll live three years after the diagnosis. If we diagnose it in the third year, you'll live five years—and we gleefully proclaim that our early diagnosis has given you a longer survival span.

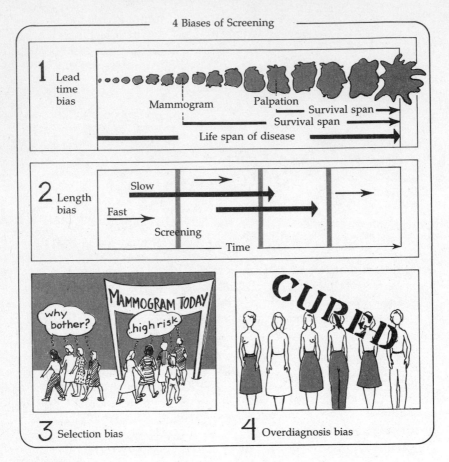

FIGURE 19-1

Actually, it hasn't—it's just given you a longer time to know you've got the disease, which may or may not be a benefit. So just looking at years of survival after diagnosis isn't enough—we need to know how many people actually die of the disease with and without early detection. Most breast cancers have been around six to eight years by the time they appear on mammogram, and most women with breast cancer survive many years, so this bias can be very misleading.

The second bias is length bias. For instance, take a test done every two years on a large number of people. Fast-growing tumors aren't around as long, so there's less time in which they can be detected. Slow-growing tumors are around longer, so you have time to find them. If, for example, one tumor takes six years to become two centimeters, and you do a test every two years, you're likely to find it before the six years are up. Another, very aggressive, tumor grows to two centimeters in nine months. You won't find it in your first test, and before you do your second, it's become a palpable lump and has been found. So screening tests select against fast-growing tumors, and catch the slow-growing ones—which have a better prognosis. It's like a nighttime security guard going around the bank every hour. The guard will catch a slow robber who takes three hours to get the job done, but the fast robber, who can do the job in 20 minutes, will be in and out before the guard shows up. The chances are that the fast robber is also the most efficient one; the guard will only get the slower, less competent criminal.

Then there's the selection bias. If you make mammograms available to all women over 50, and you don't offer any extra incentives to take the test, who's likely to take you up on your offer? For the most part, it'll be the people who perceive themselves as high-risk: they've already had breast cancer, or their mother has had breast cancer. The women who don't worry as much about getting the disease are less likely to bother getting the test. So usually the women who go for screening have a higher risk than those who don't.

Finally there's the overdiagnosis bias. You detect suspicious areas on a mammogram—they may or may not indicate cancer. Precancer (see Chapter 16) falls into this category: if it were never diagnosed, in many cases nothing would happen and you'd never know you had it. But if it's overtreated—that is, preventive mastectomies are performed wherever it's found—the cure statistics can get very inflated. If, as it currently appears, only 30 percent of precancers will ever become cancers, and mastectomies are performed on all women found to have precancer, huge numbers of women will appear to have been cured, whereas the majority—70 percent—would never have gotten cancer in the first place.

What's needed for a truly accurate study is a randomized controlled study with mortality as its endpoint, to take care of the lead time bias. If you take a group of women and pick randomly who'll get the test and who won't—that takes care of self-selection and overtreatment. If you have the same numbers of fast- and slow-growing tumors in the overall group, this counters the length bias, and ensures that both the study group and the control group have the same risks of, and the same kinds of, cancer. The studies like this are few and far between. It behooves us to examine the data supporting each modality of screening against this standard, however, if we are truly to understand its worth.

Finally, we need to contend with the myth of early detection. As we discuss in Chapter 18, the concept of "early detection" is somewhat misleading. But is it a myth? Not really: there are some cancers that we truly can detect early. The myth is the notion that every cancer has the potential to be found early by our current techniques. We are unfortunately limited by both our techniques and understanding of breast cancer. Screening is still our current best tool for changing the mortality rate of breast cancer. We need to take full advantage of it while working very hard to find something better.

BREAST SELF-EXAM

Until recently, breast self-exam—much touted as the obvious first step in screening for breast cancer—had not been scientifically tested to see if it could change the mortality rate of breast cancer. The first randomized controlled study of breast self-exam was done in Shanghai and reported in 1997.[1] In the study 267,040 women from 520 factories were randomly divided between a self-exam instruction group and a control group and followed for over five years. The women in the instruction group were given intensive training in breast self-examination, including the use of silicone breast models and personalized instruction, plus two subsequent reinforcement sessions and multiple reminders to practice the technique. Women in the control group were asked to attend training sessions on the prevention of low back pain and were given no information or training on BSE. All women were followed for the development of breast diseases and for death from breast cancer. There was a high level of participation, and the instruction group demonstrated greater proficiency in detecting lumps on a silicone model than did the control group. Approximately equal numbers of breast cancers were detected in the two groups (331 in the instruction group and 322 in the control group). The breast cancers detected in the instruction group were not diagnosed at an appreciably earlier stage or smaller size than those in the control group. The death rates from breast cancer in the two groups were exactly equal. Interestingly there was even a downside to BSE. The women in the instruction group detected more benign lesions (1,457 vs. 623) than did those in the control group. This means that BSE not only failed to benefit the women in the instruction group by finding cancers "earlier," but led them to be subjected to more biopsies than were those in the control group. The researchers will continue to follow all the women in the study to see if there is a late benefit to BSE that can be demonstrated. I must say that I think it's unlikely since the size and stage of the detected tumors were the same in each group.[2]

The only other randomized controlled study is taking place in Russia, conducted by the World Health Organization. The preliminary results from St. Petersburg alone have not shown advantages to self-exam.[3]

The results of the Shanghai study surprised many, but they were not really unexpected. Nonrandomized studies (see Chapter 12) have been inconsistent. Some women have never actually been instructed in how to do BSE, but even in those women who have been well taught there has been no effect.[4] Some studies show that cancers are found at an earlier stage (lead time bias) while others show no difference at all.[5,6] To date, all the evidence we have indicates that BSE is an ineffective tool in detecting breast cancer. By the time you feel a lump it's been there so long that whether you find it this month, next month, or four months from now won't make a critical difference. Most lumps are, as we said in Chapter 8, found by the woman herself, not while she's doing formal breast self-exam but rather while she's bathing or scratching an itch or making love.

Some doctors say that doing breast self-exam makes a woman feel more in control of her body and empowers her. That hasn't been true in my experience. I think it's the *provider* who feels better, feels less impotent and more in control. I find that the women themselves get scared to death and alienated from their bodies because they think they need to go on this monthly search-and-destroy mission. I also think the ones who do feel empowered often get a false sense of security. But if doing breast self-exam every month and not finding a lump makes you feel more comfortable, then you should do it, as long as you understand that its benefits are psychological and that it probably won't make a difference in your physical health.

Does BSE have any value at all? Possibly. Though it doesn't save lives, there may be other benefits. For example, as we mentioned in Chapter 2, it can be a way to become acquainted with your body—a pleasant and worthwhile activity. In addition, it may help create a better cosmetic result from lumpectomy, by finding the cancer a little bit earlier, when the lump isn't too large.

I have shifted my efforts from being a critic to trying to find something that will work. It is my most sincere hope that breast lavage, as described in Chapter 17, will serve this purpose and will put an end to the arguments about the utility of breast self-exam.

BREAST PHYSICAL EXAM

Breast physical exam—examination by a doctor or other medical professional—has never been studied by itself in terms of its usefulness in detecting breast cancer. There is, however, at least one good random-

ized controlled study in which both physical exam and mammography
were combined. This study is the basis of much of our understanding
of the advantages of screening. In New York in 1962 the Health Insurance Plan (HIP),[7] a health maintenance organization, chose 62,000 of its
female members between the ages of 40 and 64 and divided them into
two matched groups of 31,000 each. They then offered the women
in one group breast cancer screening, including mammography and
physical examinations, with follow-up exams and mammograms once
a year for three years. The women in the control group received their
usual care. (This was before the days of routine mammography, so it's
unlikely that many women in the control group had had mammograms.) The 31,000 women in the screened group were invited to get
mammograms; two thirds of them accepted and had at least one. To
avoid selection bias—since the women most likely to attend were those
at higher risk—all the women who were invited were included in the
statistics, not just those who actually came, which would underestimate the benefit of mammography. One third of the cancers detected
were detected on mammogram only, while two fifths were detected
by physical exam only and one fifth by both. After seven years of follow-up there was a one-third reduction in mortality in the members of
the screened group. After 14 years of follow-up this difference was
maintained,[8] and there is now also a significant difference in the mortality of the women under 50 as well. In fact, at 18 years follow-up the
decrease in deaths from breast cancer was equal in the older and younger group.[9] This was the first study to show the advantage of screening
for breast cancer, and it was done with the rather crude mammography being employed in the early '60s. It's important to remember,
however, that the HIP study included a physician's exam in the screening, and it's interesting to note that physical examination seemed to be
more effective in the younger women (40–50), while mammography
was more effective in the older group.

There was also a study done in Canada[10] that looked at whether,
in older women, mammograms added anything to a well-performed
medical physical exam. After a seven-year follow-up they found that
in women between 50 and 59 adding mammography didn't decrease
mortality any more than physical exam alone.

One problem is that most doctors haven't been trained to do physical breast exam. The breast has always been thought to be the property
of the general surgeon. So hardly any gynecologists and primary care
doctors have formal training in the breast. Yet most women with breast
problems go to their gynecologists or primary care doctors. This is the
source of a lot of problems because gynecologists and primary care
doctors, untrained in breast problems and breast cancer, often don't
know what to do. Surgeons always have had the advantage of edu-

cated fingers. They examine the breast and then do a biopsy. That way they learn what different breast problems feel like. Primary care doctors do not have this advantage. We need to be sure that every woman has access to a good clinical breast exam as part of her yearly checkup.

MAMMOGRAPHY

The third technique used for screening is mammography. We discussed mammography in Chapter 9 as a diagnostic tool for women who have breast complaints. Here we discuss it in relation to all healthy women as a tool for finding early disease. We've already discussed some of the limitations of screening studies. The only studies we can really count on to get answers are randomized controlled studies, where women are randomly assigned to get mammography or not.

There have been eight randomized controlled trials over the past 30 years, which is an impressive number. The findings are very striking. All eight studies consistently show a reduction in mortality in women between 50 and 69 of about 30 percent—nearly a third. (This means that out of every 100 women over 50 with undetected breast cancer 30 would have died had they not been screened.) This is the largest reduction in mortality we have seen in breast cancer. It overshadows by far the reduction in mortality we've seen in treatments with chemotherapy and surgery. In women over 50 there is no question that mammography screening can be lifesaving. We don't yet know how it affects women over 70, because there haven't been enough studies to tell us, but there is no reason to believe that the result wouldn't be the same. These benefits overall far outweigh the risks in having mammography (see below). We still need to stress, however, that mammography is not perfect and that a mammogram that shows nothing unusual is no guarantee that the woman doesn't have cancer.

What is so magic about the age of 50? It isn't actually 50 that matters, but rather menopause. Before menopause breast tissue tends to be denser because your breasts have to be ready to make milk at a moment's notice. After menopause breasts go into retirement and breast tissue is replaced by fat. Cancer shows up against fat tissue, but not against dense breast tissue. Further, breast cancer is more common the older you are. The combination of these two facts makes mammography postmenopausally more accurate. There is no argument that every woman over 50 should be having yearly mammography.

The controversy is about the women under 50. Of the eight randomized controlled studies (which looked at women between 40 and 74) the data are very clear: for women between 40 and 49 the trials have shown no effect on mortality after seven years of follow-up.[11] Four of the eight studies followed women for 10 to 12 years, but none found a statistically significant difference. Summary data from five of the eight trials showed a trend toward reduced breast cancer mortality (about 16%) only after a follow-up period of 10 or more years. In these studies many of the women began mammography while they were in their late forties and continued to have mammograms after age 50. Consequently, we can't be sure if the women who benefited from mammography in these studies would have had the same benefit if they had started having mammograms at 50. When they combined all of the randomized controlled trials, it was estimated that regularly screening 10,000 women between 40 and 49 would result in the extension of lives of somewhere between 0 and 10 women. About 2,500 women would have to be screened regularly in order to extend one life.[12]

One pro-early-mammography camp argues that cancers that occur between ages 40 and 50 seem to be the faster-growing ones. They feel the reason many studies are not showing the value of mammography in this age group is that the mammograms are not being done frequently enough. Thus, they say, we should close up the intervals between mammograms in those years—especially since 40 to 50 are the years when women still have a lot of dense breast tissue, which can mask a cancer. So it may make sense to have a mammogram every year between 40 and 50, and every two years after 50. This theory gained some credence from a study in San Francisco[13] which showed yearly mammography was less able to find cancers in younger women regardless of their breast density.

The other argument in favor of mammography between 40 and 50 is that none of the randomized controlled studies, except for the Canadian National Screening Study, was designed specifically for younger women. The Canadian study showed no significant effect in women over 50 and actually found an initial increase in mortality in younger women. However, because breast cancer is less frequent in this 40–50 age group, many more women would have to be added to the study to show the same difference in mortality. The Canadian study also suggested that at least one third of women under 50 have fatty breasts, which are conducive to mammography, and would therefore benefit. These proponents[14] contend that until there is a study that proves mammography is not helpful in this age group, we should continue to offer it.

The downside of mammography screening in young women has been underestimated as well. Over one fourth of invasive breast cancers are *not* detected by mammography in the 40–49-year-olds, compared to one tenth in the women over 50. Women with these cancers may be harmed if their diagnosis or treatment is delayed because of a normal or false negative mammogram in the face of a palpable lump.

On the other hand, many mammographic abnormalities may not be cancer, but will prompt additional testing and anxiety. As many as 3 out of 10 (30%) women who begin annual screening at age 40 will have an abnormal mammogram during the next decade. For every eight biopsies performed on this younger age group, one invasive and one *in situ* cancer are found. Finally, there is the risk of radiation. It is low, but becomes more significant the earlier the initial mammogram and the more mammograms you have. Radiation from yearly mammograms during ages 40–49 has been estimated as possibly causing one additional breast cancer death per 10,000 women. Women with inherited or acquired defects in DNA repair (see Chapter 13) may be even more susceptible to the risk of radiation. Based on statistical models from epidemiological studies of high-dose exposures, this risk is low. The actual risk at lower doses associated with mammography could be higher or lower. It wouldn't matter if the benefit were higher, but limited benefits (compared to risk) need to be considered.

In 1997 the age issue came to a head when the National Cancer Institute (NCI) sponsored a consensus conference. They went to great lengths to convene an unbiased panel of physicians, scientists, and the public to decide whether the recommended guidelines should be expanded to include women in their 40s. After extensive research, presentations, and debate the consensus was that there was not enough evidence to recommend universal screening and that each woman would need to decide for herself—with the help of her doctor— whether to be screened.

Although this seemed perfectly logical to me, it stirred up a hornet's nest of protest. All of the proponents of mammography screening reacted as if this recommendation was an affront to women. One mammographer actually termed it a death sentence. Paying no attention to the science or the carefully reasoned analysis of the panel, politicians began demanding that mammography screening be recommended to all women over 40. Congress passed a bill and Senator Arlen Spector threatened to hold up legislation if the NCI did not change their recommendation. Politics prevailed and the guidelines now suggest that every woman over 40 be screened. I think this is another issue of having nothing better to offer. If we had a screening technique that worked in younger women we would not be recommending a limited tool such as mammography. I hope that breast duct lavage will be that tool.

It should be pointed out that these arguments refer to the value of recommending frequent mammography as a public policy: the benefit to the individual woman may be very different.

If you have a strong family history of breast cancer, your chance of getting cancer is higher. Statistically speaking, there is more cancer, and therefore more chance of finding cancer on mammography. Perhaps a good analogy would be a loaf of raisin bread. The more raisins in the bread, the better chance you will see a raisin in an individual slice. For you, therefore, mammography screening may be worthwhile.

And some young women do have fatty breasts, which is good for mammography. There are always exceptions to the rule, so mammography screening may make a difference for some women under 50. One of my patients was a woman in her mid-40s whose cancer was detected by mammogram. She had a mastectomy, and seemed fine. But she was very concerned by the studies. "I keep hearing that mammography in women under 50 doesn't affect mortality," she said to me. "Does that mean I'm going to die?"

It didn't mean that at all. In her case the cancer was discovered very early, and was probably cured. She may have been one of the lucky ones for whom mammography was useful, or she may have been cured even if she had not had a mammogram and the mastectomy had been done after finding a lump. Not all women who develop breast cancer between 40 and 50 die from it; even women in their 20s and 30s survive breast cancer, whether it is detected as a lump or on mammogram.

There can be goals other than reduced mortality, as mentioned earlier with breast self-exam. With early mammography screening you might find a cancer that's smaller, so you'll be able to have breast conservation that will leave you without severe cosmetic damage.

I think one of the problems with our approach to screening is that we are wedded to the hypothesis that early detection matters. Even the newer techniques being proposed such as digital mammography, thermography, transcan, MRI, and nuclear medicine are based on the early-detection notion. Because of this we have lost sight of the biology of the disease. If the early-detection hypothesis were correct, then screening would work better. The fact that it doesn't should send us back to the drawing board to understand how breast cancer develops and how we can better intervene to prevent it.

SCREENING RECOMMENDATIONS

So, you want to do everything possible to protect yourself from dying of breast cancer, and from facing disfiguring surgery—what should you do? At the current time I would recommend the following: if you're very young you should begin getting acquainted with your breasts. Have your doctor examine your breasts during your regular checkups; after 40, make sure to get this done at least once a year. Consider getting a mammogram every year between 40 and 50. After 50, make sure you have a mammogram every one or two years. (See Chapter 9 for discussion of the procedure.)

Many doctors stress the importance of a "baseline" mammogram. Actually, your first mammogram could be called your baseline. What's more important is that you have serial mammograms: several a year or two apart so that comparisons can be made. This is what makes mammography the most accurate.

What I recommend is having a mammogram in your early 40s to find out what your breast tissue looks like. Some women discover with their first mammogram that they have very dense breasts, in which case it makes sense to hold off and not do regular mammograms till 50. But some women have very fatty breasts in their 40s, and for them, it might make sense to have screening mammograms in their 40s.

Then, once you're in your 50s (or whenever your breast density makes it feasible), you should have regular mammograms, every year or two, so we can compare each mammogram against the last one. Often that's how we catch a cancer: this year's mammogram has something that wasn't there last year and the year before. There are people who believe they can get one mammogram and that's it. Much as I oppose overdoing mammography, underdoing it is just as bad.

It's important to point out that this discussion is about screening mammograms done on women who have no symptoms but just want to get checked out. If you have a lump, you should have a mammogram regardless of your age. Mammography, whatever its limitations, is still the best tool we have for detecting breast cancer or determining the nature of a lump. We need to make full use of it while we try to find something even better.

20

Diagnosis and Types of Cancer

What are the symptoms that should alert you to the possibility of breast cancer? The most common is a painless lump, although some painful lumps can be cancerous as well. A thickening of the breast or a change in density also should be checked out. As we've mentioned in previous chapters, occasionally breast cancer shows up as a lump under the arm, a redness of the skin over the breast, eczema of the nipple, or dimpling of the skin. Finally, the most common finding these days is an abnormality seen on mammogram with no physical findings at all.

Once you've discovered a symptom or a lump that alerts you to the possibility of breast cancer, you should see a doctor. Start with your own primary care physician or gynecologist. If you're over 35 your doctor should send you for a mammogram. Even if the mammogram shows no abnormalities, if the symptom or lump persists ask to be referred to a surgeon or a breast specialist. In some areas of the country there are surgeons like myself who specialize in breast disease; in other areas you may be referred to a general surgeon. Don't be scared by the word "surgeon"—the fact that you're going to see a surgeon doesn't automatically mean an operation. Surgeons are the doctors best trained to diagnose breast problems. If you're unsatisfied with the answers you're getting from one surgeon, find another.

TYPES OF BIOPSY

What might the surgeon suggest? Very possibly, some form of biopsy. As we discussed in Chapter 11, biopsy covers four distinct procedures, so it's important to understand which procedure your doctor is talking about. Often patients think it means taking out a small piece of tissue, while the surgeon really means removing the whole lump. The type of biopsy depends in part on whether the lump is palpable or not (can be felt). If it is seen only on mammogram it can be approached by a stereotactic fine-needle biopsy, core biopsy, or wire localization biopsy. These all use the mammogram or ultrasound to localize the lump before sampling it (see Chapter 11). If the lump is palpable, then it can also be tested with a fine-needle aspiration (FNA) or a core biopsy. Finally, it can be entirely removed with an excisional biopsy, or a piece of it can be removed with an incisional biopsy. Discuss with your surgeon which approach is best for you and why. Sometimes FNAs or core biopsies are not offered because the hospital does not have the equipment, or the surgeon doesn't know how to do it, not because they are not the best choice. You need to know what your surgeon's criteria are in choosing the type of biopsy to perform.

If a woman came to me with a palpable or mammographic lesion, I tried to make the diagnosis with the least invasive procedure. That way I could often avoid giving her a scar or dent in the case of a benign lesion. If the lesion was cancer, we could discuss the options for treatment and proceed with the definitive operation. If no diagnosis could be made with a fine-needle or core biopsy I'd do an open biopsy.

Biopsies and treatment can be done in either one or two stages. The one-stage procedure was popular 15–25 years ago. You'd sign a form in advance, agreeing to an immediate mastectomy if cancer were found. This is what Nancy Reagan did in 1988 and it's still sometimes done today. The one-stage approach is based on the old theory that when we operate on an area with cancer we spread the cancer cells and that by removing the breast quickly we can prevent this spread. However, there's absolutely no evidence that a one-stage procedure has any effect on survival or cure rates.[1]

A two-stage procedure is one in which the biopsy is performed, usually under local anesthetic, and then, later, you're given the diagnosis. After that you can take time to discuss the possible treatments and make your decision.

The advantage of a two-stage procedure is that it gives you time to think. Being told you have breast cancer is upsetting, even if you've suspected it. You need time to adjust to the idea, to decide, with full information, perhaps including a second opinion, what you want to do. I don't think you can really make that decision before you know if you've got cancer. The hypothetical is very different from the real: what you think you'd decide *if* you have cancer may be very different from what you will decide *when* you have cancer.

For many women the thought of having cancer is so appalling that their first reaction is often, "I don't want to deal with this—just get it out of me and let me go on with my life." If you are one of these women, spend a day or two reflecting on this new reality. Your panic may subside and you may decide on a less drastic treatment than your original horror dictated. Whatever you decide, you'll have to live with your decision for the rest of your life—and that life won't be shortened by giving yourself a little time to think it over. Obviously, if you've got cancer you want it taken care of as soon as possible, and you don't want it to hang around for several months before your treatment. But the week or so you give yourself won't kill you, and it will help you to make the clearest decision possible. No woman should be put to sleep without knowing whether she'll still have her breast when she wakes up.

HOW TO INTERPRET A BIOPSY REPORT

The pathologist looking at the tissue removed in an excisional biopsy can tell whether or not breast cancer is present, and if it is, what kind of breast cancer you have. Your surgeon should select a pathologist who has had a lot of experience in diagnosing breast cancer. The language of a pathologist's report can be puzzling and intimidating, and for this reason patients should always discuss the pathology report with their surgeon. If a patient still has questions, she can ask the pathologist directly.

Most breast cancers (86%) start in the ducts, while some (12%) start in lobules at the end of the ducts. Thus your cancer will probably be described as either ductal carcinoma or lobular carcinoma (Fig. 20-2). Next, the report will state whether or not the cancer is invasive. Invasive cancers are also known as infiltrating cancers—a somewhat sinister-sounding description, which simply means the cancer has grown outside the duct or lobule where it started and into the surrounding tissue. In this case the report will read either "invasive ductal (or lobular) carcinoma" or "infiltrating ductal (lobular) carcinoma."

Since lobules and ducts are kinds of glands, and the medical term meaning "related to a gland" is *adeno,* sometimes these cancers are called *"adeno-carcinomas."* Some people are confused by this term, thinking it's a different kind of cancer. It's just a broader category—like calling someone from Los Angeles a Californian.

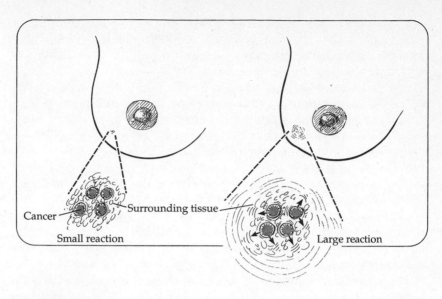

FIGURE 20-1

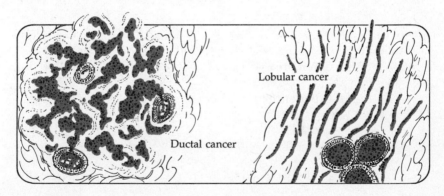

FIGURE 20-2

An infiltrating ductal cancer forms a hard, firm lump, because there is a lot of reaction caused by scar tissue (fibrosis) around the cells. This scar reaction is called desmoplasia. Infiltrating lobular cancer, on the other hand, is a little more sneaky. It sends individual cells in little fingerlike projections (papules) out into the tissues without inciting a lot of desmoplastic reaction around them, and so you may feel it as just a little thickening, rather than a hard lump (Fig. 20-2). For this reason it's harder for surgeons to tell if they've got the lobular cancer all out, because the little projections can't be felt as easily as a hard lump. Because lobular cancers elicit less scarring, they tend to grow to larger sizes (average five cm) than ductal carcinoma (average two cm) before they are detected. The prognosis is based on size, not the type of cancer. Aside from that, however, one form is no worse than the other; neither has a better or worse prognosis. There's a slightly higher tendency for lobular cancer to occur in both breasts. That is, although an infiltrating ductal cancer has about a 15 percent chance of occurring in the other breast, a lobular cancer has about a 20 percent chance—an increase in risk, but not an overwhelming one.[2]

If the cancer is not invasive, it will be called *intraductal carcinoma* or *ductal carcinoma in situ* or *lobular carcinoma in situ* or even *noninvasive carcinoma* (Fig. 20-3). These are all names for what I call precancer and were discussed in Chapter 16. Sometimes both cancer and precancer are present in one lump, and the report might read "infiltrating ductal carcinoma with an intraductal component." This finding will be discussed further in Chapter 23.

There are other names for cancers that may appear on the pathologist's report. For the most part they're variations on invasive ductal cancer, named by the pathologist according to the visual appearance of the cells under the microscope. *Tubular* cancer, in which the cancer cells look like little tubes, is very unusual—1–2 percent of breast cancers—and usually less aggressive. *Medullary carcinoma* has the color of brain tissue (the medulla). *Mucinous carcinoma* is a kind of infiltrating ductal cancer that makes mucus. *Papillary carcinoma* has cells that stick out in little papules (fingerlike projections). (See Table 20-1.) These special cancers tend to have a better prognosis than do typical invasive ductal or lobular cancers.

After deciding what kind of cancer you have, the pathologist will try to study the cells further to determine how aggressively the particular type of tumor will behave. This isn't 100 percent accurate, however; it's a little like looking at a lineup to pick out who the criminal is.

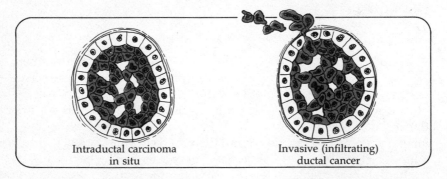

Intraductal carcinoma
in situ

Invasive (infiltrating)
ductal cancer

FIGURE 20-3

If one suspect is seedy and scruffy-looking and another is wearing a three-piece suit, you'll guess that the first one is the bad guy. But you could be wrong. Sometimes appearances can be deceiving, both in a police lineup and under the microscope.

Similarly, the pathologist who sees wild-looking ("poorly differentiated") cells will conclude that such cells are usually more aggressive, while the cells that look closer to normal ("well differentiated") are usually less aggressive (Fig. 20-4). The cells in between are called "moderately differentiated." But poorly differentiated cells aren't a sign of doom—the fact that they look wild doesn't guarantee they'll act that way. It is important to realize that most breast cancers are either moderately or poorly differentiated, but that many of the women with these cells do fine.

Another thing the pathologist will look for is how many cells are dividing, and how actively they're dividing. The most aggressive cancers tend to have a lot of cells dividing at the same time, because they're growing rapidly. Less aggressive cancers tend to have very few dividing cells. Another feature indirectly related to tumor growth and differentiation is the *nuclear grade*. The nucleus of the cell is the part that goes through cell division, so the grade gives you an idea of the degree of the growth rate and how odd-looking the nuclei are. Pathologists usually grade on a scale of 1–3 or 1–4, with the higher number being the worst (see Fig. 20-4).

Table 20-1 Types of Breast Cancer and Frequency[a]

Infiltrating ductal	70.0%
Invasive lobular	10.0
Medullary	6.0
Mucinous or colloid	3.0
Tubular	1.2
Adenocystic	0.4
Papillary	1.0
Carcinosarcoma	0.1
Paget's disease	3.0
Inflammatory	1.0
In situ breast cancer	5.0
ductal	2.5
lobular	2.5

[a]There can be combinations of any of these types.

Henderson C, Harris JR, Kinne DW, Helman S. Cancer of the breast. In DeVita VT, Jr., Helman S, Rosenberg, SA, eds., *Cancer: Principles and Practice of Oncology*, vol. 1, 3rd ed. Philadelphia: J. B. Lippincott, 1989; 1204–1206.

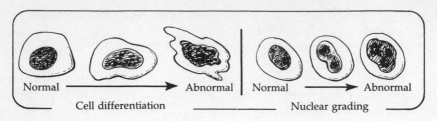

FIGURE 20-4

The pathologist will also look to see if there are any cancer cells in the middle of a blood vessel or a lymphatic vessel. If there are, it's called vascular invasion, or lymphatic invasion, and suggests that the cancer is potentially more dangerous than if it's not there. In addition, the pathologist will sometimes count the number of blood vessels associated with the tumor. This is because tumors secrete a material that causes blood vessels to grow (see Chapter 13). If there are a lot of blood vessels, it may indicate that the tumor is especially well nourished and thus especially aggressive. I noticed in my own work that if I was operating on a lump I thought was benign and there was a lot more bleeding than I would have expected, it was often the tip-off that the lump was cancerous. Another ominous sign can be "necrosis," or dead cancer cells. This usually means the cancer has outgrown its blood supply, a sign that it is growing rapidly (Fig. 20-5). All of these are methods of trying to get as much information as possible from looking at the cancer. None of them is 100 percent perfect at predicting behavior.

Sometimes all of these observations are combined as a score. One commonly used scoring system is the Bloom Richardson Score. It is based on three features: degree of tubule formation (remember, tubules are good); regularity in the size, shape, and staining character of the nuclei; and mitotic activity. Each of these gets a score of 1, 2, or 3 depending on the amount seen. The scores are then added up: 3–5 is grade one, 6–7 is grade two, 8–9 is grade three. Grade three is the highest and supposedly the most aggressive. Unfortunately all of these features are very subjective. A comparison of different pathologists' Bloom Richardson Scores on the same cancer showed they agreed only 75 percent of the time. If you see a Bloom Richardson Score on your report you will know what it is and you will also know that it is just a way to quantify how the tumor looked.

In addition, the pathologist should be able to tell you if there's cancer at the margins of the tissue that's been removed. This is done by a fairly imprecise technique. Ink is put all around the outside of the sample before it is cut up and fixed, and slides are made. If the slides show cancer cells next to the ink, this means there's cancer on the outer border. If there are cancer cells only in the middle, away from the ink, there is a clean margin (Fig. 20–6). So the report might say, "The margins are uninvolved with tumor," or "The margins are involved with tumor," or "The margins are indeterminate." If the lump has been taken out in more than one piece, we usually can't tell if the margins are clean or not. Also, we can only do representative sections of the margin; to get them all, we'd have to make thousands of slides. So when we say the margins are clear, we're only making an educated guess—we can't be 100 percent sure. (See Chapter 16 for a discussion of margins and DCIS.) What we really are trying to determine is the likelihood that some cancer still remains in the patient's breast, and if so, how much cancer.

How clearly any of these things are seen depends on the expertise of the pathologist looking at them, and how hard the pathologist looks.

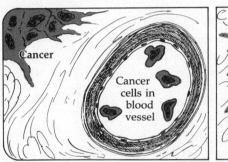
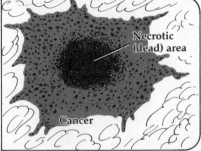

FIGURE 20-5

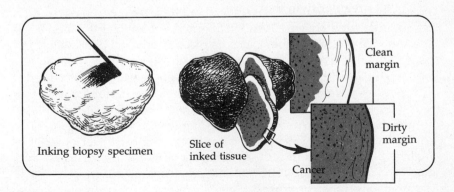

FIGURE 20-6

Someone who makes only a couple of slides and looks at them very hastily is obviously more likely to miss things than someone who makes a lot of slides and looks at them carefully. If you are at all concerned about the quality of the pathology evaluation, or even if you are not, you might want to have your slides sent to another pathologist in another institution. There is a breast pathologist with whom I work very closely, Dr. Sanford Barsky, who reviews the slides of all of the women who are seen in the Multidisciplinary Cancer Program at UCLA. Sometimes he ends up changing the diagnosis or reinterpreting a finding that might affect treatment.

Some of the things we've discussed aren't always easy to see on the slides. It can be somewhat subjective: are these cells bizarre-looking enough? Are they invading other structures? It's worth getting a second opinion. Often the pathologists themselves will ask other pathologists on the staff to look at the slides and give their opinions. If you live in a small town with a small hospital, you might want your slides sent to a big university center like UCLA, where someone sees a lot of breast pathology. You can call the university hospital's pathology department and arrange to have them look at your slides, then call your hospital and have the slides sent. Make sure it is the slides themselves they send, since that's what the second pathologist needs to see—not just the first pathologist's interpretation. You need to get the best information possible to decide what course of treatment to embark on.

BIOMARKERS

More and more we are trying to identify characteristics of tumor cells—characteristics that cannot be seen directly under the microscope but can be measured with sophisticated molecular tests—that will tell us how the tumor is behaving. We use a number of biological characteristics of the tumor to help us understand this. We have an enormous list but unfortunately we haven't yet figured out which is the best one. Every time a new fact about cancer is discovered somebody will do a test to see whether it can be a good indicator (a biomarker) of the tumor's behavior. I'll discuss here the biomarkers most frequently used.

The most common tests are the estrogen and progesterone receptor tests, which are done to find out whether the tumor is sensitive to these hormones. As we have discussed in Chapter 13, these receptors are now known to be far less simple than the tried-and-true lock-and-key analogy would imply (Fig. 20-7). What remains true is that those tumors which are lacking estrogen and progesterone receptors are not sensitive to estrogen or progesterone. It gets a lot more complex, however. Those tumors which are estrogen receptor negative but proges-

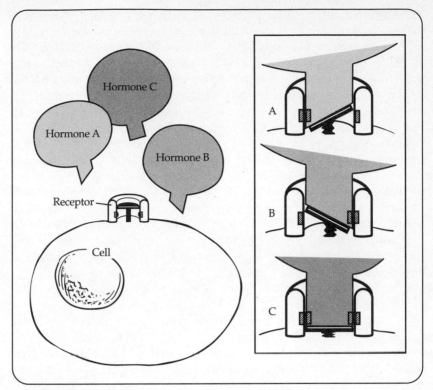

FIGURE 20-7

terone receptor positive will still respond to an esterone blocker like tamoxifen.

The implications of the hormone receptor tests are twofold. In general, tumors that are sensitive to hormones—that have receptors—are slightly slower growing and have a slightly better prognosis than tumors that aren't.[3] Generally, postmenopausal women are more likely to be estrogen receptor positive and premenopausal women are more likely to be estrogen receptor negative. Second, the test tells whether the tumor can be treated with some kind of hormonal blocking therapy. If it's not sensitive to hormones, it rarely responds to hormone blocking treatments (see Chapter 28).

Next, we attempt to figure out how rapidly the breast cancer cells are dividing, or how abnormal they are, based on the idea that the more they divide the more aggressive they must be. We do this by measuring these features in a couple of ways. One way is by *flow cytometry*,[4] measuring the amount and type of DNA (see Chapter 13). If the tumor cells have the normal amount of DNA, they're called *diploid;*

if the amount of DNA is abnormal, they're called *aneuploid*. Aneuploid tumors account for 70 percent of all breast cancer tumors. Diploid tumors behave much less aggressively because they are less abnormal. In addition, these tests can measure the percentage of cells that are dividing at any one time. This is called the *S phase fraction*. If there are a lot of cells dividing (high S phase fraction), the tumor may behave more aggressively than if there are only a few cells dividing (low S phase fraction). These markers actually give information similar to that of nuclear grade, but they're more reliable because, since they're measured by computer, they don't depend on a pathologist's subjective interpretation of how bad the cells look. Like every test, however, it has limitations. For node positive patients these tests add little new information. As we'll see in the next chapter, their main use appears to be in deciding which node negative tumors need treatment and which ones don't.

Another measurement looks for the overexpression (too many copies) of the Her-2 neu oncogene receptor. Her-2 neu is an example of one of the dominant oncogenes that contribute to cancer (see Chapter 13). Instead of being mutated, however, Her-2 neu is frequently overexpressed and amplified.[5] Her-2 neu is overexpressed in about one third of invasive cancers. Having your tumor tested for the Her-2 neu receptor is important because the test can function not only as a prognostic indicator (Her-2 neu positive tumors tend to be more aggressive) but also as an indicator of the best treatment. There are several tests that can be used for Her-2 neu overexpression and we don't know which is best. One, *immunohistochemistry* (IHC), assesses the overexpression of the Her–2 protein while the other, *fluorescence in situ hybridization* (FISH), assesses the actual gene amplification. It is the difference between measuring the effect or the cause. The initial studies of Herceptin, a monoclonal antibody to the receptor, used the IHC test[6] but work in early 2000 indicated that FISH may be more precise.[7] Herceptin is currently used in women with metastasis, and studies to determine whether it will also be useful for women as an adjuvant therapy are ongoing. (However, although almost all DCIS is Her-2 neu positive, this does not mean it should be treated with chemotherapy. It is still precancer, growing only in the duct.)

Up until now we have focused on information obtained from biomarkers that can predict which cancers are more aggressive and therefore more likely to have spread. Recently, however, we have become aware of a different use for these markers. It appears, as in the case of Her-2 neu, that some biomarkers may also be useful in predicting which treatment will work better, and how it will work. Preliminary information suggests that Her-2 neu overexpressors are more likely to respond to Adriamycin while Her-2 neu negative women may do just as well with Cytoxan, Methotrexate, and 5-FU (see Chapter 28).

There are many other markers we now know of: epidermal growth factor receptor, heat shock protein, nm23, p53.[8] I discussed some of these in Chapter 14. There are many other emerging biomarkers, and it seems that new ones are discovered every day. Most of them are elevated in cancers more likely to recur, but none is sensitive and specific enough to use routinely at the present time. Our hope is that many new markers will emerge to better predict the prognosis of a particular cancer and guide our choice of therapy. Research is now going on to determine whether combining the information from all of the biomarkers may be more accurate than using one alone. Advances in computer technology make this a feasible approach. So far it is still more of a hope than a reality. But certainly in the future these biomarkers, or new ones, will provide our most important information and will give us much more reliable information about prognosis and choice of therapy.

21

Staging: How We Guess If
Your Cancer Has Spread

The most important question is whether breast cancer has spread to other organs. This is what ultimately determines who lives and who dies. Unfortunately we have no test or scan that can reliably tell us whether breast cancer cells have gotten into, and have begun growing in, other parts of the body. Therefore we have had to use circumstantial evidence to guess how likely it is that this has happened. We do this in an attempt to determine the best therapy for any one woman—that is, just surgery for those with localized disease, saving chemotherapy for those we know have microscopic spread. Since we still don't have a method that works well, there are different approaches to this problem.

One approach is to categorize cases so that statistics can be kept and long-term survival rates for various treatments determined. This classification system, the TNM (short for tumor, nodes, and metastasis) system, is actually a holdover from the past. Although it is still used, it doesn't fit very well with our current knowledge of biology because it is based only on the size of the tumor in the breast and the number of lymph nodes involved as well as obvious spread to other organs. It does not take into consideration the behavior of the tumor or the fact that the lymph nodes are not always the main route of spread. Unfortunately we have yet to develop a biological staging system based on biomarkers (see Chapter 20) that will more accurately reflect the behavior of the tumor. Since the TNM system is still being used you might be exposed to it, so I'm including a detailed explanation here.

In this system (Fig. 21-1), the tumor is judged by how large it feels to the surgeon who initially diagnosed it. If it's between 0 and 2 centimeters, it's T-1; between 2 and 5 cm, T-2; above 5 cm, T-3 (1 cm is .39 inch). If it's ulcerating through the skin or stuck to the chest wall it's T-4. As we are diagnosing smaller and smaller tumors, subclassifications have been developed: T-1mic—microinvasion 0.1 cm or smaller in greatest dimension; T-1a, tumor between 0.1 cm and 0.5 cm; T-1b, tumor between 0.5 cm and 1 cm; T-1c, tumor between 1 cm and 2 cm.

Then the lymph nodes are examined. If there are no palpable nodes, it's N-0; if the surgeon feels nodes but thinks they're negative, it's N-1a; if they're positive it's N-1b. If they're large, and matted together, it's N-2; if they're near the collarbone it's N-3. Finally, if obvious metastasis has been discovered by any of the tests we'll describe shortly, it's M-1, and if not it's M-0.

Then all this information is combined into stage numbers. Stage 1 is a T-1 tumor with no lymph nodes. Stage 2 is a small tumor with positive lymph nodes, a tumor between 2 and 5 centimeters with positive or negative lymph nodes, or a tumor larger than 5 centimeters with negative lymph nodes. Stage 3 is a large tumor with positive lymph nodes or a tumor with "grave signs." Stage 4 is a tumor that has obvious metastasis. This staging system is continually being altered to reflect new information. The stages are calculated twice. First the surgeon does it, making a clinical estimate, and then later the pathologist looks at the tissue that has been removed under the microscope and determines the pathological stage. It has been shown that when the surgeon who has felt the lymph nodes thinks they're negative, there's about a 30 percent chance that the surgical guess is wrong, so they have to be removed and studied under the microscope to be sure of the actual stage.

In spite of the limitations of the TNM system, it still gives us a conceptual framework for categorizing each case of breast cancer so that different treatments can be compared in the same types of patients. So we still use the general stages 1 through 4 categories when describing newly diagnosed cancers.

There is a series of tests that are useful for finding large chunks of breast cancer in other parts of the body. These are called *staging tests* and shouldn't be confused with the stages of breast cancer just described. It is important to keep in mind that a cancer that starts out as a breast cancer remains a breast cancer, wherever it travels, and thus treatments used for the cancer are breast cancer treatments, not liver cancer or lung cancer treatments (very few other cancers travel *to* the

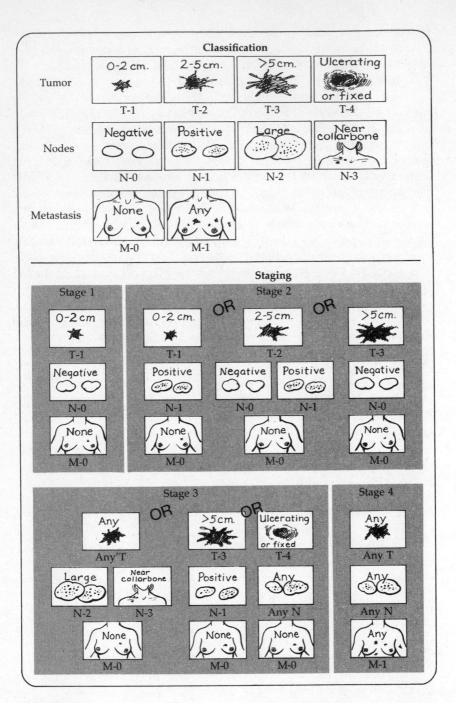

FIGURE 21-1

breast, by the way). It's a bit like what happens when a Californian moves to Paris. She's living in a new environment, but her language, her personality, her basic approach to life are still those of a Californian. She hasn't become a *Parisienne.*

To check the lungs, liver, and bones for breast cancer we do "gross" tests—so-called not because they're gross to have (although most medical tests are) but because they're used to find large chunks of cancer. We can do a chest x ray to find cancer in the lungs. We can do a blood test to see if the cancer has spread to the liver. To learn if the cancer has spread to the bones we do a more complicated test called a bone scan. A bone scan is what we call a *nuclear medicine test.* A technician injects a low level of radioactive particles into your vein, where they are selectively picked up by the bones. After the injection, you wait a few hours while the particles are traveling through the bloodstream; then you go back to the examining room where you are put under a large machine that takes a picture of your skeleton (Fig. 21-2). The machine whirs above you, reading the number of radioactive particles in your body. (The husband of one of my patients wore a Geiger counter, and right after her bone scan it started clicking whenever she came near it.) In the areas where the bone is actively metabolizing—that is, doing some-

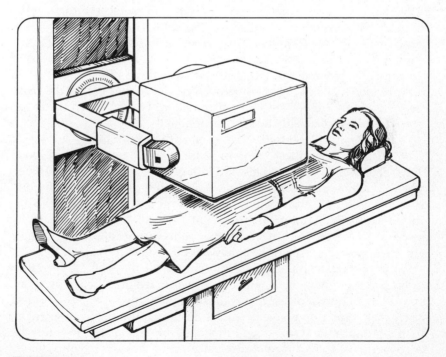

FIGURE 21-2

thing—the radioactive particles will show up much more strongly than in the more inert areas.

This doesn't necessarily mean that the bone is dealing with cancer cells, however. It can mean there's arthritis (which most of us have in small amounts anyway), a fracture that's in the process of healing, or some kind of infection. All the scan tells us is that something's happening. If there is, the next step is to x-ray the bone. This will help tell us what it is. We could just x-ray the bone to begin with, but we don't want to expose you to any more radiation than we have to.

There's a similar test for the liver, which is used if the blood test is abnormal. It's not quite as clear as a bone scan, however, because fewer radioactive particles show up in the liver when there's a metastasis. Sometimes we'll do an ultrasound test, in addition to the liver scan, to help confirm our findings.

If more information is needed, we can do a CAT scan (computerized axial tomography) on your liver, your lungs, an area of bone, or even your brain. The advantage of the CAT scan over x ray is that it doesn't just photograph you straight on, but divides your body into cross-sections that can be examined separately. For a CAT scan, you lie on a table inside a round machine, which rotates and takes pictures. It's a little more sensitive to lesions than a plain x ray, but it also exposes your body to much more radiation, so we do it only when the other tests have proved inconclusive. Finally a test called MRI (magnetic resonance imaging) (see Chapter 10) is sometimes used, especially on the brain, if more information is needed.

Frequently women ask why we don't do these other tests first if they are more sensitive. For some doctors, the reason is that the tests use increasingly higher amounts of radiation. Others avoid them because they are more costly and less available.

There are some blood tests for women with breast cancer—CEA, CA 15–3, CA 27.29. All of these are nonspecific markers found in the blood. They can be followed over time and will often go up if metastases develop. Initially we hoped these tests would tell us if there were any microscopic growth. Unfortunately, we've found that they're neither specific nor sensitive enough for that. But since they tend to go up in people with extensive metastases, they're useful in following women with metastatic disease because they help us adjust treatment.

It's important to remember the limits of all the tests. A negative finding doesn't give you a clean bill of health; it simply tells you there are no large chunks of cancer in those organs. Most people who are newly diagnosed don't have spread of this magnitude, so we no longer do these tests in the usual stage 1 or stage 2 breast cancers. If you have stage 3 or locally advanced breast cancer, or if you have symptoms in any of the organs breast cancer typically spreads to—like low back pain that started right after you found your lump and that hasn't gone away—we might do these tests. But we no longer do them routinely. They're expensive, they involve radiation, and the chances of their finding anything in a woman with early (stage 1 or 2) breast cancer is so low they just aren't worth it.[1] Some doctors still prefer to do them because they provide a baseline for seeing what those organs look like in you. If later on you develop symptoms, and if something shows up on the new blood test or x ray, the doctor can say, "Oh, yes, that's just her old arthritis," or "This is new: let's look into it more." But their utility is limited. If your doctor wants to do a test but you don't want the radiation to your body, you can say no; if your doctor doesn't want to do them and you feel more secure getting them, you can demand them.

Most cancers are found in stage 1 or 2, when the "gross tests" will almost always be negative. Yet, though more women with stage 1 breast cancer will be cured than will women with stage 2 cancers, some will still die of their disease. This is where the TNM staging system breaks down. You can have a stage 1 cancer and still have microscopic cells elsewhere in your body, or you can have a stage 2 cancer and be clear.

We desperately need a test or a scan that will determine for certain whether the microscopic breast cancer cells have spread to a particular organ. It would simplify treatment if we could say, "Yes, there's a breast cancer cell and it's in your left hip." Then we could do radiation, or chemotherapy, and afterwards do the test again to make certain we'd gotten all the cancer. But to date, no such test exists.

Since there's no foolproof method for determining the early (microscopic) stages of a cancer's spread, we have to approach it differently. We do have a number of methods of finding the likelihood of early spread—sort of trying a case on circumstantial evidence. We do this by looking for other conditions that often occur when a cancer has spread. If these conditions exist, we can guess that the cancer has spread; if they don't, we can guess that it hasn't. We go through a series of tests in different sequences to try to determine what the chances are.

The first level is based on how the cancer appears when it's diagnosed. There are certain signs and symptoms that statistically indicate a much higher chance that there are microscopic cells elsewhere. These have been incorporated into stage 3 (T-4 lesions) of the TNM system. Cushman Haagensen[2] first described what he called the "grave signs"—findings on physical exam that indicate the likelihood that microscopic cells had spread to other areas of the body (Fig. 21-3). His work was done in the 1940s before chemotherapy was used in early-

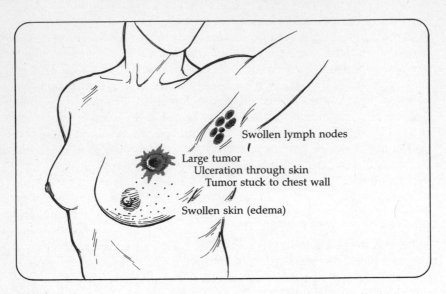

Swollen lymph nodes

Large tumor
Ulceration through skin
Tumor stuck to chest wall

Swollen skin (edema)

FIGURE 21-3

diagnosis cancer. Haagensen's plan was to determine which women could really benefit from a radical mastectomy. If there was no hope of saving a patient's life, he didn't want to cause needless suffering and destroy the quality of whatever life she had left. His system is still useful in a general way.

One sign that a cancer has probably spread is if the tumor is large—more than 5 centimeters (about 2 inches). If it's that big, there are probably microscopic cells elsewhere.

Another danger sign is swelling of the skin (edema) where the tumor is. As the skin swells, ligaments that hold the breast tissue to the skin get pulled in, and it looks like you've got little dimples on the area. Because this can create an appearance similar to that of an orange peel, it's known as *peau d'orange* (Fig. 21-4). If the tumor is ulcerating through the skin, it's ominous. If it's stuck to the muscles underneath so it doesn't move at all, that's also a bad sign. If there are lymph nodes you can feel above your collarbone (superclavicular nodes), or walnut-sized lymph nodes in your armpit, that's also dangerous. And if the skin around the lump appears red and infected, it can be inflammatory breast cancer (see Chapter 24), which is also likely to have spread.

Any one of these signs suggests a high probability that there are microscopic cancer cells elsewhere in the body. If they are present, we plan a systemic treatment (see Chapter 23) as well as a local treatment for the cancer. These tumors are called locally advanced and are often

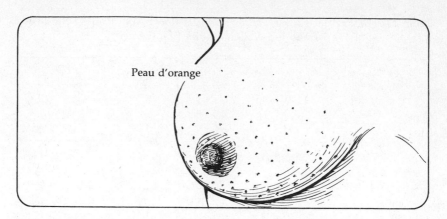

Peau d'orange

FIGURE 21-4

treated with chemotherapy rather than surgery as a first step (see Chapter 28).

Many people don't have any of these grave signs, and for them we need to go on to the next step to try and figure out the likelihood of microscopic cancer cells existing in other organs. The way we do this is to remove some axillary (armpit) lymph nodes. There are between 30 and 60 lymph nodes under the arm. We try to sample the ones most likely to show cancer cells under the microscope, and then examine them. (See Chapter 25 for this surgery.) We look at these lymph nodes because they are a good reflection of what is going on in the rest of the body. If they reveal cancer cells, we assume there's a high probability that there are cancer cells in other parts of the body. If they don't show cancer, it means there is a lower probability that there are microscopic cells elsewhere in the body. Classically pathologists have done a limited exam on all of the nodes removed. A more recent technique, called *sentinel node biopsy,* involves finding the one node the surgeon believes is most likely to have cancer cells and to examine it minutely. (Sentinel node biopsy is discussed in detail in Chapters 23 and 25.)

The lymph node evaluation doesn't give us a foolproof answer either. In about 30 percent of cases a woman with positive lymph nodes doesn't have microscopic cells elsewhere. In addition, with negative lymph nodes, 20–30 percent of breast cancers will have spread. To a certain degree the number of positive lymph nodes gives us a sense of the probability that there's spread elsewhere. With 1 or 2 positive nodes, you're less likely to have more cancer than with 10 or 15. We sometimes look at it in terms of 1 to 3, 4 to 10, and more than 10 to help us guess. However, because with any positive lymph nodes there's a

Table 21-1   Five-Year Breast Cancer Survival Rates According to the Size of the Tumor and Axillary Node Involvement

Tumor Size (cm)	Patients Surviving 5 Years		
	Negative Nodes (%)	1–3 Positive Nodes (%)	4 or More Positive Nodes (%)
< 0.5	269 (99.2)	53 (95.3)	17 (59.0)
0.5–0.9	791 (98.3)	140 (94.0)	65 (54.2)
1.0–1.9	4,668 (95.8)	1,574 (86.6)	742 (67.2)
2.0–2.9	4,010 (92.3)	1,897 (83.4)	1,375 (63.4)
3.0–3.9	2,072 (86.2)	1,185 (79.0)	1,072 (56.9)
4.0–4.9	845 (84.6)	540 (69.8)	727 (52.6)
≥ 5.0	809 (82.2)	630 (73.0)	1,259 (45.4)

Carter C, Allen C, Henson D. Relation of tumor size, lymph node status, and survival in 24,740 breast cancer cases. *Cancer* 1989; 63:181. With permission.

pretty high chance that there are cells elsewhere, we almost always treat women with that kind of spread with either tamoxifen or chemotherapy or both (see Chapter 28).

In the women with negative nodes, it's trickier. What we want is a way to figure out the identity of the 20 to 30 percent who have microscopic cells elsewhere and not overtreat the other 70 percent. We don't have a perfect technique for this. But we go on to the next stage and examine the tumor itself. We look at the features we discussed in Chapter 20 on diagnosis. We look at the size of the tumor; if it's more than 2 centimeters it has a higher chance of spread; if it's less than 1 centimeter it has a very low chance. Then we look for other factors, especially in that confusing area between 1 and 2 centimeters. We look at the biomarkers we discussed in Chapter 20—estrogen receptor, S phase, ploidy, Her-2 neu oncogene.[3] We put all of these together and make our best guess. If it looks like it's probably a fairly aggressive tumor and there's a significant chance there might be a microscopic cell somewhere in the body, then it may be worth doing chemotherapy or hormone therapy. If it looks like there's a low chance, it may not be worth it.

All of these tests are only tools that, added together, help to give us a picture of the cancer, and decide what to do (see Table 21-1). All any of these tests, and others that are being developed, can do is to give a picture of that particular tumor at one particular time—sort of like a snapshot. They cannot tell anything about how it actually acts in a particular woman.

At the end of these tests your tumor will be characterized in a description something like the following:

This is a Stage 2: 2 centimeter, node negative, estrogen recepter positive, S phase 10%, aneuploid, Her-2 neu overexpressing tumor.

This kind of evaluation is what we're currently using to make decisions regarding treatment, because it encompasses as much as we are able to know about the natural history of the disease and the biology of the tumor itself.

None of this gives us absolute knowledge. All it means is that we look at large groups of patients and say, "The majority of women with these signs have this prognosis, and are likely to have this response to this treatment." But you, the individual patient, may or may not fall into the majority category. This has a number of implications. If 80 percent of patients in your cancer category survive, you have reason for optimism—but not, unfortunately, for total rejoicing. You'll probably be in the 80 percent, but you might be in the 20 percent who don't survive. You need to be optimistic, but careful. Do everything possible to keep your advantage—careful follow-up and perhaps some of the adjunct, nonmedical techniques discussed in Chapter 29 to complement your treatment.

By the same token, if 80 percent of women in your category die, that doesn't mean you have to die. While it would make sense for you to think seriously about the possibility of your upcoming death and how you'd best want to prepare for it, it also makes sense to think in terms of being part of the 20 percent who survive. Again, it may be worth looking into nonmedical attitudinal and nutritional therapies to complement your treatment.

It's also important to note that most of the survival statistics were compiled in pre-chemotherapy days, when the only treatment was local surgery. Since chemotherapy is aimed at the entire system, it's very likely that its use will have a positive impact on the stage 3 and 4 cancers. However, since we've only been using it widely in the past 15 to 20 years, we don't yet know.

Understanding what stage your cancer is in will help your doctor suggest the treatment that seems most medically useful. It will also help you decide the treatment you want—and those may or may not be the same thing. If, for example, you have stage 4 cancer, you might decide that painful chemotherapy treatments will ruin the time you have left to live, and so choose to risk a shorter but more comfortable life span. The writer Audre Lorde, who died in 1992, explained her own reasons for making this choice in her book *A Burst of Light:* "I want as much good time as possible, and their treatments aren't going to make a hell of a lot of difference in terms of extended time. But they'll make a hell of a lot of difference in terms of my general condition and how I live my life."[4]

On the other hand, a year or two might feel like "a hell of a lot of difference" to you. You might decide that the possibility of living a little longer is worth the limited suffering chemotherapy entails. There are no right or wrong decisions here; there is only your need, and your right, to have the most accurate information possible, and to decide, based on who you are, what choices make the most sense for you.

22

Fears, Feelings, and
Ways to Cope

The first thing a woman thinks of when diagnosed with breast cancer is: "Will I die?" This is quickly followed by "Will I have to lose my breast?" Obviously breast cancer is a disease with a major psychological impact. In fact, whenever you think you have a lump, or get a mammogram, or have a biopsy, you rehearse the psychological work of having breast cancer. Although, as I have pointed out, most women don't die of breast cancer and most do not have to lose their breasts, these remain the major fears.

How does the average woman react to this terrifying diagnosis? In my experience, women go through several psychological steps in learning how to deal with breast cancer.

First there is shock. Particularly when you're relatively young and have never had a life-threatening illness before, it's difficult to believe you have something as serious as cancer. It's doubly hard to believe because, in most cases, your body hasn't given you any warning. Unlike, say, appendicitis or a heart attack, there's no pain or fever or nausea—no symptom that tells you something's going wrong inside. You or your doctor have found this painless little lump, or your routine mammogram shows something peculiar—and the next thing you know we're telling you you've got breast cancer.

Many women say this is the worst part of their journey. The initial shock can leave you feeling confused and not sure how to proceed. You are at your worst. But, once you get the medical information you need to make decisions, things will get better.

Along with shock there's a feeling of anger at your body, which has betrayed you in such an underhanded fashion. In spite of the horror you feel at the thought of losing your breast, often your first reaction is a desire to get rid of it: take the damned thing off and let me get on with my life!

While this is a perfectly understandable emotional response, it's not one you should act on. Getting your breast cut off will not make things go back to normal; your life has been changed, and it will never be the same again. You need time to let this sink in, to face the implications cancer has for you, and to make a rational, informed decision about what treatment will be best for you both physically and emotionally.

Because patients are so vulnerable at the time they're told their diagnosis, in my surgical practice I didn't like to tell them about all their options at the same time I told them they had cancer. I preferred to tell a woman she had cancer and that there were a number of treatment options that we'd discuss the next day at my office.

I began this process early on. When a patient came to me with what I thought might be a malignancy, I started talking with her right away about the possibilities, from the most hopeful to the most grim, and asked her to consider what it would be like for her in the worst possible scenario. We used the scary word: cancer. We discussed the general range of treatments we were likely to want to choose from. Then we'd talk about when I would call her with the results of her biopsy, so she could decide where she would be and who would be with her. I was taught in medical school that you should never tell a patient anything over the phone, but I found over the years that it often worked better if I did. If the patient didn't have cancer, why keep her in suspense any longer? And if she did, I preferred that she find out in her own home, or in whatever environment she'd chosen to be in beforehand.

Then if it was bad news, she didn't have to worry about being polite because she was in my office and there were all these other people around. She could cry, scream, throw things, deal with the blow in whatever way she needed to. She wouldn't have to lie awake all night hoping I wouldn't tell her something awful the next day but knowing that I would. So I would tell her on the phone, and then make an appointment to see her within 24 hours. By that time, the shock would have worn off a little bit, and she could absorb information about her options a little better.

Even when it's done this way, it can be very difficult for a patient to take it all in. For this reason I suggest that if you've been told you have breast cancer, you bring someone with you when the doctor explains your options—a spouse, a parent, a close friend. Sometimes a friend is the best idea: someone who cares a lot about you but who isn't close enough to be as devastated as you are by the news. The person is there partly to be a comfort and support, but also to be a reference later, so it's good if it's someone detached enough to remember everything that was said at the meeting, or even just someone to be a note taker while you are busy listening and trying to take in as much as possible. Such a friend is also good for asking the questions you are afraid to ask. It's a good idea to bring along a tape recorder. Then you can go over the options your surgeon has discussed with you again later on and as many times as you need to.

These days, this approach isn't all that unusual. In the past, surgeons were almost always very paternalistic: they told a woman she had cancer and she had to have a mastectomy but that when it was over she'd be cured and everything would be fine from then on. It was a lie, of course, but the patient usually believed it because she wanted to—who wouldn't?—and for the time being at least, she was reassured.

Today there's much more emphasis on doctor and patient sharing the decision-making process, and there are more options to choose from. There's also a lot more knowledge available—there are articles about breast cancer and its survival rates in both the medical and the popular press and on the Internet; you *know* you have no guarantee that everything will be fine once "daddy doctor" makes you better. All this is good, of course, but it's also very stressful. In the long run, I'm convinced you're better off when you've consciously chosen your treatment than when it's imposed on you as a matter of course. But in the short run, it's more difficult. The end result is a little more anxiety ahead of time while you are trying to make decisions about your treatment, but less depression afterwards.

Of course, different patients have different needs. Some women still want an "omniscient" doctor to tell them what to do. I was involved in a pilot study on how patients decide their treatments, and what kinds of decision making had the best psychological results. I'd expected to find that women coped better when they got a lot of information from their doctors and learned all they could about their disease, its prognosis, and the range of available treatments. But we found that this wasn't always the case. What was far more important was whether the doctor's style matched the patient's. Some women preferred to deny their cancer as far as possible, and have their doctor take care of it for them. They did better with old-fashioned paternalistic surgeons who told the women what was best for them, giving them minimal information. Others liked to feel in control of their lives, and to know all they could about their illness and its ramifications. They did better with surgeons like me, who wanted to discuss everything with them. Still others wanted a great deal of information but still preferred to defer to the doctor for decision making. There is no right or wrong style, so don't feel guilty if your needs are not the same as those of your friend or neighbor. Remember, it's about what style works best for you.

I experienced this when I was in practice. There was a well-respected, excellent breast surgeon in Boston when I was at the Faulkner. He was much more in the old-fashioned mode, and he and I would lose patients to each other all the time—sometimes we referred patients to each other. It worked out very well, and we were both happy about it, since we were both able to help people while remaining true to our own styles and philosophies.

Sometimes I would get a patient who clearly preferred not to know a lot, and over the years I'd come to recognize the signs and to respect them. I'd give such a patient enough information, but not in as much detail as I usually did, and then try to hear what she was choosing and say something like, "It seems to me that you're leaning toward mastectomy, and maybe that's the best decision for you." I still wouldn't tell her what to do, but I'd give a little more guidance than usual.

So if the first stage is shock, the second is investigating your options. (Sometimes, however, it works in reverse, and these stages can vary in order and intensity.) How extensive this investigation is varies enormously among women. For some of my patients it would consist simply in going over what I told them and discussing it with a friend. For others it involved research in medical libraries and on the Internet, and then going for second and third and fourth opinions. You can't take forever, but you don't want to hurry yourself either. In my experience, most patients can't handle prolonging this stage for more than three or four weeks.

When you're exploring the options I think it's very important to reflect seriously on what the possibility of losing a breast would mean to you. Its importance varies from woman to woman, but there is no woman for whom it doesn't have some significance. Although many women will say, "I don't care about my breast," deep down this is probably not true for most of us. A mastectomy may be the best choice for you, but it will still have a powerful effect on how you feel about yourself. For many women, the loss of a breast can mean feelings of inadequacy—she's "no longer a real woman." In her book, *First, You Cry*,[1] Betty Rollin talks about the first party she went to after her mastectomy. Although she knew she looked pretty with her clothes on, she felt like a transvestite, only playing at being a woman.

The fear of feeling this way may start long before the mastectomy—indeed, it plays a part in how the woman copes with her breast cancer from the first. Rose Kushner[2] surveyed 3,000 women with breast cancer and concluded that most women "think first of saving their breasts, as a rule, and their lives are but second thoughts."

My experience has been different. The first reaction of most of my patients has been, "I don't care about my breast—just save my life." Later, when the first shock has worn off and they've had time to think about it, their priorities remain the same, but they realize they do in fact care very much about their breast. Many women feel robbed of their sexuality when they lose a breast. Betty Rollin found that while her husband still desired her after her mastectomy, her own sexual feelings were gone. "If you feel deformed, it's hard to feel sexy," she writes. "I was dark and dry. I no longer felt lovely. Ergo, I no longer could love." Holly Peters-Golden,[3] on the other hand, points out the importance of distinguishing between the distress caused by mutilating surgery and the distress that comes from having a life-threatening disease. Certainly, in my experience with patients, the latter far outweighs the former. The fear of losing a loved one can stress a relationship and affect one or both members sexually.

Sociologist Ann Kaspar[4] studied 29 women between the ages of 29 and 72, 20 of whom had had mastectomies, and nine of whom had had lumpectomies. While, as she hastens to explain, she had no illusions that 29 women constituted a definitive study, her findings are interesting. Most of the women with mastectomies had been deeply concerned before surgery that the mastectomy would "violate their femininity." Yet, with only one exception, they reported that after the surgery it was much less traumatic than they'd anticipated, and that they'd realized that being female didn't mean having two breasts. "They got in touch with their identity as women, separate from social demands. Even the ones most determined to get reconstruction didn't feel that the plastic surgery would make them real women—they knew they already were real women," Kaspar says. She did find that anxiety was higher among the single women in her study, especially the single heterosexual women, who worried that "no man will ever want me." Those already in relationships usually found their partners were still loving and sexual, and more concerned with the women's health than their appearance.

Although the experience of these young, single, heterosexual women is consistent with my patients' experience, I've also had many other patients who had different reasons for wanting to keep their breasts. Often middle-aged women approaching or just past menopause will have very strong feelings about their breasts. They've experienced the loss of their reproductive capacity with menopause; often their children are leaving home and they are rediscovering their relationship with their spouse. This is no time for a woman to experience yet another loss around her womanhood. Elderly women too will often want breast conservation. They're already experiencing many losses and may not want to add the loss of their breasts, which have been a part of them for such a long time. Nothing makes me angrier than hearing of an elderly woman who has been told by her surgeon, "You don't need your breasts anymore; you may as well have a mastectomy." Different choices may make sense at different stages in a woman's life. Your choice should be based not only on the best medical information you can gather but also on what feels right to you. Don't let generalizations about age, sexual orientation, or vanity get in your way.

Many studies have been done recently comparing conservative surgery and mastectomy with or without immediate reconstruction, looking for differences in psychological adjustment. Interestingly, the important factor often appears to be the match between the woman and her treatment.[5] That is, the way she feels about her body, about surgery, about radiation, about having a say in her treatment, and about a multitude of other factors affects how she reacts to this new and enormous stress.

Most important for any woman faced with these decisions is the fact that she cannot make a "wrong" decision. If she is being given options it's because there are reasonable options for us to offer. Both mastectomy and lumpectomy with radiation will work equally well (see Chapter 23). It is not as though if she chooses wrong she'll die, and if she chooses right she'll live.

Along with the fears and stages of recovery, there are also a number of related issues that come up for people with cancer. One of these is the tendency to feel guilty for having cancer—a sense that you've somehow done something wrong. I found it sad yet interesting that when Nancy Reagan was interviewed on TV by Barbara Walters about her breast cancer, the then–First Lady admitted that the first thing she said to her husband after her breast surgery was "I'm sorry." People have a tendency to blame themselves for being ill anyway, and, irrational though she knows it to be, a woman will often feel she's betrayed her function as a caregiver by getting breast cancer.

In this connection, the holistic methods that we'll discuss in Chapter 29 can have their negative side. The mind–body connection is real, and its validation is very important, but it's not the only force at work in any disease. You didn't create your own cancer by eating too much sugar or thinking negative thoughts or allowing yourself to be too stressed out. I was appalled by a 1984 study that showed that 41 percent of women with breast cancer thought they brought it on themselves because of the stress in their lives.[6]

In reality, most of the studies on the relation between stress and cancer have been done on rats, and are equivocal at that—some studies show that stress is a factor in cancer, others that it's a factor in *preventing* cancer. At worst, it's only one factor, not a significant cause. I wish there *were* some simple, clear cause of cancer so I could say, "Don't do this and you won't get breast cancer." Unfortunately, it doesn't work that way. We don't have total control over our own bodies; we don't always, to use the popular New Age phrase, "create our own reality." You didn't give yourself breast cancer, and you won't help your healing by feeling guilty.

Having explored the options and their feelings, most women move into a "get on with it" stage. You know all you want to know, you've decided what you want to do, and now it's time to do it. This is the time to make your decision—you understand that you have cancer; you know the pros and cons of the different treatments; you're not happy about it but you're not still in shock.

How long the treatment lasts depends on what the treatment is. If you're getting a mastectomy, without immediate reconstruction, it may just be one or two days. If you have reconstruction, it will be several days in the hospital and a few weeks recuperating at home. If you're having wide excision and radiation, it will go on daily for six weeks, and if you're having chemotherapy in addition to your other treatments it can go on for another four to eight months. However long the treatment process lasts, it's important to have a lot of support around you, and it's important to allow yourself to feel lousy. Cancer is a life-threatening illness, and the treatments are all emotionally and physically stressful; you need to accept that and pamper yourself a bit. You don't have to be Superwoman. Get help from your friends and family—throughout the treatment. Sometimes, when you're having chemotherapy, the people who were supportive in the beginning start to dribble off. At that point, you may want to get into a breast cancer support group, where there are women who are going through, or have been through, experiences similar to what you're going through. It can be of enormous help to you. (Check with the nearest hospital or branch of the American Cancer Society.) In some parts of the country, away from big cities, it can be hard to find breast cancer groups per se, and you may not be certain about whether a mixed-gender, mixed-cancer group is appropriate for you. It's worth checking the group out, though; sometimes such groups can work well, and often many of the members are in fact women with breast cancer. You can check it out by calling the leader and getting the rundown on who is in the group, asking if your situation will allow you to relate to the others in the group. Also, you can join a support group on the Internet or a bulletin board community.

As stressful as the treatment period can be, it's an improvement over the earlier stages; you're actually doing something to combat your disease. (This feeling is often stronger when you're doing meditation, visualization, diet changes, or one of the other techniques we'll talk about in Chapter 29.) But when the treatment period is done, you're likely to find yourself in a peculiar sort of funk. This is what I see as the fourth stage: some call it the "post-treatment blues." This stage often lasts as long as the treatment itself. You're experiencing separation anxiety because the experience and preoccupation you've lived with so intensely is over, and where are you now? The routine established during your treatment has helped you feel supported, protected, and active against your cancer. Losing that feeling is hard. It's a little like being fired from a job—even one you didn't like. Rationally, you're glad it's over, but emotionally you feel lost. The caregivers (nurses, doctors, and technicians) you've come to depend on are no longer a daily part of your life. Compounding it is a reasonable fear. There's no more radiation going into your body, no more chemotherapy; without them, is the cancer starting up again? It's a scary time. This anxiety may well progress into depression, which is very common and can sneak up on you when you're least expecting it. You find yourself feeling sad and anxious; you can't sleep, or you want to sleep too much; you find you've lost interest and pleasure in people and activities that you used to enjoy. These symptoms are very normal. Often they last only a few weeks or months; but if they seem to drag on, you may want to see a counselor or therapist to help you get unstuck and go on with your life. Barbara Kalinowski, a former colleague of mine who ran two support groups at the Faulkner in Boston, has found that

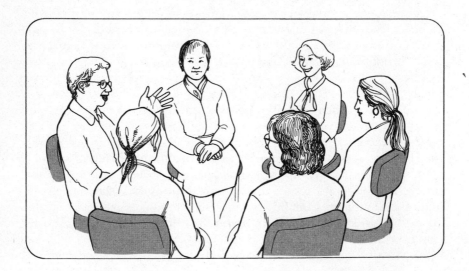

this is often one of the most helpful times for a woman to get involved with a support group. She says, "Sometimes it can be too much for a woman before this: she's working at her job, she's taking care of her kids, and she's going for treatment. Adding the extra time commitment of a support group can create even more stress. But when it's done and the depression sets in, you may really need the group."

Many women find that this period of intense feelings can be a time of emotional growth. They see it as a time to reevaluate their lives; they know their own mortality in a way they never have before. How are they living? Are they doing what they want to do for the rest of their lives? I've seen fascinating changes in some of my patients' lives during this period. One of my patients finally left a bad marriage she'd stuck with for years. Conversely, another decided it was time to make a commitment she'd avoided before—she married the man she'd been living with for a long time. A minister who lost her job because of her cancer left the ministry and got a job selling medical equipment. Another, a breast cancer nurse, left her job to work with a holistic health center. A patient whose husband once had Hodgkin's disease had her first child; faced with life-threatening illnesses, the couple wanted to confirm their faith in life and bring a new life into the world. Several of my patients began psychotherapy, not only to deal with their fears around their cancer but to look into issues they'd been coasting along with for years. They wanted to make the best of the time they had left, whether it was five years or 50 years.

This period of preoccupation and turning inward can last a long time. It's not that you're always completely depressed and out of it; you're just tired, a bit listless. Your body and mind still haven't fully healed yet.

For many women the cancer never returns, and they begin gradually to rebuild their lives. But sometimes cancer does return. Because the emotional issues of recurrence are so profound and complex, I've saved the discussion of these issues for Chapter 32.

COPING: WHAT TO TELL YOUR CHILDREN

A particularly trying issue people face is the question of what to tell their children. Again, it's an individual decision, and there are no hard-and-fast rules. I do think, in general, it's wiser to be honest with your kids, and to use the scary word "cancer." If they don't hear it from you now, they're bound to find it out some other way—they'll overhear a conversation when you assume they're out of the room, or a friend or neighbor will inadvertently say something. And when they hear it that way, in the form of a terrible secret they were never supposed to know, it will be a lot more horrifying for them. By talking about it openly with them, you can demystify it. In addition, if all goes well your children gain an opportunity to learn about survival after cancer. Kids need to know they can trust you—you don't want to do anything to violate that trust. It's a two-way communication; remember to listen to their fears. If you find it difficult to bring up the subject, there are children's books you can get that can give you a place to begin.

How you tell them, of course, will depend on the ages of the children and their own emotional vulnerability. With a little child you can say, "I have cancer, which is a dangerous disease, but we were lucky and caught it early, and the doctors are going to help me get better soon." What younger kids need to know is that you're going to be there to take care of them, that you're not suddenly going to be gone. They also need to know that the changes in your life aren't their fault. All kids get angry at their mothers, and they often say or think things like, "I wish you were dead." When suddenly Mom has a serious illness, the child may well see it as a result of those hostile words or thoughts. They must be told very directly that they did not cause the cancer by any thoughts, words, anger, dreams, wishes, etc. Your children will also be affected in other ways. You may be gone for a few days in the hospital, and will need to rest when you come home. You may be getting daily radiation treatments, which consume a lot of your time and leave you tired and lethargic afterwards. You may be having chemotherapy treatments that make you violently sick to your stomach. Your children need to know that the alteration in your behavior, and the decrease in your accessibility to them, aren't happening because you don't love them or because they've been bad and this is their punishment.

Some surgeons encourage their patients to bring young children to the examining room with them. I found that it could be very helpful for a daughter in particular to see me examining her mother. If you're being treated with radiation or chemotherapy in a center where your children are permitted to see the treatment areas, it's a good idea to bring them along once or twice. The environments aren't intimidating, and a child who doesn't know what's happening to you in the hospital can conjure up awful images of what "those people" are doing to mommy.

It is also important to be careful about changes in your older children's roles at home. You don't want to lean too heavily on them to perform the tasks you are unable to do; instead, you want to give kids things they can do that will make them feel useful. Wendy Schain, a psychologist and breast cancer survivor, and David Wellisch, a psychologist I worked with at UCLA, did a study on daughters of women who had had breast cancer. They found that the daughters who had the most psychological problems in later life were the ones who had been in puberty when their mothers were diagnosed. This was in part because their own breasts were developing at a time when their mothers' breasts were a source of problems. But interestingly enough, that wasn't the major reason for their problems. Far more damaging was the fact that they were expected to perform many of the mother's traditional household tasks. They were physically capable of this work, but they were not psychologically able to cope with the responsibility and they felt guilty about their resentment.[7] Also, it's a good idea to let their school know what's going on at home.

Most important is addressing children's two main fears: that they will not be abandoned and that they will be cared for. Hester Hill, a social worker I know who works closely with women with breast cancer, points out that it is also important not to make promises that you may not be able to keep. It is a mistake to promise, for example, that the cancer won't kill their mother. Instead, if you're asked, "Will you die?" you can reply to your children, "I expect to live for a very long time and die as an old lady. The doctors are taking good care of me, and I am taking good care of myself, and I hope to live for years and years."

Judi Hirshfield-Bartek, a clinical nurse specialist in Boston, usually recommends to couples that the partner take the kids out for some special time together. This gives them a chance to ask questions they may be afraid to ask their mother and know they'll get honest answers. A close relative or friend can also do this.

Frightening as it can be for kids to know their mother has a life-threatening illness, if you're honest and matter-of-fact with them, chances are it won't be too traumatizing. One of my patients decided when she learned about her breast cancer that she would demystify the process for her seven- and ten-year-old daughters by showing them a prosthesis (artificial breast) and explaining what it would be used for. The next day she came into my office for her appointment. When I asked her how her experiment worked, she started to giggle. "Well, they certainly weren't intimidated by it. They listened very carefully to my explanation—and then started playing frisbee with it!"

Breast cancer has particularly complex ramifications for a mother and her daughter. Aside from all the normal fears any child has to deal with, a daughter might worry about whether this will happen to her, too. It's not a wholly unfounded fear. As we discussed in Chapter 14, there is a genetic component to breast cancer. You need to reassure your daughter, explain to her that it isn't inevitable but that as she gets older she should learn about her breasts and be very conscious of the need for surveillance.

Often teenage daughters of my patients came to talk with me about their mother's breast cancer and their fears for themselves. It can be very useful to a girl to have her mother's surgeon help her put the dangers she faces into perspective, and it might be worth asking your surgeon about the possibility of such a meeting with your daughter. This may also be useful years later, if your daughter does develop problems; she's already built a good relationship with a breast specialist, and she's more likely to seek treatment with confidence and a minimum of terror.

Often daughters find themselves feeling angry at their mothers, as though the mother created her own breast cancer and in so doing made the daughter vulnerable to it. Mothers themselves often feel the same way; their feelings that they caused their own cancer expand into guilt over their daughter's increased risk. Often a patient will say to me, "What have I done to my daughter?" These feelings need to be faced and dealt with. Without openness, the cancer can become a scapegoat for all the other unresolved issues between the mother and daughter, putting the relationship at risk.[8]

COPING: FEARS OF OUR LOVED ONES

Husbands or lovers of women with breast cancer also have feelings that need to be acknowledged. They worry that she might die; they worry about how best to show their concern. Should they initiate sex, or will that be seen as callous and insensitive? Should they refrain, or will that be seen as an indication that she's no longer sexually attractive?

It's important to realize that the cancer is affecting your whole family, not just you. While you're in treatment, you're usually focused chiefly on yourself, because you have to be. But as soon as you can you need to deal with how it's affecting those closest to you. If this is difficult, sometimes it can help to go into couples therapy with your spouse, or family therapy with your spouse and children. They too are feeling frightened, angry, depressed, maybe even rejected, if all your attention is going to your illness, and they may not have as much support for their feelings as you do for yours. It's crucial to communicate with each other at this time, to work through the complex feelings you're all facing.

At the same time, you might be feeling a little apart from the people you love. You're going through something they can't really understand—only somebody else who's been there can. Breast cancer support groups can be wonderful during this time. You'll meet other women who are at various stages of the disease—including some who had it 10 or 15 years ago and are living happy, healthy lives. Often the only people you've known with breast cancer were in an advanced stage—the ones who get better often don't talk about their disease with anyone. Knowing long-term survivors can help you to realize that you're not necessarily doomed. And knowing other women who are at your stage can give you a sense of shared problems, of comradeship with people who understand what's happening to you because it's also happening to them. Indeed, you might want to look into a group even before your treatment. Hester Hill has had women who joined her group even before their surgery, so they could learn about it from the women who had already been through it.

Above all, you need to be patient with yourself. Healing, both emotionally and physically, takes time. You're entitled to that time.

SEARCHING FOR INFORMATION

Knowing that many women these days want more information, I've set up a website, www.SusanLoveMD.com, where I can post new information as it emerges. The Internet is wonderful for searching for information but you need to be a savvy surfer. If you are searching the Internet, make sure you follow a few guidelines.

1. Know who is sponsoring the site and whether they have anything to gain from the information given. For example, a site sponsored by a pharmaceutical company may have good information but be biased toward its own drugs. Some of the sites pushing alternative therapies are also selling them.
2. Know who is answering questions or giving medical advice. Is it someone you have heard of before? What are their credentials? Are they expert in breast care? You can get good advice from other women with breast cancer on the bulletin boards but you don't know if their experience is standard or if they have an ax to grind.
3. Check who wrote the information on the site and when it was last updated.
4. Look for references for scientific information.
5. If information that you get on a site disagrees with what your doctor has said, print out the page and bring it in to discuss with the doctor.

The same provisos can be applied to books and articles. I have included a list of good ones in Appendix B and there are many more being written every day.

WHAT TO LOOK FOR IN A DOCTOR AND MEDICAL TEAM

As women we are well socialized to not question authority, especially when we're sick. A good place to begin is to put together some sort of questionnaire that will help you assess your potential doctor or medical team. This doesn't have to be an actual document, but if it helps you keep your thoughts, questions, and needs organized and concise, there's nothing wrong with putting pen to paper. What are some of the things you will want to include? They may vary a bit from person to person, based on insurance coverage (or lack thereof), diagnosis, etc. The following questions will give you a good start:

Do they listen?

We all know doctors are busy, pulled in many directions, and pressed for time. When you are dealing with people you might otherwise find intimidating, you may be a bit reluctant to make demands. But remember, they are people just like you, and you can bet they'd want someone to pay close attention if they were in your shoes. Never lose sight of this fact—and don't choose a doctor who has.

Do they sit down, look you in the eye, and connect with you?

You should expect your doctors to hear you. As a way of showing they are listening and caring, it is not unusual for doctors to pull up a chair and sit face-to-face while discussing your diagnosis and options for treatment. You need to feel that your doctor sees you as a person.

Do they solicit and answer your questions?

If only one of you is doing the talking, there's a problem. You will want to make certain that your doctor not only answers any questions you may have, but also provides you with information that will allow you to make decisions, or to know where to look for the answers.

Do they show you your x rays and test reports and explain them if you ask?

Each of us has a comfort level when it comes to facing what will lie ahead in terms of surgery, adjuvant therapies, prognosis, and possibilities. You may want to know every detail. If this is the case, you should expect the doctor you select to explain tests and procedures you will be undergoing. However, you should decide in advance how much you really want to know. Some of us need the hard, fast facts; others just want a broad overview; still others want only the information they will need to take their first step. One size does not fit all, so feel free to ask about anything that comes to mind.

Do they allow you to tape the visit?

Because you may be nervous or frightened—or simply because you may be asking questions that require lengthy or complicated answers—you may want to tape-record conversations with your doctor. Don't be afraid to ask. This is a great way to make sure you aren't missing anything important. It provides you with the opportunity to review what you discussed, and also allows you to absorb what was said at your own pace, in your own time. If you run into a doctor who doesn't want to be taped, you should seriously consider whether this is someone you will feel safe and confident with, or if it's time to move on.

Do they ask you about your use of alternative and complementary therapies?

In this day and age, it is not uncommon for women with breast cancer to seek out therapies that may be considered outside the realm of Western medicine. A growing number of patients feel they need to approach the cancer on more than one level. You may try acupuncture, massage, Chinese herbs, Reiki therapy, vitamins, or many other therapies currently labeled alternative or complementary. Your doctor should want to know about these, and you will want to pay close attention to reactions when you discuss any therapies you may be trying or want to try. If you doctor dismisses these therapies without evidence that a specific therapy is harmful or ineffective, you may want to leave that doctor and find one who acknowledges that alternative treatments can help you to improve your physical and emotional well-being. Many women feel that having the option of an alternative therapy provides them with a sense of control when everything else feels like it's out of their hands. However, always be skeptical of practitioners who promise a cure, ask for large amounts of money for treatment, or make statements that simply sound too good to be true.

Do they suggest additional sources of education and support?

Ideally, your doctor will present you with brochures, pamphlets, and the names of books and other resources designed not only to assist you in making decisions about your treatment options, but also to help you regain your equilibrium. You are going to need information that will allow you to ask questions when you need to, talk to other women who have faced what you are going through, educate yourself about your specific type of breast cancer, and even have a shoulder to cry on once in a while. You should see a red flag if you are given a diagnosis, told you need surgery, and then sent home to prepare without any of the resources mentioned.

Are they threatened when you bring in information from the media to discuss?

While not every bit of information you retrieve from the Internet, magazines, newspapers, etc., may be relevant, it's imperative that your doctor be willing to analyze what you find, discuss it with you, and assist you in making decisions. Procedures, drugs, and information are changing so rapidly, it's likely you may stumble upon an article, web page, or even information in a chat room that could have a profound effect upon your treatment—and that your doctor may not even have heard about. A good doctor won't be threatened by this sort of information, but will want to interpret it for you.

Do you feel like they are partners in this journey?

While it is true that no one can travel the emotional, physical, or psychological path you will be following, it is important that your doctor(s) convey a sincere aura of understanding, support, and partnering. You should feel that any decision you reach is one both of you can agree upon, discuss honestly, and then act upon in a spirit of hope and possibility.

Do they discuss clinical trials?

A clinical trial (sometimes called a protocol or study) is designed to decide whether a new drug or procedure is an effective treatment for a disease, or has possible benefit to the patient. These trials give doctors and researchers an opportunity to gather information on the benefits, side effects, and potential applications for new drugs, as well as help them determine which doses and combinations of existing drugs are most effective.

SECOND OPINIONS

Exploring the options often means getting a second opinion; in this chapter I want to discuss the feelings second opinions evoke. Some women assume that a second opinion is just a confirmation of the treatment plan chosen. Often patients came to see me with their surgery scheduled for the next day, and were very upset if I disagreed with their doctor's plan. But that is the risk you take. As anyone reading this book knows, the treatment of breast cancer is far from straightforward. If you go for another opinion, you may well get one. When the second opinion is different from the first, a patient often assumes that this new opinion must be the right one. Further, having to think about what both doctors told her and make a decision can be extremely stressful. You feel very insecure because your life is on the line and no one seems to know what to do. But the truth is that there are choices. There are different ways to approach the problem and there is no one right answer. It's really your decision: either the first or second opinion can be right. You would like to believe that there is some objective truth: one right way to treat your disease. Unfortunately, as you are finding from reading this book, this is often not the case. You have to explore all of the possibilities until you find the one you're least uncomfortable with.

Sometimes patients are shy about seeking a second opinion—as though they're somehow insulting their doctor's professionalism. Never feel that way. You're not insulting us; you're simply seeking the most precise information possible in what may literally be a life-and-death situation. Most doctors won't be offended—and if you run into a doctor who does get miffed, don't be intimidated. Your life, and your peace of mind, are more important than your doctor's ego.

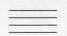

PART SIX

TREATING BREAST CANCER

23

Treatment Options:
an Overview

Over the ten years since the first edition of this book, we have seen the approach to treatment of breast cancer shift from one with surgery center stage and radiation and chemotherapy playing supporting roles, to one with chemotherapy and hormonal therapy as the leads while surgery and radiation moved into ancillary positions. This shift has accompanied a shift in thinking. Most invasive breast cancers are thought to be present for six to eight years before we can see them on a mammogram or feel them. Angiogenesis, or the growth of new blood vessels to feed the tumor, is thought to occur around year two. This means that microscopic spread has probably occurred in most tumors by the time that they are diagnosed. In some women the immune system will have taken care of these cells. As we discussed in Chapter 21, we use a variety of tests to help us guess which women still have cells elsewhere in their body, and in those women we use systemic therapy (chemotherapy or hormonal therapy) in an attempt to eliminate the cells. Local treatments, such as surgery and radiation, on the other hand are used to take care of the cancer in the breast. Some combination of these has been found to be effective for the majority of women. Although the many decisions to be made when you are newly diagnosed can feel overwhelming, it's important to realize that most of the choices have to do with variations on a theme: they involve only small differences in the chance of recurrence or survival. A diagnosis of breast cancer is not an emergency. Take your time to sort out what feels like the best approach for you.

LOCAL TREATMENTS: SURGERY AND RADIATION

The first question usually addressed is what to do about the breast. For years most surgeons did mastectomies, assuming that this drastic procedure was the most effective way to save lives. But more recently studies have proved them wrong; more is not necessarily better.

The goal of surgery in the breast is to remove or treat the cancer so that it will not come back in the breast. This can be done by taking out as much of the cancer as possible in a lumpectomy and letting radiation destroy any remaining cells. The cancer can also be removed by mastectomy, which in small tumors usually takes out enough tissue to prevent recurrence. Finally, with very large tumors we use both mastectomy, to remove as much of the tumor as possible, and radiation therapy, to take care of leftover cells. You can have a local recurrence either way—whether you have a mastectomy or a lumpectomy and radiation. People often have the misconception that if they have a mastectomy the cancer can never come back again because there's no breast left. But as I said earlier, we can never be sure if we get all the breast tissue, and it can come back again in the scar or the chest wall. I saw one patient with a very small cancer who had bilateral mastectomies because she never wanted to deal with it again, and a year later she had a recurrence in her scar. (This is rare, but occurs about 0.6% per year or 5–10% over 12 years.) She was very angry and felt she had been betrayed by her original medical team because no one had told her that this was a possibility.

The first study to compare mastectomy and breast conservation surgery was done in Italy in the 1970s. It compared radical mastectomy to quadrantectomy (the removal of one quarter of the breast) followed by radiation and found there was no difference in the survival rate between the two methods of treatment.[1] Since then, the NSABP (National Surgical Adjuvant Breast and Bowel Project) has done a study in the U.S. comparing lumpectomy alone, lumpectomy and radiation, and mastectomy, and has had similar results: lumpectomy and radiation had the same survival rate and almost the same local control rate as mastectomy. After twelve years lumpectomy alone had a 35 percent local recurrence rate; lumpectomy and radiation had a 10 percent local recurrence rate; and mastectomy had an 8 percent rate.[2] (These treatments are described at length in Chapters 25 and 27.)

The NSABP study conclusively demonstrated that in most kinds of breast cancer radiation and lumpectomy are virtually as good as mastectomy. In June 1990 a National Cancer Institute Consensus Conference concluded: "Breast conservation treatment is an appropriate method of primary therapy for the *majority* of women with Stage I and II breast cancer and is *preferable* because it provides survival equivalent to total mastectomy and axillary dissection while preserving the breast" (emphasis mine).

There are some special situations in which lumpectomy and radiation therapy might even have an edge. If your cancer is right near the breastbone or on the edge of the breast, even with a mastectomy we can't get a normal rim of tissue around the lump. However, radiation can treat the surrounding tissue. In fact, when your cancer is located there, you might consider following even a mastectomy with radiation.

On the other hand, in some situations you're better off with a mastectomy—for instance, if you have a large cancer in a small breast (although neoadjuvant chemotherapy discussed later in this chapter, may help here), or two separate cancers in the same breast, or microcalcifications spread throughout your breast.

After much study it appears that the most important factor in achieving local control is getting most of the tumor out with surgery. One way we determine whether this has happened is by evaluating the margins of what was removed (see Chapter 20). If they're free of tumor, breast conservation is fine. This can be affected by the tumor's pathology. Some kinds of tumors have the equivalent of tentacles stretching out into the breast tissue from the original lump. Ductal carcinomas with lots of DCIS (also called *extensive intraductal component,* or EIC) associated with them are often in this category. When this occurs, the margins may not be clean on the first try because the surgeon can't see or feel the "tentacles" of DCIS and cuts through them. A re-excision will sometimes take care of it. But there are some cases in which even a re-excision won't get clean margins, and a mastectomy, the ultimate wide excision, is necessary to get it all out. Infiltrating lobular carcinomas also have a tendency to be sneaky and difficult for the surgeon to find and get around (see Chapter 16). These too need a wider excision and clean margins if they are to be treated with breast conservation, and may still end up requiring a mastectomy.

On the other hand, if the cancer is a distinct lump without any of the "tentacles" that are the hallmark of extensive DCIS, then just removing it is fine. Sometimes focal (one spot) involvement of the margins is acceptable in this situation.[3] Some doctors don't understand this, and put too much emphasis on having a clean margin. The key is determining the likelihood that cancer has been left behind. In the usual type of cancer, the chance is very low, and radiation therapy can well get rid of whatever cells may remain. In fact, when lumpectomy with radiation was first employed in Boston, we didn't know that margins were important and we just took the tumor out. Reviewing these data in retrospect, we found that in tumors without EIC or lobular carcinoma our recurrence rate was only 4–6 percent over more than 10 years even though we did not have perfectly clean margins.

Another issue is whether radiation is necessary. In the NSABP study it was found that with lumpectomy alone a woman has a 35 percent chance of a local recurrence of her cancer.[4] This brings up the question of whether all women with breast cancer need radiation. If only 35 percent of women who have wide excision alone will have a recurrence, we're radiating 65 percent of women who don't need it. If we could find a way to determine which women need radiation and which don't, we could save those who don't need it and spare them the discomforts and risks of radiation.

In the hope there might be a group of patients on whom we could stop doing radiation, a study[5] I was involved in during the 1980s looked at women who fit very strict criteria, and offered them the opportunity to be treated without radiation in a very controlled context. To qualify for this study, a woman had to have a tumor less then 2 centimeters (3/4 inch), negative lymph nodes, no extensive DCIS in the tumor, no vascular or lymphatic invasion, and at least a centimeter of normal tissue around her tumor margins. We felt that by selecting out these women with relatively less dangerous cancers, we were choosing the ones who might not need radiation. We followed these women very carefully, and at the first sign of a recurrence we added further treatment. Unfortunately, we found that even in this group there was a 9.2 percent local recurrence rate in three years, compared to a 2 percent local recurrence rate in comparable patients treated with lumpectomy and radiation. Because this rate of recurrence was higher than we felt acceptable, we had to stop the study prematurely. So at least to date we haven't been able to figure out a category of women with invasive breast cancer who could safely go without radiation.

In May of 2000 the NSABP answered yet another question about local control. They reported the results from a study of node negative women with tumors less than one centimeter which had been completely excised. The women in the study were randomized to get either tamoxifen alone, radiotherapy alone or both. It was clear that tamoxifen alone was not enough to prevent local recurrences with 24% vs 11.7%. However, tamoxifen did add to the protective effect of the radiation against local recurrence—when both were used the percentage of local recurrence was only 3.6%.[6]

Mastectomy

For years the major issue in local control had been whether it's okay to do just lumpectomy and radiation instead of mastectomy. But there

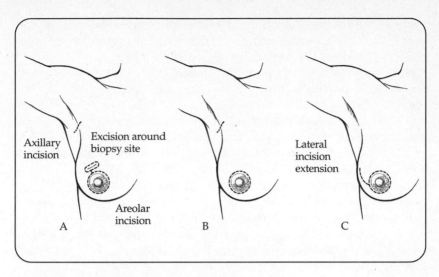

Axillary
incision

Excision around
biopsy site

Lateral
incision
extension

Areolar
incision

A

B

C

FIGURE 23-1   Skin-Sparing Mastectomy Incisions

have now been some changes in our thinking about mastectomies as well. For one thing, we always used to take out a large amount of skin when we did mastectomies, believing that would help keep the cancer from spreading. It was really a holdover from the old theory of radical mastectomy—take out as much as you can. We also liked the fact that this helped the scar to close neatly. If the surgeon leaves a lot of skin and scoops out all the breast tissue, the skin looks wrinkled and baggy. Trimming the skin creates a nice neat line across the chest. But now, as more immediate reconstructions are being done, the need to take off so much skin is being reconsidered. We've moved into the era of what's called "skin-sparing mastectomy" (Fig. 23-1). This means that instead of removing a lot of skin around the breast, surgeons will remove only the amount that's needed to take the breast off, unless the patient is *sure* she never wants reconstruction—then it's nice to be tidy. Some surgeons are experimenting again with leaving the nipple and areola when they do a mastectomy. I am a little concerned about this. The ductal systems all end up in the nipple, which means the risk of leaving disease behind if there is a lot of DCIS is significant. Nonetheless, this points out that we've begun to view mastectomy as just a very big wide excision. Getting every bit of breast tissue out isn't possible or necessary; it's getting the tumor out that really matters.

With mastectomy, whether or not it's a skin-sparing situation, we usually don't feel the need to do radiation because we believe the tumor has generally been wholly removed. But in some situations where the patient is at high risk, having cancer cells lingering in the remaining chest wall or regional lymph nodes creates a greater risk of local recurrence, and we do perform post-mastectomy radiation. Having cancer in the scar afterwards doesn't necessarily increase the patient's chances of dying (although this does signify a more aggressive cancer with a higher risk of systemic recurrence), but getting breast cancer once is upsetting enough, and preventing a recurrence is never a bad idea.

The predictors for a higher risk of local recurrence are: four or more positive axillary lymph nodes; a tumor over 5 centimeters; close margins (cancer cells at the edge of the mastectomy); and significant amounts of lympho-vascular invasion in the breast tissue. There is some controversy over whether to do radiation if there are one to three positive nodes; usually the decision will be to radiate if the doctors haven't taken out many lymph nodes. If, for example, the surgeon took out five nodes and three were positive, they wouldn't know if there were other positive nodes that hadn't been removed. If there's what's known as extra-capsular invasion—cancer cells visible outside of the lymph nodes in the removed axillary tissue—they'd also do radiation.

Post-mastectomy radiation reduces the chance of local recurrence by 50 to 75 percent (if the local recurrence rate overall is 5–10%, this makes it 3–5%). If the chance of recurrence is higher, as in the situations mentioned above, the benefit would be higher. But until lately it was not thought to have an impact on increasing survival. Two recent randomized studies in Canada and Denmark of high-risk premenopausal women with breast cancer and positive nodes showed that women treated with modern radiation therapy techniques to the chest wall and draining lymph nodes and chemotherapy, when compared with women treated only with chemotherapy, had fewer local recurrences, and the overall survival was significantly better—by about nearly 10 percent in one study, and 9 percent in the other. The overall survival was 54 percent with chemo alone, and 64 percent with both.[7,8]

Why then shouldn't everyone who gets a mastectomy and has positive lymph nodes have radiation? First, we are unsure if these two trials apply exactly to women treated in this country with different chemotherapy. Second, radiation has its own risks. Some studies show that people who had cancer on the left side and get radiation had an increase in heart disease (see Chapter 27). Radiation is getting better, since there are better techniques and more careful planning these days. But it's still more problematic in some situations than in others. Depending on the shape of the woman's chest and whether an attempt is made to radiate the internal mammary nodes, the heart and lung may be affected. Some of this depends on the skill of the radiation therapist. Ask your doctors how they feel about post-mastectomy radiation, how often they do it, and what their complication rate has been. If you are not comfortable with the answer, get a second opoinion.

Axillary Dissection

There is also the question of removing the lymph nodes under the arm. There is no evidence that axillary surgery itself affects survival, and the main purpose for doing it is to decide about adjuvant chemotherapy and to prevent recurrence in the armpit. Some surgeons have argued that if we are going to give systemic therapy to all women, node negative as well as node positive (a philosophy we discuss later in this chapter), there is no reason to dissect the lymph nodes. They feel they can save women the potential complications of this operation (see Chapter 25) by radiating the axilla (under the arm) instead. The fallacy in this argument, at least at the time of this writing, is that we are not at all sure that every woman should be treated with systemic therapy. Until we know whom to treat, or we have a better marker of prognosis than lymph nodes, I still think it is an important operation for most women. There probably is a subgroup of women, however, where the possibility of finding positive nodes is so low that it is not worth doing a lymph node dissection. This would include women with DCIS, with or without microinvasion, and those with invasive tumors less than 5 millimeters. Melvin Silverstein has shown that the chance of positive nodes in this group is less than 3 percent,[9] and many surgeons are beginning to admit that surgery is probably not necessary. Certainly the woman needs to weigh the pros and cons for herself. If she will always wonder if she was the 1 out of 100 who had a positive node and would have needed chemotherapy, maybe she should indeed have the surgery. On the other hand, if she can live with the uncertainty and less surgery, then I think it is reasonable to forego the dissection.

Luckily, in recent years, there has been a new variation on lymph node dissection that offers us a better way to find cancer spread. This is known as *sentinel node biopsy* (Fig. 23-2). The concept is pretty straightforward.[10,11] A small amount of blue dye and/or radioactivity is injected into the breast at the site of the lesion. This material then passes naturally through the nearby lymphatics to the first draining node for that area of the breast. This is the node that is also most likely to have drained any cancer cells spreading through the lymphatics from a tumor in that area. The first draining nodes (the *sentinel nodes*) are then removed and carefully studied. Since they are where escaping cancer cells are most likely to be found, they are very accurate predictors of whether there is cancer in the other lymph nodes. In other words, if the sentinel node biopsy is normal, then there's a very low chance that the surgeon will have missed a positive node. It can be done with either lumpectomy or mastectomy, and after a core or open biopsy.

Since these techniques are new, it's inevitable that their use should add dispute to an already controversial area. Who should have sentinel node biopsy, and who should have traditional node dissection, and

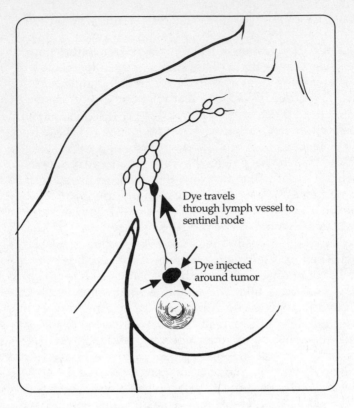

Dye travels through lymph vessel to sentinel node

Dye injected around tumor

FIGURE 23-2   Sentinel Node Biopsy

who should have both? There's some argument that every patient, whether or not she has full axillary dissection, should have sentinel node procedure done as well. The sentinel node should be located and removed, and then studied separately from the rest of the nodes. Others maintain that the sentinel node biopsy can replace full axillary dissection, saving women the complications (see Chapter 25) that such surgery may cause. This is currently being studied across the country. An argument against sentinel node biopsy is that it isn't foolproof; it still could provide a false negative. In about 5 percent of cases this happens; the sentinel node shows no cancer, and then cancer is found in the other nodes at full dissection. (Regular dissection can also miss some positive nodes.) Studies are now following women long-range to see if those who have had only sentinel biopsy where no cancer was found developed axillary recurrences later on in life. Currently the standard of care is for women who have a positive sentinel node (i.e., found to contain cancer) to go on to have a full dissection.

There are some situations in which sentinel node biopsy makes particular sense. If you have a stage I or II cancer with no palpable nodes in your armpit, it might be a wise choice, rather than having all your nodes removed. But doctors debate the upper size limit of a tumor where this is safe: some say 2 centimeters, some say 3, and some say 4.

You should always ask questions about the doctor who does the procedure. You want someone with experience, or who is working under the supervision of someone with experience, because the procedure is difficult to learn—it's been estimated that a surgeon must do between 20 and 30 cases to become really good at it.[12,13] The first few times a surgeon does it, it can be hard to find the sentinel lymph node, to inject the dye or the radioactive fluid correctly, and to know how long to wait before doing the surgery after the injection. So you probably don't want to be someone's second sentinel node biopsy case. Ask how many times the surgeon has done the procedure. In addition, ask what percentage of the time the surgeon has been able to find the sentinel node. It should be at least 85 percent (with experienced surgeons, in fact, it's 90 or 95%).[14]

Also ask about the surgeon's false negative rate. Initially when surgeons first learn this procedure they do it along with a full dissection. They take out what they think is the sentinel node, then do the regular dissection and see whether they identified the sentinel node correctly. A false negative means the sentinel node was negative but there was a positive node someplace else. The false negative rate should be under 5 percent. If a surgeon is unable, or unwilling, to give you numbers, that's a pretty good sign you should look for another surgeon. If it turns out to be the surgeon's third or fourth operation, find out who the supervising surgeon is—and get *that* surgeon's numbers.

It's also important to make sure the pathology will be done correctly. They should make many thin (1.5 mm) slices of the node. They should also do immunohistochemistry with cytokeratin, which is a way of staining for a particular protein that's found in breast cancer cells but not in lymph cells, as well as the usual stain. If they're not doing both forms of staining, find out why—and if the answer doesn't sound right to you, find someone who will do both tests.

There are some situations in which sentinel node biopsy isn't feasible. If you've had extensive breast surgery that may have disrupted the lymphatic pathways—something like breast reduction or, in some cases, silicone implants—doing sentinel node biopsy won't work. If you have nodes that are already palpable then it isn't necessary; the doctor knows where to go. If you have two lumps in different places in the breast, the sentinel nodes will be in two parts of your breast and the procedure won't work. It is less successful in older women and in women with extensive DCIS.

In some patients with severe health problems the risks of general anesthesia may outweigh the advantage of knowing the lymph node status. In these women it may be reasonable to forego this operation in favor of axillary radiation.

The discussion about axillary dissection is an ongoing one. I think in the future we'll be able to stop doing axillary dissection altogether. Once we've got a better biomarker so we can say, "This is your prognosis," we'll no longer have to subject women to the extra surgery of lymph node removal, with its side effects. At this point, however, I think it's important for every woman to question her surgeon about the necessity of the axillary dissection and make sure she's comfortable with the explanation before proceeding.

Timing of Surgery

Finally, we should mention the growing information regarding the timing of surgery in premenopausal women. There have been over 32 retrospective studies looking at this in relation to the menstrual cycle.[15,16] The researchers went back to records of women operated on 10 years earlier and tried to figure out where each woman had been in her menstrual cycle at the time of her surgery. They did this by finding out when she had her last period and then calculating a 28-day cycle. This is an imperfect method at best, given the vagaries of women's cycles, but it was the best they could do at this stage. Many found that women who were operated on in what appeared to be mid-cycle rather than at the beginning or very end of their cycle did better; other researchers did not confirm this relationship. Similar data have been found in a 1988 study showing that mice transplanted with breast cancer were cured twice as often when surgery was performed just before the animals were in heat or around the time of ovulation.[17] Of course, neither studies that observe a phenomenon nor a biological explanation are enough to establish cause and effect. The first prospective study was reported out of Guy's Hospital in November 1999.[18] The research involved 112 premenopausal women who underwent either mastectomy or lumpectomy. The patients were classified according to their phase of the menstrual cycle on the day of surgery, the size of their tumors, and whether their cancers contained receptors for estrogen or progesterone. They were followed for 10 years after surgery. At the end of the study, 45 percent of the patients who were operated on during the follicular phase (first half) of the cycle were still alive, in contrast to 75 percent of those who had surgery during the luteal phase, or second half. The menstrual cycle effect was even stronger in women who had hormone-sensitive tumors. Those whose tumors were ER positive and had surgery during the luteal phase had a 10-year survival rate of 80 percent, vs. 60 percent for those with ER-negative tumors. However, estrogen receptor status didn't appear to play a role in the outcome when women went into surgery during the follicular phase: their survival rate was 42 percent whether they had ER-positive or ER-negative tumors. Scientists have observed that factors influencing the growth of new blood vessels (VEGF) are higher in the first part of the menstrual cycle and lower in the second. This could mean that the blood vessels are leakier and more amenable to letting breast cancer escape during the manipulation of surgery.[19]

The story was much the same for progesterone receptors. Eighty-eight percent of women with PR-positive tumors and 56 percent of those with PR-negative tumors who had luteal phase surgery survived 10 years, as opposed to 44 percent of women with PR-positive or PR-negative tumors who had follicular phase surgery.

Three large studies are going on that we hope will answer this question. Meanwhile, this is one piece of information that can be used without risk. If you are a premenopausal woman with breast cancer, it certainly can't hurt to schedule your surgery during your luteal phase—and it may extend your life.

Guidelines

When I was director of the Revlon/UCLA Breast Center, I spent a year reviewing all the data with my colleagues. We came up with practice guidelines suggesting we look at every woman as a candidate for surgery that allowed breast conservation, unless she strongly preferred a mastectomy. Any woman whose cancer was picked up on a mammogram should have a post-biopsy mammogram to demonstrate that the whole tumor was removed. If she had a lumpectomy and the margins were more than focally involved, or the post-biopsy mammogram showed residual disease, or if she had EIC or infiltrating lobular carcinoma, we suggested a re-excision and axillary dissection. This step was done to gather further information on the cancer. If the new margins were clean, she was a candidate for radiation therapy. If not, she may have needed a mastectomy. The axillary node dissection would help determine the need for systemic therapy, as we discuss later. If the tumor was over 5 cm we routinely offered neoadjuvant chemotherapy in an attempt to shrink it. After three to four cycles we reevaluated the local disease. If the tumor was now gone or much smaller we would proceed with a lumpectomy. If not, we would do a mastectomy. All women who chose mastectomy were offered the option of immediate reconstruction (see Chapter 26).

Making the Choice

The first choice you may have to make involves whether you want full axillary dissection, sentinel node dissection, or both. If you want sentinel node dissection and are eligible for it, you may have to search for a doctor with experience doing it. The one thing you *don't* want to do is insist that the surgeon you're going to do a sentinel node biopsy. If your surgeon hasn't done the procedure a number of times, or doesn't feel comfortable with it, you're much better off having it done the way the surgeon's used to doing it.

But it's worth finding out who is available to you if you really want a sentinel node biopsy. In the summer of 1999 I met a 66-year-old woman who was in an HMO, and who was told by the doctor she spoke with there that he didn't do the procedure. She was very upset; an active sportswoman, she didn't want to take the chance that her golf arm might be permanently injured by the removal of too many nodes. I suggested that she ask the doctor if there was anyone at the HMO who *did* do the sentinel node biopsy. She called him, and he willingly answered that there was someone, and gave her the surgeon's name.

If your HMO doesn't have anyone, you can explain your need to them. Tell them you'd like a recommendation for someone outside of the HMO. Often they'll pay the fee for such a specialist; sometimes they'll only do this for a larger co-payment, but that may be worth it to you.

There are four clinical trials going on looking at sentinel node dissection with or without full axillary dissection, and if that's what you want, you might look into them (www.clinicaltrials.gov). There are a couple of good reasons for this. It helps us answer some of the questions we have about breast cancer. That's the noble reason. The personal reason is that the doctors working on the trial are well trained and know what they're doing, so you get quality assurance (see Chapter 12).

If you don't have palpable nodes and have a T-1 or T-2 tumor (see Chapter 21), I think it's worth having a sentinel node biopsy, even if you're also getting a full axillary biopsy. It would allow the doctor to look for which node to study most carefully.

Next is the decision about mastectomy or lumpectomy. What are some of the factors that influence a woman's choice between mastectomy or lumpectomy with radiation? There's a tendency to think that mastectomy is more aggressive, because it's more mutilating. Actually, the combination of lumpectomy and radiation is more aggressive. The doctor doing radiation will radiate all the breast tissue. The field of radiation might encompass all that tissue that the most extensive surgery misses. Some women choose mastectomy because they do not want to make the daily trips needed for radiation therapy; others may want to get it all over with as soon as possible and get back to their lives as though it never happened. It's understandable, but it doesn't work that way. It has happened, and you can never go back to your life exactly the way it was.

There are important drawbacks to mastectomy. It's less cosmetically appealing, and, even with reconstruction (see Chapter 26), it leaves you without sensation in the breast or breast area. Lumpectomy and radiation leave you with a real breast that retains its sexual sensation.

Sometimes a patient asks me what I'd do if I had breast cancer. I never tell her. I couldn't, because what I think I'd do now might be very different from what I'd actually do if I were faced with the reality. But even if I did know, what difference would it make? My choice would be based on who I am—my values, my feelings about my body, my priorities, my neuroses. It would be valid only for me. My patient comes to me for my medical expertise, but she is the expert on herself.

I've had all kinds of patients make very different unpredictable decisions, and I think it's ludicrous to make assumptions about who will want what. The real factors vary as much as women and their lifestyles vary. I'm sure there are many factors I haven't come across, but I can discuss a few I'm familiar with. For instance, there are women who choose mastectomy because of their jobs. They don't want to take any more time off from a demanding profession than necessary.

The availability of one kind of treatment or another is also a factor. In some areas there's no place nearby that offers radiation. In others, radiation is available, but it's not especially good; a radiation therapist really has to know the technique to get good results. For some women, however, their breasts are an integral part of their sexuality and identity and they are willing (and able) to go to great inconvenience to save them. One of my patients lived in a small town in the central valley of California, too far to commute to my breast center in LA. So she and her husband drove down in their mobile van and lived in the hospital parking lot until her six weeks were over. I've had patients whose cancer recurred after lumpectomy and radiation, and even though they then had to have mastectomies, they were grateful they had an extra few years with both breasts.

Regardless of the medical facts, however, you need to feel safe with your choice. Some of my patients who had lumpectomy and radiation would wake up every morning afterwards sure that the cancer had come back. They probably would have been better off with mastectomies in the first place.

The possibility of reconstruction, which we discuss at length in Chapter 26, may also play a role in a woman's decision. You might be more willing to lose a breast if it can be replaced. But you need to take into consideration the fact that a reconstructed breast is never exactly like a real one. Remember above all that it's your body and no one else's. Don't decide on the basis of what anyone else thinks is best. By all means talk to your friends and your family and your husband or lover, and think about what they say. But make your own decision. Husbands and lovers come and go, but your body is with you all your life. A truly caring mate should support whatever course you think is best for you.

SYSTEMIC TREATMENTS: CHEMOTHERAPY

After you decide about local treatment, you will need to decide about systemic therapy: chemotherapy, hormonal therapy, or both. Chemotherapy was initially used to treat leukemia, a cancer which, by definition, is present throughout the bloodstream. Later it was used to treat any metastatic cancer. The idea was that drugs circulating through the bloodstream could get to all the places a cancer cell was likely to hide. Unfortunately, it didn't always work. On further study, the researchers came to understand that the failure stemmed from two problems: there were too many cancer cells for the drugs to handle, and some cancer cells became resistant to the drugs. They then began to consider giving chemotherapy earlier and earlier, and the concept of adjuvant chemotherapy was born. Perhaps the time to give chemotherapy was right after the primary local treatment—either surgery alone or surgery and radiation—when any spread would still be microscopic. And indeed this approach seemed to work. The first studies by Gianni Bonadonna[20] and by the NSABP[21] showed that premenopausal women with positive nodes had a significant decrease in breast cancer mortality when given adjuvant chemotherapy. This set the stage for the now common practice of using systemic treatments at the time of initial diagnosis. We now give adjuvant chemotherapy to all premenopausal women with positive nodes, many with negative nodes, and many postmenopausal women.

What Is the Benefit of Chemotherapy? The Numbers

Some women want to know with as much certainty as possible the actual benefit they can get from chemotherapy. The numbers can be pretty dense, and you can skip them if you want, but I would suggest at least reading through this section once. The benefits of chemotherapy are often fewer than we think, and it is important to be realistic about it.

Chemotherapy reduces the risk of recurrence by about a third.[22]

That means that the higher chance of recurrence, the better chance that chemotherapy will work for you. If you have a 60 percent chance of recurrence, a one third risk reduction means it will reduce it by 20 percent, but if you have a 9 percent chance of recurrence the one third reduction in mortality is only 3 percent. This is an important concept to understand when trying to weigh risks and benefits.

In 1998 an overview of chemotherapy was done.[23] This study looked at all the randomized controlled studies that had been done and found that in women under 50 there was a 35 percent reduction in recurrence. In women over 50 it was about 20 percent reduction. Combined, that comes to about a third. Very few women over 70 have been in these studies, so we don't have information on this group. Overall, mortality was reduced 27 percent in women under 50 and 11 percent in women over 50.

To be useful in your own decision making, the figures need to be converted to your situation. What is the absolute change? Remember that a 30 percent proportional reduction doesn't mean that you have a 30 percent lower chance of dying from the cancer. It means, for example, that if you have a 30 percent chance to begin with, it's reduced by one third, or 10 percent. According to the latest overview, if you're under 50 and node negative, chemotherapy will change your survival from 71 percent to 78 percent—a 7 percent improvement. If you're under 50 and node positive, it would go from 42 percent to 53 percent—about an 11 percent benefit. The reason it's higher if you're node positive is that your cancer is more likely to come back, so you have a bigger benefit.

In the women between 50 and 69, there's less benefit. If you're node negative it goes from 67 percent to 69 percent, a 2 percent benefit. If you're node positive it goes from 46 percent to 49 percent, a 3 percent improvement. So although there is a benefit, it's not very big.

Recently a woman called me for my advice. She was 68, had an estrogen receptor negative tumor, and had been told by her oncologist that she should be on chemotherapy because her chance of dying in the next five years was 15 percent without chemotherapy. So she thought she might try it. I asked her if the doctor had told her what her chance of dying in the next five years was if she did take chemo. He hadn't. "I assume it means I have a 100 percent chance of surviving the next five years if I take it," she said. I told her that wasn't accurate: her chance of dying with chemo was 13 percent. She paused. "Then forget that!" she said finally. "I don't want to go through that for a 2 percent better chance!" However, some studies have shown that some women will choose chemotherapy even for a 1 percent improvement in survival. Every woman has a different view.

There's a study by S. Rajagopal[24] in which oncologists were given certain scenarios and asked whether or not they'd give chemotherapy in each scenario. What percentage of improvement in survival did they think the patient would have? Overall, they estimated a three times greater improvement than was warranted. It is important that you pin your oncologist down so that you are realistic about the benefits of chemotherapy in your case.

We are still wondering why there is a difference between postmenopausal and premenopausal women. One thought has always been that chemotherapy causes a chemical menopause in the younger woman and therefore acts much the same way that tamoxifen or ovarian ablation does. This wouldn't account for the total effect, however. The other possibility is that there is a small effect of cell kill (the same small percent seen in the postmenopausal woman) and an additional hormonal effect in the premenopausal woman, but only the cell kill effect in the postmenopausal woman. Against this theory is the fact that the chemotherapy effect may not abruptly disappear with the onset of menopause but may decrease as a woman ages. Like aging itself, it's a gradual process. The older you get, the farther into menopause, the less effective it becomes. When you're newly menopausal, it's still very likely to have some effect.

Types of Chemotherapy

If it is clear that a woman should get chemotherapy, there arises the issue of what drugs she should get. One of three combinations is usually given as adjuvant therapy for node-positive women. One is CMF—Cytoxan, methotrexate, 5-fluorouracil. The second is AC, where Adriamycin replaces the methotrexate. The third is AC followed by Taxol.

Adriamycin is one of the strongest drugs we have for metastatic breast cancer. Some doctors have concluded from this that it will probably work well as adjuvant treatment. The 1998 overview compared CMF chemotherapy with AC. There was a slight advantage to the AC—72 percent five-year survival vs. 69 percent. This benefit is usually balanced against the cardiac toxicity of Adriamycin of 1–2 percent.

There is some suggestion, although as yet not definite, that if you're a Her-2 neu overexpressor, Adriamycin works better, and if you're not, CMF works as well.[25] So it may be that if a woman's breast cancer overexpresses Her-2 neu, she will benefit most from Adriamycin at standard doses.

There's also a new drug called epirubicin, which is similar to Adriamycin. It's used with the same other drugs, so it's called CEF. One isn't any more effective than the other, but some studies suggest that epirubicin has a somewhat lower toxicity rate.

Another new category of chemotherapy drugs are the taxanes

paclitaxel (Taxol) and docetaxel (Taxotere), which were originally derived from the bark and needles of the yew tree. Initial studies were on paclitaxel and showed benefit in women with metastatic disease as well as adjuvant. In a very large study women with positive nodes were randomized to have four cycles of AC alone or four cycles of AC followed by four more of Taxol. There was an overall improvement in the women who used Taxol—a 22 percent decrease in recurrence and a 26 percent increase in mortality.[26] Overall the absolute improvement in survival was 3 percent. Docetaxel (Taxotere) has shown benefits in metastatic disease and is being tested in the adjuvant setting. Studies comparing the two drugs head-to-head are ongoing and we should have a better sense of their best uses soon.

Since there are choices to be made among different chemotherapy drugs, I think it's particularly important for the patient to enter into the decision-making process. Ask why your doctor has chosen a particular treatment regimen and ask to see studies that back it up. Find out exactly what the differences are in efficacy and in side effects. For example, some drugs are more likely to put you into menopause and thus render you infertile than others. (See Chapter 28.) Some, like Adriamycin, can be more toxic to the heart. So you may prefer to stick with the CMF. Or you may be willing to take a slightly higher risk in the hope that the stronger drug will be better. If you don't feel that you are getting straight answers from your oncologist, get a second opinion. If a clinical trial is available, consider participating in it so that we will get some answers (see Chapter 12). You are smart enough to take control of this decision.

High-Dose Chemotherapy with Stem Cell Rescue

As you can see, chemotherapy has decreased the mortality of breast cancer, but certainly not to the extent we would like. There was a theory a few years ago that the reason we didn't do very well in curing women with a lot of positive lymph nodes was that we weren't giving strong enough chemotherapy. If a little chemotherapy was good, they thought, more must be better. Some doctors believed that high-dose chemotherapy with stem cell rescue (the most recent form of bone marrow transplant) was the answer.

One of the early tests of the theory was done by Bill Peters, M.D., at Duke.[27] Peters did a nonrandomized study in women with 10 or more positive axillary lymph nodes and found that with his procedure 64 percent of patients had a five-year survival during that period. He compared this with previous studies of what had been considered standard-dose chemotherapy, which had shown 35 percent survival. Accepting this comparison at face value, clinicians were off and running. Soon this toxic therapy had become the standard of care for women with aggressive tumors, locally advanced breast cancer, and metastatic disease. Insurance companies were forced by the courts to fund it, and this gave it even better press: since insurance companies don't like to spend money, it was assumed that penny pinching was the only real reason they wouldn't support it. Sadly, that wasn't true.

The Peters study illustrates the limitations of nonrandomized studies. Comparing women in a new study with those in old ones is very much an apples-and-oranges proposition. In the historical study he used for comparison, women were all ages and in varying states of health. Some of them had responded to initial chemotherapy, while others had not. But in Peters's study, most of the women were young and healthy (essential if they were to survive the procedure), and all had whole body CT scans to rule out the presence of metastatic disease. This intensive testing assured that only the best-prognosis women with 10 or more positive lymph nodes would get a transplant. The transplant was being given to make sure the cancer was really gone, in a belts-and-suspenders approach.

What was needed was a study that took a group of similar women and randomized them into two groups: one would get high-dose chemotherapy with stem cell transplant and the other, standard chemotherapy. To his credit, Peters did this study, which was reported in the spring of 1999.[28] Unexpectedly, it showed that the standard chemotherapy did just as well as the high-dose, with fewer complications. Three other studies,[29,30] one in women with more than 10 positive nodes and two in women with metastatic disease, were also reported at that time. They, too, showed no additional benefit from high-dose chemotherapy with stem cell transplant.

One study, done in South Africa,[31] did show a benefit. But when researchers went to South Africa to see why, they found the investigator had fraudulent data.

Over 12,000 women underwent high-dose chemotherapy with stem cell rescue during the nine years it took to complete the four studies mentioned above. If all of these women had participated in randomized clinical trials, we would have had the answer quickly and could have been developing something better by now. Doctors who did the procedure outside of the studies were selling dreams rather than trying to figure out whether they worked. We can't let that happen again.

What is the downside of having this therapy? It is very toxic and expensive. To give credit where it is due, researchers have found ways to do it more safely, and the mortality rate, which used to be about 10–15 percent, is now closer to 5 percent. Still, a 1 in 20 chance that a procedure you have had done to save your life will instead kill you may not be one you want to take.

Further, the treatment has some unpleasant side effects—including shingles, lung problems, premature menopause, leukemia, and decrease in brain function. We are only beginning to study what the long-term side effects might be, as it hasn't been done long enough for us to know.

Trastuzumab (Herceptin)

Another new option is Herceptin, the antibody to the Her-2 neu oncogene (see Chapter 13). At the time of this writing it had been tested in women with metastatic disease and been shown both alone and with chemotherapy to have a beneficial effect, with improved survival along with Taxol in metastatic disease.[32,33,34] As this book went to press, studies were just being mounted to see whether it would be a reasonable adjuvant option in addition to chemotherapy for women who were overexpressors of Her-2 neu. At this time I would strongly urge any woman who is interested in trying Herceptin as an adjuvant therapy to enroll in a clinical trial so that we can quickly determine its value.

Timing

Studies are also being done on the timing of chemotherapy. Generally speaking, we tend to do the chemotherapy first and the radiation afterwards—particularly with someone with a high risk of recurrence, because we want to save her life, and radiation is more of a local cleanup. But it's not clear that delaying the radiation won't add to the risk of recurrence in the breast. There was a study done in Boston in the early '90s in which one group of women was given radiation first and the other chemo first.[35] It showed that the survival was better if chemotherapy was given first but that local control was better when radiation came first. So if a woman's chances of having microscopic cells elsewhere in the body are high, she should have chemotherapy first. If she is at low risk for systemic disease then radiation first may be fine. It is reassuring that there was no increase in breast recurrences in women who received six months of chemotherapy with AC followed by Taxol compared with AC alone for three months prior to radiation therapy.

Another issue being aggressively studied is the concept of *neoadjuvant* (or *preoperative*) chemotherapy. This means giving the chemotherapy first, before surgery, after making the diagnosis with a needle biopsy. Because chemotherapy is the most important treatment, dealing with the life-threatening element of the cancer, some of us thought that giving it first might make a difference in survival. Unfortunately, none of the studies have shown this to be true. However, we have found two other advantages. The first is that we can find out whether the chemo works or not. If the tumor starts melting away, we know the chemo is working. If it's not working, we can turn to a different chemotherapy. The NSABP study found that there was an 80 percent reduction in the tumor size, and in 36 percent of women the tumor completely disappeared.[36] This allowed doctors to do lumpectomies in 8 percent of women who would otherwise have needed mastectomies (67.8% vs. 59.8%). There's no question now that in tumors over about 3 centimeters, most surgeons will do preoperative chemotherapy. In smaller tumors, which would allow a lumpectomy anyway, many surgeons still wait to do chemotherapy after the surgery.

There has been a theory for a long time that we could pick chemotherapy the way we pick antibiotics—through sensitivity testing. With antibiotics, the doctors grow the bacteria from your infection in a petri dish that has spots of different antibiotics all over it, and then look to see which spots the bacteria grows on, and which it dies on. Then the doctor can say, "This patient's infection is sensitive to this antibiotic, but not that one, so we'll prescribe this one." This is known as *in vitro drug sensitivity testing* ("in vitro" means literally "in glass"; this refers to any experiment done outside the body).

There have been many laboratory experiments in sensitivity testing for chemotherapy, but the problem is that it's never been clear how well it translates to patients. What works in a petri dish doesn't necessarily work in a living body. There was a 1999 review of 12 prospective studies that looked at this in breast cancer.[37] They had 506 patients, 33 percent treated with chemotherapy that had been selected using in vitro drug sensitivity testing. The response rate was a little bit better—27 percent for the in vitro vs. 18 percent chosen by other means—but they didn't find any difference in survival rates. Future studies may show that there is a survival rate improvement, but for now we have no certainty of it. It may have a bigger benefit in primary disease than in metastatic disease.

There are certain drugs we can give you at the same time as radiation. If we use CMF we can do both at the same time, but we can't with AC, because Adriamycin damages the skin more and thus compounds the skin damage of the radiation.

Making the Choice

So what should you do? There is no right or wrong answer. Breast cancer is not one disease but a family of diseases. Some women have aggressive disease and others have disease that develops relatively slowly. Today with the increased use of mammography, the majority of patients (approximately 60%) are actually cured by surgery alone and do not need adjuvant treatment. It is important for each woman to get as realistic a picture as possible of the risks and benefits of any therapy so that she can make the decision that feels right for her.

Table 23-1 gives estimates of survival and the benefits of adjuvant therapy (chemotherapy, tamoxifen, or both) on 10-year survival according to age. Low risk in each age group might represent women with tumors of one centimeter or less and negative nodes; the intermediate risk group represents the typical node-negative patient; and the high-risk group typifies women with one or two positive nodes. (And remember, natural mortality in women without breast cancer is ten times higher if you are 65 than if you are 40.) The higher your risk of dying of breast cancer is, the bigger your benefit from adjuvant therapy can be.

The data are pretty clear that there is some benefit to all women from taking tamoxifen for five years if they are estrogen receptor positive. Whether the benefit is enough to convince you it is worth it is a personal decision. There does not appear to be any benefit to taking tamoxifen if you are estrogen receptor negative, and in fact there may be some harm. All premenopausal women with positive lymph nodes will benefit from chemotherapy, and many postmenopausal women will as well.

Table 23-1. Survival Estimates at 10 Years by Age and Risk of Breast Cancer Death, with and without Adjuvant Therapy

| | | Alive at 10 Yrs | | |
Hypothetical Risk of Breast Cancer Death*	Natural Mortality without Breast Cancer, Next 10 yrs (%)	No Adjuvant Therapy	Adjuvant Therapy[+]	Absolute Benefit
40 year old				
10% (low risk)	2	88	90	2
28% (intermediate risk)	2	71	77	6
57% (high risk)	2	41	51	10
65 year old				
9% (low risk)	19	73	75	2
26% (intermediate risk)	19	58	63	5
54% (high risk)	19	34	43	9

*Values shown are derived from three different risk estimates and assume exponential death with a constant hazard ratio. The differences between 40 and 65 years of age reflect deaths from other causes.

[+]Based on a 25% annual reduction in the odds of death, a reasonable estimate of the benefits of chemotherapy in premenopausal patients and tamoxifen in an estrogen receptor-positive postmenopausal patient.

Osbor DK, Ravdin PM. Adjuvant systemic therapy of primary breast cancer. In Harris JR, Lippman ME, Morrow M, Osborne CK, eds., *Diseases of the Breast*, 2nd ed. Philadelphia: J. B. Lippincott, Williams & Wilkins, 2000; 625.

For most women, many issues enter into this kind of decision. One is quality of life. If you're 80, for example, and have positive nodes, which means the cancer may come back in the next 10 years, you may decide it's worth the gamble not to do chemotherapy—or you may decide that any chance of extra time to live is worth it. If you're relatively young and have another life-threatening condition that could be exacerbated by the chemotherapy, such as a heart condition or severe kidney disease, maybe you won't feel the risk is worth it. On the other hand, you may be 50 and just postmenopausal and feel that even the chance of an extra 1 percent is worth it to you. Many women will of course be cured, even with positive nodes, but the benefits of chemotherapy in node-positive women over 10 to 15 years is substantial. Your values and beliefs will play a large part in your decision.

Women with very "good" tumors: nuclear grade 1 tumors; those with a special tumor type, such as tubular, mucinous, or papillary carcinoma; patients with ductal carcinoma in situ with and without invasion; and even patients with tumors between one and two centimeters with other good prognostic factors such as positive ER and low proliferative index have 10 year recurrence rates that range from 2 to 15 percent. Chemotherapy and tamoxifen will not improve their survival by enough to make it worth the risks.

The more difficult cases are those women with negative lymph nodes and tumors over one centimeter. We know that between 20 and 30 percent of women with negative lymph nodes will still get metastatic breast cancer and sooner or later die of it (Fig. 23-3). If we give these women chemotherapy for their primary cancer, some of them will have a delay in recurrence and improvement in survival. But 70–80 percent of women with negative lymph nodes won't ever have a recurrence, and if we give them chemotherapy we subject them to an unpleasant process that can occasionally have severe and permanent side effects—including, very rarely, leukemia.

Unfortunately we are left guessing on the basis of probabilities that are not individualized. This usually means that we overtreat, fearing that we might miss someone who could benefit.

Guidelines

All this means that a woman's decision about whether or not to have systemic treatment, and if so which treatment, is complicated.

In node-negative women with tumors of less than a centimeter, the risk of recurrence or death is so low, and the advantage of adjuvant chemotherapy or tamoxifen is so slight, that it may not be worth it. If the tumor is greater than 2 centimeters it probably is worth having systemic treatment: chemotherapy, tamoxifen, or both. If it's between 1

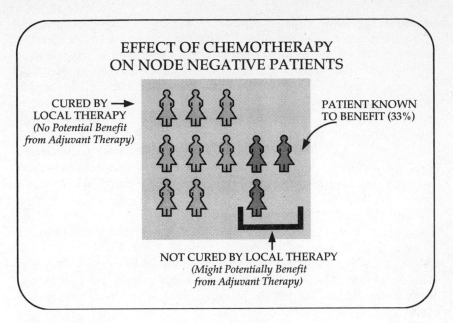

EFFECT OF CHEMOTHERAPY ON NODE NEGATIVE PATIENTS

CURED BY →
LOCAL THERAPY
(No Potential Benefit from Adjuvant Therapy)

PATIENT KNOWN
TO BENEFIT (33%)

NOT CURED BY LOCAL THERAPY
(Might Potentially Benefit from Adjuvant Therapy)

FIGURE 23-3

and 2 centimeters, it's a gray area, and that's where we use all the pathology biomarkers we discuss in Chapter 20. Unfortunately, we don't know how to add all the factors together, and you still end up having to make a guess based on the information we have.

So, at least so far, there's no perfect formula. I had one patient back in Boston who had a small tumor, negative nodes, and negative biomarkers. But she wanted chemo. Her oncologist and I both argued with her. She was adamant, and got chemotherapy. Yet a year later the cancer metastasized and she died. By all statistical predictions she should have survived, even without the chemo, and the chemo should have guaranteed her survival. This isn't meant to depress you: it often works the other way. I had a patient who was diagnosed with 17 positive nodes and had conventional chemotherapy; 13 years later she was alive and well and living in Maui. It just illustrates that we really have no certainty; to some extent, it's a crap shoot. You have to just search your heart and make your own choice.

SYSTEMIC TREATMENTS: HORMONAL THERAPY

Doctors have always been interested in the hormonal manipulation of breast cancers. In fact, the first adjuvant therapies were based on changing the body's hormonal milieu. If a premenopausal woman had a "bad" cancer, her ovaries were removed in an attempt to decrease the total amount of estrogen in her system. The idea was good, and later follow-up studies show a difference in the survival of the women who had had oophorectomy compared to those in the control group, which is as good as that for chemotherapy.[38]

Now we can actually predict who is likely to benefit from adjuvant hormonal therapy by using the estrogen and progesterone receptor test mentioned in Chapter 20. In those women whose tumors are sensitive to hormones, we can use a hormonal treatment as adjuvant therapy. We are now realizing how important these hormonal therapies really are. What they probably do, at least in part, is to change the environment around the cell (see Chapter 13). That environment can be changed in a number of different ways. One way is by stopping the source of the hormones—the ovary.

The problem with the old-fashioned method of ovary removal is that it's irreversible: if it doesn't work, we can't return your ovaries to you. So you're stuck with all the consequences of having no ovaries (see Chapter 31).

Today there are gonadotropin-releasing hormone agonists (GnRH), originally developed for endometriosis, that block the ovaries and essentially put you into a chemical menopause. The one that has been tested most for breast cancer is goserelin (also known as Zoladex). In an Australian study, women were put on Zoladex for three to five years to see if it had the same effect as oophorectomy, and found that it did.[39]

Nobody has yet studied whether the benefit remains the same if a woman takes such a drug for three to five years, stops, and menstruates again. Does the temporary menopause keep the cells dormant after the drug is discontinued, as when tamoxifen is stopped? We'll probably know that within the next few years.

All three of these modes—surgery, radiation, or chemical use—are known as *ablating* the ovaries.

There are other approaches to hormone therapy and other drugs called *aromatase inhibitors*. Aromatase is the enzyme found in the adrenal glands, fat, and muscles that converts testosterone and androstenedione into estrogen. This enzyme is responsible for much of the estrogen in postmenopausal women. In addition, recent studies[40] show that two thirds of postmenopausal women with breast cancer have aromatase in their breast tissue, giving the breast its own supply of estrogen. Blocking this enzyme can be very effective in reducing estrogen in postmenopausal women. Anastrozole (Arimidex), one of the first new aromatase inhibitors to come out, has been shown in a European study to be as good as tamoxifen in treating metastatic breast cancer and the results of a study of anastrozole vs. tamoxifen as adjuvant therapy are eagerly awaited.

Hormones can also be used in a more peripheral way. Rather than eliminate the production of estrogen, they can block it in a particular organ such as the breast. This is how tamoxifen works. It blocks the estrogen receptor in the breast and metastatic cancer cell, preventing estrogen from getting to it. This is why it has an effect in both pre- and postmenopausal women. Regardless of the total amount of estrogen circulating in the blood, tamoxifen can block it at the breast and metastatic breast cancer cell level. Studies are now under way to see whether there can be even more effect by adding one of the agents that block estrogen production (goserelin in premenopausal women or anastrozole in postmenopausal women) to tamoxifen.

Tamoxifen

Tamoxifen is a very peculiar drug. In some places, like the breast, it blocks estrogen, but in other organs it acts like estrogen. (See SERMs, Chapter 18.) Some studies show that tamoxifen causes a change in the cancer cell's normal growth factors. A normal cancer cell produces a factor called *transforming growth factor alpha* (TGF alpha), which induces growth, and an opposing factor called *transforming growth factor beta.* TGF beta is a suppressor—it acts as a brake—while TGF alpha acts as an accelerator. TGF alpha is depressed in estrogen receptor positive patients who get tamoxifen. At the same time, TGF beta is increased.[41] (Interestingly, TGF alpha doesn't get decreased in estrogen-receptor negative patients who get treated.) So tamoxifen tends to decrease the accelerator and increase the brakes—at least in estrogen receptor positive tumors.

We used to believe that tamoxifen didn't kill cells the way chemo did—it just blocked them and held them at bay. Thus we called it a "cytostatic drug" instead of a "cytotoxic drug." We thought that if you took tamoxifen for a period of time and then stopped, all those cancer cells that were in limbo would start growing again. But a 1998 overview found that for between 5 and 10 percent of women who had taken tamoxifen for five years and stopped, the reduction in death rate persisted at 10 years. Even taking it for just a year gave benefits, which lasted for up to 10 years. The longer a woman takes it, up to five years, the more the benefit. It probably changes the environment, killing cells and/or making some of them dormant (see Chapter 13). The dormancy can last until something comes along to wake the cells up. A lot of women feel they can't stop taking tamoxifen; it's their lifeline and stopping it will kill them. But that's simply not true.

In fact, taking it longer may harm them. In the past few years we've discovered that when tamoxifen is used for many years, the user can become resistant to it. The NSABP did a study randomizing women who had taken tamoxifen for five years.[42] At the end of the five years, they re-randomized the women. Half of those who were taking tamoxifen now stopped taking it, and half took it for another five years. They hoped to learn whether taking it for longer periods of time would prove even more helpful than taking it for a few years. But they discovered that 10 years seemed slightly worse. There was a small increase in cancers in the other breast, and a small increase in recurrence in the same breast. In fact, it was thought that tamoxifen can actually start feeding the cancer. It's a bit like what happens with antibiotics: if you take them for a week or two for a specific infection, it helps. If you take it for a few years, you build up a resistance, and it won't help your infections any more. The 1998 NSABP study was in node-negative women. The recommendation now is that women who are prescribed tamoxifen as part of their initial treatment should stop taking it after five years. There's less agreement about node-positive women. There's a big study going on in England called ATLAS,[43] which is looking at long-term use of tamoxifen that should answer that question. My own belief is that at this point no one taking it for adjuvant therapy should stay on it for more than five years. If you're taking it for metastatic disease, it's a different situation (see Chapter 33).

One sometimes hears the simplistic notion that tamoxifen just throws premenopausal women into menopause. Actually it doesn't. It causes a big increase in estrogen and progesterone levels.[44]

The 1998 overview shows the benefit of tamoxifen in premenopausal women. The overview studied 18,000 women with estrogen receptor positive tumors and another 8,000 with estrogen receptor negative tumors.[45] They found that in estrogen receptor negative tumors, tamoxifen really had no benefit. But in estrogen receptor positive tumors, it had a benefit across the board. Though the overall reduction in mortality was about 20 percent, the absolute improvement—the number a patient really wants to know—varied in terms of what each woman's risk was. For node-positive women, after 5 years of tamoxifen, the absolute improvement in 10 years survival was 10.9 percent (50.54 to 61.4). For node-negative women, the 10-year survival went from 73.3 percent to 78.9 percent, an increase of 5.6 percent. In women with tumors sensitive to estrogen this benefit is probably worth the risk. But it's not the 100 percent cure that some women believe it to be. When I lecture, women will often come up to me and say they're taking tamoxifen but having terrible side effects. I suggest they check with their oncologists about why they're taking it. The tendency now is for oncologists to put every estrogen receptor positive woman on it, because it benefits everyone. But it benefits by different amounts, and if you're in a category in which the benefit is only 1 or 2 percent, and it's making your life miserable, you probably won't want to stay with it. On the other hand, if you're in the 11 percent category, the suffering might be worth that chance. So it's important to ask your oncologist what benefit tamoxifen will offer you, given your specific breast cancer scenario.

The benefits seem to have no relation to age, menopausal status, or whether or not the woman has had chemotherapy as well. Before we conclude that everyone should take it we should note the recent study of node-negative women, which showed that tamoxifen can actually reduce survival in women with hormone-insensitive breast cancers.[46] Most oncologists will not recommend tamoxifen for women with estrogen receptor negative tumors.

The side effects of tamoxifen must also be considered. There is a quadrupling of endometrial cancers in women who took it for five years, although the number of cases was quite small. A study late in 1999[47] by Leslie Bernstein indicated that this risk was restricted to women who had taken estrogen (without Provera) replacement therapy in the past. Tamoxifen also increases the incidence of pulmonary emboli and phlebitis. As for other benefits, it did not decrease heart disease or colorectal cancer, as some theories once suggested, but did increase bone density a modest amount in postmenopausal women.

Tamoxifen in Women with Estrogen Receptor Negative Tumors

As we mentioned, there is no evidence that taking tamoxifen will improve your survival or decrease the chance of recurrence if your tumor is not sensitive to estrogen. This does not mean that women with ER negative tumors do much worse, only that tamoxifen does not help them. In fact a large randomized study presented in December of 1999 in San Antonio indicated that women with ER negative tumors who took tamoxifen had a higher chance of recurrence and death than those who did not take tamoxifen. This was true regardless of the fact that the tamoxifen prevented second cancers in the other breast. We don't know why this effect was seen, but it was higher in premenopausal women than postmenopausal women.[48] The NSABP reported a second study in the spring of 2000 which also showed no benefit from tamoxifen in estrogen receptor negative tumors.[49]

This raises the question of whether to take tamoxifen to reduce the risk of other conditions if you are ER negative. Tamoxifen is about as good in reducing osteoporosis risk and lowering serum cholesterol as raloxifene (Evista) is. But like raloxifene, tamoxifen has not been proved to prevent clinical fractures or heart disease. Raloxifene has never been used in women with breast cancer, so it is not a reasonable alternative to tamoxifen. C. Kent Osborne, one of the authors of the study mentioned above, stated: "The cumulative data thus suggest that adjuvant tamoxifen should be used only in patients with ER positive tumors, and, until we have results from other studies, its use as 'hormone replacement therapy' in patients with ER negative tumors should be questioned or abandoned. This argument could also extend to other selective estrogen receptor modulators (SERMs such as raloxifene) that could conceivably have effects similar to tamoxifen."[50]

I agree with Osborne completely. I think the data indicate that women who have ER negative tumors should not take tamoxifen. In light of this information, it is also likely that reloxifene is a bad idea as well.

COMBINATIONS OF CHEMOTHERAPY AND HORMONAL THERAPY

Although we have discussed chemotherapy and hormonal therapy in separate sections, they are often used together. In 1997 the NSABP did a randomized trial that compared chemotherapy plus tamoxifen to tamoxifen alone for node-negative, estrogen-receptor positive tumors. The combination was more effective (96% for CMF plus tamoxifen compared to 94% for tamoxifen alone) for survival at five years. Although they did not look at what chemotherapy alone would have done, it has been routine since then to add tamoxifen to chemotherapy in women who are estrogen receptor positive.[51]

Now researchers are asking if ovarian ablation is as good as chemotherapy and what would happen if we *added* ovarian ablation to chemotherapy: would it make it better? What if the chemo throws the patient into menopause? Is there then any reason to ablate the ovaries, since the chemotherapy has already done it?

Several studies were reported in the 1999 medical meetings looking at these questions. One Danish study compared ovarian ablation to CMF chemotherapy and found that in premenopausal node-positive, estrogen receptor positive women they were equivalent.[52] It's a good alternative for women who don't want chemo—unless, as is often the case, the reason for not wanting chemo is that they want to get pregnant.

We don't know yet, however, whether ovarian ablation is as effective as chemotherapy *plus* tamoxifen. There's an ECOG—Eastern Cooperative Group—study where they compared AC chemotherapy alone vs. AC chemotherapy with goserelin and tamoxifen vs. AC chemotherapy with goserelin in premenopausal, node-positive, estrogen receptor positive and progesterone receptor positive women.[53] These are the kinds of women most likely to respond. Those women under 40 whose estrogen levels after they took the chemotherapy were still at premenopausal level did better with ovarian ablation by goserelin and the tamoxifen did not add much. In the women over 40, the tamoxifen combination worked better when the estrogen levels after chemotherapy were postmenopausal.

So if you're in menopause and estrogen receptor positive, whether you were already there or the chemo threw you into it, tamoxifen with or without goserelin makes more sense to add to the chemo. On the other hand, if you're still menstruating after chemotherapy and you're estrogen receptor positive, progesterone receptor positive, and node positive, adding goserelin (Zoladex) alone may be worthwhile.

Whether we even need chemotherapy in the hormone-sensitive group remains to be determined.

COMPLEMENTARY TREATMENTS

We've talked about two components of treatment, systemic and local. There's a third component, which I'll touch on briefly here.

Breast cancer is caused by cancer cells existing in a particular environment (see Chapter 13). The techniques we've just discussed are methods to decrease the total number of cancer cells. But other approaches take it from the opposite end—they try to change the environment to make it less responsive to the cancer cells' efforts to get out into the body. Unfortunately, in science we haven't yet figured out a good method to do that. But the hope that we can boost the immune system is the basis of many of the so-called complementary treatments we discuss in Chapter 29. These range from visualization to diet to prayer, and it's worth your while to think about looking into these to complement whatever medical treatment you embark on. While we're not certain if they can actually affect the cancer, they will often make you feel better and empower you psychologically by giving you something that you can do as part of your own treatment.

THE FUTURE

As you can tell, things are changing all of the time in this field. Yesterday's answer may be passé today. I suggest you supplement this information with other sources and especially the Internet. On my website, www.SusanLoveMD.com, or on the NIH website, www.clinicaltrials.gov, you can find the latest studies and up-to-date information to supplement the overview we have given here.

In addition, before you decide on which treatment, or treatments, you want, I think it's always wise to consider getting a second opinion, no matter how much you trust your surgeon or oncologist's advice. The preference for a treatment is always somewhat subjective, and you're entitled to consult with more than one expert. Furthermore, special kinds of cancer might require a different approach than your doctor's, and different institutions may be involved in different research with new treatments that you might be interested in.

As we discussed in Chapter 13, the future of breast cancer treatment is not one-size-fits-all, but targeted treatments specific for the molecular biology of the tumor. Herceptin is only the first of many in this regard.

We will also alter the way we give current therapies such as chemotherapy. Having tried high doses, some researchers are now looking at very *low* doses of chemotherapy, which have been shown in mice to block angiogenesis in a way our current approach does not. There is no question in my mind that in the next edition of this book our approach will be very different than it is now. It behooves anyone newly diagnosed with breast cancer to look into the possibility of participating in a clinical trial because that is where the future is being tested right now.

24

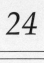

Special Cases

So far, I've been discussing the "typical" breast cancer—the small lump that forms inside a woman's breast, usually discovered by the woman herself or by her doctor, or detected in a screening mammogram. Sometimes, however, we find a cancer that manifests differently, or is unusual in its behavior.

LOCALLY ADVANCED BREAST CANCER

Once in a while, a breast cancer won't be discovered until it's fairly big—a stage 3 cancer. It will be a large tumor—larger than five centimeters (two inches), with positive lymph nodes. Or it will have one of the other features that we think give it a bad prognosis, like swelling (edema) of the skin, or a big, matted cluster of lymph nodes. It might be stuck to the chest muscle, or ulcerating through the skin (see Fig. 21-3).

These are all indications that the cancer is likely to have spread to elsewhere in your body, at least microscopically, and so when we find them we often don't do surgery as a first step. We don't need to sample your lymph nodes: we've already got the information we need. There is frequently a question of whether a wide excision is even possible. If you've got very large breasts, it might be, but if your breasts are small, we may not be able to get enough surrounding tissue out without a mastectomy. If the tumor is stuck to the muscle or ulcerating through the skin, an immediate local treatment might not be feasible at all: removing the muscle or all the skin that's ulcerated might not leave sufficient tissue to sew back together again.

All this generally suggests that we should start with a systemic rather than a local treatment, usually chemotherapy (see Chapter 28), and this is now fairly generally agreed on in the medical community. Normally the drugs used are AC (Adriamycin and Cytoxan) and/or Taxol or Taxotere. This may not eradicate the whole tumor, but if it doesn't, it can still do two important things: it can work on the cells that have spread, and it can shrink the tumor to a size that can be more easily managed with surgery or radiation.

Usually we'll continue with the chemotherapy for three to four cycles, and then reevaluate the situation. If the tumor has shrunk, we'll do a lumpectomy; if there is no change, we do a mastectomy. Even when the tumor seems to have disappeared—we can't feel it or see it on a mammogram—there may still be some cancer cells present. So we always want to at least do a lumpectomy on the spot where the tumor had been to see what's actually left. (With more imagination than is usual in surgical terminology, this procedure is called a "ghostectomy.") If the ghostectomy is clear or shows clean margins, you're a candidate for radiation. Similarly, if we can do a lumpectomy and get clean margins because the lump is small, that plus radiation is a sensible treatment. If there is still a large lump or a lot of cancer at the margins, it may be best to do a mastectomy with or without immediate reconstruction. In the case of an ulceration that doesn't leave enough skin to sew together, breast reconstruction has not only a cosmetic but also a medical advantage: reconstruction provides skin from another part of the body (see Chapter 26).

Most commonly after surgery a woman will have an additional three-to-four cycles of chemotherapy, often with paclitaxel (Taxol). Finally at the end she will get radiation therapy.

After lumpectomy or mastectomy some women with stage 3 breast cancer have received high-dose chemotherapy and stem cell rescue (bone marrow transplant, see Chapter 23). Knowing that many of these locally advanced cancers are very aggressive, many doctors felt that higher doses of chemotherapy might be better. But as we discussed in Chapter 23, in the spring of 1999 several studies reported on randomized controlled studies of high-dose chemotherapy with stem cell rescue in women at high risk of recurrence, and found that high-dose chemotherapy with stem cell transplant did not add substantially to the benefit from standard chemotherapy since the survival rates were the same. Some women have interpreted this as showing that the transplants they received were a waste. But this isn't true. The studies showed that both standard chemotherapy and high-dose chemotherapy with stem cell rescue had the same beneficial effect. However, since the stem cell rescue is accompanied by more side effects, it makes sense to stick with the standard approach. What is especially interesting about these studies is the fact that the women who received standard therapy had a much better outcome than similar women had experienced in the past. We are making progress.

Different hospitals have different preferences in treatment order and combination. Most centers do chemotherapy first and many of them will then do a mastectomy no matter what.[1] Some of them will consider breast conservation surgery if the lump becomes small enough. Then they usually follow with radiation. As we're using these combinations of treatments in this kind of breast cancer, we're actually seeing better response rates.

In many areas of the country there are protocols studying advanced cancers, trying to determine whether different combinations of drugs, or different combinations of chemotherapy, radiation, and surgery, affect survival rates. I think it's well worth considering participating in one if it's available to you (see Chapter 33).

Cancers of this sort usually fall into one of two categories, though both are generally treated the same way. Sometimes it's a very aggressive cancer that seems to have come up overnight as a large and evidently fast growing tumor (although it's been there undetectable for a while). At other times, the tumor has been present for several years and the woman has tried to pretend it wasn't there, until it's gotten huge or begun ulcerating through the skin, and she finally gets to a doctor. This latter case we call a "neglected primary"—it's not an especially aggressive cancer, just an especially frightened woman. Patients with a neglected primary cancer often do better than you might expect: if you've had an untreated cancer for five years and it hasn't killed you or obviously spread anywhere, it's clearly a slow-growing cancer.

Few studies, however, have differentiated between aggressive cancers and neglected primaries. Studies of these types of cancer taken together show a five-year survival of around 45 percent.[2] The NSABP is doing a study (number B-18) that will give us more information, but it appears now that the tumor's response to preoperative chemotherapy is the best way to predict chances for a disease-free future and overall survival rate. As you might imagine, when the tumor completely disappears in the breast and lymph nodes, the woman has a much higher response rate and does much better. If only microscopic disease is left, the patient probably still has a good chance for survival.

If you've been putting off seeing your doctor about a lump that's been growing, or if you're suddenly faced with a new large or ulcerating tumor, don't ignore it and assume you're dying—get it diagnosed and start your treatment right away. Your prognosis may not be as good as it would be with a smaller tumor, but it's not hopeless, and the sooner you begin to take care of it, the better your chances are.

INFLAMMATORY BREAST CANCER

"Inflammatory breast cancer" is a special kind of advanced breast cancer, and it's a serious one. Though we see increasing numbers of cases, it is rare, accounting for only 1 to 4 percent of all breast cancers. Overall survival is worse in women with this kind of breast cancer than in others. It's called "inflammatory" because its first symptoms are usually a redness and warmth in the skin of the breast, often without a distinct lump. Frequently the patient and even the doctor will mistake it for a simple infection and she'll be put on antibiotics. But it doesn't get better. It also doesn't get worse, and that's the tip-off: an infection will always get better or worse within a week or two—it rarely stays the same. If there's no change, the doctor should perform a biopsy of the underlying tissue to see if it's cancer. Two of my patients who have had this cancer had similar stories. One had been breast-feeding and developed what her doctor thought was lactational mastitis (see Chapter 7). It never cleared up and didn't hurt much—there was no fever or other sign of infection. It hadn't gone away or gotten worse in six months. The other patient, not breast-feeding, noticed that one breast had suddenly become larger than the other; there was also redness and swelling. In both cases, the doctors at first thought the women had infections. So if the symptoms continue after treatment, you should ask to have a biopsy done of the breast tissue and of the skin itself. With inflammatory breast cancer, you have cancer cells in the lymph vessels of your skin, which is what makes the skin red; the cancer is blocking the drainage of fluid from the skin. There was an intriguing survey on the Internet, done by G. Owen Johnson, a man whose wife had died from inflammatory breast cancer. He asked women with the disease a number of questions about it. Most of the women said they wished they had known that when redness of the breast skin doesn't respond to antibiotics it might be inflammatory cancer. Probably their doctors were not breast specialists, and didn't know about this unusual breast cancer.

Inflammatory breast cancer is the only kind of breast cancer that virtually everyone agrees doesn't call for mastectomy as its sole primary treatment. Because it involves the lymphatic vessels of the skin as well as the breast tissue, and the skin is sewn back together after a mastectomy, doing a mastectomy will leave a great chance of a recurrence in the skin. So we go directly to chemotherapy before we even think about local treatment.

A study published in 1998 shows that the incidence of inflammatory breast cancer doubled from 1970 and 1992.[3] In white women, it went from 0.3 to 0.7 in a thousand, and in African American women it went from 0.6 to 1.1. (Other races weren't included in the study.) This is reason for concern, but it's still a small number. Women with inflammatory breast cancer tend to be significantly younger than those with other breast cancers, and African Americans with this cancer tend to be younger than whites.

The three-year survival rate from inflammatory breast cancer has improved in recent years. The study published in 1998 shows an increase in survival of 10 percent (42% survival, vs. 32% earlier), while other forms of breast cancer survival only increased 5 percent (from 80 to 85%). Since the study was done in 1998, the rates may well be even higher by now, as we increasingly use more of a multimodality approach—chemotherapy, surgery, and radiation.

As with advanced cancers, we start with three or four cycles of AC with or without Taxol or Taxotere. Then we'll do a local treatment—usually mastectomy. Despite the studies mentioned previously (see Chapter 23) there are still specialists who feel that high-dose chemotherapy with stem cell rescue might have an advantage in this situation. None of the randomized studies reported out thus far focused on inflammatory breast cancer, and women with inflammatory breast cancer were not included in the 10 or more positive randomized studies discussed above. Any woman considering a stem cell transplant should be in a clinical trial.

After the mastectomy, most women will receive four more cycles of chemotherapy followed by radiation therapy to the chest wall. Serious though it can be, inflammatory breast cancer is still an extremely variable disease.

THE UNKNOWN PRIMARY

"The unknown primary" sounds a bit like the title of a murder mystery; actually, it's the name we give another kind of mystery—a breast cancer that we can't find in the breast. This is a rare form of breast cancer, accounting for less than 5 percent of cases. Someone shows up with an enlarged lymph node, usually in the armpit. It's biopsied and we find breast cancer cells, but there are no breast lumps. So we send the woman off for a mammogram, but that's not a great tool in this case: often it won't show any questionable areas. We know the cancer's there and has spread to the nodes, but how do you treat a cancer you can't find?

In the old days, doctors simply did a mastectomy on everyone in this situation and discovered cancer in the breast in between 60 and 70 percent of the cases, depending on how thoroughly the pathologist examined the breast tissue.[4] Now mammography is likely to show a density in the breasts of such patients, and there are fewer women with truly unknown (or undetected) primaries. A 1997 study from Vanderbilt suggests that the use of MRI and perhaps PET scan (see Chapter 10) can increase the ability of doctors to find the primary cancer. MRI is more sensitive than mammography, and the PET scan can show the metabolism of the cancer. (MRI is available in more places than PET scan.) If the doctors can find the primary cancer, then the patient has the option of getting lumpectomy and radiation rather than a mastectomy.

In those situations where no breast lesion can be found, the treatment is more controversial. There's no doubt that a mastectomy would get rid of the cancer, but we have to ask if it's necessary, given that the primary cancer is so tiny we can't even detect it. It can be devastating to a woman to have a mastectomy and then learn that the primary cancer didn't show up in the tissue after all, and she's had her breast removed for nothing. Many doctors think radiation should be sufficient. Others strongly disagree, insisting that, since there's no way to pinpoint the exact location of the cancer for the radiation therapist, a mastectomy is called for. And many radiation therapists don't like doing radiation in these cases, because they can't give the usual boost of radiation (see Chapter 27) to the actual site of the tumor.

If a mastectomy is overkill and radiation is chancy, what can you do? Some doctors think you should have chemotherapy, then wait and see if something shows up in the breast, rather than do any local therapy right away. In fact, since positive lymph nodes indicate a high chance of cancer cells elsewhere in the body, most doctors now will start with chemotherapy, whatever local treatment they do later.

But it can be a little scary to leave it at that, hoping the chemotherapy has wiped out the original cancer. So some doctors recommend an upper-outer quadrantectomy.[5] Since many cancers are located in that area of the breast, there's a good possibility that the mysterious tumor is there. Others favor doing multiple fine-needle aspirates to try and find the tumor—truly a needle-in-the-haystack approach, but sometimes an effective one.

Every case of unknown primary is different. I've had two interesting cases. One was a woman with a strong family history of breast cancer. She was very thin and small breasted, and her breasts weren't lumpy; it would seem that any lump, however small, would be easy to find. She had an enlarged node in her armpit, and the node was found to be cancerous. I did nine fine-needle aspirates in different areas of her breast and found cancer in four of them. I did fine-needle aspirates in the other breast as well, and one of these revealed cancer, so we decided to remove both breasts. It turned out that in the breast on the side with the enlarged node she had a fairly widespread cancer that hadn't formed lumps but had snaked through the breast tissue.

In the other case, I did fine-needle aspirates again. This time they were negative, but the patient had had a positive lymph node, so we had to do something. My patient emphatically didn't want a mastectomy. She was somewhat psychic, and was convinced that the cancer was in the upper-outer quadrant. Since that's the site of many cancers anyway, a quadrantectomy seemed a good idea to both of us. After removing the tissue, I turned it upside down, and there, on the under surface, was the lump. Both she and I were greatly relieved. Because we'd found the location of the cancer she was able to have radiation, and to keep her breast. In other women I've treated, we've never found the primary at all. Recently a woman called me to ask for advice. She was 68, and had been diagnosed with an unknown primary. Her surgeon was insisting that she have a mastectomy, but she really didn't want it. I suggested an MRI, and spoke to her surgeon about it. He was reluctant because she had had implants and he felt that imaging techniques wouldn't work. I told him that MRI actually worked very well with implants. Since this is a fairly recent discovery he hadn't known that, and was glad to hear it. She had an MRI, and it did in fact reveal the cancer. It was a four-centimeter tumor that had draped itself around the implant. Because of this position, it was necessary to do the mastectomy after all. But at least the woman knew that the operation was indeed necessary, and not a possibly fruitless hunting expedition.

It's interesting to note that, contrary to what you might expect, the survival rate in cancers that show up in the nodes but not in the breast is actually a bit better than it is for cancers that show up as both a breast lump and an enlarged node.[6]

It's unlikely that you'll have this kind of cancer, but if you do, it's important to think about what treatment you'll be most comfortable with. If your surgeon comes down with a hard line and tells you there's one sure way to deal with it, be suspicious and insist on a second opinion.

PAGET'S DISEASE OF THE BREAST

Dr. Paget was an active gentleman, and he's gotten his name on any number of diseases: there's a Paget's disease of the bone and a Paget's disease of the eyelids, as well as a Paget's disease of the breast. The diseases have no relation to one another, except for their discoverer.

Paget's disease of the breast is a form of breast cancer that shows up in the nipple, as an itchiness and scaling that doesn't get better. It's often mistaken for excema of the nipple—a far more common occurrence. Paget's disease is almost never found in both breasts (bilateral), so if you've got itching and scaling on both nipples, you've probably got a fairly harmless skin condition. However, if it doesn't get better, you should get it checked out, whether it's on one or both nipples.

First you'll need to get a mammogram to make sure there's no cancer in the breast itself. Then you should get the skin on the nipple biopsied. This can be done in the doctor's office with local anesthetic; it's called a "punch biopsy," and involves removing only about a millimeter or two of skin. If it's Paget's, the pathologist will see little cancer cells growing up into the skin of the nipple—that's what makes the skin flake and get itchy. Sometimes it's associated with a cancer inside the breasts; sometimes not. It's often associated with ductal carcinoma in situ (see Chapter 16).

There are probably two variants of Paget's disease: one associated with an invasive cancer in the breast and one that involves only the nipple. The former would be treated as any invasive cancer would. If the invasive cancer lump is far from the nipple, a mastectomy may be necessary to get both areas out; otherwise wide excision and radiation is a reasonable alternative.

Paget's disease that involves only the nipple has a better prognosis than regular breast cancer.[7] It doesn't tend to be too aggressive, and usually the lymph nodes turn out to be negative. Until recently most doctors assumed that you needed a mastectomy—they seemed to think that if you couldn't keep your nipple, your breast didn't matter.[8] Most women, of course, know better.

This has been a campaign of mine, and a few years ago some of us managed to convince the rest of the medical establishment that all that was needed was to remove the nipple and areola, and that many women prefer to keep the rest of the breast if they can.[9,10] True, your breast looks a bit funny after the nipple's been removed—but it is still there. An artificial nipple can be made by a plastic surgeon (see Chapter 26). Many women, however, don't mind the way the breast looks, as long as they look natural in a bra. Some of my patients with this kind of Paget's disease chose plastic surgery, and some didn't bother with it.

CYSTOSARCOMA PHYLLOIDES

The most dramatic thing about this kind of cancer is its name. It's usually fairly mild and takes the form of a malignant fibroadenoma (see Chapter 8). It shows up as a large lump in the breast—it's usually lemon-sized by the time it's detected. It feels like a regular fibro-adenoma—smooth and round—but under the microscope some of the fibrous cells that make up the fibroadenoma are bizarre-looking, cancerous cells. It's usually not a very aggressive cancer. It rarely metastasizes; if it recurs at all, it tends to recur only in the breast. In the past it was usually treated with wide excision, removing the lump and a rim of normal tissue around it.[11] More recently, however, we've learned that all it needs is simply to be scooped out. This is made possible by the fact that the tumor has its own casing around it, allowing it to be neatly removed, like a pecan from its shell. This is far less mutilating to the breast than wide excision, and studies have shown it to work remarkably well. One study showed a 6.4 percent recurrence rate.[12] In another series of 24 patients there was only a 4 percent recurrence.[13] Cystosarcoma phylloides doesn't require radiation, and we usually won't check the lymph nodes since it so rarely metastasizes. We'll watch you closely to see if it recurs, and if it does, another wide excision will usually take care of it. I had one patient who came to see me because her cystosarcoma phylloides had recurred three times, and her surgeon told her she'd have to have a mastectomy because it kept coming back. I told her I thought we should wait and see if it did come back, and in the six years I followed her, it hadn't.

The medical literature will sometimes talk about a "benign" versus "malignant" cystosarcoma phylloides, based on a subjective interpretation of how cancerous they think the cells are. The implication is that malignant cystosarcomas will behave more aggressively. Although there are rare cystosarcomas that do metastasize (5%) and ultimately kill the patient, it is hard to predict this accurately in advance. Most surgeons will suggest a more aggressive approach (mastectomy) if the pathologist feels that it's "malignant." These cancers are sufficiently rare that you may well want a second breast pathologist's opinion before embarking on any more aggressive therapeutic approach.

CANCER OF BOTH BREASTS

Once in a great while a woman will be diagnosed as having a cancer in each breast at the same time. Typically this will be discovered when, finding a lump in one breast, she gets a mammogram to find out what's going on there, and learns there's also a lump in the other breast. A biopsy shows them both to be cancer.

They're probably both primary cancers; one isn't a metastasis of the other. So they're both treated the same way: we do a lumpectomy, or mastectomy, and lymph node dissection on one and then the other side. Usually the surgeon will first dissect the lymph nodes on the side that appears worst, so that, if the nodes are positive and will require chemotherapy, the other nodes won't necessarily have to be dissected if the second cancer has a low likelihood of spreading to the nodes. Unfortunately, the surgeon's guess isn't always right. I recently had a patient who had three cancers: she had a lump in the top of her right breast, and the mammogram showed two densities in the bottom of the left breast. They'd all been biopsied with needles. She really wanted to keep her breasts, so I did a wide excision of the right breast and sampled the lymph nodes, and they were fine. Then I did a wide excision of the two cancers in the left breast, and on the left side she had positive lymph nodes. You can have radiation treatment on both breasts at the same time, but the radiation therapist has to be very careful that the treatment doesn't overlap and cause a burn in the middle area.

It isn't necessary to do the same treatment on both breasts. You might decide on a mastectomy on one side and wide excision plus radiation on the other, for example. It is important to note that your prognosis is only as bad as the worst of the two tumors—not doubly as bad as either one.

CANCER IN THE OTHER BREAST

Sometimes a woman who has had cancer in one breast will turn up with cancer in her other breast. Usually this isn't a recurrence or a metastasis; it's a brand new cancer. It's possible for breast cancer to metastasize from one breast to the other, but it's rare. A new primary cancer has a different significance than a metastasis. What it suggests is that your breast tissue, for whatever reason, is prone to develop cancer, so you developed one on one side and then several years later the other side followed along. As with any new cancer, it's biopsied and removed, your lymph nodes are dissected, and you're treated. Your prognosis isn't made any worse because you developed the second breast cancer; it's as bad as the worst of your two cancers. You can still have breast conservation; you don't have to have a mastectomy if you don't want it. People who have second cancers are more likely to have a hereditary predisposition to breast cancer (see Chapter 14). Some women are so scared of getting cancer in the other breast that they consider having a prophylactic mastectomy to prevent it (see Chapter 18).

BREAST CANCER IN VERY YOUNG WOMEN

Sometimes a cancer is unusual, not in itself, but in the situation in which it occurs. As we noted earlier, breast cancer is most common in women over 50, and there are many cases in women in their 40s. It's far more rare in women under 40, but it does occur. We tend to be particularly shocked when it occurs in a young woman. Usually in this situation it's detected as a lump, since we generally don't do screening mammography in young women for all the reasons we discussed in Chapter 19.

Very often a young woman gets misdiagnosed. She detects a lump, or a thickening, and she's told it's just lumpy breasts, or "fibrocystic disease," and it's followed for a while until doctors realize it's something serious. Although this can be horrifying, in fact it's quite understandable, since the vast majority of lumps in women under 35 are totally benign, and the risk of cancer is very low. The fact that cancer is not diagnosed immediately doesn't mean that the young patient will die; as we've said, most breast cancers have been around 8 to 10 years, and whether it's diagnosed the minute you find it or six months later isn't the critical factor. I think we're so horrified when a young woman gets breast cancer that there's a disproportionate number of law suits against doctors for failing to find breast cancer in this population, because they're often misdiagnosed and because it's such a gut-wrenching situation. But in most cases the doctors are not negligent. Still, we do need to teach doctors that young women can develop breast cancer and that doctors should remain vigilant.

The youngest patient I diagnosed was 23. She was on her honeymoon and discovered a lump. We diagnosed her as having cancer; she had a positive node, and she underwent radiation and chemotherapy. Ten years later she developed a local recurrence that required a mastectomy.

Many doctors believe that breast cancer in a young woman is more aggressive than in older ones. Two studies have recently shed some light on this theory. Both studies showed that the mortality from breast cancer was higher in women who had been pregnant in the past four years.[14,15] The risk was highest right after a pregnancy, and decreased with each year, going back to normal after four years. Since young women are more likely to have been recently pregnant (25% of all breast cancers in women younger than 35 are associated with pregnancy),[16] they will show more of this effect. This suggests that it may not be the woman's age itself that affects aggressiveness but the changes in her immune system (necessary so that her body won't reject the fetus) and hormones that go with pregnancy.

Breast cancer in younger women is more likely to be hereditary.[17] That makes sense—if you've inherited a mutation, and you only need one or two more mutations to get cancer, you're one step closer, and you're likely to get there faster, whereas if you "acquire" breast cancer, you still need to get all of the mutations. That doesn't work all the time. Like older women, the majority of younger women with breast cancer have no family history. But if you have breast cancer in your family you're more likely to get it at a younger age than if you don't.

Overall, there is no evidence that breast cancer in a woman under 35 matched for prognostic features (see Chapter 20) is any more aggressive than a cancer in an older woman. Younger women do, however, have a higher incidence of poor prognostic features such as negative estrogen receptors, poor differentiation, and high proliferative (growth) rates. Still, a young woman and an older woman with the same tumors will have the same general prognosis.[18]

With younger women, there's some question about whether it's safe to do lumpectomy and radiation. The concern is twofold. One is that we don't know what the long-term—40- to 60-year—risks of radiation are. The other is that there appears to be a higher local recurrence rate reported in young women who get lumpectomy and radiation than in women in their 40s and 50s.[19] However, recent studies show that there's also a higher local recurrence after mastectomy in that group.[20] The treatment for breast cancer in young women is pretty much the same as for older women, with the option of either breast conservation surgery with radiation or mastectomy with or without reconstruction.

Interestingly, chemotherapy works better in younger than in older women. We've decreased the death rate for breast cancer through our treatment in this subgroup more than in any other. There are problems with chemotherapy, however. Often it will put a young woman into menopause. The really young woman—in her 20s or early 30s—is less likely to have that happen than the woman in her late 30s or early 40s. The closer you are to your natural menopause the more likely it is that it will push you over (see Chapter 31). So the much younger woman will probably get her period back after the treatment course is finished. If that happens, she'll still be fertile.

Because of the likelihood of chemotherapy-induced menopause, some women have considered preserving their eggs before the treatment so they can still have children later. There are problems with that, however. With the current state of technology, you can't preserve an egg alone, but can only save an embryo. Unfertilized eggs won't keep frozen, but the fertilized egg will. So you must choose your sperm donor or partner.

The second problem is that in order to make the eggs grow and harvest them, you have to be given a lot of hormones. And doctors are often reluctant to give those high doses of hormones to someone with breast cancer. I generally don't encourage doing that, unless my patient is so anxious to have her own baby that she's willing to risk anything. Several of my patients have looked into it, but it's so daunting that none of them have gone through with it. Most women feel that their survival is of utmost importance and that they can explore other modes of parenting once their treatment is done.

When a young woman has breast cancer, there's an increased risk for her mother, as well as her sisters and daughters, and they should all be monitored closely.

Finding the right support group can be difficult for the younger woman. Such groups are usually made up of women in their 50s and older, and she can feel very out of place. (Check out the www.SusanLoveMD.com website for support groups for younger women.) Most hospitals are making an effort to have support groups for young women, because the issues are often quite different. There are several books now on dating after a mastectomy, which is a concern to single women of all ages, as are all the psychosocial issues we discuss in Chapters 22 and 30.

The incidence of breast cancer in the other breast is about 5 to 8 percent per year, which usually maximizes out to about 10 to 15 percent. However, women with BRCA1 or BRCA2 mutations can have a much higher chance of developing a second breast cancer in the same or other breast. Since younger women have many more years to get cancer in the opposite breast, their risk is slightly higher than that of older women. Because of this, some doctors may advise young women to have prophylactic mastectomy of the other breast.

BREAST CANCER IN ELDERLY WOMEN

Just as very young women can get breast cancer, so can very old women—women over 85—and they have some of the same issues very young women do. Neither end of the extreme always fits our general modes. There are studies[21] showing that older women aren't treated as aggressively—there's a tendency not to give them all the options for treatment—to sort of say, "Well, they're old; they don't really want chemotherapy." I think a special effort has to be made to make sure that that's what the patient wants, and not have the physicians make their own assumptions.

In addition, there's a tendency to do mastectomies on older women, without offering them breast conservation treatments, assuming that at that age a woman doesn't care as much about her looks. Some doctors will tell an older woman that six weeks of radiation therapy will be too much for her, making mastectomy sound less arduous than lumpectomy plus radiation. But radiation isn't really all that hard to go through, and as we said in Chapter 23, for some older women, just as for their younger friends, it's far better than the emotional trauma of mastectomy.

Not only do many doctors neglect to mention lumpectomy/radiation, they also neglect to offer reconstruction to the older woman upon whom they've urged mastectomy, again assuming that she won't care enough about her looks to want it. And again, that assumption may be totally off base. I can remember one patient in her mid-80s with very large, droopy breasts, who had always wanted to have reduction but thought it was too dangerous. She got a cancer at the upper end of one of her breasts. She wanted breast conservation; she didn't want a mastectomy. But it seemed foolhardy to us to radiate all this breast that didn't show cancer. So after discussing it with her, we did a lumpectomy, and bilateral reductions, and then did radiation. She was delighted; when the radiation was done she went off on a cruise and found a new boyfriend.

So you can't make any assumptions.

There's a move, particularly in the United Kingdom, to treat older women with breast cancer—women 70 or over—with tamoxifen alone, rather than with surgery. There are two studies in which women were divided into groups, getting either surgery and tamoxifen or tamoxifen alone. They found that about a third of the women responded to tamoxifen alone: their tumors shrank and sometimes even disappeared. In one study of 113 women,[22] the cancer disappeared in 38, got smaller in 17, didn't change in 34, and got worse in 24. Thus, almost a third of women might have been spared a mastectomy. The long-term data regarding local recurrence and metastasis are not yet available.

The other study[23] found that in 34 months there was no difference in survival rate or quality of life between women who had surgery plus tamoxifen and women who had tamoxifen alone. More of the women who had had tamoxifen alone had to have surgery later, in contrast to those who had had surgery in the first place. The doctors who did the study argue that when an older woman has breast cancer she should be put on tamoxifen alone, and then if that doesn't work at the end of three to six months she can be operated on. That saves a third of the women from the dangers and discomforts of surgery. It also suggests that if you're older and are fragile, and you don't want to go through surgery, it's reasonable to start you off on tamoxifen alone and hope you can continue to avoid surgery. But long-term data aren't in yet.

Part of the problem in studying women over 70 is that we really can't evaluate long-term survival, since there are so many other illnesses that elderly people die from. And not all elderly women are frail. I had a 95-year-old patient in Boston who wasn't especially frail at all—in fact, she was very active. She developed breast cancer. I did a lumpectomy and put her on tamoxifen. Unfortunately, she couldn't tolerate the tamoxifen, and she stopped it. She was fine for about a year and a half; then her cancer recurred locally. I did another lumpectomy, and this time I really tried to get her to stick with the tamoxifen, and she did for a while. The last I heard she was still going strong. So when we look at how to treat "old" women, we need to look at how frail they really are: it will vary greatly. People who live into their 90s tend to be pretty healthy, or they wouldn't live to that age. We can't just assume, as many doctors do, they'll be dead in a year or so, and forget it—sometimes they live to over 100.

CANCER IN PREGNANCY

Once in a very great while a patient develops breast cancer while she's either pregnant or breast-feeding. We used to think that such a cancer was especially aggressive, and that the pregnancy-related hormones fired up the cancer and made it worse.

The studies are contradictory. Most studies have shown that, stage by stage, it's no worse than any other breast cancer. The problem is that it usually isn't discovered right away. When you're pregnant, your breasts are going through a lot of normal changes, which can mask a more dangerous change. For one thing, they're much lumpier and thicker than usual. Similarly, when you're breast-feeding, as we discussed at length in Chapter 3, you tend to have all kinds of benign lumps and blocked ducts, and you may not notice a change that ordinarily would alarm you. Infections are common when you're breast-feeding and can mask inflammatory breast cancer, so the physician may also find diagnosis of inflammatory breast cancer difficult.

Two studies done in the early 1990s which we discussed earlier in this chapter suggest that there may be something to the old theories. They found that women who were diagnosed with breast cancer while pregnant or within four years thereafter did indeed have a higher mortality rate.[24,25] As more women are having later pregnancies at the age where breast cancer becomes more common, this may become a bigger issue.

Treatment is also a problem. What we can do about your cancer depends on what stage of pregnancy you're in. If you're in the first trimester, you might want to consider therapeutic abortion, depending on your beliefs about abortion and how much this particular pregnancy means to you. It is important to add, however, that there is no evidence that women who abort their fetuses have a better prognosis. It's just easier to proceed with treatment. If you continue with the pregnancy, treatment options are somewhat limited. We wouldn't give you radiation in the first trimester because it can injure the fetus, and we're quite leery about chemotherapy, since the fetus's organs are being formed at this time and the data suggest a high rate of fetal malformation with chemotherapy in the first trimester. For the same reason, we don't want to give you general anesthetic, which rules out a mastectomy. We can do a biopsy or a wide excision under local anesthetic. But if further treatment is called for, like a mastectomy or chemotherapy, we usually try to wait until the second trimester.

In the second trimester, since the fetus's organs are already formed and it's safer to use general anesthetic, we can do a mastectomy. We would rather not risk radiation. In recent years, studies have shown that chemotherapy can be used safely in the second and third trimesters. So far, in these studies the babies' health has appeared to be fine. The problem is that we won't know for many years if there are complications later in the child's life. If you're in your third trimester, we could do a lumpectomy, or, if need be, a mastectomy, and possibly chemotherapy, then wait for further treatment like radiation and/or tamoxifen until the child is born. We can begin chemotherapy if it's important to get going right away. If you are close to your due date, your obstetrician can keep testing and, as soon as the baby can be expected to survive outside the womb, can induce labor, do a cesarean section, and then start you on chemotherapy and radiation after delivery.

My neighbor in Los Angeles was diagnosed with breast cancer when she was pregnant with her seventh child. Most of the physicians told her to abort and she had trouble convincing them that she wanted her seventh child just as much as the first. She underwent a mastectomy in the second trimester and did well. Because she had many positive nodes she received chemotherapy during her third trimester. Her delivery went well, and she said for years afterward that this seventh child was the smartest of all, which she attributed to chemotherapy.

In the mid-1990s I saw a woman who had been diagnosed 20 years earlier, when she was seven months pregnant. She had undergone a radical mastectomy and then had radiation with Cobalt while she was pregnant. She said she had to have a dose monitor in her vagina to keep track of the amount of radiation her fetus was receiving. Nonetheless she carried the baby to term and both were fine 20 years later.

Breast cancer during lactation isn't quite as complicated, since you can always stop breast-feeding and start your child on formula. Radiation will probably make breast-feeding impossible, and you won't want to breast-feed if you're on chemotherapy, since the baby will swallow the chemicals.

We're not sure yet if lactation affects the cancer itself. I've had two patients whose breast cancer showed up while they were lactating. Both were treated, both stopped breast-feeding, and both did well without a recurrence for several years. After much debate both women decided to get pregnant again. One had a recurrence during the second pregnancy; the other had a second primary develop while lactating.

This leads me to the question of whether, if a cancer shows up while a woman is pregnant or lactating, there is a higher risk of a recurrence in another pregnancy. Obviously we can't do a randomized study, and it's too unusual an occurrence to draw any conclusions. Our evidence is purely anecdotal. For now, all I can suggest to someone who has developed breast cancer while pregnant or lactating is to consider seriously not having another pregnancy, in case it affects the chance of a recurrence. (See Chapter 30 on the question of pregnancy after having breast cancer, and Chapter 3 in regard to breast-feeding after having breast cancer.)

An article by breast surgeon, Jeanne Petrek in 1997[26] discussed the question of pregnancy after breast cancer. She looked into a number of published series (articles by doctors reviewing their own cases over a period of time) and found that breast cancer survival didn't change with a subsequent pregnancy. But because there were a number of possible biases (see Chapter 12), the results are really inconclusive. It's possible that the doctors selected their patients in such a way that they told only the women who were likely to be cured that pregnancy would be safe, and discouraged the others. Or it may be that getting cancer while you're pregnant has a different effect on your body than getting it afterwards. Petrek's point, and I think it's a wise one, is that we don't really know the answer yet. She's begun a large, multi-centered trial at Sloan Kettering. This will look at a number of issues concerning breast cancer and reproduction, and should give us some of the answers we need.

WOMEN WITH IMPLANTS

There's no evidence that women with implants have a higher vulnerability to breast cancer than other women, and some evidence that it may actually be lower.[27] Sometimes it's detected on mammogram, and sometimes the lump is palpable. It's diagnosed in the same way as any breast cancer—with a biopsy. We may be able to do a needle biopsy, depending on where the lump is—we don't want to stick a needle into the sack and spread the silicone, or saline, loose in the breast.

The treatment options are the same. You can have lumpectomy and radiation.[28] You can radiate with the implant in place. There is a higher incidence of encapsulation (see Chapter 5), but other than that there's no problem. You might think that cutting into the breast would break the silicone cover, but there are a couple of ways around that. One of the things we can do is use the electrocautery instead of the scalpel, and that can't cut into the implant.

If you had injections, back in the 1960s when they were legal, the same applies. It's even harder with implants to detect cancer on mammogram, since it's hard to tell what's silicone and what's something else. So you need to go to a good place where they can very carefully monitor you. And it's very important to have the mammograms serially, where they compare one year to another, because that's what can tip you off: one of these lumps that you were calling silicone is growing. You can have lumpectomy and radiation.

BREAST CANCER IN MEN

This book addresses breast cancer in women, and there's a reason for that. It is the most common malignancy in women, and very rare among men, accounting for less than 1 percent of male cancers. Many of the men who get it seem to have a family history on their father's or their mother's side.[29] There's also a theory that it's connected to gynecomastia—femalelike breasts (see Chapter 1), either in the present or during the man's puberty, but so far we have no proof of this. We do have proof that men with Klinefelter's syndrome, a chromosomal problem in which not enough testosterone is produced, are susceptible to breast cancer.[30]

For a time there was some concern that men who got estrogen treatments for prostate cancer would be more vulnerable to breast cancer, but this doesn't seem to be the case. What can happen is that the prostate cancer itself can metastasize to the breast.[31]

Breast cancer in men shows itself in all the ways it does in women—usually as a lump—but it tends to be discovered at a much later time because men aren't usually as conscious of their breasts as women are of theirs. The treatments are the same as well. The cosmetic implications are somewhat different for them. On the one hand, they don't tend to be invested in breasts as crucial to their sexuality the way women are. On the other hand, they're far more often in situations where their naked chests are visible: it can be more awkward for a man to have a scar, to lack a nipple, or to have a deformed chest, than it is for a woman. So, like a woman, a man might prefer lumpectomy and radiation to mastectomy. The one extra consideration is hair. After radiation therapy a man will lose most of his chest hair on that side. If he is very hairy, a mastectomy with the scar hidden in hair might prove more cosmetic. Depending on where the tumor is, the nipple can often be conserved. If he loses the nipple, a plastic surgeon can give him an artificial one. When I worked at UCLA, a golfer with a small breast cancer came to me. He was very distressed that the only option he had been given was a mastectomy. After a lumpectomy and radiation, he was very happy and felt more normal on the course.

Treatment in terms of chemotherapy and axillary nodes are exactly the same as for women. Interestingly, tamoxifen works in men. Why an estrogen blocker works in a man, I don't know. But it does tell us that the way tamoxifen works isn't as simple as it once seemed to be.

DCIS (ductal carcinoma in situ) is even more rare in men than is breast cancer. In 1999 the Armed Forces Institute of Pathology did a study on male DCIS.[32] They found 280 cases of pure DCIS and 759 of invasive. They studied the pure DCIS cases. They found that it existed in older rather than younger men. It was different from DCIS in women (see Chapter 16) in that it was more frequently the low-grade papillary version than either cribiform or the high-grade comedo kind. High-grade DCIS was especially rare. Occasional cases showed necrosis. The men were treated with wide excision alone without radiation for this low-grade DCIS.

I recently got an e-mail from a man who had DCIS. He had been given a mastectomy and then radiation. Then he was told he'd have to be put on tamoxifen. He wanted to know if tamoxifen could harm him.

It's unlikely that it would have. There are lots of data on men taking tamoxifen, and it doesn't harm them. They can get hot flashes, but they can't get vaginal dryness or endometrial cancer, or any male version of those.

But this man didn't need it. He probably only needed a mastectomy without radiation. The only data for tamoxifen with DCIS show a very small benefit, and that occurs only with women who had lumpectomy and radiation, not mastectomy. The doctors were probably inexperienced in male breast cancer, and thought it wisest to use every treatment possible.

Usually, however, when a man has a breast lump, it isn't cancer, it's unilateral gynecomastia, which can happen anytime in a man's life, especially if he's been on some of the drugs used to treat heart conditions or hypertension or smokes marijuana. It's never a cyst or fibroadenoma—men don't get those.

OTHER CANCERS

When I arrived at UCLA in 1992, within the first week or two I got a call to see a patient who had a breast lump. It was soft and smooth, and on the side of her breast. It felt like a cyst, but I tried to aspirate it and that didn't do any good. Then she had a mammogram and an ultrasound, which confirmed that the lump was solid. We took the lump out under local anesthesia, and indeed it was malignant. When I talked to her afterwards, I broke one of my cardinal rules—never make absolute promises. I told her that, though it was unfortunate that her tumor was malignant, it was a small tumor and I could guarantee that she wouldn't have to get chemotherapy: since she was postmenopausal, the most she'd need would be tamoxifen.

Then we looked at it more closely under the microscope, and it turned out that it wasn't a breast cancer at all—it was lymphoma, a lymph node cancer in the breast. The way to treat lymphoma is with chemotherapy. The tale has two morals. One, never break your own wisest rules. And two, things aren't always what they seem. It's ironic that my first breast cancer patient at UCLA didn't have breast cancer at all. (I'm glad to report that she responded well to the treatment and is doing fine.)

So occasionally you can have other kinds of cancer in the breast. Since the breast contains several kinds of tissue besides breast tissue, any of the cancers associated with those kinds of tissue can appear in the breast. In addition to lymphoma (since there are lymph nodes), these include a cancerous fat tumor (liposarcoma) and a blood-vessel tumor (angiosarcoma). You can also have a melanoma—a skin cancer. Connective tissue in the breast, as elsewhere, can become cancerous. Usually these cancers are treated the same way they'd be treated in any other part of the body—the tissue is excised, and radiation and chemotherapy follow (the chemicals are different from those used to treat breast cancer).

When another form of cancer shows up in the breast, we know it isn't breast cancer from the pathologist's report. As I've discussed earlier, each kind of cancer has its own distinct characteristics, and we rarely mistake one kind for another. We choose treatment for the particular cancer rather than breast cancer treatment. We didn't, for example, do an axillary section on my lymphoma patient.

It's important to remember that having breast cancer doesn't immunize you from other forms of cancer. You have the same chances as anyone else of getting other cancers. I've had a couple of patients with breast cancer who were also heavy smokers. They were treated for their breast cancer, continued smoking, and ended up with lung cancer. A bout with any kind of cancer can provide a useful time to consider altering your lifestyle in ways that promote overall health.

25

Surgery

Almost every form of breast cancer will involve some surgery—the initial biopsy, and probably a mastectomy or a partial mastectomy (lumpectomy) as well. It's always a frightening thought, but demystifying the process can be helpful. We've already discussed some surgery in previous chapters (5 and 11); in this chapter we will go over what you can expect from your surgeon and your operation for breast cancer. I will be fairly explicit because I think the more information you have, the less scared you will be. If you find surgical details unpleasant, you may want to skip some parts.

When I was in practice, I would talk with the patient a few days ahead of time and explain exactly what I'd do in the operation, and what risks and possible complications were involved. I would draw her pictures and show her photographs, so she'd know what to expect. (If your doctor doesn't do that, you can check my and other websites for photos and descriptions.)

As with any operation, patients are asked before the surgery to sign a consent form. This can be a little scary, especially if you read all the fine print, because it asks you to state that you're aware that you can die from the surgery or suffer permanent brain damage from the anesthetic. This doesn't mean that these things are likely to happen, or that by signing the form you're letting the doctors off the hook if something *does* happen. Rather, it's a guarantee that you've been told about the procedure and its risk and that you still want to have the operation. (Obviously you have to balance for yourself the risk involved in the operation against the risks of not having it.)

It's very important that you do know the risks. You should never permit yourself to be rushed through the signing of the consent form. You should be given the form well before you go in for surgery—it's hard to read small print when you're about to be wheeled into the operating room. You need to have plenty of time to ask the surgeon any questions about risks and complications. If anything confuses you at all, be sure to ask.

For the bigger operations (mastectomies and flap reconstruction) I often recommend that the patient donate a couple of pints of her own blood a week or two prior to the procedure. Transfusions are rarely necessary in breast surgery but it's a nice secure feeling for the patient to know that if she does need blood she can get the safest type possible, her own. If your surgeon doesn't offer this, you should ask. The Red Cross is more than happy to assist in this procedure.

Your surgeon will tell you to stop taking aspirin, aspirin-containing products, or nonsteroidal anti-inflammatory drugs at least two weeks before surgery. All of these interfere with clotting and will therefore cause more bleeding in surgery. If someone has taken a drug of this type we will do a "bleeding time" (a test that tells how fast your blood clots) prior to surgery to make sure it's safe to proceed. If not, we postpone the surgery for a week or two until the clotting returns to normal. It is important to tell both your surgeon *and* anesthesiologist about all drugs, vitamins, and herbs you are taking so they can check for interactions.

As we discussed in Chapter 23, the timing of surgery may also be important. I would recommend that premenopausal women try to time their surgery for right after ovulation (early luteal phase) if possible.

ANESTHESIA

There are a variety of anesthetics that we can use in various procedures. There's local anesthesia, which we described in Chapter 11; there's general anesthesia, which we describe below; and there's a kind that falls in between, that puts you into a kind of twilight sleep in which you're somewhat aware of what's happening but you really don't care. (This was also described in Chapter 11.)

There are other anesthetics that are midway between local and general. A nerve block can sometimes be useful. But a nerve block works only in an area controlled by a single nerve and in which the controlling nerve is easily accessible. Since the breast area involves a number of nerves, we can't use it for major breast surgery.

There's also the spinal—more extensive than the nerve block, but less extensive than general anesthetic. Local anesthetic is put into the spinal fluid where it bathes the spinal column, making all the nerves below the area go numb. Unfortunately, it can't be used above the waist, since it would numb the nerves that control breathing and heartbeat. The epidural works similarly, and has similar limitations.

Local anesthesia doesn't usually work for extensive breast surgery; the amount of local anesthesia you'd need to block out the pain would be toxic. This is because most breast cancer surgery beyond the biopsy stage requires that we take out lymph nodes in your armpits, and all the nerves that go to your armpit go also to your hand. The sentinel node biopsy may well change this problem.

In the old days, general anesthesia just meant ether, but in recent years it's become a very complex and sophisticated combination of drugs. The first element in any general anesthetic combination is something to induce sleep quickly—usually propofol. This drug is given intravenously, and puts you out immediately. Its effects last only about 15 minutes, so it's followed with a combination of other drugs. Sometimes the anesthesiologist will use a combination of narcotics to prevent pain, gas to keep you unconscious, and a muscle paralyzer to keep you from coughing or otherwise moving during the operation. Since the muscle paralyzer prevents breathing, it's necessary to put a tube down your throat and into your windpipe to keep your airway open, and hook you up to a breathing machine to assure that you get enough oxygen into your body during the operation. Sometimes they skip the paralysis and put a tube into your throat, letting you breathe yourself. Sometimes rather than use the narcotics they'll just use gas; some kinds of gas can keep you asleep and get rid of pain.

Which of these various agents are used, and in what combination, will be chosen only after consultation with the individual patient. Your medical history will make a big difference here. If you have asthma, for example, a drug that opens up the airways is more suitable so that you don't get an attack under anesthesia. If you have a heart condition, a drug that doesn't aggravate the heart but has a calming effect on it will be chosen.

Since anesthesia and its administration are so sophisticated and precise, most hospitals will have you talk with the anesthesiologist before the operation. Anesthesiologists are well-trained doctors who've gone through at least three years of specialized training after their internships. Your anesthesiologist will take your medical history, looking for things in that history that might suggest using, or not using, various of the anesthetic agents. She or he will ask about chronic diseases you may have, past experiences with anesthetic, etc., and only after thoroughly exploring all this with you, will decide what to use in your operation. This interview is very important since as much of the risk of any operation is in the anesthesia and its administration as is in the surgery. When you talk to the anesthesiologist, ask questions, and give any information you think might be of importance. Many hospitals also have nurse anesthetists who help administer anesthesia under an M.D.'s supervision.

Before you're put to sleep you're hooked up to a variety of monitoring devices. There's an automatic blood pressure cuff. There's an EKG monitoring your heart rate. Sometimes a little clip or piece of tape is put on your finger, toe, or earlobe to measure the amount of oxygen in your blood. If the operation is a lengthy one, a catheter is put in your bladder to measure the amount of urine output and make sure you're not dehydrated. So your bodily functions are all carefully monitored.

Once you're on the operating table, you're asleep very quickly. Many people who haven't had surgery for 30 or 40 years remember the old days of ether, and are nervous about the unpleasant sensations they recall while going under. But sodium pentathol works much differently, and most patients report it as a very pleasant experience. You may experience a garliclike taste at the back of your mouth just before you go under, and you may yawn. Propofol may burn as it goes into your arm. Then you're asleep. Don't worry: in spite of all the television melodrama, you're not likely to reveal all your deep, dark secrets under sodium pentothal.

How you wake up from the operation will depend, again, on what drugs have been used. With some drugs an antidote can be given to end the drug's effects. So if, for example, you've been given a muscle paralyzer, a drug can restore your muscle mobility. But if you've been given gas to put you to sleep, you have to wait slightly longer till the gas wears off. As soon as they think you're awake enough to breathe on your own the tube is removed. Occasionally you'll be vaguely aware that this is happening, but usually you're still too out of it to notice. You stay a little fuzzy for a while. When the surgery is over, you're taken to the recovery room where a nurse remains with you, monitoring your blood pressure and pulse every 10 or 15 minutes until you're fully awake and stable.

Patients often feel cold when they first wake up. Particularly in a big operation, when you haven't been covered up, you've lost body heat; in addition, the intravenous (IV) fluids going into you are cold. Some of the drugs can create nausea, and you may feel sick when you first wake up. This was succinctly described by a recovery room nurse I once saw on a TV show. She was asked what patients usually say when they first come out of anesthesia, and it was clear the host was expecting something profound or moving. Instead, she replied, "They say, 'I think I'm going to be sick'—and then they are."

You may find that you wake up crying, or shivering, but only rarely do patients wake up in great pain. You'll probably fade in and out for a while, and then you'll be fully awake. But expect to be groggy and out of it for a while. It's several hours before most of the drugs are out of your system, and a day or more till they're all gone. If it's day surgery, you'll probably want to just go home and go to bed; if you're still in the hospital, you'll sleep it all off there.

Even apart from the surgery, anesthesia itself is a great strain on your body, and it will cause some degree of exhaustion for at least four or five days. People often don't realize this, especially if the surgery itself is very painful: they attribute all their exhaustion to the pain of the operation. But anything that puts great stress on your body—surgery, a heart attack, an acute asthma attack, or anesthetics that interfere with your body's functions—will have a lingering effect. It's as if your body takes all its energy to mobilize for the big stress, and doesn't have any left over for everyday life for a while. You need to respect that, and give yourself time to recuperate from the stress of both the surgery and the anesthetic.

There are, of course, risks involved in using general anesthetic, but it's important to keep them in perspective. With the refinements in anesthesia in recent years, the risks are extremely low (about one death in 200,000 cases).

Depending on how complicated the operation is, you can now have surgery in which you're admitted to the hospital the day before, or on the same day you have your surgery. In some cases you can even have day surgery—"outpatient" surgery. In the last few years I was practicing I tended to do lumpectomy with axillary dissection only on an outpatient basis; so my patient had her two hours of surgery, spent another few hours in the recovery room, and then got to go home. I frequently did mastectomies as day surgery or just an overnight stay. Since the rate of infection is twice as high among women who stay in the hospital, I think leaving as soon as possible is a good idea. (I understand the concerns of many patients that managed care companies try to save money by sending people home too soon, but in some cases, leaving the hospital as soon as possible really can be best for the patient.) Many women prefer going home right away, while others feel more comfortable staying in the hospital for a couple of days. A patient who has a mastectomy and immediate reconstruction will be in the hospital for about two to five days. If your surgeon wants to send you home earlier than you feel comfortable with, discuss your problems with him or her and see if you can arrange a longer stay.

When the surgery is being done under general anesthesia, all the pre-op procedures are the same, whether it's day surgery or whether you stay in the hospital for a number of days. "Twilight sleep" procedures still require the same pre-op preparations, since they need to be monitored, just as general anesthesia does.

PRELIMINARY PROCEDURES

In the operating room, before you are anesthetized, the anesthesiologist will be setting up, and the nurses will put EKG leads and an automatic blood pressure cuff on you. Often we use something called "pneumatic boots"—plastic boots that pump up and down massaging your calves during the operation to prevent clots from forming during the time you are immobile. (Fig. 25-1). A grounding plate is put on your skin to ground the electrocautery and protect you from shock. The IV is put in, and then you're given propofol. During this time your surgeon may or may not be with you. Some surgeons prefer a more personal contact beforehand; others maintain a professional distance. I used to like to establish a connection with my patient beforehand, so I'd go into the operating room and, while all these procedures were taking place, I'd stay there with my patient and hold her hand. My patient was scared, and usually I was the only person there she knew. This contact also helped me confirm my commitment to the patient as an individual who had offered her trust to me.

Once my patient was asleep, I'd do what every other surgeon does: I would go out to scrub (wash my hands). With personal contact established, I liked to use this time to distance—I needed to be an objective craftsperson to do the best job possible.

After scrubbing, the surgeon goes back into the operating room. The area of your body that's going to be worked on is painted over with a disinfectant, drapes are put around you to prevent infection, and the operation is under way.

All of the procedures I've just described are done regardless of what kind of operation you're having. What varies, obviously, is the process of the particular operation. Now I'll describe what happens in each different breast cancer operation, starting with the simplest and moving on to the more complex. (Biopsies were described in Chapter 11 and reconstruction will be in Chapter 26.)

Most surgical operations have traditionally been done with a scalpel or scissors. More recently, electrocautery (a type of electric knife) has been used with less blood loss. The newest technique is laser surgery,

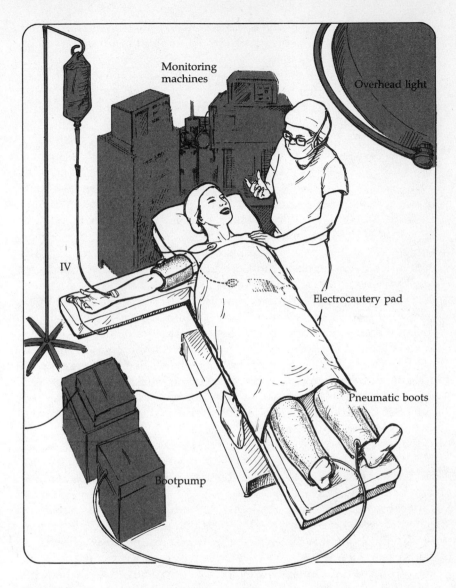

FIGURE 25-1

which is being used more and more for breast operations.[1] Some people have the misconception that using the laser means we don't have to make an incision; we just vaporize the tissues. It's not that easy. We still need to make an incision. Although there have been claims of less postoperative pain and less tumor recurrence, there are no good randomized studies as of yet. I think the laser may have a place in the future of breast surgery, but you need to realize that it isn't some Star Trek magical zapper; it's just another tool to aid the surgeon in doing the operation.

PARTIAL MASTECTOMY AND AXILLARY DISSECTION

In the past, there was only one operation done for breast cancer: mastectomy. Now, however, you can choose instead an operation that removes the lump and part of the surrounding tissue, combined with postoperative radiation (see Chapter 27). Partial mastectomy, lumpectomy, wide excision, segmental mastectomy, and quadrantectomy are all names for this type of operation and are used virtually synonymously (Fig. 25-2). What each term means depends on the surgeon who's using it. Except for quadrantectomy, none of the terms suggests how much tissue will be removed, and often surgeons use "quadrantectomy" when they don't necessarily mean they'll remove a fourth of the breast. With a partial mastectomy, the "part" removed can be 1 percent or 50 percent of the breast tissue. "Lumpectomy" depends on the size of the lump. "Wide excision" just says that you'll cut away tissue around the lump—it doesn't say how much you'll cut. "Segmental" sounds like the breast comes in little segments, like an orange. But it doesn't, and the segment removed can be any size. Your surgeon will use whatever term appeals most to her or him. I like "partial mastectomy" at the moment, because it's the term that insurance companies seem most comfortable with.

If you're opting for surgery that involves taking out part but not all of the breast tissue, you need to make sure your surgeon explains very precisely how much tissue will be removed, and what you're going to look like afterwards.

Because this is a relatively new procedure, standard techniques haven't been worked out yet. One thing that's been determined is that we should choose the direction of the incision based on which area of the breast contains the cancer.[2] In addition, the area of the breast involved should determine the way the tissue is removed and whether it is sewn back together. After years of being a breast surgeon I discovered something that should have been obvious long ago, but had never occurred to me. Women look at their breasts when they're standing in front of a mirror; surgeons look at the breasts when the patient is lying flat on her back. So the surgeon's impression of the best cosmetic effect may not be the same as the patient's. Plastic surgeons, at the end of an operation on the breast, will typically sit the patient up to see how the breast looks with gravity acting on it. But it's not something other surgeons tend to think of. For example, Langer's lines, which are standard classical surgical teaching, are supposed to be the lines of skin tension

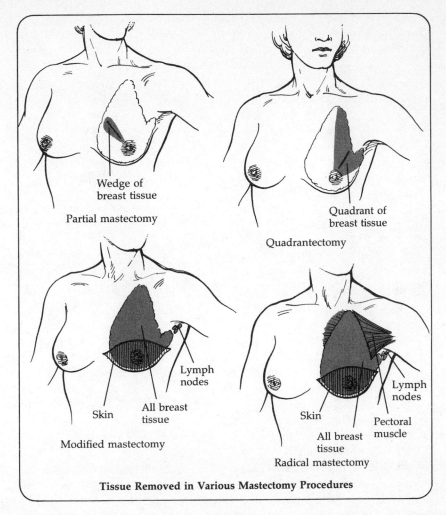

Wedge of
breast tissue

Partial mastectomy

Quadrant of
breast tissue

Quadrantectomy

Lymph
nodes

Skin   All breast
tissue

Modified mastectomy

Lymph
nodes

Skin

Pectoral
muscle

All breast
tissue

Radical mastectomy

Tissue Removed in Various Mastectomy Procedures

FIGURE 25-2

that show us where to best make the incision so that the scar will have as little visibility as possible. The pictures of Langer's lines for the breast look like a target—a bull's-eye with concentric circles (Fig. 25-3). But when you think about the breast of a woman standing upright, that doesn't work: the breast is in a U-shape, not a circular shape, as the breast is being pulled down by gravity. So the way we used to make incisions is probably wrong. Most breast surgeons and many general surgeons now understand the changes in the skin with position. Ask your surgeon if you are unsure.

When I was at the Faulkner Breast Centre in Boston, we did a study asking patients what they felt were the most significant aspects of the

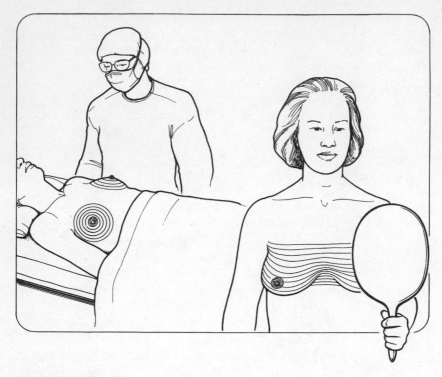

FIGURE 25-3

cosmetic results. My bias going into the study was that the most important thing for the patient would be that we sew her breast tissue back together again in such a way that her breast wouldn't have a dent. It would be a smaller breast, but it would be the right shape. The study showed that I was wrong. What was most important to the patient was size of the breast and the nipple placement. Shape was less important.[3]

When you think about it, it makes sense. If you have one breast one size smaller than the other, it's hard to buy a bra that fits at all, or clothing that fits properly. But it's much easier if you've got a breast that's the right size but has a dent in it, because you can push the edges of the dent together inside the bra cup. So I stopped sewing the breast tissue together and instead sewed just the subcutaneous tissue—the fat and the skin. That would leave the size as close as possible to the other breast.

Another thing we realized is that if the surgeon does a horizontal incision, above or even below the nipple, it changes the nipple position, pulling it in the direction of the incision. The same thing happens with a vertical incision: the nipple gets pulled to the side, or toward the middle of the chest. A radial incision will leave the nipple position unchanged. But that too is imperfect. Radial incisions are likely to be very visible in a bathing suit or a low-cut blouse, particularly if they're on the upper part of your breast. So as the patient, you have to decide which is more important: would you rather have your nipples lined up symmetrically, or would you rather have a scar that won't show above your bathing suit? The answer to that varies from woman to woman. These are the kinds of questions that we're just starting to look at in terms of breast conservation. We now have an atlas to demonstrate the best techniques for all surgeons.[4]

With partial mastectomies, as with most surgical procedures, different surgeons have slightly different approaches. Some like to keep the patients in the hospital for one or two days. I always preferred to do a partial mastectomy and lymph node surgery as day surgery.

The operation itself, however, is pretty standard. It begins with carefully monitored general anesthetic. The surgeon usually starts by taking out the breast tissue in a wedge, like a piece of pie, all the way down to the level of the muscle (Fig. 25-4). That piece is given intact to

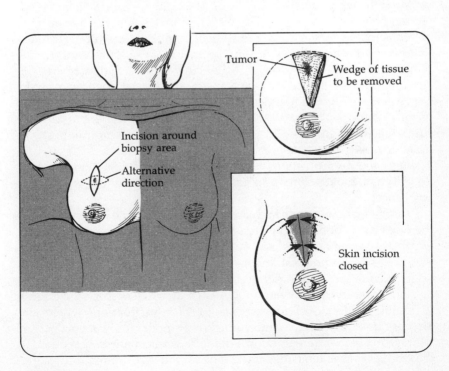

FIGURE 25-4

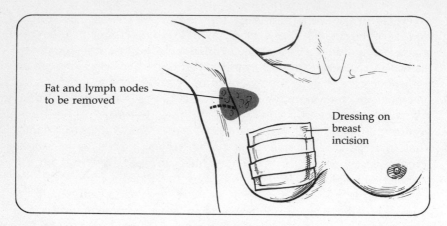

Fat and lymph nodes to be removed

Dressing on breast incision

FIGURE 25-5

the pathologist, oriented with sutures. Then the tissue and skin are sutured together. Some surgeons put drains into the breast to collect fluid
afterwards. I found this unnecessary, and rarely did it.

When the breast surgery itself is finished, the surgeon will begin operating on the lymph nodes (Fig. 25-5). An incision is made about two
inches across the armpit, and the surgeon removes the wad of fat in the
hollow of your armpit which contains many of the lymph nodes. The
lymph nodes, as I said earlier, are glands—sometimes they're swollen
and big, but usually they're very small and embedded in fat. We take
out a section of the fat, defined by certain anatomical boundaries, that
usually contains at least 10 to 15 lymph nodes. We hope, but can't be
sure, that we've included in this fat the significant lymph nodes. The
tissue is sent to the pathologist, who examines the fat and tries to find
as many of the lymph nodes as possible. The pathologist then cuts each
node in half, makes slides and examines each of them to see if there is
any cancer.

This is where we see the advantage of sentinel node biopsy. We find
the one or two nodes that are most likely to have cancer, so we don't
worry that we may miss a node that's over in a corner somewhere.
And since the pathologist knows that this is the node to check, it will
be checked out much more thoroughly than the many nodes in a regular node dissection (see Chapter 23). Thus there's less room for error.

Sentinel node biopsy alone is most useful in situations where you
are very unlikely to have cancer in a lymph node. It gives you the advantage of being sure without the complications of a full dissection. In
the rare case when a positive node is identified on examination, the patient can be recalled and undergo a full dissection at a later date to

make sure it was the only one. The reason it's important to have the rest of the nodes out when the sentinel node is positive is that there's likely to be cancer in some of the other nodes and they need to be treated with either surgery or radiation.

The procedure for a sentinel node biopsy is still relatively new and the technical details are still being figured out. There are those who favor using blue dye, those who favor a radioactive tracer, and those who prefer to do both. Many of the doctors who do the procedure do both. Blue dye can be given at the time of the surgery itself, because it spreads to the nodes pretty quickly: the doctor can inject the blue dye as soon as the patient is asleep. By contrast, the radioactive tracer must be given at least three hours ahead of time, since it takes that long to get from the tumor to the lymph node. It's usually injected under local anesthetic, around where the tumor is or was.

If you have had an injection of the radioactive tracer, the doctors have no trouble finding the node—the gamma counter tells them where to make the incision. Once the incision has been made, they can then see a blue lymph vessel leading to the lymph node, and track it.

Infrequently, the sentinal node will be not in the patient's armpit but up in her chest, beneath the sternum, and here the radioactive tracer has a definite advantage. The absence of radioactivity in the armpit will lead the doctor to check for it elsewhere. The usefulness of removing lymph nodes from under the breastbone is still controversial, and surgeons need to weigh the pros and cons. It doesn't change a woman's survival rate, but it may affect her decision about whether or not to have chemotherapy.

It's always a good idea to ask your doctor what kind of procedure is being done on you. One woman I know of had sentinel biopsy done and didn't even know it. She had a lumpectomy and node removal under general anesthetic, and assumed that nothing unusual was being done. They removed only four nodes—all of which were tested with the usual method, all showing no spread. She left the hospital certain they had gotten out all the cancer. "They told me they were 90 percent sure," she said, "but they'd call me in a few days with the rest of the results." The rest of the results came from the additional scrutiny given the sentinel node, in which they did in fact find more breast cancer. Though she felt "devastated," she at least had more accurate information on which to base her decisions.

Most doctors, however, will tell you what procedures they're planning. Barbara, a woman I met while she was volunteering for my nipple fluid studies (see Chapter 17), was happy to have both the sentinel node biopsy and a full axillary dissection because she knew that with sentinel node biopsy as part of the process, they would remove fewer lymph nodes. As a flight attendant she was particularly concerned about this, since she was afraid that with many nodes removed, she was likely to have lymphedema (swelling of the arm), which would probably be exacerbated by the constant changes of air pressure involved in her job. So far she has had no swelling since the procedure.

First her doctor injected the radioactive dye before the surgery. "I lay on the table, and the camera doing a lymphoscintraphy scan came down at me. It looked like a huge diving bell," she says. "When the nuclear medicine was shot in, it was painful." They waited five minutes after the anesthetic, then put the dye into one breast. Because they were doing both breasts, the procedure took about an hour. She was lying down on a gurney, and every 10 minutes the camera would take another picture to see if the tracer had moved to a lymph node yet. "This diving-bell camera was practically in my face, and I couldn't move at all," she says. "But at least it wasn't as bad as the MRI, where I *really* couldn't move. Here at least I could scratch my nose if I had to in between pictures!"

The surgery itself lasted several hours, and she stayed overnight in the hospital. "At 9 p.m., I had to go to the john, and the nurse helped me. My pee was a bright cobalt blue. I had known about it, but the poor nurse hadn't and she was really shocked." The blue dye was being eliminated from her body. Although there was also some blue in her breasts, that took about a month to clear out.

They took out a number of nodes—9 in her right breast and 15 in her left. They had done a test called *keratin immunohistochemical stain* on the sentinel nodes and found micrometastases.

The operation on her nodes left her with several weeks of discomfort. "I felt like I had a wad of scotch tape under each armpit," she recalls. "For about two weeks, I couldn't stand my arm and chest skin meeting." By the end of a month the discomfort left, and it was never bad enough to make her take the painkillers the doctors had given her.

Sometimes a patient will want to have her nodes radiated, rather than taken out. There are data showing that radiating negative nodes works as well as removing them in terms of preventing the cancer from coming back in the nodes. The important thing is to find out whether there *is* cancer in the nodes, because to date that's our best way of guessing whether cancer has begun to spread into the rest of the body.

Some women will have more nodes than others. Every now and then a patient will ask me, "How come you got seventeen lymph nodes in me and only seven in my friend?" We are all built differently. The existence of that difference was brought to my attention one time after I'd done a routine axillary dissection. A new pathologist was dissecting out the nodes. She amazed me by finding 40 in a specimen that usually would contain 15. She had just looked harder than usual. However, the total number of nodes is less important than the number that are positive. The most important thing is for the surgeon to remove the tissue that should contain the nodes. There have been studies showing that the chance of missing a positive lymph node if we remove the tissue in the lower two levels of the armpit is less than 5 percent.[5]

Many surgeons put a drain in the axillary incision afterwards, but again, I preferred not to—there's not enough fluid to worry about, in my experience.[6] I would put a little long-acting local anesthetic into the wound, so my patient didn't wake up in pain later, and then sew up the incision.

The operation takes from one to three hours altogether. You wake up in the recovery room and, according to your surgeon's preference, you can go home that night or in a day or two. As I said, I usually preferred to send patients home that day, unless they had some medical condition that might be aggravated by anesthesia—severe asthma, heart problems, etc.

When you go home you'll have a small dressing on your incision. I would use dissolvable sutures inside the skin and Steristrips on the skin, so my patient could take a shower or bath or go swimming without worry. Though there were no sutures to take out, I did like to see my patients ten days to two weeks after the surgery to trim the knots of the sutures as well as to monitor their progress. An earlier visit can be scheduled to discuss pathology results.

RISKS AND COMPLICATIONS OF PARTIAL MASTECTOMY

There may be some loss of sensation in your breast after a partial mastectomy, depending on the size of the lump removed. If it's a large lump, there may be a permanent numb spot, but there won't be the total loss of sensation that results from a mastectomy.

Your breast may be different in size and shape than it was before, and consequently it will probably be somewhat different from your remaining breast. How great the difference is depends on how much tissue was removed and how skillfully the surgery was done. If your breasts have become asymmetrical to an extent that disturbs you, you can get partial mastectomy breast pads called shells to wear in your bra. You can also get reconstructive surgery: a small flap of your own tissue is put in to fill things out (see Chapter 26). Or, depending on how large your breasts are to begin with, you can get the other breast reduced to create a more symmetrical appearance. Usually, however, that won't be necessary. If you have a small lump, and medium or large breasts, it's often hard to tell afterwards which breast was operated on, except for the scar.

The possible complications resulting from lymph node surgery are more serious. There's a nerve—and sometimes two or three nerves—going through the middle of the fat that has been removed. This nerve gives you sensation in the back part of your armpit. It doesn't affect the way your arm works, but it does affect sensation. If that nerve is cut, you'll have a patch of numbness in the back part of your arm (Fig. 25-6). Many surgeons cut the nerve, because it's difficult to save, and they don't think sensation in the armpit is very important anyway. Of course, most surgeons are men—they've never shaved their armpits, and they don't know how awkward it can be when you can't feel the area you're shaving. Most breast surgeons and many general surgeons try to save the nerve. Even if the surgeon does save it, it may get stretched in the process and give you decreased sensation either temporarily or permanently. If the sensation is gone for more than a few months, the loss is probably permanent. (If this happens to you, you might want to give up shaving your armpits, or to use an electric shaver rather than a razor, which is more likely to cut the skin and cause bleeding.)

Another complication, one that's unusual, is fluid under the armpit. Most women get some swelling, but some will get so much that it looks like they've got a grapefruit under their armpits. When it gets to this point, the fluid usually is aspirated (drawn off).

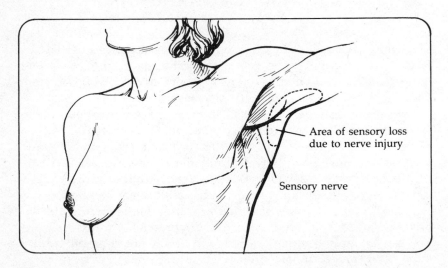

Area of sensory loss due to nerve injury

Sensory nerve

FIGURE 25-6

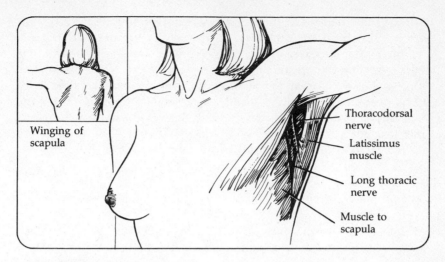

Winging of scapula

Thoracodorsal nerve

Latissimus muscle

Long thoracic nerve

Muscle to scapula

FIGURE 25-7

Very rarely, a patient gets a hematoma from surgery and can remain sore and dramatically bruised for several weeks afterwards. The surgical dressing tape may cause a rash, known as "tape burn."

Another early problem can be phlebitis in one of the arm veins. This usually shows up three or four days after surgery. The woman says, "I felt wonderful after the operation and now I have this tight feeling under my arm that goes down to the elbow and sometimes even to the wrist. And I can see a cord. The pain is worse and I can't move my arm nearly as well as I could before." This is an inflammation of the basilic vein. It is not serious but it's bothersome. The best treatment is ice and aspirin or a lymphatic. It will go away within several days to a week.

The major complication, but fortunately an uncommon one, is swelling of the arm, a condition called *lymphedema,* which we discuss in chapter 30.

Another rare complication of lymph node surgery involves the motor nerves (Fig. 25-7). These are different from the sensory nerves. Two motor nerves can be injured by lymph node surgery. One of them—the long thoracic nerve—goes to the muscle that holds your shoulder blade against your back when you hold your arm straight out. If that nerve is injured, your shoulder blade, instead of remaining flat, will stick out like a wing when you hold your arm out. Hence it's called a "winged scapula." (There are other causes of winged scapula as well; sometimes it's a congenital condition.) If you're not athletic, it probably won't affect you very much in your daily activities, but it affects activities like serving in tennis or pitching a baseball.

Permanent winged scapula cases are extremely rare; if the condition is temporary, it should go away in a few weeks or months. In order to cause a permanent winged scapula, the surgeon would have to cut completely through the nerve at a high level.

The other nerve is called the thoracodorsal nerve, and it goes to the latissimus muscle. Damage to this nerve is rare and less noticeable than the winged scapula. It will probably give you some sensation of tiredness in the arm, which won't work quite as well as it did before, but it won't give you any glaring problem.

At Home after Partial Mastectomy

Your surgeon may put your arm in a sling to prevent your moving it around and pulling the incision apart. I never liked to do this; I think the earlier you start moving your arm around normally the less chance there is that it will get stiff. Keeping the arm in a sling will cause it to stiffen, even if you haven't had an operation. If your arm is kept immobile for any length of time, you'll need physical therapy to help you start using it again. But if you do use your arm normally right away, you probably won't need physical therapy (see Chapter 30). I found that my patients were sufficiently sore that they didn't tend to fling their arms about anyway. You shouldn't lift anything more than about five pounds with that arm for several days, but then you can use it pretty normally afterwards.

Once you're sent home, the biggest problem, as we said, is that you're exhausted. Respect that tiredness; you've just been through major surgery, anesthesia, and an emotionally difficult experience. The exhaustion often comes and goes suddenly. You'll feel fine, and go out shopping; when you get home you'll suddenly feel completely wiped out and need to sleep. It will take several days before you feel fully recovered.

You'll have some pain, but probably not a lot. Like most doctors, I'd give my patients pain medication—usually Vicodin or codeine—when they went home, but the majority of them didn't even finish off the prescription. There are occasionally people who have a lot of pain, and if that's the case it's a good idea to let the doctor know, because it's often a sign of something wrong, like postoperative bleeding or a hematoma.

After a lumpectomy, you should wear a good, strong, support bra day and night for about a week—it hurts when your breast jiggles. Another trick my patients have taught me, particularly my patients with larger breasts, is that if you want to lie on your side, you can lie on the

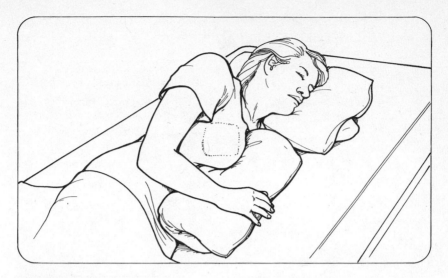

FIGURE 25-8

side that wasn't operated on and hold a pillow between your breasts: the pillow cushions the breast that's been operated on (Fig. 25-8).

The pathology results will usually be available within a couple of days. The surgeon can then tell you what the margins were like and what was actually in your breast tissue and, most important, whether there was any cancer in the lymph nodes. On the basis of the pathology report, you'll discuss the next steps, and whether there is a need for adjuvant therapy.

TOTAL MASTECTOMY

In spite of the availability of partial mastectomy and radiation, which conserve the breast, most women in this country still get total mastectomies as their initial therapy for breast cancer.

"Total mastectomy" should not be confused with "radical mastectomy." The latter, once the norm, is of interest now for historical reasons only. The surgical procedure was basically the same as that for the modified radical (described below), but, obviously, more extensive. In addition to removing the whole breast the surgeon removed the pectoralis major and pectoralis minor muscles (see Figure 25-9). All of the lymph nodes in the axillary area (up to the collarbone) were removed as well. It was far more deforming than the mastectomy we do now.

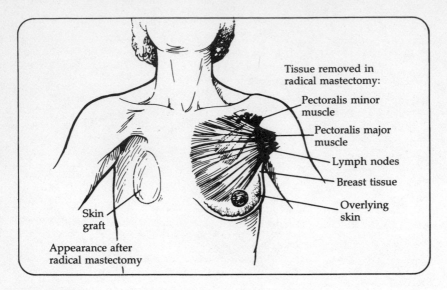

Tissue removed in radical mastectomy:

Pectoralis minor muscle

Pectoralis major muscle

Lymph nodes

Breast tissue

Overlying skin

Skin graft

Appearance after radical mastectomy

FIGURE 25-9

There's virtually no situation any more in which it's necessary. For very large tumors we almost always use neo-adjuvant chemotherapy to shrink them before we do surgery (see Chapter 28). In other cases, the tumor is stuck to the muscle, so the muscle has to be removed in order to get the tumor out. (In very rare cases, the cancer will actually have spread into the muscle itself.) We used to do radical mastectomies in all of these cases, but now we just take a wedge of muscle right under the tumor and leave the rest.

"Total mastectomy," the name we usually give the form of mastectomy used today, is a bit of a misnomer, since we can never be certain the operation is total. Our goal is to remove all the breast tissue, but we can't ever be sure we've done that. We remove as much of the breast tissue as we can and some of the lymph nodes. It usually takes between two and five hours.

The breast tissue, as we discussed earlier, extends from the collarbone down to the edge of the ribs and from the breastbone out to the muscle in the back of the armpit. The surgeon wants to get as much of that breast tissue out as possible. So we start with an elliptical incision that includes the nipple and whatever scar you have from the biopsy; exactly where it is depends on where your biopsy scar is (Fig. 25-10). We take that skin out. With the increasing popularity of immediate reconstruction, surgeons have taken to removing as little skin as possible ("skin sparing"). Next we tunnel underneath the skin all the way up to the collarbone, then down to the border of the ribs, from the middle of the sternum, and out to the muscle behind your armpit. Once the dissection is done, we peel the breast off, leaving the muscle behind.

When the breast is fully removed, we reach up under the skin to the armpit and remove some of the lymph nodes, as we do for the axillary dissection described earlier. We send the breast tissue and the attached fat with nodes to the pathologist, who examines it and begins the process of fixing it to make slides. Meanwhile we sew together the flaps of skin around the incision. You end up completely flat (or, if you're very thin, slightly concave), with a scar going across the middle of that side

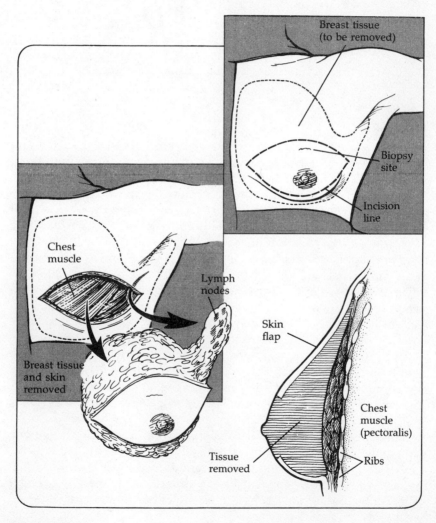

FIGURE 25-10

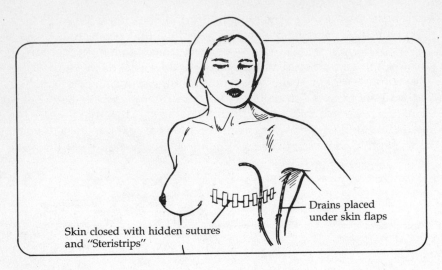

Skin closed with hidden sutures and "Steristrips"

Drains placed under skin flaps

FIGURE 25-11

of your chest. The skin doesn't completely stick down right away, and the body doesn't like empty spaces, so the area will fill up with fluid. To prevent this, we put some drains in—soft, plastic tubes with little holes in them, coming out of the skin below the scar (Fig. 25-11). They help create suction that holds the skin down against the muscle till it heals. Fluid will come out of these drains—it's just tissue fluid, the kind you get in a blister. Initially there'll be a little blood in the fluid, but after about 24 hours it will be clear.

If you've decided to have immediate breast reconstruction (see Chapter 26), the plastic surgeon will either come in after the mastectomy is finished but before the skin is sewn up and do the reconstruction, or be part of the team from the beginning, raising the flap while the surgeon is doing the mastectomy.

As in other operations, the pathology results will be available in a couple of days. This tells you what the breast tissue looked like and, more importantly, if there is any cancer in the nodes. If there are any indications of systemic spread you'll want to discuss adjuvant systemic treatment (see Chapter 28).

Different surgeons have different styles in postoperative treatment. I'd usually put a big, bulky wraparound dressing on my patients because it helped them feel protected from the world for a while. You'll probably stay in the hospital at least overnight. When there's no longer much fluid coming out of the drains—in about three or four days—we'll take the drains out and change the dressing. We used to keep people in the hospital till all the drains came out—nowadays patients sometimes go home and come back later to get the drains removed.

While you're in the hospital, someone from Reach to Recovery or a similar group may come to see you with what's called a "going-home prosthesis." In some places it is free, in others insurance companies will pay for it if it's ordered while you're still in the hospital, but not if you wait till you're home. Insurance policies vary; make sure you check out what yours will cover. (See Chapter 26 for a discussion of prostheses.) For bilateral mastectomy patients there are soft camisoles with pockets for the prostheses.

Some women want to see the wound right away; some prefer to put off looking at it for a week or two. Either way is fine; you need to decide what will make you feel best. But it's important that you look at it at some point. It's amazing how, if you're determined to avoid looking at your body, you can do so when you shower, get dressed, even when you make love. That's okay for a while, but this is the body you're going to be living with, and you need to see it and accept it.

Many of my patients liked me to be with them the first time they saw their scar. This way I could offer emotional support and also answer any questions they had right away. If you would like your surgeon with you when you first look at your chest, ask.

Others prefer to be alone when they first look at the scar. Some want to see it alone before showing it to their husband or lover. Again, there's no right or wrong way to face it, as long as you do face it. In my experience, most women are relieved that it doesn't look as bad as they feared it would.

Numbness around the chest wall is one of the more unfortunate results of the operation. The breast's nerve supply has been cut. So the area around the scar of the mastectomy will be permanently numb. Some sensitivity remains around the outer borders of the area on which your breast was located. Sometimes the breast area is not entirely numb, however; you can tell if someone's touching you. Unfortunately, this usually isn't a pleasant sensitivity. It can be very uncomfortable, like the sensation that you feel when your foot's asleep and starts coming back again, with a tingly feeling. This is known as dysesthesia, and, while it may lessen in severity, it will remain with you. Often people who've had mastectomies don't like their scars being touched because it brings about this slight unpleasant sensation. Some women will recover sensation over a long time.

Some women also experience phantom breast symptoms—like the amputee who still feels itchiness in the toes that are no longer there. The mastectomy patient may feel her nipple itch, or her breast ache, as though it were still there. All this means is that the brain hasn't yet realized what's happened to the body. The nerve supply from the breast grows along a certain path in the spinal cord and goes to a certain area of the brain. The brain has been trained over the years that a signal from this path means, for example, that the nipple is itching. When the nipple's been removed, the signal may get generated in a different place further along the path, but the brain cells think it should be coming from the nipple, and that's the information they give you. This will gradually improve as your brain becomes reprogrammed.

Audre Lorde described some of the feelings wonderfully in her book *The Cancer Journals:* "fixed pains and moveable pains, deep pains and surface pains, strong pains and weak pains. There were stabs and throbs and burns, gripes and tickles and itches."[7] In addition, some women will feel a tightness around the chest as the healing starts. This will ease up over time, and all the weird sensations will start to settle down.

Risks and Complications of Total Mastectomy

Like any operation, the mastectomy has some risks. In the process of removing the breast tissue we've severed a number of blood vessels. The only ones left are those that go the whole length of the flap of skin left when the tissue underneath is removed. These vessels can barely get to the ends of the flap. Sometimes this doesn't give us enough of a blood supply, and it doesn't heal right; a little area of skin dies and forms a scab (Fig. 25-12). Once the wound has healed, the scab falls off. It's usually not a very serious complication. If a big enough area of skin is involved, or there's an infection, the surgeon may have to trim the dead tissue so the body can heal the wound.

A second possible complication occurs when fluid continues to collect under the scar after the drains are removed. You'll know this is happening because there's a swelling around the incision; sometimes you'll hear a slosh when you're walking, or you'll simply feel the fluid on your chest. If it's a small amount of fluid you can just leave it alone and it will eventually go away by itself. If there's a lot of fluid, you can have it aspirated with a needle: it won't hurt, since the area's numb, and it usually doesn't even require local anesthesia. (We try to avoid too many aspirations, though, since there's always the slight risk of transmitting infection through the needle.) Again, this isn't a serious complication, but it can be an annoying one. Surgery is never fun. But it's often necessary, and if you know what to expect ahead of time, you can reduce the stress and fear surrounding it.

The risks from the lymph node removal—loss of sensation, phlebitis, lymphedema or swelling, and winged scapula—are the same as for

Two possible complications . . .

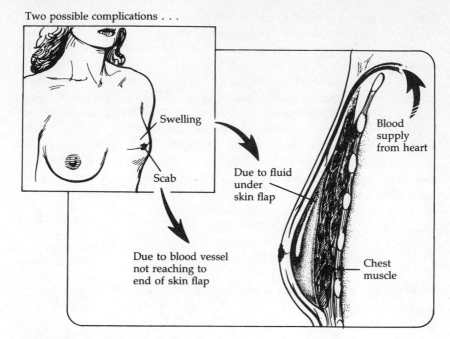

Swelling

Scab

Due to fluid under skin flap

Due to blood vessel not reaching to end of skin flap

Blood supply from heart

Chest muscle

FIGURE 25-12

partial mastectomy and axillary dissection. Again, it's important to move your arm around and keep it from stiffening. Ellen Mahoney, a breast surgeon in Northern California whom I admire, tells her patients to keep their hand behind their head while reading or watching TV postoperatively to stretch the scar.

Many doctors and nurses will send you home with extensive instructions regarding care of your arm after surgery. They are trying to prevent infections, which are more likely to occur when lymph nodes are gone. So they will insist that you never garden without gloves because you might get pricked by a thorn, or that you never reach into a hot oven, or cut your cuticles, or have injections in that arm. Be sensible: you want to reduce the risk of infection, but a minor infection isn't going to kill you, and there's no need to live your life in terror of pinpricks. Be reasonably careful, and if you do get an infection, get to your doctor as soon as possible and have it taken care of, because it's important to try and prevent lymphedema. Although you should try to avoid significant trauma to the involved arm (having blood drawn, blood pressure cuffs), this is not as vital as it was in the days of radical mastectomy. Probably the most important prevention is avoiding heavy lifting with your arm hanging down for a period of time—don't carry a suitcase or briefcase. Try to get your groceries delivered instead of carrying them yourself; if that's not feasible, get one of those little grocery carts and wheel them home. Get suitcases with wheels if you do any traveling.

Theoretically, at least, sentinel node biopsies cause fewer complications. There haven't actually been studies showing that there's less likelihood of a swollen arm, but it seems likely. Much, however, will probably depend on how good the doctor is at finding the node and on where the node is. If it's close to the surface, there will be much less surgery. But if it's deep inside, or far over to the left or right, the doctor may have to be doing a lot of digging to get to it, and that may cause more complications. And since it's done with less anesthetic, there will be fewer problems related to anesthesia.

Exercise After Mastectomy

Exercise is important after your treatment, and not only in terms of lymphedema. Again, doctors can often be overrestrictive. After you've had a mastectomy or a lymph node sampling, your surgeon may tell

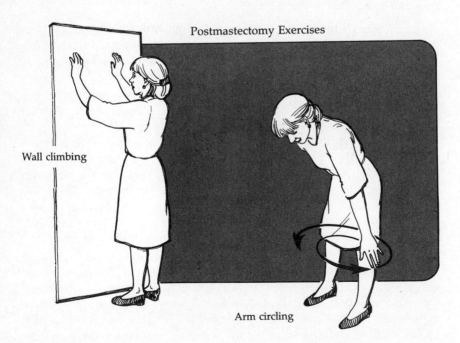

Postmastectomy Exercises

Wall climbing

Arm circling

FIGURE 25-13

you not to move your arm at all. There's a lot of controversy about how protective of the area you should be.

If you do keep your arm very still at first, you'll probably find your shoulder extremely stiff when you start moving around. That's to be expected—if you take someone who's in perfect health and put her arm in a sling for a week, she'll end up with a stiff shoulder.

Certain exercises, however, can help your shoulder (Fig. 25-13). One is called "climbing the walls." It involves walking your fingers up the wall, stretching a little bit farther each time. You can do it while you're watching TV or talking on the phone. The other one involves leaning over and making bigger and bigger circles with your arm. Swimming is also an excellent exercise.

If your arm remains very stiff after two or three weeks, ask your doctor to refer you to a physical therapist. Only about 10 to 15 percent of my patients needed physical therapy. It's very important to get your shoulder flexible again, and soon; otherwise you can end up with a condition called "frozen shoulder," which is difficult to treat success-fully. If you already have shoulder problems, see a physical therapist preoperatively for advice.

Any sport or exercise you did before your cancer, you can do now—and you should, if you want to. If you've been a fairly sedentary per-son, you might want to change that. You might also want to examine your eating habits, and health habits in general. Often people who have suffered life-threatening illnesses are more aware of the impor-tance of health than they were before, and want to invest energy into maintaining their health as much as they can.

26

Prosthesis and Reconstruction

If you've had a mastectomy, the first decision you'll probably want to deal with is whether, and how, to create the appearance of a breast. Most women take it for granted that they have to appear to the outside world as though they had both breasts. For years, there was only one way to do that—through a prosthesis, a sort of elaborate "falsie" designed for women with mastectomies (Fig. 26-1). Nowadays, there is also another option, the "reconstruction" of an artificial breast mound and nipple that will, to a greater or lesser extent, have the appearance of a real one.

Before you decide on one of these options you might want to consider a third possibility—not disguising your mastectomy at all. It's not a choice many women make, but there are a few who do choose it, without regrets. One of my patients thought about her options, then concluded that "a prosthesis sounded too uncomfortable, and reconstruction hasn't been around long enough to see what long-term effects it can have. And then I decided I was comfortable with the way I look." She goes to work, jogs in a loose T-shirt, and feels that "it's other people's problem if they're uncomfortable with it." Once in a while, she feels a need to look more "normal"—especially when she has important meetings with new business associates. Her solution is to stuff

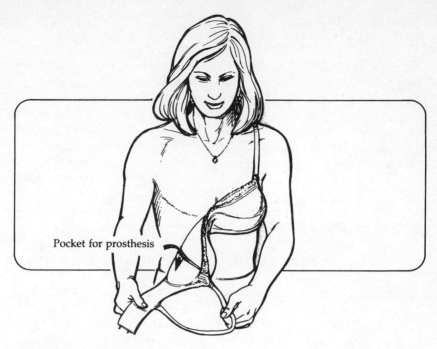

Pocket for prosthesis

FIGURE 26-1

shoulder pads from her dresses into her bra. "I never liked shoulder pads anyway," she laughs. "Now I get to put them to good use!" For other women, refusing to create the illusion of a breast is part of their feminist beliefs. Artist Matushka has created photographs of herself in a cutaway gown, showing not her remaining breast but the mastectomy scar. One photograph was on the cover of *The New York Times Magazine.* The effect is harsh and defiant, choosing to show the world what the disease of breast cancer does to a woman's body. Writer Deena Metzger,[1] whose book *Tree* addresses her cancer, has a photograph with a different approach: she softens the effect of the amputation by covering the scar with a beautiful, evocative tattoo of a tree, creating a new beauty where the beauty of her breast once was.

Having the self-confidence to feel comfortable without the appearance of a breast is wonderful, but most of us are products of our culture and need to feel that we are cosmetically acceptable to the outside world. In some cases there are actual penalties for failing to appear "normal." If nonconformity will cost you your job, for example, you're likely to want to wear a prosthesis (or "breast form," as it's also called) at least part of the time.

PROSTHESES

The option of wearing a prosthesis will probably be offered to you right away. In most areas of the country the hospital will arrange for someone to visit you to talk to you about prostheses while you're still in the hospital—your visitor will be either from Reach to Recovery (see Appendix B) or from a firm that sells prostheses. You can get a temporary prosthesis and then shop around for your permanent one. The prosthesis fits into a pocket in your bra. Usually you can buy them in medical supply houses or in fancy lingerie stores. Each environment has its advantages and disadvantages—in the former, you may be put off by the implications of mutilation, the wheelchairs, and artificial limbs; in the latter you might feel painfully reminded of the breast you no longer have. Your doctor or the American Cancer Society can help you find places to buy your prosthesis, or you can ask friends who've had mastectomies.

There are stores that will custom-make a prosthesis for you; it's expensive, and your insurance company may not pay for it, but it might be worth it to you to get a totally precise match. (In general, it's a good idea to check with your insurance company before buying your prosthesis anyway; different companies have different quirks, and you want to be sure of what your own expenses will and won't be.) If you're on Medicare, they'll pay for a prosthesis every year or two years—with a prescription. (Why you need a prescription for a prosthesis, I don't know—I've never met a woman who bought one for the fun of it—but the ways of bureaucracies are mysterious.) There are also specific forms for swimming, though most of the better prostheses are made of silicone and are thus waterproof to begin with.

If you live in a rural area where there are no lingerie shops or medical supply stores that carry prostheses, or if you find it too painful to approach a salesperson about buying one, several mail order catalogues also offer them, in a range of prices. I've seen them advertised in both women's wear catalogues and catalogues that specialize in health products for older people. These catalogues also sell mastectomy bras for the forms. You can also get them on the Internet; check out our website, www.SusanLoveMD.com. You can also find bathing suits tailored for the woman with a mastectomy from such catalogues as Land's End.

Prostheses come in a range of prices, with varying quality. If you haven't insurance to pay for your prosthesis, or if you're undecided yet as to whether you want a prosthesis or reconstruction, you'll probably want the least expensive form available, at least temporarily. Catalogues and many stores offer forms for as low as $15, and mastectomy bras for around $10.

Y-ME, a volunteer organization of breast cancer survivors (see Appendix B), will send prostheses, as well as wigs, to women who need them to deal with chemotherapy-induced hair loss, if they have the size required in stock, for a nominal fee.

Prostheses are made in different sizes, and they're also made for different operations. If you've had a radical mastectomy you can get a fuller prosthesis than if you've had a simple mastectomy. If you've had a wide excision that's left you noticeably asymmetrical, you can get a small "filler," or shell, that will fit comfortably in your bra. In the past, prostheses didn't have nipples, and this has caused some problems for women whose remaining breast had a prominent nipple. (Betty Rollin in her book *First, You Cry*,[2] has a very funny description of her efforts to make her own "nipple" out of cloth buttons.) Fortunately, that's changed: any prosthesis you buy will have a nipple, and you can get a separate nipple to attach to it if your own nipple is more prominent than the one on the prosthesis.

Some situations may affect what is the right prosthesis for you. Certain kinds of disabilities, for example, can make a particular prosthesis create further discomfort. Judith Rogers, an activist in Breast Health Access for Disabilities who has mild cerebral palsy, found that her first prothesis caused problems. "It was good in terms of matching the size of my remaining breast," she says. "But it was bad for my shoulder: it was too heavy for me. It pulled down, harming my muscles and increasing the effects of lymphedema." When she got rid of it and got a lighter one, she had less pain. You need to take into consideration all the factors involving your particular body and mind when you choose a prosthesis, and take your time deciding, if need be.

RECONSTRUCTION

Another option is reconstruction—the creation, by a plastic surgeon, of a new and natural-appearing breast. Breast reconstruction has made a big difference both physically and emotionally for many women who have had mastectomies. But it's important to understand its limits before you decide to have it done.

What's constructed is not a real breast. When it's well done, it will look real, but it will never have full sensation, as a breast does. Any surgeon who tells you "We're going to take off your breast and give you a new one, and it'll be as good as new" is either naive or dishonest. Sometimes they'll tell you that the new breast "feels normal"—at best, a half-truth. It will feel normal to the hand that's touching it, but it will have little sensation itself. However, feeling is only about one-half skin sensation and at least one-half cerebral. You may have some "feeling" return, but it will never feel completely normal to you. As one of my patients told me, you need to have time to bond with your new breast.

Is it worth doing, then? For many women, yes. It can make you feel more normal, to yourself and other people, since it looks like a breast. It can make you feel more balanced. And it can make your life a little easier—you can wear a T-shirt or a housedress and not worry about putting on a bra. If the doorbell rings while you're still in your bathrobe, you don't have to deal with whether or not you want the mail carrier to see your unevenness. It makes it easier to buy bathing suits and other "revealing" clothes. In *Why Me?* Rose Kushner explains why she decided to have reconstruction done. She was alone in a hotel room one night when she was awakened by the sound of the fire alarm and the smell of smoke. She jumped out of bed, threw on her clothing, grabbed her glasses, and ran. Downstairs in the lobby with the other guests, she realized that only she had gotten dressed; the others were all in their robes. Then she realized why: "This 'well-adjusted' mastectomee wasn't going anywhere publicly with one breast."[3]

A reconstruction can help some women put their cancer experiences behind them. As one of my patients said, "When I was wearing my prosthesis every day, when I looked at my body and it was concave where there had been a breast, I felt that I was a cancer patient, that I was living with that every single day. With the reconstruction I feel that I'm healthy again, that I can go on with my life." Another patient says that after her mastectomy, "I always felt the hollows under my arm. After my reconstruction, I put my arms down, and something was there. That's when the tears came; it was splendid to have that back."

On the other hand, it isn't necessarily right for everybody. One of my patients regretted her decision to have reconstruction. Displeased with the appearance of her reconstructed breast, she also felt that getting the reconstruction functioned as a form of denial. "It caused me to postpone the mourning I had to do over losing a breast," she says. "Instead of mourning the loss of a breast, I was thinking in terms of getting a breast. So it wasn't until the process was over, and I saw my new breast, which wasn't like my other breast, that it hit me that I'd lost a breast. If I had the decision to make now, I don't think I'd have reconstruction."

The best reconstructions look like real breasts—but not all operations are the best, and some look real only through bras or clothing.

Reconstructive surgery is done in a number of ways. There are two basic kinds—those using artificial substances and those using your own body. Within these categories, there are also variations. In the first category is the implant, which can be either silicone or saline (salt water). There has been much controversy about silicone, which we've discussed at length in Chapter 5. Although it was banned in 1992 by the FDA for use in breast enlargement, women who choose it for breast reconstruction still have access to it—at least as of this writing.

Although there have been two million implants used over the last 30 years there is still very little information about their long-term effects. The government study discussed in Chapter 5 is designed to change that. When the implant is done for breast reconstruction, there is no concern about interfering with mammography, and there is no evidence that implants interfere with the detection of recurrences.[4]

The procedure for both silicone and saline is the same. The disadvantage of the saline is that it may feel more like water than flesh and when it leaks the reconstruction completely collapses. The advantage is that when it does leak, it's harmless saline going into your body, and not silicone, with its possible dangers. We should note, however, that it is still encased in a silicone envelope. If the solid silicone is a problem (as of now we have no data) the move to saline will not eliminate it. The same holds true for other envelope substances now being used in experiments.

The implant is placed behind the pectoralis muscle and the skin is sewn together, which will give you a bulge (Fig. 26-2). The silicone has some weight and bounce to it, which will help it feel real. The problem is that it can't give you a very large breast because it's behind the muscle pushing everything forward and everything has to close over the top of it, so you're limited in size. Also the implant-reconstructed breast tends to stay firm, while your other breast may not. The implant won't gain and lose weight with you either. It works best in smaller-breasted women, or on women who have had bilateral mastectomies and are happy with small breasts. It's easier to do than any of the other operations. With the implant, your hospital stay won't be longer than usual. If you're having it done some time after your mastectomy, the hospital stay will be about two to three days.

My plastic surgeon colleague, Dr. William Shaw, has found in his practice that there are certain categories of women for whom implants are often a better choice than the other forms of reconstruction we discuss later. "For an elderly woman who wants something better than a prosthesis, something she can comfortably wear a bra and clothes over, it may make more sense. She is unlikely to be concerned about the problems 15 or 20 years down the line, and it's an easier operation than the others." At the other end of the spectrum is the younger woman with preschool children at home. "Often I find that a woman in this sit-

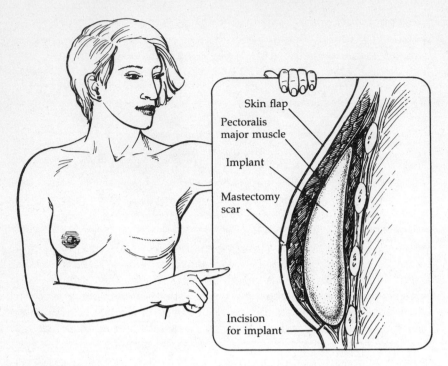

Skin flap

Pectoralis
major muscle

Implant

Mastectomy
scar

Incision
for implant

FIGURE 26-2

uation is most concerned with spending all the time she can with her
family—and five days longer in the hospital plus the recovery from a
flap surgery can make a big difference. Five or ten years later, she may
want to come back and have a flap operation—but for now she just
wants something to get by with."

A variation on the implant is the expander. A hollow, empty sack is
placed behind the muscle and everything is sewn closed. There's a little tube and a little valve on the sack, and gradually over the course of
three to six months the doctor injects more and more saline into it,
which stretches the skin out (Fig. 26-3). When it's become the size you
want, the sack is removed and replaced with a permanent saline or silicone sack. The disadvantage is that the process drags out over several
months, and while the skin and muscle are stretching, it can be uncomfortable. The expander will probably add no more days to your hospital stay, or, if done separately, it will keep you in the hospital about two
or three days.

In surgery there's always the danger of postoperative infection.
With the expander or an implant it can be more difficult to treat; since
they are foreign to your body any infection will not heal. One of my

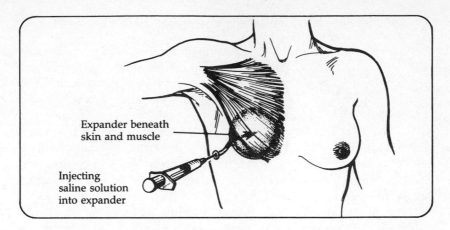

Expander beneath
skin and muscle

Injecting
saline solution
into expander

FIGURE 26-3

patients had a very bad infection and had to have the expander removed. Moreover, implants and expanders are more likely than other
procedures to necessitate your having something done to the other
breast to make it match. They're going to give you a nice, perfect, 17-
year-old's breast, and you're probably not a nice, perfect 17-year-old.
Since the reconstructed breast doesn't sag much, it may be higher than
you want it to be. One of my patients who was very unhappy with
her operation found this particularly displeasing. "The reconstructed
breast didn't look like my real breast, and it was much higher," she
says. "I had to start wearing a bra, which I don't like at all." So when
plastic surgeons tell you implants are the easiest form of reconstruction, requiring the least amount of surgery, it's true as far as it goes, but
you need to consider that it may end up involving more surgery, on the
other breast.

Because of this, it's important to let the plastic surgeon know what
size you want to be. I had a flat-chested patient who wanted an implant. She wanted to stay flat-chested; that was what she was used to
being. But the plastic surgeon had a difficult time believing that; he
was conditioned to thinking all women wanted large breasts. He kept
trying to persuade her to let him give her a larger implant and to enlarge her other breast to match it. Another of my patients had had silicone implants and the implant on one side had encapsulated. But she
liked the hard, firm, rocklike texture of that breast, and when she had a
mastectomy on the other breast, she wanted the reconstructed breast to
match the encapsulated one. The plastic surgeon again had a hard time
with that—it wasn't what women were supposed to want. If you know
what you want and your plastic surgeon argues with you, argue back

451

or change plastic surgeons. It's your body, not the surgeon's, and it's you who will live with that body.

When the operation works well and the patient's expectations are realistic, implants can make a wonderful difference in her life. As one of my patients says, "I forget it's there—it's a part of me now. It's a little harder than my other breast, but otherwise great: I don't have to worry about what I wear."

Dr. Shaw warns of one other hazard. As we discussed in Chapter 5, implants don't always last forever. For the woman who has had implants to enlarge her breasts, needing them replaced can be upsetting enough. For the mastectomee, it can be devastating. "It's like losing the breast all over again," he says. Such patients almost always need the flap reconstruction described below, since the fact that they have had problems with the implant suggests that they're likely to have further problems later on. "If you have problems with implants, I might take the implant out and do it again. I might even do it a second or third time. But the fourth time, I wouldn't. I don't think I can be any smarter the fourth time than I was, or the other surgeon was, the first three times." So patients need to weigh the comparative ease of the implant surgery against the inconvenience and emotional consequences of possible later surgeries.

I don't particularly favor either the implants or the expanders, though of course I would support whatever my patient wanted. But because of the inferior cosmetic effects, the mismatch with the other breast, the possibility of needing them replaced in the future, and the possible health problems with silicone, I don't personally think it's the wisest choice.

There are several procedures using your own tissue, and that's what I tend to favor. In the myocutaneous flap, a flap of skin, muscle, and fat is taken from another part of your body and moved. It's better than the silicone implant in the sense that it's your own tissue, and because you've got extra skin, it can make a bigger breast and a more natural droop. You may feel more normal externally, since it's real tissue, skin, and fat, though it will still have little sensation.

There are two different techniques for the myocutaneous flap. One is the pedicle, or attached flap (Fig. 26-4). Here the tissue is removed except for its feeding artery and vein, which remain attached, almost like a leash. The site from which the tissue was removed is sewn closed. The new little island of skin and muscle is then tunneled under the skin into the mastectomy wound. Since the blood vessels aren't cut, the blood supply remains.

The more recent operation is the "free flap," one of whose pioneers is Dr. Shaw. "Like all the other plastic surgeons, I did the tunnel procedure in the beginning. But then there were patients I couldn't do the

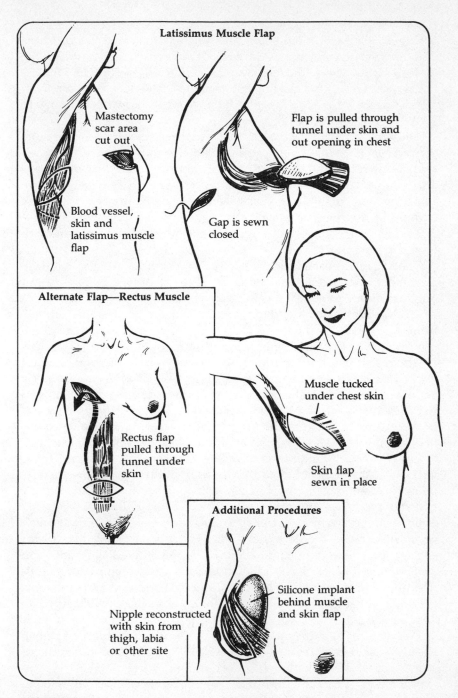

Latissimus Muscle Flap

Mastectomy scar area cut out

Flap is pulled through tunnel under skin and out opening in chest

Blood vessel, skin and latissimus muscle flap

Gap is sewn closed

Alternate Flap—Rectus Muscle

Muscle tucked under chest skin

Rectus flap pulled through tunnel under skin

Skin flap sewn in place

Additional Procedures

Nipple reconstructed with skin from thigh, labia or other site

Silicone implant behind muscle and skin flap

FIGURE 26-4

tunnel procedure on, because they'd had a gall bladder operation that cut across the upper muscle, or something like that. With the free flap, you don't have to disrupt the abdomen as much." In the free flap, the tissue is removed and the feeding artery and vein are cut. Then the tissue is moved to a new location and the artery and vein are sewn to an artery or vein in the armpit, with a microscope to allow the surgeons to see what they are doing.

The free flap is not limited to the abdomen. Free flaps can be done by transplanting tissue from other parts of the body to make a breast—such as from the buttock area (gluteal flap), from the hip area (deep circumflex iliac flap) from the lateral thigh (the tensor fascia lata flap), from the inner thigh (the gracilis flap), or from the opposite back (latissimus free flap). This means you can have a flap even if your abdomen has been scarred and take advantage of whatever abundance nature has granted you.

The advantage of the pedicle flap is that it's easier to do, so there are more plastic surgeons who can do it. A disadvantage is that we can only use tissue from locations that can stretch to the breast—the abdomen or the back. The other disadvantage is that in making the "tunnel" from where that tissue is to the breast, we have to disturb all the tissue en route, so we're disturbing a lot of your body surface. What this means is that you'll have a lot of long-term complications that aren't terribly serious but can be pretty uncomfortable. If we take it from the abdomen, your abdominal muscle will no longer be as strong and you won't be able to do things like sit-ups. One of my patients now has to wear a panty girdle all the time, to help support her weakened abdominal muscle. Another has found that since the operation the area around her upper abdomen is so sensitive that she can't wear anything with a waistband. I should add, however, that these problems are relatively rare, and most of my patients who have had the procedure have had few problems, and much satisfaction. If the tissue is taken from your back there will be fewer problems, although you may weaken your back somewhat. This may interfere with shoulder strength for special sports like mountain climbing or competitive swimming. You also may need more physical therapy. Some women have a lot of stiffness and pain after this flap because it throws their whole shoulder girdle off. In either case, you'll have a scar on the area from which the flap has been taken.

With the free flap, the operation is much harder because the surgeon has to be skilled at sewing blood vessels together under the microscope (Fig. 26-5). Most plastic surgeons aren't expert at it. However, in expert hands, the complications are much fewer, because the tissue in between doesn't have to be disturbed; less tissue is taken out, and it's simply removed and sewn closed. Further, because the tissue is re-

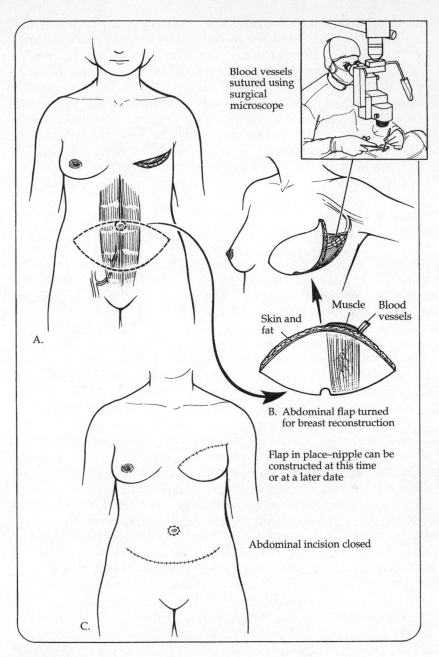

Blood vessels
sutured using
surgical
microscope

A.

Muscle   Blood
vessels

Skin and
fat

B. Abdominal flap turned
   for breast reconstruction

Flap in place–nipple can be
constructed at this time
or at a later date

Abdominal incision closed

C.

FIGURE 26-5

moved rather than tunneled through the body, it doesn't have to be taken from the back or the abdomen; it can come from anyplace there's anything extra. It can come from your buttocks, the saddle bags on your thighs, or anyplace else (Fig. 26-6). It's about five to eight hours of surgery, and you'll probably be in the hospital for four to seven days. If the blood supply gets messed up, part of the flap can die off, and further surgery will be necessary. The patient I mentioned earlier, who had gotten an infection from her silicone expanders, was unable to have either the latissimus or rectus procedure, because of medical problems she had had in her back and abdomen. The free-gluteous flap was the only alternative she had left, and, though it was difficult surgery involving a long healing period, she feels it was well worth the pain and inconvenience involved.

When I was practicing at UCLA I worked with Dr. Shaw—the best expert in the country—on this procedure, and we had great results. In this kind of situation I favor free flaps for reconstruction. It's really been the "Cadillac" operation, and it's not available everywhere. But this is beginning to change. Dr. Shaw says the free flap is being increasingly used in the United States.

In the last two or three years a new variation of the free flap was introduced by Dr. Robert Allen of New Orleans, the so-called perforator flap. Instead of taking some muscle with the free flap, the surgeon dissects the arteries that perforate through the muscle to the skin, and thus spares the muscle completely. It was found that, with a sufficient number of perforators to support the skin and fat, one does not need to take any muscle at all. While there may be obvious theoretical advantages to not taking muscle, this approach does add some tedious dissection through the muscle and possibly a small risk of complications related to this portion of the dissection. Thus, in the end, it becomes a practical decision as to whether it's worthwhile to do the extra dissection to save a little bit of muscle. According to Dr. Shaw, the concept of the perforator flap has been very helpful in focusing our attention on the perforators (the perforating arteries) rather than the amount of muscle. As a result, there's a tendency to take less and less muscle and do what's called a "muscle sparing" free flap. Sometimes it's obvious that there are large perforators which would make dissection fairly easy; then it's worthwhile to do a perforator flap. If the perforator vessel runs in the muscle for a long distance, then it may not be worth the trouble involved, says Dr. Shaw. The issue of back problems in the TRAM (trans rectus abdominus muscle) flap is not significant in most cases. In fact, there are patients who claim their back problems have improved after the abdomen is tightened by the TRAM flap operation. With the current "muscle sparing" flap techniques, it's unlikely that the abdominal wall function is altered enough to increase the number of back problems.

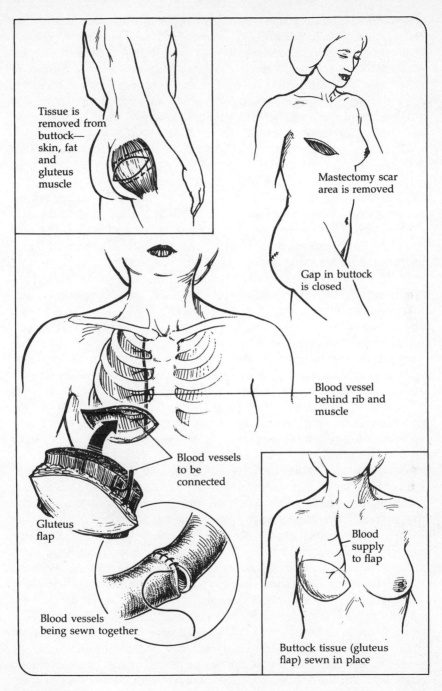

Tissue is removed from buttock—skin, fat and gluteus muscle

Mastectomy scar area is removed

Gap in buttock is closed

Blood vessel behind rib and muscle

Blood vessels to be connected

Gluteus flap

Blood vessels being sewn together

Blood supply to flap

Buttock tissue (gluteus flap) sewn in place

FIGURE 26-6

Another alternative is to do a combination operation, using the latissimus flap and a silicone implant behind it (see Fig. 26-4). This can be useful because of problems with the abdominal area. The reasons for choosing latissimus flap and silicone implants are twofold: it is technically a little bit easier and does not require microsurgery, so it can be done by more surgeons; and sometimes the abdomen is not suitable because of insufficient volume in a very thin patient or previous surgery (abdominoplasty or TRAM flap).

With this flap, you'll probably be in the hospital for four or five days; the stitches will be out in two to three weeks, and by five or six weeks, you'll be ready for a fully active lifestyle again.

As I noted earlier, both versions of the flap procedure require highly trained plastic surgeons. There aren't that many of those surgeons around, and it might be virtually impossible for you to find the one you need. There are far more plastic surgeons in the country who can do the simpler procedures of the implant or expander.

To decide what's best for you, discuss it with your surgeon and separately with a plastic surgeon. They will look at you and your body, see how your body hangs together and how your breasts look before your surgery, and tell you what kind of procedure they think would be best for you. Make sure you ask them which procedures they are familiar with and do regularly. Often a woman has come to me who has been told she's not a candidate for a flap, when in reality the plastic surgeon she saw just doesn't know how to do the operation.

My Boston colleague Robert Goldwyn, who has done many reconstructions, points out something crucial: you should always be shown pictures of the best and the worst results your plastic surgeon has had. Some doctors will show women only the best results—an act he compares to false advertising. It's important for you to know the limits of what the procedure can do for you, and the risks you run of having far-from-ideal results. Dr. Shaw concurs, and emphasizes the importance of demanding absolute honesty from your plastic surgeon.

Any of these procedures can be done immediately, or at some later time. The advantage of having it done immediately is that you don't have to face another operation later; your regular surgeon performs your mastectomy and then, while you're still under anesthesia, the plastic surgeon comes in and does the reconstruction. In my experience, many women don't have reconstruction because they don't want to go through more surgery. The disadvantages are that it's a longer time in the operating room (usually about six to eight hours) and it's harder to schedule, since you have to get the surgeon and the plastic surgeon at the same time. When reconstruction is done immediately the surgeon often performs a skin-sparing mastectomy (see Chapter 25). This makes it easier for the plastic surgeon to close the incision over the implant or flap.

At UCLA, while I did the mastectomy, the plastic surgery team was working on the flap in the abdomen. (If the tissue was taken from the buttocks or back, I operated with the patient lying on her side.) By the time I'd finished the mastectomy they were ready to start moving the flap up. Through this teamwork approach, we were able to get the time down to about four or five hours.

When we were done, the patient was taken to the "flap room," a three-bed room that's sort of an intensive care unit for the flap—not for the patient, for the flap. The concern was that something would happen in the area where the blood vessels were sewn together, and the blood supply would get blocked, which would cause the flap to turn black and die. So they carefully monitored the flap with temperature probes taped to the flap, and if the flap started getting cold, it alerted the surgeons that the blood supply might be compromised.

Whether you've had your surgery at a facility like the UCLA center or not, you'll come out of anesthesia feeling like a Mack truck just hit you. You've had hours of surgery on both your breast and your abdomen, back, or buttocks. There's continuous pain medication you can get through an IV with a button you can press so that you can control the timing. You're kept in bed rest for one to two days, and you have a catheter so you don't have to get up and go to the bathroom. By about the third or fourth day you start feeling a little better, and you can get out of bed and walk around a bit. You're usually in the hospital about four to six days altogether. There are drains placed in the abdominal scars as well as in the chest. Usually you won't have much pain in your chest, which will feel numb, but your abdomen, or the other area the tissue has been taken from, will hurt a lot.

So it's certainly an ordeal to go through. The ordeal continues for a time, in a milder form—you'll probably end up getting a second operation for final touch-ups, and to make a nipple if you want one. Sometimes after the operation there will be a little too much tissue one place or another, so they do some fine-tuning. It won't hurt because it's numb.

But it's usually worth it. You do recuperate after a while—we've even done it on elderly women who have other medical problems, and it's worked for them. The cosmetic effects are superior.

If the free TRAM is the operation you want, you should take the time to research and find out who in your area can do it. If there's no one in your area, and you still want that form of reconstruction, you can always wait, have the mastectomy first, and then go find the right plastic surgeon when your treatment is done.

It's also possible that you won't be sure at first whether you want reconstruction. Both Dr. Shaw and Dr. Goldwyn say that some premastectomy patients they see are too upset by the cancer and the prospect of a mastectomy to make yet another major decision at the time. When they come across this kind of ambivalence, they suggest the patient have her mastectomy, take whatever time she needs to deal with it, and then, when she feels ready, come back if she still wants reconstruction.

According to Dr. Shaw, reconstruction is much better organized and understood by the patient these days. Also, diagnosis of breast cancer is accepted by patients in a much less frightened and more rational way and women today are better informed about breast cancer. Dr. Shaw notes a change in the last 20 years: many women, he says, actually welcome the opportunity to discuss reconstruction and long-term appearance immediately. There are obviously some who cannot handle the additional decision-making related to reconstruction, but they're becoming a minority.

Many plastic surgeons don't like to do immediate reconstruction because it's a new procedure and they're leery of it. If you want it done and the surgeon tries to argue you out of it, don't give up—just look for a surgeon who's had experience and is comfortable with it.

There is no time limit for reconstruction. In fact, current techniques have made it a better option than it used to be. If you had a mastectomy in the past and are now thinking about reconstruction, you should feel encouraged. Even with a radical mastectomy, reconstruction is still possible. Or if you'd decided against reconstruction, and now want to reconsider, that's also fine. (I've had patients who've had their mastectomies in the winter and didn't want reconstruction, and then decided in the summer, when they wanted to wear bathing suits and sundresses, that maybe it was a good idea after all.) Women with bilateral mastectomies can have both sides reconstructed—and to any reasonable size they'd like. If you were an A cup and always wanted to be a C, now you can do it!

Once the new breast is on, you can also get a nipple made. We don't do it right away because the surgeon needs to be sure it's in the right place. There's a lot of swelling after reconstructive surgery, so we need to wait till that's gone down and the nipple is placed on the breast as it will look permanently. It will look "real," and match the color of your original nipple. Sometimes the skin from your inner thigh is used, since it's darker than breast skin. Sometimes a surgeon can just make a nipple from the tissue in the flap and tattoo an areola. Whether or not you want to bother with the nipple depends on why you want the reconstruction. If it's just for convenience, you may decide against it. If you want the new breast to look as real as possible, you'll probably want the nipple. Again, it's your decision—you're the one who'll go through the surgery, and you're the one who'll live with the results. I've had a couple of patients who, before they had the nipple put on, showed their reconstruction to anyone who was curious—then once the nipple was on, they didn't want to show it. Somehow it felt more like a real breast, and displaying it seemed suddenly immodest.

Breast reconstruction depends on the patient's goal. Some women are very concerned about symmetry; many others aren't. Do you want to look good in your clothes, or is it important that a new lover won't even know you've had surgery? Do you want to have your remaining breast altered to achieve a more perfect match? These are not foolish concerns, and you should never hesitate to look for what you want out of guilt over "vanity." You've been through an unpleasant and life-changing experience; you're entitled to do what you can to make its aftermath as comfortable as possible for yourself. Talk with your plastic surgeon about all the possibilities, and decide what's best for you. Dr. Shaw warns against looking for one universal operation that's best for every patient. "One of the mistakes surgeons and patients both make is to act as if breast reconstruction is some kind of product you can compare objectively—what's the best airplane? But one thing I've learned over the years is that there's no one operation that's best for everyone."

Today, a reasonably good breast reconstruction can be achieved after mastectomy using expanders and implants or with one's own tissue from the abdomen, buttocks, back, or thighs. To achieve symmetry between the nonmastectomy breast and the reconstructed breast, however, sometimes requires alteration of the normal breast—to reshape, reduce, or enlarge it. In cases of a large, droopy breast on the normal side, various reduction techniques can be utilized to make that breast smaller to match the reconstructed breast. If the breast volume is satisfactory, then the breast can be reshaped by "mastopexy" techniques to lift the nipple and reshape the breast. Occasionally, when the normal breast is too small, it may be augmented by placing an implant behind the muscle. This should be done cautiously because the implant-augmented breast tends to be firmer without the natural droop, thus presenting a potential problem for achieving symmetry if the opposite is done with one's own tissue. Also, one needs to be careful about potential problems in the follow-up of this breast in terms of palpation or mammography. In high-risk patients, this would not be a good idea.

Whatever you decide, check with your insurance company. Some companies will pay for either a prosthesis or reconstruction but not one and then the other, and that might affect your decision.

The Unacceptable Reconstruction

Sometimes reconstruction isn't entirely successful—it may not give you the look you want or it may be a source of pain or medical problems. It can be a source of unpleasant sensations ranging from pins and needles, to burning, to sharp pain. You may just find it hard to adapt to the feel of an implant. An implant may seem solid, even rocklike, to the touch. The breast's hardness certainly isn't due to the saline implant but to the scar tissue that has formed around it, encasing it in a tough capsule.

Sometimes plastic surgeons focus on crafting "the perfect breast," not on replicating the patient's natural breast. Even when an implant matches the breast, the new breast is often heavier, because the implant and scar tissue weigh more than breast tissue. The result is often a breast that is too big, or feels too big.

Because surgeons see women lying on an operating table, they see breasts from a different perspective than do the women, who usually see themselves standing before a mirror. As a result they may misjudge the way a breast will fall when the woman is on her feet (see Chapter 5). If it is a good match for her other breast, which appears flatter when she is lying on her back, it will probably be smaller when the woman stands up.

Occasionally, the new nipple (which is not a true nipple but is tissue that has been taken from another part of the body or that has been tattooed to resemble a nipple) is higher or lower than the nipple on the other breast. If the nipple is applied while the reconstructed tissue is still swollen from the surgery, it may no longer match when the swelling goes down.

You don't have to simply resign yourself to your problem. A plastic surgeon can cut away hard scar tissue and replace implants, exchange an implant for a flap, reduce or enlarge a breast, or lift and reorient nipples.

Technology is improving, and so are surgical techniques, as experience with the procedure—and the demand for it—grows. Get a referral to a plastic surgeon from a friend or your breast surgeon, explain your problem, and have the plastic surgeon outline a plan for correcting it. If possible, get a second opinion. Again, ask for pictures of the plastic surgeon's best and worst outcomes.

Occasionally, if the skin has been altered by radiation, or is not elastic enough to make additional reconstructive surgery advisable, the best course may be to remove the implant and get a prosthesis instead.

Partial Reconstruction After Lumpectomy

When a patient has a poor result from wide excision, many times a reasonable result can still be achieved by one of two methods. If the breast is large enough in overall volume the surgeon can often "rearrange" the breast tissue and perform a customized "mastopexy" to reshape the breast. This usually involves lifting the nipple up and moving the breast tissue around some to fill in the depressed areas. Usually, a similar procedure with a slight reduction is needed in the opposite breast to achieve symmetry. Other times, the problem of a distorted, depressed breast after wide excision can be corrected by replacing some volume back into that depressed area. That is usually done by taking a flap of tissue from under the arm and then transposing it into the defect or taking part of the latissimus muscle and the skin and fat over it and moving it into the defect. In this way the reconstructed breast is made up entirely with the patient's own tissue; therefore, it can easily be examined by palpation or mammogram.

Women who have had a large amount of tissue removed and have a poor cosmetic result can have a delayed partial reconstruction. The cosmetic results are good, and we have found that the flap tissue doesn't obstruct a mammogram. The one thing you shouldn't do—and this is very important—is to get a small silicone or saline implant put in the remaining breast tissue. We can't mammogram through an implant. If the woman has a recurrence it's likely to be in the same area—the area that's obscured with the implant. When women have an implant for augmentation there are techniques we can use to push the implant back and take a mammogram. When an implant is used to fill out the breast after a lumpectomy, it is in the middle of the breast tissue so it is always in the way. A flap, however, uses the body's own tissue, which is mostly fat, so it won't block the mammogram.

Contralateral Mastectomy for Symmetry

There is another possible alternative, one that some women request. If your only aesthetic concern is asymmetry, you can have both breasts removed. While this destroys a perfectly healthy breast, it does make it possible to wear loose shirts without wearing a bra. I had only one patient who chose this route, and she had to fight with her insurance company to get them to pay for the removal of the healthy breast. She told them that since they paid for reconstruction for symmetry they should pay for a contralateral mastectomy for symmetry. I would warn any woman considering this option that she should think of it only in cosmetic terms: it won't guarantee that she'll never again have breast cancer (see Chapter 23), although it may decrease her risk.

27

Radiation Therapy

The idea of radiation therapy may make you nervous. After all, radiation can cause cancer, and the last thing you want is to find yourself in danger of even more cancer: you've got quite enough now, thank you. But the doses given in radiation therapy rarely cause cancer, and often cure it. We've discussed this at length in Chapter 23.

As a form of local control (treatment of an original cancer), radiation is more effective in some kinds of cancer than in others; it's been very effective with breast cancer.

Radiation is often used in conjunction with surgery, so you might have had a lumpectomy (or even a mastectomy) before your radiation. It works best when it has comparatively few cells to attack—it's least effective on large chunks of cancer. So we try, if possible, to do the surgery first, getting rid of most of the tumor surgically and then cleaning up what's left with radiation.

In the old days, we used cobalt as a source of radiation. Most places now use radiation generated by electricity in machines called linear accelerators. The edges of the beam from this type of machine are "sharper." Also, the treatment is planned more precisely, with newer planning machines called simulators. Even so, there is still internal scatter, which can affect other spots. Some women who have been treated for Hodgkin's disease now have breast cancer. Though it's unfortunate, radiation therapy is important treatment and if the Hodgkin's had gone untreated the women probably would have died long ago. In any event, this presents a challenge for breast conservation.

In the early days of radiation, women who were radiated after a mastectomy for breast cancer often developed other problems because of the radiation. If the machine is aimed straight-on at the breast, the lungs also get radiated and, if it's the left breast, so does the heart. Some studies show that women whose left breasts were radiated after they had mastectomies had a higher incidence of heart disease 20 years later than other women—including women whose right breasts were radiated.[1]

We've come a long way since those days. We've refined the process of administering radiation so that it's possible to treat the breast tissue while sparing most of the adjacent normal tissue. We administer the radiation in tangents to the breast, so that it goes through the breast tissue of one breast and out into air, and much less gets into your heart or lung (Fig. 27-1).

Like surgery, radiation is a localized treatment. (Chemotherapy, given through an injection or a pill, goes through your bloodstream and affects your entire body.) It's aimed at a very specific area and affects only that area. It's usually administered by a machine called a linear accelerator, which accelerates charged particles and shoots them at

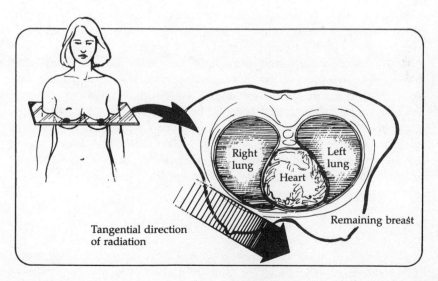

Right lung Left lung Heart Remaining breast

Tangential direction of radiation

FIGURE 27-1

a target that generates photons. These photons are aimed directly at the body part they're intended for, as a beam. The beam is sharpened in the head of the machine to minimize scatter.

As we discussed in Chapter 23, radiation complements lumpectomy as an alternative to mastectomy. Sometimes it is also used with mastectomy. The original treatment used for breast cancer was mastectomy. But the early surgeons soon began to notice that some patients still didn't do well. There were certain predictors for which patients did badly, based on the grave signs we discussed in Chapter 21: very large tumors, a lot of positive lymph nodes, involvement of the skin. So in these cases postoperative radiation was used after the mastectomy. For a long time, in the 1960s and 1970s, most women who had mastectomies and also had danger signs, especially positive lymph nodes, would get cobalt—the form of radiation used then. You hear some real horror stories from those days—burns to the esophagus, skin burns, etc. Then we did a study to see how well it was working. We discovered that it wasn't; the survival rate remained the same. We were decreasing local recurrence—recurrence in the chest wall or the scar—but this didn't seem to cure anyone. The cancer had already spread.

When it became clear that the problem was really systemic, we began using adjuvant chemotherapy, and that did affect cure rates. So postmastectomy radiation was dropped. We decided to radiate only women who actually had a recurrence in the chest wall. It was thought that in most women chemotherapy itself would work to prevent local recurrence.

But over the past 15 or 20 years, as adjuvant chemotherapy has improved survival, we're seeing more local recurrences. Chemotherapy, which does so well at stopping cancer that's spread outside the immediate area, doesn't help the immediate area itself. Even women who had stem cell rescue or bone marrow transplants—the process that gives the highest dose of chemotherapy—still had a high local recurrence. So now most of the protocols for bone marrow transplant include both mastectomy and radiation. There's a move back to doing postmastectomy radiation in certain groups of patients—those most at risk for recurrence after mastectomy, such as the ones with over four positive nodes, lymphatic vascular invasion, or a large tumor.

INITIAL CONSULTATION

Radiation oncologists (who are always M.D.'s) like to see patients soon after the biopsy—ideally while they still have the lump, to get a firsthand sense of the tumor. At UCLA we would all see the patients as a team. Sometimes the initial consultation would be in the radiation therapy department and involve a team approach, including a specially trained radiation nurse who inquired into the patient's needs, taking into account her emotional response to her cancer. The consultation involved a physical exam as well as conversation with the patient.

This first visit to a radiation oncologist doesn't mean you'll necessarily have radiation treatments. The radiation oncologist will talk with you and get your medical history, do an examination, review your x rays and slides from any surgery you may have had done, and talk with your primary doctor, your surgeon, and your medical oncologist if you have one. They will then come up with a recommendation. Make sure you are offered options. Ask the question: what is my risk of local recurrence with and without radiation therapy? If the choice of radiation does seem appropriate to you, you'll be sent for a planning session and whatever x rays are needed after surgery (see Chapters 25 and 26), if any has been done.

There are issues that may enter into the decision about whether or not to use radiation. One is that if you have large breasts the equipment they have may or may not be able to accommodate them. You may need to find a center that has the correct equipment. Breast size should *not* be a criterion for excluding radiation.

Another issue is that a bit of the lung gets radiated, and if you have chronic lung disease, that can be dangerous. So with patients who have conditions like chronic obstructive pulmonary disease or emphysema we often do the planning session (see below) just to do the measurements—to see how much lung will be affected and whether or not it will be safe for them to have radiation therapy. By having the woman lie on her stomach, they are able to spare more lung tissue.

Women with collagen vascular diseases like lupus or scleroderma, can have increased skin reaction in response to radiation, so they are usually not good candidates either.

Previous radiation to the chest is usually a contraindication to breast radiation. Your radiation oncologist should carefully review your previous treatment records to assess whether it's safe to give you breast radiation.

In any of these cases, when the potential risks of radiation are greater than the potential gains, a mastectomy should be done rather than lumpectomy and radiation.

Since radiation therapy after mastectomy is done primarily to prevent a recurrence in the chest wall or scar, there is a choice as to whether to do it now or later. In those women who have conditions precluding radiation therapy, it may be better to wait and attempt it only if there is a local recurrence.

THE PLANNING SESSION

Usually you'll wait at least two weeks after surgery before the planning session, to make sure everything's healed and you can get your arm up over your head comfortably.

The session takes about an hour. You put on a johnny and lie on a table with your arm lifted and resting on a form above your head. Over you there's a machine, similar to the radiation machine, called a "simulator" (Fig. 27-2). It doesn't actually give radiation, but it uses the same energy as a chest x-ray machine. You are imaged in the same position you'll keep for treatments. A lot of measurements and technical x rays are taken to map where your ribs are in relation to your breast tissue, where your heart is in relation to your ribs, etc., figuring out precisely how that area of your body looks (Fig. 27-3). Depending on what area of your body is going to be radiated, you may also be sent for x rays, a CAT scan, or ultrasound to get more information. Then they'll put all the information into a computer, which calculates specifically the angles at which the area of your body should be radiated. In some cases they'll actually make a mold for you to hold your arm in, so that you'll

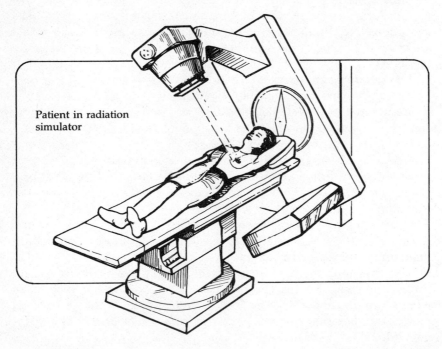

Patient in radiation simulator

FIGURE 27-2

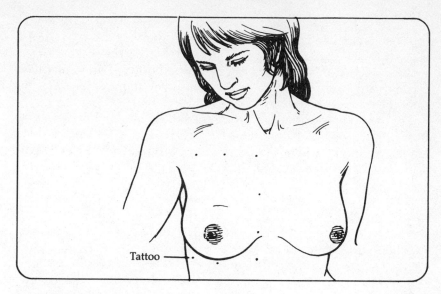

Tattoo

FIGURE 27-3

be in the same position every day. Women with very large breasts are sometimes treated lying on their stomach.

Before the treatments start, the radiation oncologist will mark out the area of the breast that's going to be treated. In most cases it is only the breast. Sometimes it's the breast and lymph nodes. You should be aware that the breast and the lymph node areas will be treated from different angles, thus covering a fairly large area of your chest. Many doctors use tattoos, which are permanent little blue dots, to outline the area to be radiated (see Fig. 27-3). There are a couple of reasons for that. One is to be sure that during the treatment they use the same "landmarks" and position you exactly the same way every time. The other is to make sure that in the future a radiation oncologist will know you've had radiation in that area, since you can only be radiated once on any given spot. So if, for example, you get cancer in the other breast, and the area is near that of the previous cancer, the tattoo mark will tell the radiation oncologist where the field that can be radiated ends. I found them useful because often when I was doing a follow-up exam on a patient whose surgery wasn't terribly extensive, I couldn't remember which breast was treated—it can be a year or so after the last exam. So I looked for the tattoo, and that let me know.

Although the dots may be cosmetically displeasing, they're not going to turn you into Lydia the Tattooed Lady—they're tiny and, depending on your skin coloring, can be invisible. One radiation nurse I

469

know says, "I've had patients call me up and say, 'I've washed my tat-toos off—I can't find them!'" Some doctors use Magic Markers, espe-cially if the patient is adamant about not having tattoos; the problem with this is that the markings can be washed off, and you don't have this guidance for the doctors working with you in the future. You can limit the number of tattoos to four.

The tattooing can be somewhat uncomfortable, like pinpricks, or bee stings at worst. The other discomfort patients sometimes feel is a stiff arm; especially after recent surgery it can be awkward to lie with your arm above your head for 20 minutes.

THE TREATMENTS

Radiation treatments are scheduled, paced out, once a day, for a given number of weeks. Time-consuming though this is, it's necessary, since if you get too much radiation all at once your skin will have a bad reac-tion and it increases the complications. The treatment schedule varies from place to place. Usually it's given in two parts. First, the breast as a whole is radiated, from the collarbone to the ribs and the breastbone to the side, making sure all the area is treated, including, if necessary, lymph nodes. This is the major part of the treatment, and will last about five weeks, often using about 4500–5000 rads or centigrays of radiation (a chest x ray is a fraction of a rad). If there are microscopic cancer cells in the breast, this should get rid of them. After this, the "boost" (described later) is given. In the spring of 2000 a provocative study from Canada compared three weeks of radiation to the tradi-tional six. With 4.6 years of follow-up there was no difference in the two groups. If these results can be replicated we may soon be complet-ing radiation much faster.[2]

How soon after the planning session the treatment begins varies from hospital to hospital, depending on how many radiation patients there are, how much room is in the radiation department, and how large the staff is. Sometimes it will be between two weeks and a month, and often patients worry that the delay will cause the cancer to spread. Though the wait doesn't pose any real danger of the cancer worsening, it can be emotionally hard on the patient.

There may be delays for other reasons. Depending on the status of the lymph nodes, you may be getting chemotherapy first, and your doctors may not want you to get both treatments at the same time. As we mentioned earlier, with some drugs, such as CMF (see Chap-ter 23), you can have chemo and radiation together; with others, like Adriamycin, you usually have the chemo first and then the radiation. Sometimes they're given in a sandwichlike sequence: chemotherapy, then radiation, then more chemotherapy.

There are important skin-care guidelines to follow during your treatment. You should use a mild soap, such as Ivory, Pears, or Neutrogena. During the course of your treatment don't use soaps with fragrance, deodorants, or any kind of metal. All of these can interact with the radiation, and it's important to avoid them. Don't use deodorant on the side that's being treated; almost all deodorants have lots of aluminum. Through the course of the treatment you can use a light dusting of cornstarch as a deodorant; it's usually pretty effective, though it varies from patient to patient. But don't use talcum powder.

When you go for your first treatment, it's wise to bring someone with you for support. You're facing the unknown, and that's usually scary. Most patients don't feel the need to have someone with them after the first session.

For the treatment itself, you'll change into a johnny from the waist up. It's wise to wear something two-piece so you only have to remove your upper clothing. You can wear earrings or bracelets, but no neck jewelry. After you've changed, you'll be taken into a waiting room; the wait may be longish, and varies from place to place and day to day, so you may want to bring a good book or your Walkman. Then you're taken into the treatment room. You're only there for about 10 minutes, and most of that time is spent with the technologist setting up the machine and getting you ready. There's a table that looks like a regular examining table and, above it, the radiation machine (Fig. 27-4). You lie down on the table, and a plastic or Styrofoam form is placed under your head. This has an armrest above your head, in which you'll hold your arm during the treatment. When you're set up, the technologist leaves the room and turns on the machine. The radiation isn't given all at once; it's done a number of times from different angles—twice if only the breast is radiated, more if lymph nodes are also being treated. The technician will position you, leave, turn on the machine for a little less than a minute, come back in, reposition the machine, and go out again. If you're claustrophobic, you may find lying under the machine a little uncomfortable, but it doesn't last long, and the machine itself never moves down toward you.

Radiation therapy units have cameras, so they can see you while you're being treated, and an intercom system, so that if you're anxious and need to talk with the technologist, you can. If a friend or family member comes with you, many hospitals allow them in the room outside the treatment room. They can watch on the monitor and are able to hear you through the intercom. The most important thing for you to do during the treatment is to keep still. You can breathe normally, but don't move otherwise.

Your blood may be drawn during the course of the treatments—once at the beginning of the therapy process, or maybe once a few weeks later, to make sure there's no drop in your blood count. This

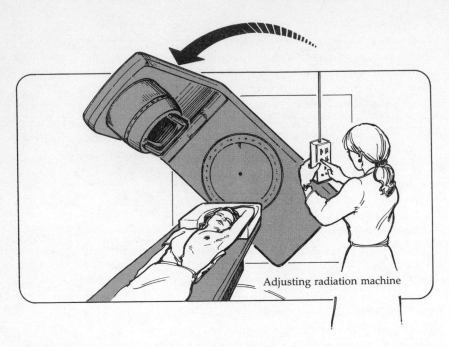

Adjusting radiation machine

FIGURE 27-4

usually isn't a problem with breast cancer, since there's not much bone marrow treated, but we do it to check, especially in patients who have had chemotherapy.

THE BOOST

After a course of radiation to treat your breast, you'll be given a boost—an extra amount of radiation on the spot where the tumor was. The boost is done in one of two ways. The more recent, and more frequently used, boost is done by the electron beam. Electrons are a special kind of charged particle that gives off energy that doesn't penetrate very deeply, so it's good if the original tumor wasn't very deep. The electron boost is given by a machine; it's aimed at the area where the tumor was. It doesn't require hospitalization.

The other type of boost is a radioactive implant (brachytherapy), inserted either under general anesthetic or under local anesthetic and some kind of sedation (Fig. 27-5). This had been used more often in the past, but is now being reconsidered as the only treatment for small tumors. Thin plastic tubing hooked like thread into a needle is drawn through the breast where the biopsy was done. Then the tubing is left in and the needle withdrawn. The number of tubes varies; sometimes

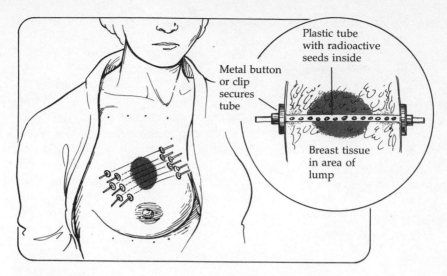

Plastic tube
with radioactive
seeds inside

Metal button
or clip
secures
tube

Breast tissue
in area of
lump

FIGURE 27-5

they are inserted in two layers. Small radioactive pellets called iridium seeds, which give off high energy for a very short distance, are put into the tubes, "boosting" the immediate area of the biopsy. This implant is left in for about 36–48 hours. It varies depending on how active the seeds are, how big your breast is, and how big the tumor is.

This radiation can be picked up by people around you, although not in large doses. Normally, that's no problem, but for some people, like pregnant women, exposure to even that much radiation could be dangerous, so you can't be out in crowds during the time the tubing is in. Thus you're usually kept in the hospital with a sign on the door saying "Caution: radioactive." At the end of about 36 hours, both the radioactive sources and the tubes are removed, a process that requires no anesthesia, and, unless there's some other reason for you to stay hospitalized, you can go home.

Whether the electron boost or the implant boost or no boost is used depends on a variety of factors—the amount of surgery you had, the size of your tumor, the size of your breast, and the equipment available to your radiation oncologist. Some oncologists have no electron machine available; some haven't had training in the implant procedure; some simply prefer one treatment to the other.

When both options are available, the doctor will often choose one based on the amount of surgery that's been done. When we first started doing lumpectomy and radiation we tended just to take out the lump and then radiate the breast to clean up the margins, and then we used the implant. Now the trend is to do more surgery, taking out more tissue to obtain clean margins, and to use a boost, the electron beam.

What most people find hardest to deal with is the time the treatments take. They last for six weeks in total, five days a week. If your workplace and home are fairly near the hospital, you may be able to come right before or after work. Otherwise, you may have to cut into the middle of the workday, or take time off from your job. Some mothers use babysitters; others bring their children to the hospital, along with a friend who stays with them while the mother has her treatment. If your children are old enough to be curious, or are scared at not knowing what's going on, you might want to have them wait in the room directly outside the treatment room, where you'll be visible on two monitors and can talk with them through an intercom. This can demystify the process and alleviate the children's fear.

SIDE EFFECTS

The side effects of radiation depend on the part of the body that's being treated. If it's the breast and you have soft bones you may have asymptomatic rib fractures, which you won't feel but which will show up on x ray. Depending on how your chest is built, a little of the radiation may get to your lung and give you a cough. Your radiation oncologist will tell you about all the possible side effects before your treatment starts. Also, it's a good idea to ask to talk to someone who has already been treated.

You'll usually have some kind of mild "sunburn" effect. The severity varies considerably from patient to patient—one person will get a severe skin rash while another will barely be bothered at all. Unlike the case with sunburn, fairness of skin isn't relevant.

The other major symptom virtually every radiation therapy patient has is tiredness. I used to think this was because of the amount of time involved in the treatment, but there's more and more evidence that, like anesthesia (see Chapter 25), radiation itself creates tiredness. The body seems to be using up all its resources to cope with the radiation, and doesn't have much energy for anything else. The fatigue usually gets worse toward the end of the treatment, and its severity depends on what else is going on in your life, so you'll probably want to cut back on your activities somewhat if at all possible. The fatigue may last several months after the treatment has finished, and it may even begin after the course of treatment is over.

The extent of the fatigue varies greatly. One of my patients, a lawyer, had no problem working a full day, but says she "didn't feel like going out for dinner after work." For others, the fatigue is extremely unpleasant. One of my patients compared hers to the effects of infectious hepatitis, which she'd had years before. "The symptoms sound very nondescript," she says, "but I felt really rotten. I was tired all the time—not the tiredness you feel after a hard day's work, which I've always found fairly pleasant. My body just felt wrong—like I was always coming down with the flu. Some days I couldn't function at all—I had to keep a cot at my job." She also experienced peculiar appetite changes. "My body kept craving lemon, spinach, and roast beef—I ate them constantly, and I couldn't make myself eat anything else."

When the breast is being radiated, it may sometimes swell and get more sensitive; if you're used to sleeping on your stomach, you may find that uncomfortable. As we discussed in the last chapter, one trick is to hold a pillow between your breasts and sleep on the side that hasn't been treated. This sensitivity, like the other side effects, can take months to disappear, and you may find that breast especially sore or sensitive when you're premenstrual.

Interestingly, few of my patients get depressed during radiation, but many get depressed afterwards—possibly because, time-consuming as the treatments are, there is a sense of activity, of doing something to fight the cancer, and when it's done, there's a sense of letdown. This really shouldn't be too surprising. It happens in dozens of other intense situations, like the classical postpartum depression, or the feelings that occur when any time-consuming structure in your life is over—a job you've worked at, the end of a school term. This may be the time to get involved in a support group, if you haven't already done so. You'll have a little more time since you're not going to the treatments, and the company of others who know how you're feeling may help you get through these emotions.

Often the skin feels a little bit thicker right after radiation, and sometimes it's darker colored; that will gradually resolve itself over time. The nipple may get crusty, but that too will go away as the skin regenerates. This can take up to six months, and in the meantime you'll look like you've been out sunbathing with one breast exposed.

If there's been a lot of radiation to the armpit, it will compound whatever scarring the surgery caused, and the combination can also increase your risk of lymphedema (see Chapter 30). Another, rare, side effect of radiation to the armpits is problems with the nerves that go from the arm to the hand, causing some numbness in the fingertips.

Aside from skin reaction and tiredness, there are some later side effects. Some women get costochondritis, which is a kind of arthritis that causes inflammation of the space between the breasts where the ribs and breastbone connect (Fig. 27-6). The pain can be scary—you wonder if your cancer has spread. It's easy to reassure yourself, though. Push your fingers down right at that junction; if it hurts, it's

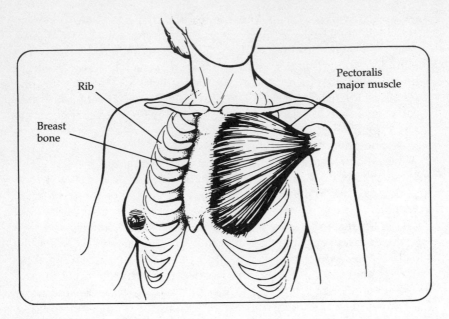

FIGURE 27-6

costochondritis, and can be treated with aspirin and anti-arthritis medicines. It will go away in a few weeks.

When the treatments are over you'll continue to get some tenderness and soreness in your breast, which will gradually go away. But it will never feel completely normal again. You'll continue to have some sharp, shooting pains from time to time—how often varies greatly from woman to woman.

Often patients worry about being radioactive—that they'll harm other people. They ask, "Can I hug my grandchild? Can I pick up my kids?" Once the treatment is over, and you leave the treatment room, you can be close to anyone (the implants described earlier are an exception). It's like lying in the sun—once you're out of it, the effects remain, but the sunlight isn't inside you, and can't be transmitted to anyone else.

Finally, but thank goodness rarely, radiation can cause second cancers. These are usually a different kind of cancer, a sarcoma, and don't occur for at least five years after radiaton therapy. Our best guess is that, for every 1,000 five-year survivors of wide excision and radiation, about two will develop a radiation-induced sarcoma over the next 10 years.[3] As we mentioned in Chapter 25, a rare kind of sarcoma can develop after a mastectomy if a woman develops a badly swollen arm. Both situations are very unusual. I've never seen either one myself.

Above a certain dosage, radiation given again will damage normal tissue. So if you have breast cancer and it recurs in the same breast, you can't have it radiated again. If you have the tattoos we mentioned previously, they will make sure future doctors know you've had radiation treatment in that area.

The decision on how best to use lumpectomy and radiation will depend on which procedure has the best medical results, as well as the best cosmetic results. Usually lumpectomy followed by radiation creates the best cosmetic results.

After your treatment is completed, your radiation oncologist will continue to see you, as will your surgeon. In addition to making certain there are no new tumors, the radiation oncologist is watching for signs of complications from the radiation, and the surgeon for signs of surgical complications. These complications are rare, and radiation remains one of our most valuable tools in the treatment of local breast cancer.

THE FUTURE

As with all the field of breast cancer treatment there are several new approaches to radiation therapy in the works. Dr. Silvia Formenti at NYU is researching whether in selected postmenopausal women with very small breast cancers (less than two cm) that have been completely removed by surgery, getting radiation two to three times a day in a very focal way is as safe. This approach could decrease the time needed to undergo therapy from six weeks to one or two (5 vs. 30 radiation sessions). Others are looking at just boosting the bed of the tumor with implants, without the extenal beam radiation. This too would shorten the time needed. In addition, some researchers are trying to figure out how to make tissue more sensitive to radiation so that less can be used. The trend toward bigger surgical resections with clean margins has meant that we can explore shorter, more concentrated radiation approaches.

28

Systemic Treatments

The hallmark of systemic therapies is their ability to affect the whole body and not just one local area. The systemic treatments used for breast cancer include chemotherapy, hormonal therapy, and antibody therapy.

Chemotherapy has gotten a lot of bad press, and it's a pity, because it's one of the most powerful weapons against cancer that we have. It literally means the use of chemicals to treat disease. As we use it, however, it usually refers only to the use of cytotoxic chemicals (those that kill cells).

How does chemotherapy work? As discussed in Chapter 13, each cell goes through several steps in the process of cell division, or reproduction. Chemotherapy drugs interfere with this process so that the cells can't divide. As a result, they die. Different drugs are used in this process at different points, so often more than one kind of drug is used at a time (Fig. 28-1). Unfortunately this effect on cell division is not very selective. It acts on all cells that are rapidly dividing—including hair cells and, more importantly, bone marrow cells, as well as cancer cells. The bone marrow produces red blood cells, white blood cells, and platelets on a continuous basis (Fig. 28-2). Chemotherapy slows this production down. When we give chemotherapy, then, we have to be careful not to stop the production altogether. This is one of the rea-

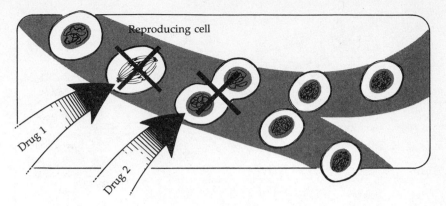

FIGURE 28-1

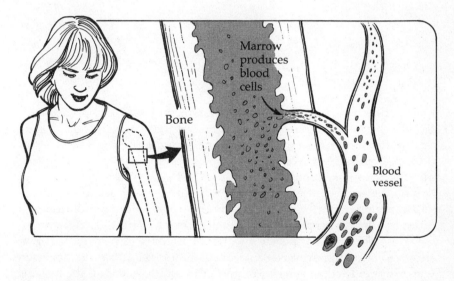

FIGURE 28-2

sons chemotherapy is given in cycles, with a time lapse between treatments to allow the bone marrow to recover.

Another reason the drugs are given in cycles is that not all the cancer cells are dividing at any one time. The first treatment will kill one group of cells; then three weeks later there will be a new set of cancer cells starting to divide, and the drugs will knock them out, too (Fig. 28-3). The idea is to decrease the total number of cancer cells to a number small enough for your immune system to take care of, without wiping out the immune system while we're at it. When we first started giving

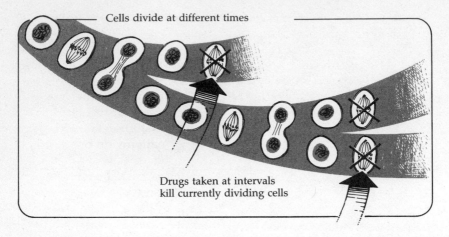

Cells divide at different times

Drugs taken at intervals
kill currently dividing cells

FIGURE 28-3

adjuvant chemotherapy after breast surgery, we gave the treatments over a two-year period. Later studies showed that six months was as good as a year, which was as good as two.[1] The extra treatment may have actually harmed the immune system without having any additional effect on the cancer. There probably is a certain key dosage or duration beyond which an additional drug is useless, but it hasn't been determined yet. We know now that for some patients, just three months of adjuvant chemotherapy may be best.

Another kind of systemic therapy is the use of hormones or hormonal manipulations to change the body's own output of hormones in order to affect the growth of hormonally sensitive tumors. This can include surgical procedures such as oophorectomy (removing the ovaries), radiating the ovaries, using drugs that block hormones, or even using hormones themselves. We don't fully understand all the reasons these hormonal treatments work, but there is no question that they do work well in certain patients. Since hormone therapy affects only hormonally sensitive tissues, its side effects are more limited than those of chemotherapy. It doesn't kill other growing cells, such as hair and bone marrow. Hormone therapies can kill tumor cells by depriving them of the estrogen they require to live. Without estrogen, some tumor cells will commit suicide (apoptosis). Antibody therapies such as trastuzumab (Herceptin) are also being used to treat cancers which overexpress Her-2 neu (see Chapter 23).

Systemic therapies are used at two different points in the natural history of breast cancer. The first is at the time of diagnosis, when it's called adjuvant therapy. The second is at the time of recurrence elsewhere in the body, when the cancer has metastasized. We will discuss the latter in Chapter 32.

When there is a possibility that you'll need systemic therapy, you'll want an appointment with a medical oncologist, or cancer specialist, who specializes in systemic treatment. After talking with you at length, and reviewing your records, the doctor will decide what systemic program you need and what your options are. These options may vary from place to place. There are general guidelines for breast cancer treatment, drawn up by a group of nationwide breast cancer specialists. At UCLA we developed our own specific guidelines to cover many situations. The field is always changing, however, and it is important that you check with several doctors before you settle on your treatment. You'll want the advantage of the most up-to-date information. Check the Internet for the latest recommendations. You may also want to become involved in a protocol or clinical trial (see Chapter 12).

There are many well-trained medical oncologists throughout the country now, and you can usually get very good treatment close to home. You may, however, get a second opinion about chemotherapy or hormone therapy at a cancer center before you start. (See Appendix C for a list of comprehensive cancer centers.) Sometimes the cancer center and your local medical oncologist can work together in designing and supplementing your treatment, giving you the best of both worlds.

Your doctor or medical team will also discuss with you the role of systemic treatment in your overall treatment, the expected toxicity, and how the side effects will be managed. Before you make a decision together with the doctor and sign a consent form, all these things must be made very clear to you. (See Chapter 23 for how to pick a good doctor or team.)

The time spent on this depends on the institution and the particular doctor or nurse you're dealing with. Ideally, you'll spend an hour or so, since the information is extremely detailed. Susan McKenney, a nurse practitioner I used to work with at the Dana Farber Cancer Institute, also gives the patient a written description of everything she needs to know. "I like to translate the information from a didactic, medical form to a written, easily understandable explanation that she can take home and look over at her own convenience; often this is the consent form for a protocol. It's hard to take that much in at one time, and the patient is often overwhelmed—she's dealing with the unknown. I've had a patient sit with me for a hour and the next week when she comes in for her treatment, she can't tell me the names of the drugs she's going to get." Sometimes oncologists will spend a lot of time explaining chemotherapy but relatively little on the side effects, risks, and complications of hormonal therapy such as tamoxifen. Make sure you understand exactly what drugs you are getting, how you will be getting them and what side effects you can expect, and what can be done to prevent or lessen the side effects.

In addition, says McKenney, it's difficult for a patient to feel that chemotherapy or hormone therapy is really going to help her, because she's being told about all the unpleasant things it may do to her in the process. She needs time to assimilate the information about the side effects she'll have to deal with, and written information helps her do this.

You might also want to review the Wellness Community Physician/Patient Statement in Appendix D and discuss it with your doctor.

In Chapter 23 we talked about the decision-making process and options for adjuvant therapy at length. Now we look at the actual experience of receiving chemotherapy or hormone therapy.

ADJUVANT CHEMOTHERAPY

Once you've signed a consent form for chemotherapy, you'll be scheduled to come in for your treatment. It may be in a clinic, your doctor's office, or, rarely, in a hospital. A blood sample is usually taken to check your blood count before your treatment, to help the doctor or nurse know whether your body is capable of taking chemotherapy—and as a baseline for comparison later. Your initial dose is determined by your body surface area (height and weight). This is a good (but not perfect) guess at what the optimally safe and effective dose of chemotherapy is for you.

The bone marrow's recovery rate helps the doctor adjust the dosage of drugs—a process known as titration. We check to see if the marrow has recovered by doing a blood count. A high blood count means that the dose of chemotherapy is probably too low for you, and you'll be given more. If your count is too low then the dose is probably too high and needs to be lowered. Sometimes when the count is too low you have to wait for a day or two before treatment to allow your bone marrow more time to recover. When giving adjuvant chemotherapy, your oncologist should be very reluctant to administer anything but the standard dosage. Dose reduction (lowering) should only be undertaken for severe, life-threatening toxicities because it is the standard doses that have been shown to be effective.

Think of the bone marrow as a factory churning out red blood cells, white blood cells, and platelets. Chemotherapy injures half the factory's employees, and the factory doesn't work as well till they're all recovered. Recently, however, we've discovered some drugs that help accelerate the recovery of the patient's bone marrow—keeping all the workers healthy so the factory can get back on track.

The major drug we have for this is GCSF (granulocyte colony stimulating factor), a natural product you normally have in your blood. Its function is to stimulate the bone marrow to make more white blood cells in times of stress or infection, when you need to build up your immune system. Now we've found a way to utilize this in chemotherapy treatment.[2] It's a natural product, which we made from bacteria through genetic engineering. We found that when we give it to someone, it whips up their bone marrow, so that instead of having a normal white blood cell count of 10,000, they have 40 or 50 thousand. So now when a woman's white blood cell count becomes too low we give her GCSF in an injection and it hastens the bone marrow's recovery. It's like operating on those injured factory workers and getting them back to work. GCSF is thus able to reduce the time it takes your bone marrow to recover after chemotherapy. Because it's important for full doses of adjuvant chemotherapy to be given, and as close to on time as possible, your oncologist should consider adding GCSF to your chemotherapy if your blood counts are delayed in recovering.

Blood counts are taken throughout the course of your therapy, generally weekly for 10 to 14 days after each treatment. When your white blood count is low you have an increased risk of infection, although interestingly enough this doesn't usually include colds; if your platelets are very low you are at an increased risk of bleeding (luckily this is quite rare). Increasingly, oncologists are using antibiotics to prevent you from getting an infection when blood counts are low. If you do this, you can often skip the midcycle blood count as you are already protected from infection.

If your treatment begins the day the blood count is taken, you'll have to wait for 15 to 45 minutes for it to begin. In any event, you'll probably have to wait while the drugs are being mixed, though again this will depend on the practice in your institution. Though the wait may be annoying, it can also be an advantage: often this is an opportunity for women to talk to each other and find support in being together. (If you would prefer some time alone, however, you might want to bring a book, magazine, or Walkman with you.)

Chemotherapy treatments are usually given every three weeks, in 21-day cycles, or in 28-day cycles. If it's a 21-day cycle you may come in for an injection every three weeks. On a 28-day cycle, you come in for treatment on day 1 and day 8, and then go two weeks with no therapy. That's two weeks with therapy and two weeks off. During this time your treatment may be all intravenous, or a combination of intravenous medicine and pill, taken orally at home. The treatments can last anywhere from 12 weeks to six months to a year.

Treatment areas vary from hospital to hospital. Sometimes there's an entire floor for oncology patients, and sometimes just a separate area of a larger floor. Chemotherapy can also be given in a private doctor's office. Everyone is aware of the anxiety level of the patients and will try to make the area as comfortable as possible. Since the process doesn't involve machines, it doesn't look as intimidating as the radiation area. The room will be comfortably lit, and often has television sets or stereos in it. You may have a room to yourself, or be sitting with several other patients who are getting their treatments. You'll sit in a comfortable lounge chair for the procedure (Fig. 28-4). Many patients bring a book or a Walkman. If your treatment is a long one, you might want to invest in one of those tiny, checkbook-sized TVs and watch your favorite talk show or soap opera. Or, if you have easily transportable paperwork for your job, you can work while the treatment is in progress. If you like having a friend or family member with you, most hospitals and doctors will permit that.

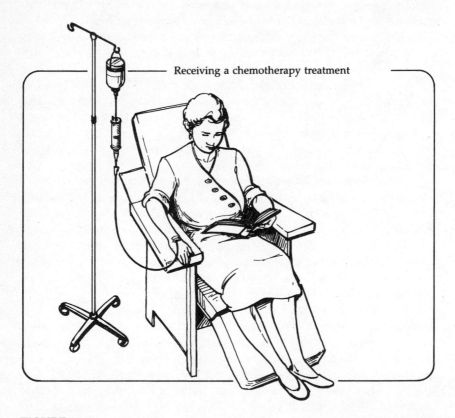

Receiving a chemotherapy treatment

FIGURE 28-4

The length of time a treatment takes, and the intervals at which treatments are given, will vary depending on the type of drugs, the institution giving you the treatment, and the protocol being used. Several different combinations of drugs may be used, each requiring a different time length for administration; in addition, you will likely be given extra fluid as well as medications to control nausea and vomiting. Sometimes a treatment will last 10 minutes; sometimes it will last three or four hours.

The treatments are given either by your medical oncologist or by a specially trained nurse. There's nothing particularly painful about the treatment itself, which feels like any IV procedure. The chemicals come in different colors—in breast cancer, the drugs we use are usually clear, yellow, and red.

You usually don't feel the medications going inside you, though some patients do feel cold, if the fluids are run very fast or if they're cold to begin with, and if the patient's body is especially sensitive to cold. The doctor or nurse will always be there with you, and they're both highly trained specialists in chemotherapy. Sometimes the drugs irritate veins and cause them to clot off and scar (sclerose) during the course of the treatment. This can make it very hard to get needles into the veins.

There's a procedure to overcome this that has existed for some time, but in recent years we're doing it far more frequently than we used to. This is the use of what we call a central access device, a portacath—a catheter-type device placed under the skin into a major blood vessel in the upper chest (Fig. 28-5). Needles can go in and out of that device and spare the patient the discomfort of having peripheral veins (the ones close to the surface, which are normally used for needles) stuck. It's important to make sure the catheter is inserted in the side of the body away from the affected breast, in case you might eventually have a mastectomy or need radiation therapy. This involves a surgical procedure, usually done under local anesthetic. It can be a bit uncomfortable, but it's a trade-off. Patients like the fact that they don't have to get stuck with a new needle each treatment, but on the other hand it can feel a little strange for a while to have a catheter under your skin. The other problem is that the catheter is a foreign body, and on rare occasions can cause an infection. It also needs to be flushed every so often with a blood thinner, to prevent a clot. For most women, the decision to use or not use a catheter is reasonable either way, but it is essential for a patient who has a lot of trouble with her veins, and for a patient who is getting a bone marrow transplant (discussed later in this chapter).

There are seven drugs commonly given as adjuvant chemotherapy for breast cancer: cyclophosphamide (Cytoxan) (C), methotrexate (M),

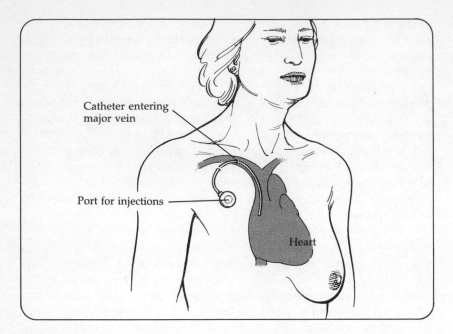

Catheter entering
major vein

Port for injections

Heart

FIGURE 28-5

5-fluorouracil (F), Adriamycin (A), or epirubicin (E); and paclitaxel
(Taxol) or docetaxel (Taxotere) (T). These are usually given in combinations, CMF or AC followed by T. Other drugs (hormones) such as
tamoxifen and sometimes Zoladex or Lupron may be added in young
women who are still menstruating.

Side Effects of Chemotherapy

Side effects vary according to the drugs used. (See Appendix A for a
detailed list of some of the drugs most commonly used against breast
cancer and their side effects.) The most immediate potential side effect
concerns Adriamycin, which can leak out of the vein and cause a very
severe skin burn that could require skin grafting. For this reason, it's
generally given in a very specific way: avoiding weak veins, and running in the IV with lots of fluids, so that if it should leak out it won't
cause as much harm.

A more common side effect is nausea and vomiting. Overall about
20 percent of women who get CMF, and more of the women who receive AC, will complain of nausea and vomiting. Usually the nausea
doesn't start until four to six hours after the injection. It can last any-

where from a few hours to two days or more, and can come in waves at varying time intervals, or remain constant the whole time—again, this happens differently for each person, and we can't predict in advance how it will work for you.

We've got a lot of new drugs to treat nausea, including powerful ones like Zofran, Kytril, and Anzemet. These drugs work extremely well for most people, so the days of constant horrible nausea and vomiting are becoming history. Unlike the older anti-nausea drugs, Zofran, Kytril, and Anzemet don't make you feel spacey or depressed and out of it. I used to have patients who felt so awful on the anti-nausea drugs that they preferred toughing it out, so they could be functional when they weren't throwing up. One of my patients who underwent chemotherapy told me that whenever she ran into any of the doctors or nurses who worked with her she got waves of nausea for years after her treatment ended, even though the doctors and nurses had been very helpful and supportive. These days most oncologists have women take nausea pills on a specific schedule to *prevent* the nausea and vomiting, such as twice a day for three days starting the night of chemotherapy.

Because the thought of chemotherapy can be frightening, it is a good idea to bring someone with you for your first treatment to see how well it goes and, if you've come by car, to do the driving if necessary. Then if the first treatment goes well and you feel all right afterwards, you may not need anyone for the following ones. Usually, if you start off feeling all right and your anti-nausea drugs are effective, you'll probably get through the rest of the treatments with relative comfort.

In addition to the drugs, some hospitals, like the Beth Israel Deaconess in Boston, incorporate such anti-stress mechanisms as visualization, imagery, and relaxation techniques into their treatment program. They have found that these are often very effective. If your hospital or doctor doesn't offer such techniques, you might want to try some of the ones discussed in Chapter 29, or read some of the books suggested in Appendix B. Many of the techniques are simple and easy for you to teach yourself. In addition, many adult education centers and holistic health institutes in cities and towns all over the country have visualization programs. Acupuncture and Chinese herbs, also discussed in Chapter 29, have also proved to be effective in nausea relief.

Sometimes chemotherapy causes you to lose your appetite (anorexia, which is different from anorexia nervosa). In spite of this and the nausea, 21 percent of women will have some weight gain while on treatment—gains of between 5 and 15 pounds.[3] Food may taste different to you, and some chemicals interact badly with certain foods, though both loss of appetite and chemical interaction are less common with breast cancer drugs than with others. The National Cancer Institute puts out a helpful recipe booklet for people whose eating is affected by their chemotherapy. You may also experience peculiar odors. Barbara Kalinowski, who co-facilitates a support group for women with breast cancer in Boston, describes one woman who talked of constantly walking through her house opening windows so she could get rid of the odor, which she described as similar to the smell of a new car.

Fifty-seven percent of premenopausal women will have hot flashes while on adjuvant chemotherapy. The drugs can create a chemically induced menopause, with hormonal changes, hot flashes, emotional mood swings, and no periods.

An article in the *Journal of Clinical Oncology* suggests that the strongest predictors of whether you're going to go through menopause with treatment are age and type of chemotherapy.[4,5] The closer you are to natural menopause, the higher your risk. The average age of menopause is 51. A woman of 45 who receives chemotherapy has an 80 percent likelihood of going into menopause as a result, which is much greater than is the case with tamoxifen. A 35-year-old woman has a 20 percent chance of becoming postmenopausal. Many women don't know this ahead of time, and suddenly have to deal with something unexpected in the midst of their treatment.

With CMF (cyclophosphamide, methotrexate, 5-fluorouracil) given for six months, the risk of premature menopause is approximately 35 percent in women younger than 40 vs. 90 percent in women older than 40. In contrast, less that 15 percent of women younger than 40 who receive four cycles of AC (Adriamycin and cyclophosphamide), and 60 percent of those over 40, will become menopausal.[6,7] Overall, it is the cumulative dose of cyclophosphamide that is strongly related to premature menopause. It is not known what effect the recent addition of taxanes (Taxol and Taxotere) to AC will have on the ovaries. Although roughly half of the women younger than 40 may regain some menstrual function, the percentage is much lower in older women. There is some evidence in animals that putting the ovaries into reversible menopause with Lupron during chemotherapy might be more protective,[8,9] but it has not been tested yet in women.

If you do experience early menopause, you will of course be infertile. If your period comes back you can still conceive. Since it's difficult to tell which group you're in you must use mechanical birth control while on treatment if you're heterosexually active, since the chemotherapy drugs will severely injure a first trimester fetus. (See Chapter 31 for a further discussion of the treatment of menopausal symptoms.)

Chemotherapy treatments used in breast cancer, as in many other cancers, often cause either partial or total hair loss. This is somewhat predictable according to the drugs used and the duration of treatment. Women who get Adriamycin as part of their treatment always lose their hair, usually fairly soon after the onset of treatment. On the other hand, women who receive CMF only sometimes lose their hair; hair loss occurs about three weeks after treatments have begun, and the hair doesn't fall out all at once. You'll wake up one morning and find a large amount of hair on your pillow or in the shower, or you'll be combing your hair, and notice a lot of hair in the comb. This is almost always traumatic for patients, so it's probably wise to buy a wig before your treatment starts. It's best to go to a hairdresser or wig salon at the start of treatment, so the hairdresser knows what your hair usually looks like and how you like to wear it—it makes for a better match. Often, women receiving CMF end up not having to use the wig. (You can always donate it to a local breast resource center.) But patients who haven't prepared in advance for the hair loss have a difficult time emotionally if it does occur.

Remember, though, it isn't only the hair on your head that falls out. Pubic hair, eyelashes and eyebrows, leg and arm hair—some or all of the hair on your body will fall out, although in most women the eyelashes and eyebrows only thin a bit. Most of the time that isn't too much of problem cosmetically—you can thicken your eyebrows with pencil, for example—but it can be startling if you're not prepared for it.

It may take a while after the treatments have ended for your hair to grow back. Usually a little down begins to form even before your treatments have ended, and within six weeks you should have some hair growing in, though the time depends on how fast your hair normally grows. Often it comes back with a different texture—curly if it's been straight, but eventually the curl relaxes and your hair most often returns to normal after several haircuts. It may come back in a different color, most commonly gray or black.

Some women experience sexual problems, often related to the frequently occurring vaginal dryness related to menopause. The chemotherapy lowers your blood counts, which can cause infection. And you may suddenly encounter problems with your diaphragm or an IUD due to dryness. In addition there are the physical and psychological effects of the treatment. It's harder to feel sexy when you are tired and bald. This is an important time to communicate with your partner about each of your feelings and needs and to try and find a comforting compromise. (See Chapter 30 for a discussion of sexual issues and breast cancer.)

Fuzzy thinking and fatigue are common side effects (see Chapter 30) that are just beginning to be acknowledged. Other common side effects include mouth sores, conjunctivitis, runny eyes and nose, diarrhea, and constipation. You may have bleeding from your gums or nose, or in your stool or urine, though this is unusual. You may get headaches. Any of these can be mild or severe, or anything in between.

The long-term side effects include chronic bone marrow suppression and second cancers, especially leukemias. This risk is certainly small—half a percent in the NSABP series—and probably worth the benefit of the treatment, but it's important to remember that, rarely, there may be a long-term side effect.[10]

Adriamycin in particular can be toxic to the heart. We believe that it's dose-related, and is rare with four to six cycles of Adriamycin, but it's possible that there are also long-term cardiac effects that we don't yet know about. For example, some of the people who were treated with Adriamycin several years ago[11] for childhood cancers are experiencing heart failure and need heart transplants. We're only beginning to consider this now because in the past we used Adriamycin only for metastatic cancers, and those patients usually died of the cancer within a few years. Now that we're using it more frequently for women with negative lymph nodes, the patients may well be alive in 20 or 30 years, and we may see more side effects than we did before. It is important not to assume that a drug or treatment that is relatively safe at the time will be safe over the long haul. However, recent long-term studies of Adriamycin in women with breast cancer show that few have heart problems more than 10 years after treatment.[12] One of my former patients ended up with a heart transplant because of heart disease she'd developed after being treated with Adriamycin. Overall, the risk of having a heart problem due to the Adriamycin is about one in 200 treated women. I'm not suggesting that we abandon all use of Adriamycin for adjuvant treatment—my patient, after all, survived long enough to get her heart ailment. Adriamycin is one of the best drugs we have to treat breast cancer. If it is indicated it should certainly be used. But we should not use it indiscriminately in women who are not at such high risk.

Taxol, or paclitaxel, can cause a reversible dose-dependent cumulative *neuropathy*. This is a pins-and-needles sensation, often in the hands and feet, which can get worse with each dose but is generally ultimately reversible. Taxol can cause hand-foot syndrome, an itchy rash on the palms of the hands and the soles of the feet. It can also cause an allergic reaction, but giving women preventive medication in their IV prior to the Taxol is highly effective in preventing this. Taxol can also cause eye problems. Docetaxel (Taxotere) also can cause the neuropathy but is generally milder than paclitaxel. Taxotere also causes a unique syndrome of swelling and fluid retention; fortunately, this is reversible but it takes a long time.

Though there's no way to know in advance for certain how you'll react to your treatments (every woman is unique), your doctor or nurse can tell you how people who've been treated with the drugs you're on have done in the past.

While it's important to be prepared for the possible side effects, it's equally important not to assume you'll have all, or even any, of them. This assumption can intensify, and sometimes even create, the symptoms. Sometimes people who see the side effects as a sign that their illness is getting worse can contribute to their own negative feelings. Bernie Siegel,[13] the doctor who has worked so intensively with mental techniques to reduce pain and help heal diseases, reports in his book *Love, Medicine, and Miracles* on a study done in England in which a group of men were given a placebo and told it was a chemotherapy treatment. Thirty percent of the men lost their hair! Positive thinking and—importantly—exercise, as well as keeping up your normal activities, can actually significantly reduce the side effects of chemotherapy.

Most chemotherapy treatments are given on an outpatient basis. You will soon know whether you are going to feel sick and, if so, on which day the nausea hits and how bad it is. Most women are able to continue their normal lives and their work schedules with minor adjustments while receiving treatments. You won't feel great, but you'll be functional. In 2000, adjuvant breast cancer chemotherapy should be tolerable and you should be able to function well. If it's not, ask your doctor or nurse for strategies to reduce the side effects. Many options are available.

It may, however, be a good time to take up your friends' offers of help. A ride to your treatment can be wonderful: both for the company and the release from worry about traffic and parking. Child care may well give you a breather in a stressful time, as can offers to cook dinner or clean the house. Most friends and family members really do want to help, and this may well be the best time to use all their support.

Don't expect to feel perfect the minute your last treatment is over. Your body has been under a great stress and needs time to recuperate. It often takes six months or even a year before you feel perfectly normal again. It will happen, however, so don't despair. (See Chapter 30 for a discussion of rehabilitation after breast cancer.)

ADJUVANT HORMONAL THERAPY

Hormonal therapies are generally easier to take with fewer side effects than chemotherapy. The best known and most widely used is tamoxifen. In terms of its administration, tamoxifen is the simplest of the breast cancer therapies. You don't need to go anywhere or have anything done to you—you simply take a pill. Tamoxifen is usually taken as a single pill (20 mg) or as two 10-mg tablets. It is better to take the two pills together so you don't forget the second one.

Because we look at tamoxifen in relation to chemotherapy we tend to minimize its side effects. And indeed, compared to chemotherapy, its side effects are fairly mild. But they do exist, and for some women they can be quite significant, including phlebitis (blood clots), pulmonary emboli, visual problems, depression, nausea and vomiting, vaginal discharge and hot flashes. All of these are rare except for the hot flashes. A lot of women who have these symptoms ask me if they could be caused by the tamoxifen. When I say yes, they say, "Thank God—I thought I was going crazy because my doctor said I wouldn't have side effects."

It's wrong to assume tamoxifen should always be used because it's comfortable and risk-free. First, as my colleague Dr. Craig Henderson is fond of saying, a nontoxic therapy is not justified just because it's nontoxic. Second, and probably more important, we don't actually know that it *is* nontoxic. Tamoxifen is not without some risks, albeit small ones.

The most common of the side effects are hot flashes—and they occur in about 50 percent of women on tamoxifen. They can be severe or mild, just like any hot flashes. They eventually go away, but "eventually" may mean years. New drugs like Effexor can be very helpful in reducing the number and intensity of these hot flashes.[14] Other alternative choices are discussed in Chapter 29.

About 30 percent of women on tamoxifen will get major gynecological discomforts—anything from vaginal discharge to severe vaginal dryness.

A small percentage of women get severely depressed. It can be insidious, very slow in onset, so you don't realize it's happening until you're in the midst of a horrible depression. When you get off the tamoxifen, the depression lifts. It may be that this is more prevalent in women who are prone to PMS and postpartum depression—susceptible to hormonal mood swings. Antidepressants can be very effective in treating depression in women who really need the tamoxifen to reduce their risk of recurrence.

There's some evidence that tamoxifen may, in unusual cases, increase *thrombophlebitis*, a form of phlebitis in the leg in which the vein gets irritated and forms clots.[15] This is rare but can be very dangerous as the blood clot can travel to the lung (pulmonary embolus) and can even be fatal. It is important to let your doctor know right away if you develop leg swelling and pain while walking.

The most serious side effect of tamoxifen is uterine cancer. A large NSABP study looking at the use of tamoxifen found a cumulative risk of 1.2–1.6/1000 patient years.[16] The risk is higher the longer the women are on the drug. This is not surprising, since the uterus is one of the places where tamoxifen acts like estrogen, and thus, like estrogen alone, can cause uterine cancer. For women who have had hysterectomies this isn't a problem, but it's a risk to others. A 1999 study published in the *Journal of the National Cancer Institute* has delved into the uterine cancer risk and clarified it enormously.[17] They found that most women on tamoxifen have no increased risk of uterine cancer at all no matter how long they take it. The ones at risk are those who have taken estrogen replacement therapy (ERT) (without a progestin like Provera) in the near or distant past.

This makes sense. These days no one with a uterus would take estrogen without Provera, because we know it causes uterine cancer. In the past, however, we weren't so smart. It is those women who were on ERT, even if they stopped 10 years ago, who still have a propensity for uterine cancer. Add tamoxifen to this primed uterus, especially in a woman who is overweight, and you have a problem.

The study compared 324 women who had developed endometrial (uterine) cancer to 671 women who had not. It confirmed a 52 percent higher chance of getting endometrial cancer if you took tamoxifen than if you didn't. (Remember, this just means that the risk is half again as high. If the risk is 1 in 1,000 women as is commonly accepted, it becomes 1.52 in 1,000 women.) The risk increases by 18 percent per year of use. By two years, the risk has doubled, and if you take it for more than five years the risk is almost four times as high (3.72). This sounds bad, but remember that the overall risk of developing uterine cancer with the standard five years of tamoxifen use is about 1 percent. The vast majority of the time, the uterine cancers are curable with a hysterectomy. Women who have *not* been on ERT are even less likely to get uterine cancer.

A second, though less significant, confounding factor was body weight. It is known that women who are overweight have an increased risk of getting uterine cancer postmenopausally, probably caused by the increased estrogen that's made by fat. In this study, overweight women who had taken ERT and then took tamoxifen had the highest risk of getting uterine cancer. Heavier women on tamoxifen who had never taken ERT showed no increased risk. But thin women who had taken ERT had a higher risk of uterine cancer on tamoxifen.

If you're taking tamoxifen to treat your cancer and were previously on estrogen therapy without a progestin, you shouldn't stop the drug, but rather make sure you're closely monitored by your gynecologist. If you experience abnormal bleeding, report it immediately to your doctor.

There has been much discussion in the breast cancer field about how this monitoring should be dealt with. Some are recommending endometrial biopsies or vaginal ultrasounds on all women on tamoxifen. I think this is a bit much, especially with the recent data mentioned above. In addition, recent studies have shown that vaginal ultrasounds are not particularly helpful in distinguishing the rare uterine cancers from the swelling of the uterine lining which can occur with tamoxifen.[18] I think a routine gynecological exam once a year is probably adequate, but anyone with bleeding should be evaluated. Some gynecologists prescribe progesterone with tamoxifen on the theory that since progesterone protects the uterus from cancer in women on Premarin it should be used here as well. The trouble is that we have no data on the safety of progesterone in women with breast cancer. I would be very reluctant to add yet another unknown drug to the mix, especially with the new data showing that progesterone added to estrogen as HRT increased the risk of breast cancer (see Chapter 15).

In rats, tamoxifen causes liver cancer. But that doesn't tell us too much, since in rats almost any estrogen causes liver cancer. Liver cancer has never been tied to tamoxifen use in women in spite of exhaustive research. Some women can have an increase in their liver blood tests which goes away once they stop taking tamoxifen. Many women on tamoxifen experience some eye problems, including blurry vision and, less commonly, cataracts. There's some concern that in premenopausal women, because tamoxifen stimulates the ovaries and increases estrogen and progesterone levels, it may increase the incidence of ovarian cysts and stimulate ovulation while blocking estrogen in the breast. This means that if you're heterosexually active, it is imperative that you use some type of effective barrier contraceptive while taking the drug. Tamoxifen can damage a fetus and it is very important not to get pregnant while taking the drug.

It's interesting to note that there are several bonuses in spite of its side effects. Tamoxifen improves your high-density lipoproteins and your low-density lipoproteins, which may make you less likely to get heart disease.[19] Tamoxifen certainly doesn't make osteoporosis worse—most often it makes it better in postmenopausal women, and sometimes it stablizes it,[20] much like raloxifene.

The most important thing about tamoxifen is that it treats the cancer you have, and it reduces your chance of getting cancer in the opposite breast by 50 percent; that is, from 15 to 7.5 percent. So considering all these pros and cons, it is worth taking unless you have had problems with blood clots in the past.

As we discussed in Chapter 23, the current data suggest you take tamoxifen for five years and then stop. Much to everyone's surprise, the benefits of decreasing the chance your cancer might come back and decreasing second cancers continue even after you have stopped the drug. Tamoxifen is therefore likely to kill cancer cells or, more probably, put them into a dormant state.

At one time there was the suggestion that in premenopausal women tamoxifen had to induce menopause. If their periods didn't stop we'd double the dose. There's no evidence, however, that a higher dose works any better. In fact, tamoxifen doesn't put premenopausal women into menopause at all; on the contrary, it increases estrogen and progesterone in their bloodstreams.[21] A woman of 45 is only slightly more likely to go into menopause than other women her age. One poor women came in to see us at UCLA; she had had chemotherapy and then her oncologist had started her on tamoxifen. When her period didn't stop he doubled and then tripled her dose. Her side effects were horrific and her period got heavier. He told her she would have to have her ovaries taken out since they were not responding to the tamoxifen. Since tamoxifen is a stimulant and not a depressant to premenopausal ovaries, it was he who was confused. We just dropped her tamoxifen dose to normal and she did fine.

It takes six weeks for tamoxifen to get out of your system when you stop. So if you miss a pill one day, it isn't the end of the world. Just go ahead and resume taking your tamoxifen the next day.

Toremifene, a drug that has been approved by the FDA for treatment of metastatic disease, is sometimes used in place of tamoxifen, especially for women who are intolerant of tamoxifen. Raloxifene is a SERM (see Chapter 18) that has been shown to decrease breast cancer in postmenopausal women with low bone density. Since these women are at low risk of breast cancer, it is not clear if it would have the same effect in women with breast cancer or those who are at high risk. One study of 14 women with metastatic breast cancer showed no effect from raloxifene.[22] A second study showed an 18 percent response rate in metastatic disease.[23] At this time it is definitely *not* an alternative to tamoxifen as adjuvant treatment of breast cancer.

Until recently only tamoxifen was being given as an adjuvant hormonal treatment. As we mentioned in Chapter 23, Zoladex (goserelin) and Arimidex (anastrozole) have recently been studied in the adjuvant setting. Zoladex, which puts you into a reversible menopause, is given by a monthly injection. It has the side effects of menopause complete with hot flashes. Arimidex is a tablet taken once a day, with few or no side effects, but its benefit in the adjuvant setting has yet to be demonstrated. We await the results of a large clinical trial comparing the effectiveness of tamoxifen vs. Arimidex or both together.

29

Complementary and Alternative Treatments

Twenty years ago, if you told people you were doing daily meditation to help cure your cancer, or closing your eyes and visualizing your cancer cells as dirt stains and your immune system as a scrub brush washing them away, they'd have assumed your disease had driven you completely crazy. Some people still would. But today, many cancer patients are combining these techniques with their regular treatments, often with their doctor's blessing, and sometimes with their doctor's participation. A 2000 study in the *Journal of the National Cancer Institute* looked at four ethnic groups (Caucasian, Latina, African American, and Chinese) and found that about one half used at least one type of alternative.[1] African Americans most often used spiritual healing (36%); Chinese used herbal remedies (22%); Latinas used dietary therapies (30%) and spiritual healing (26%); and Caucasians used dietary methods (35%) and physical methods (21%) such as massage and acupuncture.

Therapies involving particular diets, vitamins, and herbs are becoming increasingly popular. Almost all of these therapies are based on theories about the role of the immune system in fighting off disease, and the need to strengthen that system (see Chapter 18). Unfortunately, up to now, none of these therapies has been proved to have an effect on the immune system. But they do bear examining, and may have other benefits.

With increasing attention being paid to "other than standard Western therapy," the categories have become more formalized. Barry Casselith, a researcher at Memorial Sloan Kettering Hospital, came up with a useful distinction at the 1999 Oncology Symposium on Alternative and Complementary Treatment. (The existence of such a conference is in itself a sign that the medical establishment is slowly moving into a more open-minded approach to healing.) Dr. Casselith defines alternatives as methods promoted to treat cancer and used instead of mainstream therapies. By contrast, she says, complementary (or adjunctive) therapies are those meant to treat symptoms and improve quality of life; they are given in conjunction with mainstream therapy. Validation of this distinction has come from the renaming of the Office of Alternative Medicine, which is now called the Center for Complementary and Alternative Medicine.

Among alternatives, Casselith includes high-dose vitamin therapy, antineoplastons, macrobiotic diet, herbal remedies, metabolic therapies and detoxification, and some healers with special abilities. The crucial point of concern is that people turn to *it* instead of standard therapy. They do it in part, she says, because they want more control over their treatment, they want to strengthen their body and spirit (both of which they believe will be weakened by chemotherapy), and they find such approaches more supportive psychologically than the treatment offered at hospitals. About 8–10 percent of cancer patients whose diagnosis is confirmed by tissue biopsy decide not to use mainstream therapy and immediately seek alternative care.[2] Many people simply distrust the government and the medical establishment, concerned that these institutions care only about medications that have been proved by Western science. The huge increase in food supplements, however, many marketed by traditional pharmaceutical companies, suggests that the "medical industrial complex" cares more about profits than whether medications have been proved by Western science. Some people are convinced that there is a cancer conspiracy—they believe there really is a cure for cancer but we're not telling people, because the drug companies want to make money. But this too fails to hold up under scrutiny. While it is true that there is a whole industry built up around cancer research and treatment, it is also true that it can easily shift if and when a cure occurs—as it did when the polio vaccine was invented.

In contrast to alternative therapies, Dr. Cassileth defines complementary treatments as supportive care used to decrease symptoms and to enhance the quality of a person's life, along with mainstream care.

These tend to be less expensive than "alternative" treatments, and usually they're medically safe. Complementary therapies include: meditation, counseling, diet, herbal supplements, yoga, certain teas, massage, Reiki healing, acupuncture, and acupressure. None of these is considered a means of curing cancer but only of working with the medical treatment. Often surgery, chemotherapy, and the knowledge that you have cancer can bring on mild depression and anxiety, for example, and studies have shown that the herb St. John's wort can help moderate depression, while another herb, Kava Kava, can help with moderate anxiety.

The use of complementary therapies is often based on certain other beliefs, which, although they have a grain of truth, may not be totally accurate. One such belief is that the body has self-healing properties. This is true—but only to a point. There certainly is a mind–body connection but there are also forces beyond our control. Another belief is that certain things can increase the immune system and help cure a cancer. Again, there's some truth in this, but there's no magic bullet that will zip up your immune system enough to cure cancer by itself.

I think it's very important to be looking at complementary, rather than alternative, treatments if you have breast cancer. For all its limitations, Western medicine is still probably the most important component of any successful effort to cure cancer or to put it into significant remission.

COMPLEMENTARY THERAPIES

Mental Techniques

There are a number of techniques that seem to work because of the "placebo effect." The placebo effect is what takes place when your mind, in effect, tells your body that it's getting a certain healing substance, and your body responds as though it were true.

For years, placebos have been used to test the effectiveness of new drugs. If, for example, we're looking to see if substance X relieves symptom Y, we take 100 randomly chosen subjects, and give 50 pills containing substance X and 50 apparently identical pills without substance X. None of the subjects knows who is really getting substance X. When we look for the results, we discover that 49 of the 50 subjects who took the substance X pills no longer suffer from symptom Y, while only 10 of the other 50 are relieved of their symptom. We now have good reason to believe that substance X indeed does cure symptom Y. But what accounts for the 10 subjects who didn't really take substance X and yet were cured? They thought they were taking it, and it had the same effect on their symptom as if they were actually taking it. In other words, your belief that a particular substance, or withdrawal from a particular substance, will relieve your condition may, in itself, cause it to do so.

This doesn't mean you're gullible or stupid or imagining things; it means that the mind affects the body in ways we don't yet fully understand, and that you're fortunate enough that the body–mind interaction is working in your favor. Norman Cousins, the *Saturday Review* editor whose *Anatomy of an Illness* recounts his recovery from a connective tissue disorder, devoted much of his book to the placebo effect. "The history of medication," he writes, "is far more the history of the placebo effect than of intrinsically valuable relevant drugs," pointing to the success doctors in ancient times had with such "treatments" as bloodletting with leaches and giving their patients powdered unicorn horns. He calls the placebo "the doctor who resides within," who "translates the will to live into a physical reality."[3] If a sugar pill can reduce swelling and eliminate pain in substantial numbers of people, perhaps that same effect can be brought about directly and consciously by the mind. This is the theory behind most mental healing techniques.

There is increasing evidence of this mind–body connection. David Spiegel ran a support group for women with newly diagnosed metastatic breast cancer and showed that the women who participated in the support group lived, on average, 18 months longer than those who did not.[4] F. Fawzy at UCLA did an experiment with people who had melanoma. He randomly assigned half of them to participate in a six-week group with stress reduction and support. He was able to show that the immune system's weapons, natural killer cells in the blood, were higher in the patients who were part of the support group. He also found that these patients had fewer recurrences at six years.[5]

Prayer

The most obvious mental technique is one that's probably very familiar to you—prayer. For centuries, people of all religions have believed in the power of prayer—and for some of them it seems to have worked. In spite of the fraudulence of some charismatic healers, many are sincere; and the faith people bring to them may bring about their own healing.

Estelle Disch, a Boston-area therapist who has worked with many cancer patients, is not herself a believer in Christian theology, but she has seen the belief work for others. "A deeply religious Catholic woman I know has bad colon cancer," she says, "and she goes to every charismatic healing service she can find. I firmly believe her faith has kept her alive. If you're praying for health, on some level you're seeing yourself as healthy, and I believe that makes a difference." Believing that there is a power that can make you well—whether that's God, or your surgeon, or your own will—can help you to get well. History is full of accounts of miracles, and while we have no laboratory proof that these accounts are accurate, there are simply too many of them to dismiss. No doubt some "miracles" are a fraud, and some self-delusion, but I'm convinced that some are indeed exactly what they claim to be, and that faith, of whatever sort, has played a part in their occurrence. I often pray for my patients, hoping to harness whatever forces I can to help them achieve the result that is best for them.

In the mid-1990s two separate groups of researchers pulled together collections of scientific studies on the effectiveness of prayer, and the results are thought-provoking, to say the least. Paul N. Duckro, a professor of psychiatry and human behavior at the Saint Louis University School of Medicine, looked at experimental studies conducted over 20 years and found striking examples of the effectiveness of prayer.[6] One study looked at 18 children with leukemia, divided into two groups. Families from a distant Protestant church were given the names of 10 of the children and asked to pray for them without their knowledge. Fifteen months later seven of the ten were alive, while only two of the eight children in the control group were alive. Larry Dossey, former chief of staff at Medical City Dallas Hospital, reported on similar studies in his book *Healing Words.*[7] In one study discussed, a randomized double-blind trial of 393 heart patients at San Francisco General Hospital, half the patients were prayed for daily and half weren't. None of the patients, their doctors, or their nurses knew who was being prayed for and who wasn't. The patients who received the prayers had fewer complications and needed fewer antibiotics.

Meditation and Visualization

Meditation has been a very serious part of almost every major religion in history. While there are many forms of meditation, the ones most commonly used in conjunction with healing work are variants of that very simple one in which the person sits in a comfortable position, eyes closed, focusing on the inhaling and exhaling of breath, and chanting a "mantra," a particular word or phrase. The Eastern "ohm" is fine if you like it, but it usually doesn't have much meaning for Americans, and you might do better to use a phrase consistent with your own beliefs—"peace," for example, or a brief phrase from a prayer used in your religion.

Herbert Benson, an M.D. who has extensively studied various forms of nonmedical healing, describes this particular form of meditation as "the Relaxation Response." He used it as the basis of his work as director of Behavioral Medicine at Beth Israel. He and his colleagues run a number of groups for people with a variety of diseases. The technique gives the mind a rest and then a chance to deal with the issues that being ill raises. Physiological responses occur when you elicit the relaxation response. These include a decrease in pulse, blood pressure, respiration rate, oxygen consumption, and overall metabolism. These physiological responses contribute to stress reduction.

Most programs that use meditation combine it with visualization, or imagery. This too is an ancient technique, discovered in recent years by "New Age" devotees. It's used for a variety of purposes, from finding a parking space to curing cancer. Its basis is the belief that if you create strong mental pictures of what you want, while affirming to yourself that you can and will get it, you can make virtually anything happen.

The pioneers of visualization in disease treatment were the then-husband-and-wife team of Carl and Stephanie Simonton (an oncologist and a psychologist). *Getting Well Again,* their 1978 book which was reissued in 1992,[8] has influenced many cancer patients as well as doctors and psychologists. In it they recount their experiences with "exceptional cancer patients"—those who recover in spite of a negative prognosis—and maintain that their visualization techniques have significantly extended patients' lives.

Though Bernie Siegel (discussed earlier), the Simontons, and others claim their techniques have cured cancer, the evidence is chiefly what we call "anecdotal"—that is, stories of individuals or groups of individuals, rather than studies set up in controlled situations. This doesn't mean visualization can't cure cancer or prolong cancer patients' lives; it simply means that so far we have no firm proof that it does.

What studies have proved, however, is that visualization and meditation combined can reduce pain and the uncomfortable side effects of cancer treatments—we've already discussed this a bit in Chapters 27 and 28. This in itself is impressive and, combined with the possibility that it might affect the outcome of the disease, makes a meditation-visualization program well worth trying.

How does visualization work? Typically you do a meditation-relaxation exercise first to become fully relaxed and receptive to the imagery that came to you. Then you begin to visualize your cancer in terms of some concrete image—gray blobs inside your breast (or whatever area you're dealing with). Then you picture your white blood cells, or your radiation or chemotherapy treatments, as forces countering the cells (Fig. 29-1).

The Simontons have favored violent images—soldiers attacking the cells, or sharks destroying them. These images, however, aren't always

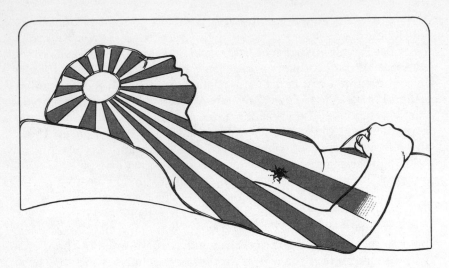

FIGURE 29-1

right for everyone. A friend with metastatic breast cancer felt much better singing her cells a lullaby to put them to sleep.

Most people do relaxation and visualization images as part of a group, working on a regular basis with the group, and doing the exercises daily between group meetings. If there is no such group near you—and even if there is—you can learn the techniques on your own. I've had patients who've used the techniques in groups and by themselves. One of my patients started off in a group, and found it helpful in the beginning. "But what I got out of it mostly was the techniques, which I use at home on my own. I'm not much of a joiner, I guess." She is convinced that the techniques have been a useful part of her healing and have helped her deal with the anxieties her cancer caused. "Cancer is no longer the first thing I think of in the morning and the last thing I think of when I go to bed."

Similar to visualization, and often used in conjunction with it, are affirmations. These are statements affirming one's value and one's intentions, recited aloud if possible, mentally if necessary. Like visualization, they can be used for any goal, from wealth to spiritual growth, and they're often used for health. One of my patients had a list of her favorites, which include "I am now willing to become free of all pain and illness," "I am now renewing my body's ability to heal itself," and "I now let the light from above heal me with love." Others prefer to frame their affirmations in terms of choice: "I choose health."

I'm told by people who work with affirmations that it's important to frame them positively rather than negatively—not "I am not staying ill" but "I am growing more and more healthy each day."

They also suggest that affirmations should be repeated regularly, and frequently. You can say them while you're taking your shower, walking to your car, or unloading your groceries. Unlike many of the other mental practices, they needn't take time from a busy schedule. Susan Troyan, one of my surgical colleagues in Boston, has patients bring in positive sayings which are read during their surgery. She says that whether or not it helps healing, it gives women a much needed sense of control.

Laughter

Reader's Digest has for many years had a section of humor called "Laughter, the Best Medicine." They meant it metaphorically, but when Norman Cousins set about to cure himself of his neurological illness, he took it literally. "I discovered that ten minutes of genuine belly laughter had an anesthetic effect and would give me at least two hours of pain-free sleep," he wrote.[9] There appears to be some medical basis for this: laughter can stimulate endorphins—chemicals that act like narcotics in the brain.

Some of my patients have found that laughter is an important part of their healing process. One woman had breast cancer twice, and, along with her medical treatments and her meditation, she worked laughter into her regime. "I told people I wanted to laugh. Friends send me funny books, cut out cartoons, call me and say funny things," she said. Though she eventually died from her cancer, her multileveled approach to fighting it gave her the strength she needed to live her life fully to the end—including helping launch the breast cancer political movement we discuss in Chapter 34 .

Certainly giving yourself time not to think about your cancer, just escaping into zany humor, can be emotionally very healing. Be sure to pick the things that make you laugh. Cousins enjoyed Marx Brothers movies and *Candid Camera* TV shows. You might prefer stand-up comedians such as Jerry Seinfeld, or P. G. Wodehouse novels, or *I Love Lucy* reruns—whatever makes you laugh out loud and hold your sides, totally absorbing you into its delightful nonsense.

Psychic Healing

Before you scoff at the idea of psychic healing, remember that it's respected by some intelligent people. In his hospital in the African jungle, Albert Schweitzer often consulted with a witch doctor whose work he respected.[10] Much of charismatic Christian healing involves laying-on-of-hands, a classical psychic healing technique. And the relatively new "therapeutic touch," designed by nurses in the U.S., uses a similar approach.

I haven't had much experience with psychic healers in terms of my own patients, but there is a fair amount of anecdotal evidence about cures through psychic healing, and my co-author, severely asthmatic, had a brief but dramatic improvement after a few sessions with a healer. She's not certain whether this was the result of the healer's power or of her own mind, and she doesn't care: "What I care about is breathing, and he helped me do it," she says.

Certainly if the placebo effect has any validity there's no reason psychic healing can't trigger it. As long as you're not paying exorbitant sums to a psychic who guarantees a cure, a few sessions with a psychic healer won't do you any harm—and it might do some good.

Sometimes psychic healing isn't even done in person—healers and even ordinary people "send healing energy." Again, according to anecdotal evidence, it sometimes seems to help. One of my Jewish patients had a Catholic nun as a fellow patient at the time of her mastectomy. "Sister Cecile got all the nuns in her convent praying for me," recounts my patient. "I know that helped. Every time I've had surgery I've gotten people from every religion, every belief system, working for me—prayer, positive vibrations, whatever. I'd say, 'I'm going into surgery at 8 o'clock this Thursday, and I need your positive thoughts.'"

Whatever else such healing thoughts can do, they can achieve a twofold benefit. For the patient, it is a reminder of all the love and support that's out there for her—from friends, from loved ones, even from strangers. And for those who love her, it can alleviate some of the terrible sense of helplessness they feel in the face of a loved one's suffering. For the most part, your friends can't operate on you or administer your chemotherapy, but they can pray or send healing thoughts.

Unfortunately psychic healing has barely been studied at all by scientists, but Herbert Benson, in his *Beyond the Relaxation Response*, cites studies done in Canada by Dr. Bernard Grad that suggest the possibility that such healing, even when the subject isn't aware it's being done, may actually have an effect on illness.[11] (This echoes the studies on prayer mentioned earlier, and suggests that the placebo effect alone isn't enough to account for the effects of either prayer or psychic healing.) Hopefully, when doctors become less territorial about their healing abilities, more and more research will be done in this area.

Something else in the psychic realm to which people attribute healing powers are crystals and other stones. Many believe these can affect different parts of your physical and emotional health, and that using them to meditate, wearing them as jewelry, or simply keeping them around can help you remain healthy, or restore health if you're ill.[12] As far as I know, no scientific studies have been done on the healing power of stones, but that doesn't mean they can't work. Some of my patients have great faith in them, and I like to keep a small collection of amethysts in my office.

My co-author, who has done some research on the popularity of healing stones, speaks of them this way: "In an age when many people don't believe in a personal God, but do believe in some kind of higher power, crystals can function like the Catholic rosary or the Jewish mezuzuh. They provide a concrete symbol of your own belief in your ability to heal, but they don't tie that belief into a particular theology. And the fact that different stones are connected to different healing functions links them with the Catholic saints." According to her research, amethyst is seen as an all-purpose healer, while sugalite and tiger's eye are considered particularly effective with cancer, and moonstone is seen as helpful in the healing of women's cancers. "But almost everyone who works with stones will tell you that the most important thing is that you feel strongly drawn to a particular stone, and that its power comes as much from your connection to it as from any outside definition of its particular function."

Some patients bring their healing stones to radiation, chemotherapy, or other frightening or unpleasant treatments; they can be very soothing. One of my patients had her favorite crystal taped to her hand during surgery. Another carried her sugalite with her to her chemotherapy treatments, and held it to the parts of her body that the chemicals most negatively affected.

My co-author recommends a touch of common sense in regard to healing stones. "If a salesperson tells you that a $100 crystal is more powerful than a $10 one, you might want to take your business elsewhere. Stones aren't capitalists; if they really can heal, I don't think their ability will be limited by their price-tag or their karat count."

Diet, Vitamins, Herbs, and Acupuncture

All the treatments I've discussed so far use purely mental or spiritual techniques—they don't involve putting any physical substance into the body. Some forms of nontraditional treatments use herbs, vitamins, or other substances, as well as particular diets believed to heal cancer.

Studies show that women who eat a diet high in fruits and vegetables may have a decreased occurrence of breast cancer, and others show that women who are obese at the time of diagnosis have a poorer prognosis (see Chapter 18). So there's scientific evidence that would support changing your diet to a low-fat diet, and also losing weight once you are diagnosed. There is a large national study called the Women's Intervention Nutrition Study (WINS) that has randomized postmenopausal women to either eat a long-term, very low-fat diet or continue with their usual fare. This study should answer the question regarding dietary change after treatment. In addition to changing the composition of their diet, women might also want to decrease the portions.

Data show that people who are already heavy or who gain weight with their treatment have a worse chance of survival. Thus it's important to help people avoid gaining weight and to lose it if they're overweight already.

Unfortunately many proponents of dietary therapy go too far. They take the observational data suggesting that certain dietary components can decrease risk and assume that that means they can also cure cancer.

There are many diets recommended for cancer in general, and some for breast cancer in particular, most of which are low in fat, high in fruits and vegetables. They usually suggest avoiding processed foods, sugar, alcohol, and beef and chicken treated with hormones. If you decide to attempt a nutrition approach to healing your cancer, you should work very closely with your nutritionist and your physician both to create your particular diet and to coordinate it with your other treatments.

Macrobiotic diets have been extremely popular with many who believe that cancer can be cured or prevented through nutrition. They can be considered either complementary or alternative. Based on a Zen philosophy too complex to begin to describe here, macrobiotics emphasize whole grains, miso soup, fresh vegetables, and beans, with little fruit (only the fruit grown in your own region) and no sugar. Michio Kushi's *The Cancer Prevention Diet*[13] explains the diet in detail, and has specific suggestions for breast cancer patients, including 50–60 percent of whole grain cereals, 5–10 percent of tamari or miso soup, 20–30 percent cooked vegetables, 5 percent small beans, and 5 percent "sea vegetables." He rules out fats, iced foods or drinks, and a number of fruits. Unfortunately Kushi recommends that patients refrain from chemotherapy, radiation, or surgery. This, especially in cancer that is not yet metastatic, can be dangerous, even tragic.

The diet itself, while generally a healthful one, can, if too strictly followed, cause some problems for a patient undergoing chemotherapy or radiation, or recovering from surgery. It's low in calories and in protein, and when your body is depleted from these processes, that can be dangerous. If you're on a macrobiotic diet while undergoing medical treatments, make certain it's not causing medical problems—and perhaps, at least while you're being treated, you might want to modify the diet somewhat.

For many Western palates, a macrobiotic diet can be odd and unappetizing. If it's unpalatable to you, it probably won't do you any good.

If a state of well-being is an essential part of getting well, as the concepts I discussed earlier in this chapter suggest, regularly eating foods you loathe can be counterproductive.

Changing one's diet, however, can be an active way to participate in one's own recovery. A patient of mine who started her macrobiotic diet when she was diagnosed with cancer is certain it played some part in her healing, and she continues on a modified macrobiotic diet. "It's part of how I changed my life around in the wake of learning about my cancer, part of taking control of my body again," she says. She finds the diet comfortable and helpful.

Some branches of complementary healing involve treatments not usually defined as medicine. One of these is the ancient Chinese science of acupuncture, which sees healing in terms of "meridians," energy channels that run through the body. Special needles are inserted into the meridians. Acupuncturists have worked with breast cancer patients, usually in conjunction with Western medical treatments.

Marie Cargill, a Boston-area practitioner of Traditional Chinese Medicine (TCM), has used acupuncture with breast cancer patients. "What they've been using in China is a combination of Western treatments—surgery, radiation, chemotherapy—and Traditional Chinese Medicine," she says. "The oncologist sees a limited part. The patient is in and out, in and out, and then at the end, the patient is let go except for periodic follow-up. But meanwhile, we have a patient trying to survive. What patients do in China—and what I try to encourage here—is to put themselves under the care of a TCM practitioner all the way through the whole process." Acupuncture, she says, can strengthen the body overall, as surgery, radiation, and systemic treatments cause weakening.

Cargill and many other practitioners of TCM like to combine acupuncture with Chinese healing herbs. "We usually recommend the person start herbs a few days to a week before chemotherapy or radiation, which will allay almost all the side effects, and then continue all the way through, and stay under the care indefinitely." That way the herbs can fight whatever cancer cells may still be in the body. If the cancer is advanced, or there are other health problems as well, Cargill especially recommends combining acupuncture and herbs—"acupuncture two or three times a week, at least to begin with." She tells of a patient who had both AIDS and metastatic breast cancer. "We had no illusions at that point that we could save her life, but the acupuncture and the herbs helped the quality of her life enormously." Both acupuncture and herbs, she says, can work in a threefold level. They can help relieve all the side effects of radiation and chemotherapy—nausea, hair loss, fatigue, loss of appetite. "Cracking toxin herbs" fight the cancer itself and supplement the work of the other treatments.

Other herbs help build the immune system, which chemotherapy breaks down. There are particular herbs for breast cancer, which are different from herbs used for other cancers. In addition, there are herbs to work on the depression and anxiety that often accompany life-threatening illness.

Unfortunately, it can be hard in this country to find Chinese herbs and herbal practitioners outside of a big city. Some patients find a practitioner through a friend or acquaintance, visit the practitioner once for an initial examination, and then work with the practitioner over the phone. Though Cargill feels the combination of acupuncture and herbs is the best approach, she says that acupuncture alone can work well, if it's used frequently enough. She also suggests that women with a family history of breast cancer should start taking herbs when they're young and take them throughout their lives.

There are studies being done on some herbal remedies, and the results are encouraging. According to Barry Cassileth, several mushroom-derived compounds are approved for cancer therapy in Japan.[14] PC-SPES, a combination of eight herbs used in Traditional Chinese Medicine has been demonstrated to be useful for prostate cancer.[15] Another Traditional Chinese Medicine formula of 19 vegetables increased the survival of 12 patients with late-stage non–small cell lung cancer. In addition, the nontoxic vegetable brew significantly improved the quality of life.[16] Helene Smith, a researcher from San Francisco who developed metastatic breast cancer, pushed for a study of an individualized Tibetan herbal formula. Although she died of breast cancer, the study is being done. This is all the more remarkable because it required approval from the FDA and the University. It is a model for the fact that these alternative therapies can be studied and tested and indeed deserve to be.

Homeopathy

Another area of holistic healing is homeopathy, which practitioners describe as a method of self-healing stimulated by very small doses of those drugs that would produce in a healthy individual symptoms like those of the disease being treated. The drugs are chosen by the patient with the assistance of a homeopathic practitioner, who may or may not also be an M.D. The substances are all legal, and over-the-counter; you can take them on your own, but it's wiser to consult with someone who's trained and can suggest remedies suited to your problem and your overall health history. Common homeopathic substances include belladonna and bryonia. Ted Chapman, a homeopathic M.D. in Boston, has worked with patients who have breast cancer. He emphasizes that homeopathy doesn't cure cancer, and he doesn't recommend it in place of medical treatment. "Doctors work on the end product of the disease, and they come in from the outside. We're working from the inside, on what makes you vulnerable to your disease in the first place." Like many other adjunctive therapies, homeopathy is thought to work on the immune system, working to strengthen the patient's mind and body. It's helpful in alleviating some of the side effects of radiation or chemotherapy by giving tiny amounts of substances that can provoke these symptoms. The only negative side effect of homeopathy, says Dr. Chapman, is a brief aggravation of your symptoms—pain, fever, etc.—before they begin to regress.

Bioelectromagnetics

Magnets are popular with many people for the treatment of a number of diseases. The theory is that magnetic fields penetrate the body and heal damaged tissues, including cancers. There are no good scientific studies supporting this claim. Wearing magnets is probably not dangerous, however, and can have a beneficial mental effect for people who believe in them. And while their efficacy hasn't been proved, it hasn't to date been disproved either.

ALTERNATIVE TREATMENTS

Some treatments have been proposed to take the place of medical treatments. Most of them have not been studied in any scientifically rigorous way and their risks and complications are largely unknown. I mention them to be complete, but I don't endorse their use.

The best known of these is laetrile, a substance made from apricot pits. It hasn't been shown to work in any randomized, controlled studies, but it has a fair amount of nonscientific support. It's illegal in the U.S., and is currently being used in clinics in Mexico. Unfortunately its method of action has been misrepresented. Those who advocate its use claim that the cyanide it contains will be broken down by normal cells and not by cancer cells, thus causing the latter to die. This is not true, since neither type of cell can break down the cyanide. There have been reports of deaths from cyanide poisoning in patients taking laetrile.[17]

Another treatment is immuno-augmentative therapy, which was invented by Lawrence Burton, who practices in the Bahamas since it is illegal in the U.S. It is an individualized treatment considered by its advocates to restore natural immune defenses against all forms of cancer.

Metabolic therapies with detoxification are widely offered in Mexico, especially in Tijuana. One variant, the Gerson treatment, claims to counteract liver damage caused by chemotherapy with a low-salt, high-potassium diet, coffee enemas, and a gallon of fruit and vegetable juice daily. Other recipes are used at other clinics. The Gonzalez regimen includes a restrictive diet, pancreatic enzymes, and coffee enemas and has had some success with inoperable pancreatic cancer.[18] The National Cancer Institute is now sponsoring a randomized clinical trial at the Rosenthal Center for Complementary and Alternative Medicine at Columbia University.

Stanislaw Burzynski has developed antineoplaston therapy, which is available at his clinic in Houston, Texas. Although there have been anecdotal reports on its efficacy, it has yet to be proved. Chemically antineoplastons consist of phenyl acetate, a metabolite of phenylalanine that is being studied for potential anticancer activity by researchers at the National Cancer Institute and elsewhere.[19,20,21]

Shark cartilage was very popular for a time as a cancer treatment, based on its antiangiogenic properties. The problem is that the protein molecules are too large to be absorbed. A study looking at its efficacy showed no benefit.[22]

CanCell is a remedy developed by James Sheridan in 1936. It is composed of common chemicals and is apparently nontoxic. Despite many patient testimonials it has not been tested in a clinical trial.[23] Essiac is another popular herbal cancer alternative used in Canada and the U.S. It is made up of burdock, turkey rhubarb, sorrel, and slippery elm. Although data supporting its anticancer effects are lacking and it is illegal in Canada, it is available in health food stores in the U.S. Iscador is a derivative of mistletoe and is widely used in Europe. Data supporting its utility in cancer treatment have not been published.

Research

The Center for Complementary and Alternative Medicine is doing studies on melatonin, ginseng, mistletoe, and oleander for the treatment of breast cancer. The latter appears to have an antiangiogenesis factor. The Center is also studying shark cartilage. Ironically, these studies are being generated by people in traditional medicine. Most of the companies that make these products aren't trying to get them studied. Many of the alternative practitioners say they don't have the money to do the studies. They do, however, charge a lot for their treatments. The National Institutes of Health will help them with the necessary studies if they are truly interested. It now has a division of alternative medicine set up to help study some of these techniques. Perhaps

I'm being cynical, but I can't help wondering if they have an investment in *not* having them studied.

Many time-tested herbal and diet-based therapies are now being studied for their abilities to induce or extend remission. At the same time the absence of government regulation of supplements means that there are scores of unproved remedies or inadequate dosages of proved ones on the shelves of the pharmacies and grocery stores of the United States. This makes it very difficult for consumers to know what is safe to use. I do believe strongly that all treatments—be they bone marrow transplants or laetrile—need to be held to the same standard and should be adequately studied in randomized controlled trials.

Many people go to the Web for information on alternative and complementary healing, as well as on traditional medicine. This can be a good tool, but you need to know how to use it. Check a few things. Is the organization giving the information well known—have you heard of it before? Can you tell who's sponsoring the site, and what their qualifications are? Is it for profit or not for profit? Is the information dated and referenced? Are there data for safety and efficacy, or just anecdotes? Remember that anyone can have a website. On www.SusanLoveMD.com we offer links to many of the reliable sites, and will be doing clinical studies of many of these herbs.

If you are interested in researching any unproved cancer therapy I suggest that, in addition to the material you get from the therapy's advocates, you go to your local American Cancer Society Division Office or check quackwatch.com. They keep statements on these treatments that are fair and will describe for you exactly what is involved, as well as the known risks, side effects, opinion of the medical establishment, and any lawsuits that have been filed. Make sure you are really informed.

While I don't recommend patients take on a treatment that excludes the use of traditional treatments, I do feel this is a highly personal decision. What risks any of us will take for what reasons depends very much on who we are and what our values are.

There are, in fact, situations when refusing traditional treatment isn't really much of a risk. There are some cancers, and some stages in the development of other cancers, when the treatments we have simply aren't very helpful. If your prognosis isn't good, and chemotherapy isn't likely to extend your life for any length of time, you may well consider that the discomforts of the treatment aren't worth the slight chance that it will cure you, and that an alternative treatment offers both better survival hope and more comfort during the remainder of your life. Audre Lorde, the poet and political activist whose *Cancer Journals* described her experiences with breast cancer, later published a book of essays, *A Burst of Light*.[24] In the title essay she describes how, when she learned her cancer had metastasized to her liver, she decided to forego chemotherapy and use homeopathic methods instead. When the tumor in her liver was first discovered, in February 1984, she refused even to have it biopsied, fearing the surgery would spread the cancer cells—a common, although not very realistic, fear. Instead, while in Berlin teaching classes, she went to a homeopathic doctor who treated her with injections of Iscador (mistletoe). Later, she continued this treatment at a homeopathic clinic in Switzerland. When a sonogram later demonstrated that she did indeed have metastatic cancer, her doctor told her, accurately, that chemotherapy could add only about a year to her life. She decided to stick with her homeopathic healing, adding visualization and meditation to the process, and determinedly living her life to the fullest. She lived until November 1992—an impressive achievement with liver metastasis, and who's to say that it wasn't because she chose a treatment that she believed in, and that allowed her to remain as active as possible, doing the work to which she was so passionately committed?

As much as I wish it were otherwise, traditional medical treatments are imperfect. They are often successful, and should not be lightly discarded. But they can be supplemented, in ways we have good reason to believe may increase some patients' survival rates. Whether any of these ways is right for you, I can't say. But I recommend that you look into them, and take from them what seems helpful to you. I like the attitude of one of my patients, a 46-year-old woman whose cancer metastasized to her bone marrow, and who did remarkably well for several years. A devout Catholic, she cherished the advice of a nun who told her to "work as though everything depended on you, and pray as though everything depended on God." She had surgery and tamoxifen therapy. She also went on a macrobiotic diet, later reinforcing it with a diet of linseed oil and cottage cheese recommended by a holistic doctor in Germany. She took a mind–body course at Beth Israel, and one of Bernie Siegel's workshops, and continued a regular meditation and visualization program. Whenever a church had a healing service, she went to it—"Catholic or Protestant, I go wherever I'll get healed," she said. She went to Lourdes with her aunt, who also had cancer ("I stayed for three days," she says. "It was a very emotional, very draining, experience—my aunt's tumor disappeared"). She carried an amethyst with her, and was interested in crystals. "Because I'm Catholic, my friends gave me a rosary made of crystal, which I carry with me all the time, so I've got the healing power of the rosary and of the crystal combined. I'm not settling for just one thing."

Though she ultimately died from her cancer, her health improved during the year she began integrating these methods into her healing work. In spite of the cancer in her bones, she went mountain climbing and cross-country skiing—and dancing.

I don't know which component of this patient's healing work did the most good, but I do know that her commitment to taking control of her healing process turned a terrifying experience into a triumphant challenge. She gave herself every chance to survive, and to live a quality existence—which she did to the end. Not everyone, of course, will have the time or energy to follow all the routes she has, but everyone can learn from her example and make a wholehearted commitment to life.

PART SEVEN

LIVING WITH BREAST CANCER

30

Life After Breast Cancer

You've had breast cancer, you've been treated for it, and now it's time to get on with your life. But your life has changed now, and you have to adjust to your new situation on a number of levels. One of my patients told me that "it's like your life breaks into a million pieces and when you put the pieces back together they don't quite fit exactly the same."

THE FOLLOW-UP

For one thing, you'll have to be dealing medically with the fact of your cancer for a long time. Usually the surgeon and/or other specialists who did your primary treatment—your mastectomy or wide excision—will follow you at regular intervals for a period of time. Sometimes coming to these appointments is a reminder of what you have been through.

At UCLA there is a follow-up program in which patients are seen every six months for the first two years and every year after that. The program includes not just exams and mammograms but also physical therapy, nutritional counseling, psychosocial support, and involvement in research.

In follow-up examinations there are a few things the doctors are looking for. In the breast or mastectomy scar they look for lumps. They check the neck and the area above the collarbone for lumps that might indicate a lymph node, and feel under both arms. Once a year or once every six months they'll do a mammogram.

In addition, they question the woman very carefully about how she's feeling physically. They check to see if she's had persistent and unusual pain in her legs or back, or a persistent dry cough, or any of the other symptoms described at length in Chapter 32. In general, if you have a new symptom that doesn't go away in a week or two, check it out. Usually that's what most patients do anyway.

Patients are often surprised when their doctor doesn't find anything on their follow-up exam; they've been waiting for the cancer to pop up again, and tend to be very anxious about examinations. Often because they're especially worried on the anniversary of their original diagnosis, an examination will serve a psychological purpose as well as a medical one by alleviating their fears. Doctors seldom find something on a follow-up that the patient hasn't already noticed.

Not all symptoms mean the cancer has spread. Women who have had cancer may also acquire other diseases as they age. Having had cancer does not make one immune to arthritis or diabetes, for example. Aside from ordinary, nonrelated problems, patients experience changes as a result of the treatment for their cancer. Part of the reason it's important to have frequent checkups is that a breast that's been radiated undergoes a lot of changes. There will be a lumpy area under the scar and perhaps some skin firmness and/or puckering. By keeping track on a regular basis the doctor can assure the patient that the changes she's experiencing are related to the treatment—and if there's a different, more ominous change, the doctor can distinguish it from the others.

For the same reasons your surgeon will probably want you to have mammograms every six months for a year or two, and then once a year. In addition to monitoring the treated breast, the doctor will watch your other breast for the possible development of a new cancer, since women with cancer in one breast have an increased risk of getting it in the other. The untreated breast should be x-rayed every year. This eventuality is not inevitable; the risk is about 1 percent per year, or an average of 15 percent over a lifetime.[1] (See Chapter 24 for a discussion of the second primary cancer.) There are some types of breast cancer that indicate a greater propensity for a second breast cancer to develop. Cancers with a lot of lobular carcinoma *in situ* (see Chapter 20) have been thought to fit into this category.[2] Even in this situation, however, the increased risk to the second breast is about double, or 2 percent per year, a cumulative lifetime risk of 30 percent. Obviously the younger you are and the longer you live the greater the chance you have to develop a second cancer. If this is too scary for you, you may want to consider a preventive mastectomy on the other side, but I find that most women prefer close follow-up to such a drastic step. If you're considering this, it's important to remember that a mastectomy almost never removes all the breast tissue in your body and therefore can't guarantee that you won't develop breast cancer again.

In addition to your regular doctor, you may be followed by your whole team—your radiation oncologist and/or your medical oncologist might also want to check on you regularly. Some patients find this a little overwhelming, and don't want to spend all that time trekking back and forth to doctors. More typically, you'll be followed by one of the members of the team, or even by your local family doctor, if she or he has some experience with breast cancer. Your HMO may affect which kind of follow-up is available. In the near future we'll be training primary care doctors in how to follow breast cancer patients, so if something occurs that may be dangerous, they'll know to refer you to a specialist.

Some doctors still do blood tests every three to six months, including not only your blood count (CBC) but also specific tests (for example, a CEA, CA 15–3, or CA 27.29), as well as liver blood tests which they hope will catch metastatic disease at the earliest point. They don't always succeed. Most of these tests are not very sensitive or specific. They go up when there is metastatic disease but they also go up for other conditions. Not only are they limited in their ability to find metastasis early, but there's no evidence that such detection does you any good.[3] As we note in Chapter 32, we still have no guaranteed way of curing metastatic disease—though we can relieve symptoms and perhaps add a few years to your life. There's no evidence that treating metastatic disease before it shows symptoms will give you more time than treating it after the symptoms have surfaced;[4] and in terms of quality of life, knowing sooner that you have a metastasis probably doesn't do you much good. So these tests can actually interfere with quality of life without affecting its length. Even when they turn out negative, you still might have a metastasis that is too small to show up on the tests. This also holds true for the routine use of bone scans, chest x rays, CAT scans, and liver blood tests.

The only test useful in terms of longevity is the mammogram, which shows if there's a local recurrence in the breast or a cancer in the other breast. So unless you're taking part in a protocol that requires regular testing, you may not want to have the other tests.

With breast cancer, unlike some other cancers, we can't be sure that if it hasn't recurred within a few years, it won't. It's usually a slow-growing cancer, and there are people who have had recurrences 10 or even 20 years after the original diagnosis. In some ways this is similar to a chronic disease. You are never quite sure if or when it will come back again.

Time does, however, affect the *likelihood* of recurrence—the longer you go without a recurrence, the less likely you are to have one. So going 10 years without the cancer coming back should give you reason for optimism, if not certainty.

Since problems resulting from treatment can come up years afterwards, it's important to keep records of the treatment and to have continued contact with somebody who knows about the delayed effects of treatment. An oncologist colleague of mine from Los Angeles, Dr. Patricia Ganz, says, "I've seen women 10 or 15 years after their treatment who have no records of what happened years ago. And we've had to try and reconstruct their history. Survivors need to have knowledge about what they were treated with, so they can remind their family doctor or tell any new doctor about it, and have medical records to show them."

At the end of the treatment period you go back to your normal activities; you look fine and, physically, you feel fine. Everybody's relieved that things are back to normal again—everybody but you. You may still be very nervous. Physical problems that wouldn't have bothered you before now seem ominous. That slight headache that two years ago you would have dismissed as tension—has the cancer metastasized to your brain? And what does the bruise on your arm mean—have you got leukemia? You're now in the "I can't trust my body" stage. Well, why should you trust your body? It betrayed you once, and you know it can do it again. Every time you go for a checkup, every time you get a blood test, you're terrified. In my experience with patients, this stage usually lasts two or three years, until you've had enough innocent headaches and bruises, enough reassuring checkups and blood tests, to feel somewhat trusting of your body again.

And then, just when you are settling down and starting to forget about it, something pops up in the paper or on the news about a risk factor or new treatment, and it all comes back to you. You start wondering if it was the alcohol or birth control pills (or whatever happens to be on today's "hit list") that caused your cancer. Or you regret the decision you made, thinking, "With this new information maybe I should have done things differently." Remember, what is past is past. You can't change the way you lived your life in the past based on new information just coming to light today. And you have to comfort yourself with the realization that you probably got the best treatment that was available at the time you were diagnosed. If there are improvements in treatments now, that's wonderful—but you can't waste your energy on what might have been. Read the newspapers and keep informed if you're interested, but don't use it to torture yourself about what might have been. Gradually you will regain your perspective.

Though life will never be completely the same, you'll stop living in terms of your cancer. The fears and memories will come back occasionally—maybe at your yearly checkups, maybe on the anniversary of your diagnosis, maybe when you find out a friend had a recurrence. But they'll be part of your life, not the center of it.

LIFESTYLE CHANGES

Often people who have suffered life-threatening illnesses are more aware of the importance of health than they were before, and want to invest energy in maintaining their health as much as they can. They often opt for specific lifestyle changes.

Any sport or exercise you did before your cancer you can do now— and you should, if you want to. If you've been a fairly sedentary person, you might want to change that. As we mentioned in Chapter 18, it's been shown that exercise helps prevent breast cancer. It can't help but benefit women after their diagnosis. Not only will it make you feel better but it will help you regain a sense of control over your body.

You might also want to examine your eating habits and health habits in general. At UCLA researchers are currently participating in a national study looking at the effect of a very low-fat diet on postmenopausal women who have been treated for breast cancer. As we discussed in Chapter 29, nutrition is an important component in healing.

HEALING THE MIND

Obviously, not all aftereffects of breast cancer are physical (see Chapter 22). You've had a life-threatening illness, and one that affects your sense of permanence. You feel more fragile. Emotional healing techniques are more varied and individual than physical ones, but there are many that have proved helpful to my patients and other women with breast cancer.

Often women keep a journal of their experiences to refer to later and to help them cope with their feelings. Some take their healing out beyond themselves—reaching out to other women who are going through what they've been through. Writers like Audre Lorde, Betty Rollin, Rose Kushner, and Katherine Russel Rich have written about the experience (see Appendix B for a list of first person books). Actress Ann Jillian wrote and starred in a TV movie about her battle with breast cancer, in the hope of helping other women. Years ago, when breast cancer was still considered somehow shameful, public figures like Shirley Temple Black, Happy Rockefeller, and Betty Ford spoke out in the mass media about their experiences, hoping to encourage women to examine their breasts and have any suspicious lump checked out immediately.

It's not only famous women, or women in glamorous occupations, who can help other women with breast cancer. Two of my patients are psychotherapists who now specialize in breast cancer therapy. Another has begun doing breast cancer workshops at her corporation. A sales clerk might want to work in a store selling prostheses, since she now has a special understanding that might help her customers.

If your profession isn't one that can be adapted to some form of working with breast cancer, or if you don't feel drawn toward spending your work life dealing with the disease, you can still help other women—and thus yourself—on a volunteer basis. For example, you might want to get involved with Reach for Recovery (see Appendix B), or some similar group that works with breast cancer patients. You know how frightened you were when you were first diagnosed. The presence of someone who's survived the disease can be enormously reassuring to a newly diagnosed woman who only knew people who died from it.

You can also become involved in political action, like the work done by the National Breast Cancer Coalition (see Chapter 34). You can define the level of your participation according to your own energy, time constraints, and degree of commitment: anything from an occasional letter to your congressperson to organizing demonstrations and fundraising events. Jane Reese Colbourne, a former vice president of the Coalition, found that in her own experience political activism had been "a very good way to channel anger at the fact that you've had this disease. For me, it was the next step after a support group. Talking about it with other women was important—but I wanted to do something about it."

Finally, make sure you don't feel ashamed of what you've been through. Cancer still carries a stigma in our culture, and breast cancer can have especially difficult associations. You need to demystify it to yourself, and to others. You don't have to dwell on it, but it's not a good idea to repress it either. You need to have friends you can talk freely to about your disease and your feelings about it; you need to know you can include it in casual conversation, that you don't have to avoid saying, "Oh, yes, that was around the time I was in the hospital for my mastectomy."

SEX

One of the least discussed subjects about life after breast cancer is sexuality. Your surgeon won't bring it up if you don't; in fact most surgeons will assume that if you're not complaining, everything must be fine. Yet most women find sex hard to talk about—especially when it concerns feelings, perhaps only half recognized themselves, about losing both their sexual attractiveness and their own libidos when they lose a part of their bodies so strongly associated with sexuality. Doctors need to learn how to open the subject delicately, in a way that doesn't feel intrusive to the woman and yet makes it clear that she has a safe place to discuss issues around sexuality that have arisen for her. I remember one surgeon who had referred a patient to me on his retirement. He said that after her mastectomy she had surprised everyone with her rapid recovery and exclaimed over how well she had "dealt with it." I took over the case, and in my first conversation with her I found out that, however well adjusted she seemed on the surface, she had not yet looked at her scar—and this was five years after the operation. She had never resumed sex with her husband and even dressed and undressed in the closet so he couldn't see her.

Many women have difficulties with sex and intimacy following a breast cancer diagnosis. Aside from feeling that your body has betrayed you, there is a feeling of invasion from the treatments. All these strangers have been poking and prodding you for weeks; you may almost feel as though you've been violated, and you forget that your body can provide you with pleasure. It takes a while to feel good and in control of your body again. You need to communicate these feelings to your partner so he or she can help you in your healing.

Some women find that after surgery, whether mastectomy or lumpectomy, a sexual relationship becomes even more important in helping them regain their sense of worth and wholeness. There may, however, be changes. One patient of mine who had had bilateral mastectomies felt that all the erotic sensations she had formerly had in her breasts had "moved south," and that her orgasms were doubly good. Other women miss the stimulation from a lost breast so much that they don't want their other breast touched during sex. Dr. Patricia Ganz, who has both worked with and studied the problems of women with breast cancer, talks about the problems women who have had lumpectomy and radiation may experience: "Especially with women who had radiation a number of years ago, they often find the breast isn't as soft and beautiful as it was before the radiation." These changes in the conserved breast can carry over into their sexual relationships.

Some of the changes may be more practical than emotional. Your arm or shoulder may not be as strong on the side of your surgery, and this can make certain positions more difficult during intercourse, such as kneeling above your partner. You may feel uncomfortable lying on the side of the surgery for many months. It is important that you communicate with your partner so that together you can explore new ways of lovemaking that you both enjoy.

Chemical menopause (see Chapter 31) can also affect a woman's sexuality. Menopause, like aging itself, often lessens sexual desire, and when that combines with other breast cancer issues a woman can find that her libido is abruptly and seriously lessened. Studies are now being done to see whether the libido loss of women with chemically induced menopause is more severe than that of women who have experienced menopause normally.

Dr. Ganz adds that it's difficult to separate out the physiological and emotional aspects of libido loss. "Sex is at least partly in the brain," she says, "and the hormones circulating in the body affect the brain and thus sexual arousal. Psychological distress can affect hormones; we've found in our work that women who have a lot of psychological distress have more sexual dysfunction."

It is important to note that there are no aspects of sexual intimacy that will cause cancer or increase the chance of recurrence. Nor can cancer be "caught" by sucking on a nipple. Barbara Kalinowski, who once co-led support groups with me at the Faulkner in Boston, finds that "sometimes women who have had lumpectomy and radiation have a fantasy that the breast still has cancer in it, and don't want it fondled because they fear it will shake things up and send the cancer cells through the rest of the body." Even when your intellect knows such fears are groundless, your emotions may still accept them—and that's bound to have an effect on both partners' sexual pleasure.

Sheila Kitzinger[5] in her book *Woman's Experience of Sex* says that some women have told her that an important part of their healing process was having a brief affair. They said it was all well and good for a husband of 35 years to still love them without a breast, but they needed the confirmation that they were still sexually attractive to feel whole again. That might work for you—though it could also put a severe strain on your marriage. At the very least, however, you'll want to be in touch with whatever feelings you're having about sex, and decide which ones to act on and which ones to simply fantasize about.

This brings up another issue. If you are single and dating, should you tell or not? Again, this is an individual decision. Some women will tell a prospective lover way in advance, preferring to have it out in the open before the moment of passion. Others will wait until the last instant when there is no turning back to disclose their secret (never a

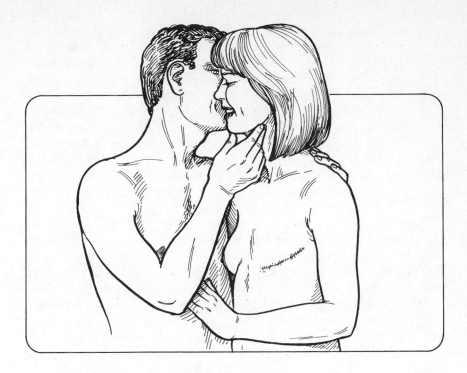

good idea). For the woman who has had only a small lumpectomy, or who has had mastectomy and a very attractive and natural-looking reconstruction, the need to tell a casual lover about her situation may or may not arise. However, in a long-term relationship, it's important to be honest. For the woman whose surgery leaves visible alteration, dating can be a matter of concern. Yet it doesn't mean you have to resign yourself to a life of celibacy. Barbara Kalinowski found that several women in her support groups were able to form successful, new romantic relationships shortly after the surgery was over. She recalls one woman who had never married and who had a mastectomy with reconstruction in her 50s. "I got a call from her a couple of years ago. She was as giggly and happy as a teenager. 'Guess what!' she told me. 'I'm getting married!' They were planning a honeymoon in Paris and she was ecstatic." Another woman from one of Kalinowski's groups had been happily married to a man who had been wonderful to her during her treatments. Two years later he died of a heart attack. Soon after his death she met a widower and they fell in love. "They decided not to wait," Kalinowski says, "because they both knew how chancy life was. She told me, 'We both learned that we don't want to wait for anything anymore.'"

Working out these issues and feeling comfortable with yourself are all part of the healing process. If you find it difficult or if you get stuck on some issue you may well want to try some counseling. A diagnosis of breast cancer reminds you that life can be short and you certainly want to live it as fully as you can.

Many women worry about whether their partner will be turned off by their condition and new body. There are, of course, many horror stories of husbands and significant others who opted out of having sex or who walked out entirely. And I am sure it happens. The impact of cancer can be as devastating to the partner as to the patient herself. Partners may feel angry, ashamed, and vulnerable to illness themselves. Their lives and dreams have been changed, but they typically get less support. They feel guilty complaining when they are not the one having to undergo treatment. Some people have problems dealing with serious illness, and others may use it as an excuse to get out of a relationship they thought was not working. Most important is the quality of the relationship and the level of communication. Work by David Wellisch[6] at UCLA indicated that the involvement of the husband in the decision-making process, hospital visitation, early viewing of the scars, and early resumption of sexual activity was important for optimal functioning of couples. Open dialogue is critical in this process, and it applies to nonmarried and lesbian couples as well.

Another study[7] found that patients' and their partners' levels of adjustment were significantly related; if one partner was experiencing difficulties in adjustment, the other was also likely to be having problems. It is important that difficulties in communication and sex be addressed promptly. Patricia Ganz[8] found that most sexual issues were resolved by one year and that if they were not they were never resolved. Counseling—where you can talk about your feelings in a protective environment—can be important in preventing serious problems. Hoping a situation will get better on its own rarely works; in fact, it causes the problem to become chronic. Request help for such problems as decreased libido and vaginal dryness; you might even consider seeing a sex therapist.

PHYSICAL ADJUSTMENTS

More women are now living for many years after breast cancer treatments. This is, of course, a wonderful development. But it brings to these survivors a particular set of problems we seldom had to deal with in the past—problems that are the result of the treatments themselves.

Long-Term Side Effects of Surgery and Radiation

Unfortunately, your body doesn't always feel like it did before your cancer began. Radiation can cause some delayed problems. There's a side effect that can occur between three and six months after you've finished your treatment. The muscle that goes above and behind your breast, the pectoralis major muscle (see Fig. 27–6), will get extremely sore. That's because the radiation has caused some inflammation of the muscle, and as it begins to regenerate and get back to normal, it can get sore and stiff, just as it would if you threw it out using it in some strong athletic activity. Again, most women think it's the cancer spreading—especially since the radiation's been over for months and they're not thinking in terms of new side effects from it. If you grab that muscle between your fingers it will feel extremely sore.

Many women find they have a stiff or frozen shoulder a month after breast surgery. Arm and shoulder problems are more a consequence of lymph node dissection than the operation on the breast. When your armpit hurts it's natural to want to avoid disturbing it by keeping your arm immobilized, but when you don't use your arm your shoulder muscles grow weak and the tendons and ligaments tighten. You may find you have difficulty reaching; it's very painful to raise your hand above your head. When you don't use your arm for too long a time you risk developing frozen shoulder—a condition in which the joint becomes locked. Frozen shoulder can be more difficult to treat than a stiff shoulder, and it sometimes requires surgery. This isn't an inescapable consequence of the procedure: it can be prevented, and if necessary reversed. Start with gentle exercises, like climbing the wall with your fingers and circling your arms as soon as you feel able (see Chapter 25). The YWCA has a wonderful exercise program (Encore) which focuses on helping women recover. Swimming is also good because it doesn't put weight on the arm. You can resume any exercise routine you enjoyed doing in the past.

If exercising on your own isn't successful, a physical therapist can assess what you are capable of doing and where you need help, and can devise a program to increase your strength and flexibility. This therapist can train you to do exercises properly so that you don't get hurt trying to do them yourself. Insurance plans often cover physical therapy after breast surgery, so be sure to ask.

Massage has effects similar to those of exercise. It can help relax tight tendons to get your shoulder back into commission. Acupuncture is another possibility. Although it has been tested for only a few applications in Western medicine, it hasn't been demonstrated to cause harm. There is some evidence it can help to relieve lower back pain, so it may also help shoulder stiffness, although there are no scientific data to that effect.

Scarring is an inevitable consequence of breast surgery, one you may have given little thought to beforehand. Initially, many women are so intent upon saving their life that they have little time to address how their body will look once they are through with therapy. Of course, the look of the scar depends not only on the extent of surgery, but on your skin, your body type, the size of your breast, and the type of surgery you had. To avoid being surprised by the way your body looks after surgery, ask your doctor to let you see pictures of women who have had a similar operation, go to our website and look at the "show me" collection, or read books on the subject (see Appendix B). There are several things you can do to make the scar more acceptable to you, from working with the surgeon to prevent surprises to having plastic surgery on the scar afterwards.

After mastectomy, it can take more than a year for the incision to heal completely. It's sometimes difficult to know whether a problem is temporary or whether it will be with you long-term. Either way, you might want to discuss problems that seem significant or unusual with your surgeon. It's also important to remember that you don't need to wait a year to have additional surgery or procedures to correct the problems.

The scar may be raised, seemingly filled with extra skin. This is often referred to as a keloid scar. It is a result of an overly aggressive effort by the body's immune system to heal the wound. The body keeps filling the scar with collagen long after the wound has closed. The tendency to form keloid scars is probably inherited, and there is little that can be done to prevent them. A plastic surgeon may be able to improve the appearance of your scar. There is nothing wrong with being concerned about your physical appearance. You've been through a very unpleasant and life-changing experience; you're entitled to do what you can to make its aftermath as comfortable as possible for yourself. Talk to a plastic surgeon about all the possibilities and decide what's best for you.

A mastectomy leaves a fairly large wound. When the surgeon pulls the skin and underlying tissue together to close it, the surface of the chest is drawn taut. In contrast, the surrounding tissue under the arm may seem baggy and excessive and hang over your bra. If fat is a major component of the extra tissue under the arm, it can be removed through liposuction. Excess skin can also be eliminated without increasing scarring.

Even a lumpectomy can cause considerable change in the breast you've saved. It may look foreign and disturbing to you; it may have a dent, look shrunken, or appear to be pulled to one side. As pointed out in Chapter 25, if the surgeon sutures the fat and skin separately there will be a depression because the fat does not fill out the entire area under the skin, but the breast will still be about the same size as the other one. If your breasts are large the change may be barely noticeable; if they are small, a substantial portion of your breast may be missing. If the surgeon brings the edges of the incision in the fat and skin together there will be no dent, but your breast will be smaller than the other one. When tissue is removed, it can also change the position of the nipple, giving the breast a lopsided look. The direction of the incision has a lot to do with the position of the nipple, pulling it in the direction of the incision. For example, a vertical incision may drag it toward the middle of the chest or the armpit; a horizontal incision can relocate it to a position higher or lower than formerly.

If you are still troubled by the look of your breast months or years after surgery, you can always have a reconstructive procedure. A plastic surgeon can discuss various techniques to realign nipples, reshape breasts, and make the breasts more symmetrical. For example, if you have large breasts you may want to consider having reduction surgery done on the healthy breast to make it a better match for the one on which the lumpectomy was performed. Or if you find that the lumpectomy has raised the nipple, you may want a breast lift on the other side to even things out. Be sure to ask to see pictures of other breast cancer patients the surgeon has treated. If your main objective is to look good in clothing, a mini-prosthesis, called a shell, may be the answer.

Long-term problems may result from the surgery as well. While most women experience some pain in the weeks after surgery, especially mastectomy, many will have such pain for years afterwards. It can begin years after the operation. Forty-nine percent of patients who have operations for breast cancer say they have some sort of ongoing pain or change in sensation, and 10 percent say it interferes with their daily lives.[9] The biggest complaint is "aching," experienced by 44 to 47 percent of the women who say they have pain. Many others describe it as a "stabbing" pain. "Shooting," "sharp," "tiring," and "throbbing" are other descriptions. They feel the pain in the mastectomy scar, the arm, even the muscle under the breast. I've known a number of women who had this problem and it really affects their lives badly.

We don't know precisely what causes the pain, but it seems clear that it involves damage to the *intercostalbrachial* nerve, the nerve that causes numbness in the arm, and which is usually cut during lymph node surgery . It's also related to the intensity of a woman's postoperative pain. Again, we don't know what that means; it could be that these women have low pain thresholds, or it could be that they had the earlier pain because the intercostalbrachial nerve was injured.

C. B. Wallace studied pain that women experienced a year after different kinds of breast surgery.[10] Lumpectomy alone resulted in pain among 31 percent of subjects. Mastectomy plus reconstruction caused pain in 49 percent of the women. Women who had had breast reconstruction varied: those who had implants under the muscle had pain in 15 percent of cases, whereas those who had them above the muscle had pain 21 percent of the time. Mastectomy alone caused pain through the armpit and arm: 82 percent of women had pain under their arms three months after a mastectomy, and in 16 percent, it lasted at least six months. Sometimes the pain was so bad the woman couldn't move her arm, and she got "frozen shoulder" (discussed earlier in this chapter). Women who had had breast reduction suffered later pain in 22 percent of cases, and 40 percent of women who had breast augmentation had pain. One study[11] shows that more careful surgical techniques reduce the amount of chronic pain. They found there were fewer pain problems from operations performed in centers that did lots of surgery than in those that didn't. It makes sense: an inexperienced surgeon is more likely to injure nerves.

This kind of pain has been treated with *myofascial release,* a form of massage.[12] Among my patients acupuncture has helped a great deal. Another pain study[13] suggests that if the pain is caused by damaged nerves, antidepressants can relieve it; this has no relation to the patient's frame of mind but to the specific way such drugs work on nerves. Most large hospitals have pain specialists whom you can consult.

Lymphedema

A major long-term complication is swelling of the arm, a condition called lymphedema, which can result from removal of the lymph nodes. It can be so slight that you notice it only because your rings are gradually feeling too tight on your fingers, or so severe that your arm is huge, even elephantine (Fig. 30–1). It can be temporary or permanent. It can happen immediately, or years after your operation. What causes it to happen? Basically, lymphedema—sometimes called "milk arm"—is a plumbing problem. Normally, the lymph fluid is carried through the lymph vessels, passes through the lymph nodes, and gets dumped back into the bloodstream, near the heart. The lymph nodes act like a strainer, removing foreign material and bacteria. So if you have surgery in the area and it scars over, some of the holes are blocked

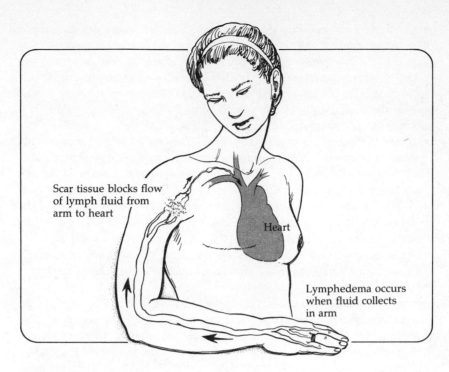

Scar tissue blocks flow
of lymph fluid from
arm to heart

Heart

Lymphedema occurs
when fluid collects
in arm

FIGURE 30-1

and the drainage can't work as effectively. The fluid doesn't drain out as well as it needs to, and everything backs up and swells. Protein leaks into the tissue and then scars, causing the condition to become chronic. This used to be much more common—we'd see it in about 30 percent of cases—because more extensive surgery was done. Nowadays, since we remove less tissue, it happens only in about 10 percent of mastectomies, according to current studies. I think, however, that this figure is a bit low, and that if we measured every patient carefully in the follow-up visits we'd find the mild cases are a lot more common, and that for whatever reason the women don't tell their doctors about it.

Most women are cautioned about hand and arm care after surgery with the hope that they can prevent lymphedema from happening in the first place. There are no data supporting these recommendations, however. One study comparing women who had had bilateral mastectomies and axillary dissections to those who only had surgery on one side showed no difference in the incidence of lymphedema.[14] Most of them continued to have blood pressures done and blood drawn from one of their arms, suggesting that those procedures are not as dangerous as we might have thought. New studies are being done to try to determine whether the classical precautions are really necessary.

Lymphedema proceeds through stages. First is the latency stage where the arm is not swollen, but as a result of surgery there is a reduced capacity for transporting lymph fluid. As long as there are no undue stresses on the system all will be well. The next stage, stage 1, is reversible, soft swelling. The skin is still normal and the swelling can be relieved by elevating your arm. Stage 2 is no longer spontaneously reversible because there are fibrous changes in the tissues that make your arm feel hard. In this stage there are frequent infections, which exacerbate the situation. The final stage is "lymphostatic elephantiasis." This is an extreme increase in volume and texture of your arm, with typical skin changes, including deep skin folds. As one of the experts in lymphedema treatment said, "Since there is no cure for lymphedema the goal of therapy is to reduce the swelling and maintain the reduction"—in other words, to bring lymphedema back to a state of latency.

One of the best ways to accomplish this goal is a treatment first devised in Germany called "complete decongestive physiotherapy." Numerous observational studies have established its effectiveness, which is well acknowledged in Europe and, increasingly, in the U.S.[15,16] It is usually done by a physical therapist and involves four steps.

1. Skin and nail care that may also include topical and systemic antifungal drugs (with the skin free of infection before treatment)
2. Manual lymph drainage, a special technique of compression
3. Compression therapy using bandaging
4. Decongestive exercises

The treatment is done in two phases. The first phase is an attempt to mobilize the accumulated protein-rich fluid and to start to break up the chronic scarring. This phase is intense and can last four weeks—ideally, treatment is given twice a day five days a week. The next phase, which immediately follows, includes compression garments and bandaging at night. Although this is a great new treatment, it is also expensive and time-consuming. The best results come when the patient is in stage 1. If you are considering it, make sure you find a physical therapist or doctor who has been trained in the technique. The National Lymphedema Network (www.lymphnet.org) can help you locate one in your neighborhood.

Other therapies include elevating your arm to help reduce some of the swelling. Physical therapy and exercise can help in early cases. There are long support gloves, similar to the stockings they make for varicose veins, which, though unesthetic, can reduce the swelling. (Ask for Class II [30–40 mm Hg] or Class III [40–50 mg Hg] support.) Although in Australia they initially reported good results with the group of drugs called benzopyrones[17] such as coumarin, more recent randomized controlled studies have shown them to have no value.[18]

My theory about lymphedema is that we're probably approaching it backwards. The tendency has been to tell you to go home and elevate the arm if you have a little bit of swelling, to put on an elastic arm-stocking if you have a lot of swelling, and to use the pump if you have an extreme amount of swelling. But by the time you use the pump, your tissues have been so stretched out they've lost all their normal elasticity. It's like putting on a pair of panty hose you wore all day yesterday. What then happens is that as soon as you get off the pump more fluid fills all this loose skin up again.

I think we should act aggressively when we find a small amount of swelling—use physical therapy, manual massage, the pump—and try to reverse it. Then we'd probably be able to reverse the process in more people, because they'd still have the elasticity in their skin. There have been a number of operations for lymphedema, but none of them has been very effective.

Lymphedema has been vastly underestimated by the medical profession. The difficulties of women with lymphedema, physically and psychologically, are enormous. Anne Coscarelli, Director of the Rhonda Fleming Mann Resource Center for Women with Cancer at UCLA, feels that the medical profession underestimates the psychological stress of having lymphedema. It is a constant reminder that "the ordeal is not over," and the fact that it has to be "managed" is a reminder that you can't get back to your old life. On top of this, it generates less support from caregivers and family because it is not life-threatening. Most women suffering from lymphedema benefit greatly from talking to others about the experience either in a support group or on a bulletin board on the Internet. In 1995 at UCLA we started what I think was the first lymphedema support group, in an attempt to address some of these problems. The only way to prevent lymphedema is to stop doing axillary dissections. Luckily, that day is on the horizon (See Chapter 25).

Cellulitis

Cellulitis is an infection of the skin. It occurs more commonly in places on the body that have diminished access to the immune system, such as areas of swelling or areas that have been radiated. It can start from any small infection and rapidly spread, often with a red streak up the arm or redness of the arm and/or breast. There is usually a fever as well. Although this type of infection can sometimes be treated with oral antibiotics, more often than not it requires hospitalization for intravenous drugs. Some women who are prone to recurrent attacks of cellulitis find it useful to ask the doctor for a prescription for an antibiotic to carry around with them so they can start taking it if there is the least sign of impending infection. In a series from Memphis, Tennessee, 1 percent of the lumpectomy and radiation patients had cellulitis of the breast.

LONG-TERM SIDE EFFECTS OF CHEMOTHERAPY

In the past, chemotherapy was used only to treat metastasis. Oncologists at that time weren't thinking about long-term effects; their hope was to keep the patient living a few years longer than she would without the treatment. If she lived long enough to deal with long-term effects, she and her doctors were happy. As we've become able to detect micrometastases, and to use chemotherapy on people whose cancers haven't yet significantly spread, this has changed. A woman treated with chemotherapy may now live for many years, and the issues surrounding her long-term well-being are important. Only now are we beginning to grasp the implications of this development.

As we mentioned in Chapter 28, often one of the major long-term side effects of chemotherapy in younger women is premature menopause. Because this is such a big issue I've devoted a whole chapter to it (see Chapter 31).

"Chemo" Brain

There are many other aftereffects of chemotherapy which we're just beginning to acknowledge, either because they're more subtle or because they take longer to materialize. For example, studies show decreased cognitive function (what patients call "chemo brain"). Unfortunately, doctors basically have dismissed women with this problem, telling them they're "lucky to be alive." Well, the women know they're lucky, but since they *are* alive, they want to be as sharp as they can be.

Finally, however, chemo brain is getting the research it needs. Is this the result of the chemotherapy itself, or of the premature menopause brought on by chemotherapy in younger women? A study in the 1995 *Psycho-oncology* looked at cognitive function in a group of 28 stage 1 and 2 breast cancer patients between 3 and 8 months after they'd finished having CMF chemotherapy.[19] Seventy-five percent scored two standard deviations below test norms that had been published on healthy people, based on one or more of 16 measures.

Unfortunately, the study didn't have a control group, so it left a lot of questions unanswered. Nor did it show how this group of women tested before chemotherapy. Since depression can also cause decreased brain function, critics wondered if the alterations were the result of the likely mental state of someone facing life-threatening illness, rather than the chemotherapy itself. But a later study from the Netherlands, done in 1999, did have a control group, and found similar results.[20] They took 39 breast cancer patients treated with the CMF drug combination (see Chapter 28), some of whom had been treated also with tamoxifen for three years and some of whom hadn't, and looked at them two years after the treatments were finished. The control group of 34 patients, whose ages were matched with those of the main group, were lymph node negative patients who had had surgery but no chemotherapy. In their cases as well it was about two years after the end of treatment. They found that the patients who had been on CMF reported significantly more problems with concentration: 36 percent, vs. 6 percent in the control group. They also reported more memory problems: 21 percent vs. 3 percent.

They did neuropsychological tests on the women, and here too there was a large difference. Twenty-eight percent of patients treated with chemotherapy, vs. 12 in the control group, had significant impairment of cognitive function in a broad range of areas—mental flexibility, speed of taking in information, visual memory, and motor function. What's fascinating is that there was no relationship between the reported complaints and the neuropsychological test results. The women who complained of symptoms weren't necessarily those who showed impairment on the tests, and those who showed impairment on the tests hadn't always noticed it in their functioning lives. There's no way to know why this is the case. (It may be that the women who complained had higher cognitive skills in the first place and thus noticed the problem more readily, but their reduced capacity still left them in an "unimpaired" category.)

Tamoxifen use made no difference, in either the reports or the tests. Nor did whether or not the woman was in menopause (so it can't be attributed to cognitive problems caused by menopause). The women who reported the problems often had anxiety and/or depression, but neither showed up as a factor in the tests. Nor did fatigue or time since treatment.

Another study showed that high-dose chemotherapy with stem cell rescue has an even worse effect on cognitive function than does standard chemotherapy. This evidence of dose-related damage seems convincing.

I doubt that most oncologists warn women who are considering chemotherapy that they may lose a significant part of their brain function. For someone who needs the treatment to survive, it's worth it, but in cases where chemotherapy offers only a miniscule survival improvement, it may not be.

Fatigue

An interesting study looked at fatigue after chemotherapy. (Anyone who's had chemotherapy knows about such fatigue; now we doctors are catching up to the patients!) The women who had chemotherapy suffered 61 percent more fatigue than the women in the control group.[21] I think of it as "the poop-out syndrome." Your body is still trying to heal, and usually we've underestimated how long it takes to get back to normal after your body has been assaulted by surgery, radiation, and chemotherapy. One patient says it takes as long to get back to normal as it took to get the treatment: if you have six months of chemotherapy, you have six months of fatigue from it.

There are two ways you can approach this fatigue: drugs and exercise. Much of the fatigue while on chemotherapy and after is caused by anemia. This can be treated by transfusions or by erythropoietin (Epogen), a drug that stimulates the bone marrow to produce more red blood cells.[22]

Several studies show that aerobic exercise decreases the fatigue.[23,24,25] This may be hard to force on yourself—the last thing you feel like doing when you're exhausted is exercise! But it's worth pushing yourself. Probably it works by increasing endorphins.

Weight Gain

Although the cause of weight gain with chemotherapy is not clear, one study revealed that 50 percent of patients gained more than 10 pounds.[26] This was independent of type of chemotherapy, age, and menopausal status, although the women who gained weight did have a decrease in activity. This is another argument for exercise. There are some data suggesting that overweight women have a higher mortality than lean ones.[27] This has increased interest in nutritional and exercise programs for survivors.

Bone Loss

To begin with, women with high bone density have a higher risk of breast cancer. The problem is that once younger women undergo chemotherapy and are thrown into premature menopause their bone density drops. This appears to be related to menopause and not to chemotherapy per se, as opposed to the fuzzy thinking discussed above. Tamoxifen and, to a lesser extent, toremifene work well to maintain bone although they don't build it. They have about the same effect as raloxifene (Evista), improving bone density by 2–3 percent. For women not on tamoxifen, clondronate has been used in Europe with chemotherapy; it seems to block bone loss as long as it is taken. This is a bisphosphonate drug, a cousin to alendronate (Fosamax), and is available only in Europe. It would make sense to consider Fosamax if your bone density is particularly low.

Heart Disease

As mentioned in Chapter 28, the major concern in heart disease comes from the use of Adriamycin. The danger is related to the dose of the drug and the duration of its use, as well as to underlying risk factors such as chest wall radiation and age. Heart disease can be acute and transient with arrythmias and no symptoms, or chronic with damage to the heart muscle and congestive heart failure. At the usual doses of Adriamycin, about 1 percent of women will get heart failure. Mitoxantrone, a drug sometimes used for metastasis, has also been shown to cause heart failure, especially when used alone at high doses.

PREGNANCY

If you are still menstruating, a question that nearly always comes up is whether or not you should risk getting pregnant once you've had breast cancer. There are two areas to consider—the ethical implications and the health-related implications.

In the not too distant past doctors (usually male) tended to impose their own value judgments on patients and to tell them not to get pregnant until at least five years after having breast cancer. If you survived five years, they reasoned, there was a good chance you'd won your bout with breast cancer; otherwise, they didn't want you bringing a child you couldn't raise into the world.

This is a moral decision for the patient to make, not the doctor, and there are two equally valid ways to look at it. Some women do indeed feel they don't want to have a child if they're not reasonably sure they'll be around to raise it. Others feel that even if they do die in a few years they'll be able to give a child the love and care it needs in its early years; they want to pass on their genes before they die. Consideration of a husband's or partner's ability to nurture a child will weigh on the decision as well.

Having a child is never a decision to make lightly, and having a life-threatening illness complicates it further. Think it through carefully and get the thoughts of people whose opinions you respect—and then make your decision.

Can getting pregnant decrease your chances of surviving breast cancer? I wish I knew. Although there are no randomized studies, cancer centers that have reported on the outcome of women who have had pregnancies following breast cancer have shown no difference in survival.[28,29]

We do know that getting pregnant won't cause the cancer to spread; either it has spread or it hasn't before you've gotten pregnant. But if you had a tumor that left microscopic cells in your body, it's possible that pregnancy, with its attendant hormones, could make them grow faster than they would have if you weren't pregnant. This could decrease the time you have left, so that, for example, if you would have died of breast cancer four years from now, you'll die in three years instead.

So the question is, do you want to take that risk? If you've had a lot of positive nodes, or a very aggressive tumor, or some other factor that increases the likelihood of micrometastases, you'll want to take that into consideration. It may be worth the risk to you, or it might not. Again, that's a very individual decision.

If you get pregnant, how will your breasts react? If you've had a mastectomy, obviously nothing will happen on the chest area where your breast was, but your other breast will go through all the usual pregnancy changes we discussed in Chapter 3. If you've had lumpectomy and radiation, the nonradiated breast will probably go through the normal changes. Radiation damages some of the milk-producing parts of the breast, so the radiated breast, while it will grow somewhat larger, won't keep pace with the other breast, and will have little or no milk production. You can nurse on one side only if you want. The only problem with that is increased asymmetry; the milk-producing breast will grow, and may stay larger even after you've finished breast-feeding. If this disturbs you a great deal you can have the larger breast reduced later through plastic surgery (see Chapter 5). One of my patients got pregnant shortly after she finished her radiation treatments, and successfully breast-fed the baby. But one breast ended up twice as large as the other. Knowing she wanted another child, she waited till after her next pregnancy to get the breast reduced.

It's probably a good idea to wait till a year or so after your treatment to get pregnant. It's a stressful process and you won't want to add morning sickness to the nausea you're likely to get from the chemicals.

On the other hand, I had a patient who inadvertently got pregnant right after she'd finished her chemotherapy. After talking it over with her husband and her caregivers, she decided to have the baby—who's now a perfectly healthy little girl.

We have been talking about having a child after breast cancer when you are still fertile, of course. Another issue, which comes up more often now in the age of assisted reproduction, is whether it is safe to have a child using in vitro fertilization (IVF) or donor eggs. Both have been successful in women after treatment for breast cancer.[30,31] The question, however, is whether they are safe. Both therapies involve treatment with cyclical estrogen and progestins to prepare the uterus; IVF also involves drugs to stimulate ovulation. Just as we don't know whether pregnancy after breast cancer is safe, we don't know whether assisted pregnancy is safe. As the numbers of young women who are breast cancer survivors increase, we need more studies to answer these questions.

The decision is up to you. If the stress of dealing with cancer and its uncertainties is too great, you may not want to have a child. On the other hand, if you do want to have a child, perhaps creating a new life can help you to cope with the knowledge of mortality that a life-threatening illness carries with it—a reminder that even death isn't the end.

INSURANCE AND GETTING A JOB

Unfortunately, medical and emotional problems aren't the only ones you'll have to face. There is what often amounts to discrimination against people with cancer. There are some precautions everyone with cancer needs to take.

In the first place, be sure you don't let your insurance lapse. Your company can't drop your policy because of your illness, so you're safe on that score. But many insurance companies won't take on someone who's had a life-threatening illness, and others will take you on but exclude coverage in the area of your illness. If you change jobs and go from one company's coverage to another, you'll probably be all right (but make certain of this before you accept the new job). If you quit for a while, make sure you keep up your insurance on your own. It's costly, but not nearly as costly as not being covered if you have a recurrence.

Life insurance and disability insurance are also harder to get if you've had breast cancer. More and more cancer survivors are fighting to get this changed, and it should get better in the future. But for now, be very alert.

One of the hardest questions is whether or not to tell employers and coworkers about your cancer. There are pros and cons either way. Federal law prohibits federal employers, or employers who get a federal grant or federal financial assistance, from discriminating against the handicapped or anyone mistakenly thought to be handicapped. The Americans with Disabilities Act (ADA), which was passed in 1992 and amended in 1994, extends this concept to the private sector. Any employer with 15 or more employees is prohibited from discriminating against qualified applicants and employees because of any disability. Cancer and other diseases are considered disabilities under the terms of this legislation. The employer must also make reasonable accommodations to the disability—for example, if you have trouble reaching a high shelf because of pain from your mastectomy your employer must make material accessible on a lower shelf, or even build you a lower shelf if that's at all feasible.

Still, many women fear employers will find subtle ways to discriminate against them if their cancer is discovered. One of my fellow breast cancer activists tells a great story of how she handled the loss of her job after her mastectomy, before the ADA was passed. Furious, she stormed into her boss's office, reached into her dress, pulled out her prosthesis, and slapped it on his desk. As he gaped at her in horror, she snapped, "Sir, you are confused—I had a mastectomy, not a lobotomy!" Then she calmly walked out, leaving her boss to buzz his secretary and ask her to remove the prosthesis.

However, there is also the possibility that your boss and coworkers will offer you increased support if you are open. It is a dilemma that is probably best solved on an individual basis. There is more and more attention being given to cancer survivors in the workplace, and you may well be able to find a career counseling center that can give you good advice.

If you are looking for a new job there is even more difficulty. Some companies are reluctant to hire someone with cancer. This too is illegal under the ADA, but there is always the fear that an employer will find another excuse not to hire you. You might want to be open about your cancer because you don't want to work for someone with that attitude. On the other hand, you might need the job too much to risk being turned down. But if you don't tell them and then end up missing a lot of time for medical appointments or sickness, you could run into problems that might have been avoided if you'd been frank in the beginning. It's a tough problem, and there are no easy answers. We have included some references and reading about cancer and the workplace in Appendix B.

31

Dealing with
Menopausal Symptoms

We have discussed the problems with hormone "replacement" therapy and menopause in Chapter 15, and looked at who is likely to be
thrown into menopause by chemotherapy in Chapter 28. Now we'll focus on what the woman who has had breast cancer (or is at high risk)
can do about menopausal symptoms.

A woman can arrive at menopause in one of three ways: naturally—
simply by living long enough—surgically, by having her ovaries removed, and chemically, through chemotherapy. This is as true for the
woman with breast cancer as it is for everyone else.

Someone treated with a mastectomy but not chemotherapy or
tamoxifen might find that she goes into natural menopause right on
cue. Or she could be thrown into menopause by a hysterectomy that
includes oophorectomy (ovaries removed) for bleeding or some other
problem unrelated to her cancer. In these situations her symptoms will
be the same as those for women who have not had breast cancer
(which means they can range from nonexistent to severe). The only difference will be that the estrogen question will loom larger for her than
for someone who is not at any particular risk of breast cancer or recurrence.

She may be thrown into menopause by chemotherapy. Or she may have been taking hormone replacement therapy and been told abruptly to stop. The symptoms that arise in these situations will be doubly hard to sort out since chemotherapy and tamoxifen add their own symptoms or side effects to the mix. Similarly, a woman may be prescribed Zoladex, which creates a state of reversible menopause.

With natural menopause the ovaries continue to produce hormones albeit at a much lower level. Obviously a woman who has gone through surgical menopause—removal of her ovaries—has no ovarian production of hormones afterwards, although her fat and adrenal glands may produce some very small level of estrogen, as well as testosterone and androstenedione, which are converted by fat, muscle, and breast tissue into estrogen. What we don't know, however, is what happens with women who have chemical menopause. Does the chemotherapy completely destroy the ovaries so they never produce anything again? Or does it simply throw the woman into regular menopause, so she gets postmenopausal levels of hormone production? We do know that women around 30 who get chemotherapy often go into temporary menopause, and get their periods back (see Chapter 28). This might mean that the chemicals don't totally wipe out the ovaries' capacity to produce hormones, but simply push the middle-aged woman in the direction she's already heading. So it may be that these women who are apparently thrown into permanent menopause still have some ovarian hormone production, or it may mean that some of them do and some don't. This is an area we simply need to study more.

There are really two aspects of menopause that a woman needs to consider. The first and often the most apparent one is that symptoms can come with a sudden or even an erratic change in hormones. These symptoms, as we discussed in Chapter 15, are usually transient, lasting for two to three years on average. They need to be treated specifically, and there is a large menu of options.

The second is the way menopause has been portrayed, as the cause of diseases that occur in later life, most particularly heart disease and osteoporosis. There are several global approaches to these problems; and then there are specific remedies for specific symptoms and prevention of specific diseases. Before I launch into an analysis of the pros and cons of the options, I think it is important to point out that doing nothing is an acceptable choice. You don't have to treat or manage menopause unless it is interfering with your life. I will review the three other overall approaches that women with breast cancer might consider: hormone replacement therapy (HRT), soy protein, and natural progesterone.

HORMONE REPLACEMENT THERAPY

As discussed in Chapter 15, the problems of old age are not restricted to menopausal women and may not be caused by low estrogen per se. Nonetheless we have been led to believe that estrogen is necessary to prevent them. When you've had breast cancer, however, concerns about using hormone therapy to prevent other diseases are even more important.

There are a number of levels to this. For one thing, the chance of your getting a recurrence of a disease to which you now know you're vulnerable, and vulnerable at any age, is measured against the chance of your living long enough to get diseases that typically happen in old age. The average age for a hip fracture is 80. The average age for a first heart attack is 74. The average age for Alzheimer's is mid-80s. Should breast cancer shorten your life, these diseases may not be of concern.

Because hormone therapy as prevention is being sold so heavily to the baby boomers, women who have had breast cancer feel especially drawn to it. They're already dealing with a terrible assault on their health, and they want to do all they can to keep healthy in every way. But ironically, they're the ones for whom such drugs may be dangerous, and it's important to evaluate benefit vs. risk.

Some oncologists are beginning to consider trying estrogen in women who have had breast cancer. They reason that there are no data demonstrating that it is dangerous for women with breast cancer, and that the benefits may outweigh the risks. They are correct that the data on the dangers of HRT in breast cancer survivors are almost nonexistent, but so are the data on its safety! They may also not have looked critically at the data supporting the use of hormone therapy postmenopausally and are assuming that the statements they hear regarding its ability to prevent heart disease are correct. Although there have been several small nonrandomized series of women on estrogen after breast cancer reporting no increased recurrences, it is much too soon to tell if this approach is safe.[1,2]

As I have been writing this edition I have been struck with the fact that we are preventing breast cancer with antiestrogens (tamoxifen) and treating breast cancer by putting women into menopause. Pregnancy increases both the risk of getting breast cancer and the aggressiveness of the cancer, and the use of HRT shows a slightly increased risk of getting it. It makes no sense to me to give estrogen to a woman who has already demonstrated a vulnerability to a breast cancer. This is especially true since the benefits of long-term postmenopausal hormone use are far from proven.

It is important for the woman with breast cancer to examine all the information and develop her own plan. So in the following two sections I'll review two options in addition to HRT (these are also useful for any woman who wants to avoid additional estrogen).

SOY PROTEIN: A NATURAL SERM?

When I lecture on either menopausal hormones or breast cancer the question I get asked most is about soy. Soy is a food source of isoflavones. Sometimes it is called a phytoestrogen. This is a poor word choice. Although soy acts like estrogen in some organs it blocks estrogen in others—so it's more like a phytoSERM (selective estrogen receptor modulator; see Chapter 18) than a pure estrogen. In addition, it has many effects other than its hormonal ones. It blocks tumor cells in a petri dish regardless of whether or not they're sensitive to estrogen. We are only beginning to study the properties of this natural substance.

The first clue that soy might reduce breast cancer came from observational studies of women in various parts of the world. The studies discovered that women in Japan have much less breast cancer than in the U.S. and many of the European countries—and one of the big differences between Japan and Western countries is that their diet is heavy in soy. These observational data (see Chapter 12) cannot prove cause and effect. Nonetheless it is enough to spur other studies.

More specific observational data continued to support the hypothesis. In a study in Minnesota in December 1998,[3] 12 healthy premenopausal women, half of whom were given a diet high in soy, were studied. The ones with the soy diet had a decreased excretion of estrogens. Another study[4] in premenopausal women found that a soy diet reduced estrogen and adrenal androgens and made the menstrual cycle last a bit longer—which, as I pointed out in Chapter 15, decreases breast cancer risk. They believe this may be why soy seems to reduce breast cancer.

Which takes us to the mice. When they gave soy to prepubescent mice, the rodents' breast tissue started maturing and differentiating the way it does in pregnancy. This suggests that one way soy may decrease breast cancer is by maturing breast tissue in teenagers much the way a pregnancy might. On the other hand, there is evidence that soy increases the growth of cells in the breast. In monkeys estrogen stimulated both the ducts and the lobules. Soy did too, although there was a little less stimulation in the lobules and a lot less in the ducts. When estrogen and soy were given together, soy blocked the effect of the estrogen, although there was still some stimulation. In one study of premenopausal women with both benign and malignant disease, the subjects were given either soy or a placebo for two weeks before surgery.[5] At the time of surgery the researchers obtained some cells from the tissue that had been removed. They found an increase in cell growth in the lobules after 14 days of taking soy. Similarly, in a study of nipple aspirate fluid (see Chapter 17), women who had eaten a diet high in soy and were either premenopausal or took estrogen replacement therapy showed an increase in proliferating cells.[6] Some physicians have concluded from this data that soy causes breast cancer. That's an awfully big leap.

It's important to remember that breast stimulation doesn't equal cancer. Soy seems to act in a couple of different ways. Its weak estrogen properties may cause breast cells to grow. On the other hand, its other properties of blocking invasion and angiogenesis (growth of new blood vessels) may be more important in preventing breast cancer. In petri dishes and in animal models, soy definitely inhibits breast cancer growth. And a recent study out of Sanford Barsky's lab at UCLA shows that it has this effect on cancer cells that are both estrogen receptor positive and negative.[7] Clearly soy is more than just a plant estrogen.

Occasionally a woman with breast cancer says to me, "My tumor is estrogen receptor positive: does that mean I can't take soy?" I reassure her that soy is not estrogen—it is an isoflavone and has many effects. I do not think there is a risk in having one serving of soy a day. I often get asked whether a woman who's taking tamoxifen can also take soy, or if the soy counteracts the tamoxifen. Here too the news seems to be good. A study in mice with chemically induced cancers showed that soy inhibited the tumor incidence, and when they added tamoxifen, the combination reduced both incidence of tumors and the number of tumors that did develop.[8] So it appears, at least in this study, that soy and tamoxifen work synergistically. There's no evidence that they counteract each other.

With the discovery of estrogen receptor beta, we have seen soy's similarities to the SERM. Researchers have found that soy appears to fit into the beta receptor, rather than estrogen receptor alpha. Soy's usefulness in helping to prevent a number of conditions has been demonstrated in studies not only in rats but in humans and in their closest animal counterparts, monkeys. There have been several randomized controlled studies on hot flashes and soy, showing a reduction in hot flashes not only in countries where soy is a large part of the diet, like China and Japan, but also in the West.[9]

In addition, soy not only decreases LDL cholesterol (the bad kind), but increases the good cholesterol, HDL, significantly. And unlike Premarin, which increases triglycerides, soy decreases them.[10] It also increases bone density.

In terms of the uterus, there is no evidence that soy causes uterine cell stimulation, so there is no reason to suspect it causes uterine cancer.[11] Some researchers believe estrogen can help the brain, though it's far from proven. One of the mechanisms it is believed to protect is the center for learning and memory. A group of rats with the cozy title of "retired breeder rats" were hysterectomized, then given either purified estradiol or soy and tested for neurological proteins in the blood. Both estrogen and soy improved these factors, in exactly the same way.[12]

Overall the data on soy are good, and it's probably safe for women with breast cancer, but the final answers aren't in yet. You will have to decide for yourself whether to try it. If you do, try eating one serving (40 grams) of soy protein. I am confident enough to have a soy drink for breakfast every day, which has vastly decreased my hot flashes, fuzzy thinking, and sleepiness. (Then again, maybe they would have stopped anyway.)

How should you take the soy? Ideally you should eat it as tofu, soy beans, or soy milk. There are a number of cookbooks around that show how to cook with soy. (It also helps prevent prostate cancer and so is good for the whole family). If you do not have time to cook, then try one of the soy protein powders such as Healthy Source or Revival. What you do not want to do is take soy capsules or capsules of isoflavones or genestein. Although these two are definitely ingredients of soy, we do not know which one is more important. Nor do we know whether they work the same in isolation as they do when they are in food. Also, it is much easier to overdose on soy in capsule form than as tofu. Always remember moderation.

NATURAL PROGESTERONE CREAM

Popular books like *What Your Doctor May Not Tell You About Menopause: The Breakthrough Book on Natural Progesterone* by John Lee have promoted natural progesterone cream as a safe alternative for menopausal women with breast cancer. There are several aspects of the "natural progesterone cream" story that need to be differentiated. First of all, although it is natural to have estrogen, testosterone, and androstenedione produced by the ovaries postmenopausally, there is no progesterone produced. Estrogen only has to be balanced by progesterone when it is at premenopausal levels in the uterus. The postmenopausal woman does not need replacement progesterone—or estrogen for that matter—nor is there any requirement for the remaining estrogen to be balanced. Menopause is normal. Our bodies need high levels of hormones to reproduce, and then at menopause they shift down to lower levels which are, for the most part, still adequate to help prevent osteoporosis, heart disease, and other illnesses of old age.

Estrogen alone and estrogen with either progesterone or progestin (progestin refers to any kind of progestational agent, whether progesterone or Provera) will decrease hot flashes, as will natural progesterone cream, as demonstrated in a recent randomized controlled trial.[13] Short-term use (two to three years) of these hormones postmenopausally for symptom relief in high-risk women is probably safe.

The next question is whether progesterone is safe and efficacious for symptoms other than hot flashes. In the only randomized controlled studies that I am aware of, natural progesterone cream alone showed no benefit for bone density.[14,15] The PEPI study,[16] which compared estrogen alone, estrogen and natural progesterone, estrogen and Provera cyclically, and estrogen and Provera continuously showed that progestins (both Provera and progesterone) reduced the beneficial effects of estrogen on cholesterol. Provera was worse than progesterone, but progesterone was worse than estrogen alone. Another interesting finding was that all of the estrogen and progestin combinations, including natural progesterone, showed an increased mammographic density in almost a third of women. As we mentioned in Chapter 20 mammographic density has been shown in many studies to indicate an increase in breast cancer risk. In addition, the women taking both estrogen and a progestin (Provera or progesterone) had more breast pain, a sign of breast stimulation.[17] Both of these findings correlate with the findings of a recent study of premarin and Provera that showed adding Provera to the estrogen increased the risk of breast cancer in postmenopausal women eightfold.[18] In addition, progesterone in petri dishes causes breast cancer cells to proliferate or grow.

But things get more complicated. It matters whether you give progesterone with estrogen or alone. In cell culture progesterone primes the cells and gets them ready to grow; then estrogen causes the growth. It may be that progesterone alone gets the cells ready but doesn't actually cause them to grow if there are no stimulants around (estrogen is not the only one).[19] Thus there is a chance that progesterone without estrogen in a postmenopausal woman may neither increase nor decrease breast cancer. When I asked one of the foremost researchers in the field of progesterone in the breast, Kate Horwitz at the University of Colorado, she said it was possible but only hypothetically. The dose of progesterone and the method of giving it, as well as the schedule, can have very different effects, she said, and it is not clear which, if any, are safe. For example, one study done in France looked at the use of a cream of 19-nortestosterone (a synthetic progestin) in premenopausal women and found a decrease in breast cancer risk, while all of the other progestins had no such effect.[20]

Are the over-the-counter creams safe? Not clear. Although there are published reports on the levels of progesterone in the creams, they are not required to be standardized, so one batch could have one level and the next something different. The absorption of the creams depends in part on which part of the body they are applied to. Luckily there is a commercially available natural progesterone pill called Prometrium, which is probably a safer way to take it.

At this point I think we can safely say that progesterone cream will decrease hot flashes and that its effect on the breast is unknown. When given with estrogen it increases breast cancer risk, but when given alone it may be neutral, that is, it may not increase or decrease breast cancer risk. It does not have any beneficial effect on the bones when given alone.

PREVENTION: OSTEOPOROSIS

We discussed the issues of bone density in Chapter 15. Although women with breast cancer tend to have less osteoporosis, chemotherapy may lead to an increase in bone loss. A woman who has had breast cancer should have a bone density test following her treatment and then again in a year. Note that one test tells you only what your bones look like now. It will not tell you whether you are actively losing bone. It could be that your bone density has always been low. You are being compared to the average 35-year-old and that may or may not be a fair comparison. Bone loss occurs slowly enough that waiting a year will not lead you to crumble in the meantime. The current treatments we have only block bone loss, so if you are not actively losing bone they will not work. If the two tests show that you are actively losing bone, you may want to try one of the drugs which block bone loss. If not, you should concentrate on maintaining the bone you have in the best way you can.

How do you do this? The first step is to make sure you have enough calcium and vitamin D. Studies have shown that calcium and vitamin D decrease fractures even though they don't have a great effect on bone density. So if you're concerned about osteoporosis, take 1,500 milligrams of dietary calcium and 400 to 800 international units of vitamin D daily. If you smoke, give it up. In addition, exercise is vital. It should include weight bearing as well as strength training. Studies have shown an increase in bone density and a decrease in fractures in women who train with weights.

If you are losing bone or have osteoporosis, the best choice is alendronate, whose brand name is Fosamax. This drug has been shown in randomized double-blind studies to increase bone density by 8 percent and to decrease fractures in the hip and spine. It is of much less value in women who just have osteopenia (low bone density) rather than actual osteoporosis, especially if they are not actively losing bone. In Europe, clondronate has been shown to decrease bone metastasis.[21] Women on pamidronate (a cousin of Fosamax) had less cancer spread to the bone. This phenomenon is currently being studied further.

Other drugs being used include Calcitonin, which is given as a nasal spray and is especially helpful for women with fractures of the spine. Although raloxifene (Evista) has been approved for osteoporosis,[22] it is only about half as good as Fosamax in increasing bone density and decreasing fractures (see Chapter 30). In addition, it has not been studied in women with breast cancer or even women at high risk. It is not a good choice for the breast cancer survivor—at least not until we have further safety data.

There's a drug being used currently in Europe called Tibilone,[23] a synthetic steroid that acts in some ways like estrogen, progestin, and androgens. It's been shown to have good effects on hot flashes and also to help prevent osteoporosis. It has not been tested in women with breast cancer at this time.

Ipriflavone, a drug based on isoflavones (like soy), has been shown in randomized controlled studies to decrease osteoporosis.[24] It is now available in health food stores. Since it is an isoflavone and not an estrogen, there is no reason it shouldn't be safe in women with breast cancer. But again, we don't know.

Finally, is there ever a time when it makes sense for a survivor of breast cancer to take estrogen in order to prevent osteoporotic fractures? I don't think so, but if you were to consider it you should know that you don't have to start at menopause. Since you're unlikely to get osteoporotic fractures in your 50s, maybe that isn't the time to start estrogen. The pharmaceutical companies have pushed the idea that starting at 50 will prevent bone loss at menopause. But bone loss is not the only factor. And the estrogen holds back bone loss only while you're taking it. If you take it at 50 and stop at 55, when you're 80 your bones will be the same as they'd be if you'd never taken it at all.

On the other hand, recent studies have shown that you can catch up later, when it's likely to matter.[25] You can lose some bone at 50, start taking estrogen at 65 or 70, and have almost the same benefit at 80 as you would have had taking it for 30 years. Then, if the estrogen does cause breast cancer, it probably won't start until you're 80 or older, and by the time it would kill you you'd probably have died of something else. (If you plan to live to 120, start the estrogen at 105!)

Furthermore, at whatever time you take hormones to prevent or contain osteoporosis, you should take a smaller dosage than the usual "one size fits all" that doctors tend to prescribe—.625 milligram. That's a good dosage for getting rid of symptoms at age 50, but it's overkill for osteoporosis prevention. At least one study, by Bruce

Ettinger, suggests that .3 milligram is enough.[26] Lower doses are less risky.

There is so much research currently going on in this field that we will soon be able to rebuild bone, and the notion of using a nonspecific drug like estrogen will seem nonsensical.

PREVENTION: HEART DISEASE

As we discussed in chapter 15, we haven't proved that there actually is any benefit to the heart from taking estrogen. The studies with tamoxifen and raloxifene have demonstrated a decrease in cholesterol but no comparable improvement in heart disease mortality. An NIH-sponsored study by David Herrington[27] was recently reported by Reuters. No benefit was found from Premarin and combination HRT in women with heart disease (over four years), confirming the HERS study. And, as this book went to press, data from the first two years of the Women's Health Initiative showed a small *increase* in heart attacks and strokes in the women on HRT. Nonetheless, heart disease is the biggest killer of women and merits some attention to the available means of prevention. There are several ways to help prevent heart disease. If you smoke, give it up; it's a major contributor to heart attacks. Watch your weight; if you're overweight, lose weight with a sensible eating and exercise plan. If you have diabetes, be extra careful to follow your treatment regimen. If you have high blood pressure or high cholesterol, have them treated with specific drugs. The statins, or cholesterol-lowering drugs, have been shown in randomized controlled double-blind studies to lower cholesterol and decrease deaths from heart disease. With these kinds of data it seem crazy to consider estrogen, which has not yet been tested for prevention.

Avoid eating a lot of fats, particularly animal fats. A very low-fat diet—10 percent of your diet—can prevent and even reverse hardening of the arteries. Avoid eating much red meat, and eat more fish, or follow a vegetarian diet (with few or no animal fats, such as those found in cheese). Exercise is the best "drug" for your heart—and for practically everything else that might ail you. If you're old enough to be reading this chapter, don't go overboard right away: consult your doctor and start a good, reasonably paced program that will get you up to 30 minutes of aerobic exercise a day—and that includes fast walking, swimming, even dancing. Recent studies have shown that avoiding isolation and participating in social activities also decreases heart disease.

In fact, heart disease is much more a factor of lifestyle than estrogen. In the Nurses' Health Study,[28] the women who did not smoke, were not obese, and had normal cholesterol had no cardiac benefit from taking estrogen though others did.

TREATMENT FOR PERIMENOPAUSAL SYMPTOMS

Although there are sometimes symptoms during the postmenopausal years, most of the symptoms that cause discomfort come in the perimenopausal years, when your body is preparing to move into menopause. These symptoms also occur in women who are suddenly thrown into menopause.

Hot Flashes

A behavioral approach can help. For one thing, you can avoid triggers. These vary greatly among individual women, but you can soon figure out what yours are by keeping a daily "hot flash diary." Spicy foods, caffeine, stressful situations, and hot drinks are among the more common triggers. Once you've identified them you can choose to avoid them. Sleep in a cool room; carry a hand fan (I carry one in my briefcase); dress in cotton and in layers; try paced respiration exercises (practicing deep, slow abdominal breathing); try acupuncture; eat a serving of soy foods and ground flax seeds daily; walk, swim, dance, or bike-ride every day for 30 minutes or more. If none of this helps, try vitamin E (800 mg) or the herb black cohosh (Remifemin), or create a support group.

But do these work? There are data from randomized controlled studies supporting acupuncture and paced respiration. In addition, there are good data from randomized controlled double-blind studies on black cohosh, using both Premarin and a placebo as the controls. These studies found that the herb reduces hot flashes, and also helps vaginal dryness. Many researchers in the U.S. aren't aware of these studies because they were done in Germany.[29,30] There are randomized placebo-based data on dietary soy (*not* isoflavone pills) and hot flashes as well.

A group at the Mayo Clinic has done a good study of menopausal symptom relief in women who have had breast cancer, which can also be of use for all women.[31] This group, the North Center Cancer Treatment Group (NCCTG), studied more than 650 women with breast cancer and reported a number of findings. First, they found that a placebo alone appeared to cause a 20 to 25 percent reduction of symptoms in four weeks. (This may show a psychological component to hot flashes, but it may also simply reflect the nature of hot flashes themselves: they tend to come and go anyway. My own example is fairly common, and serves to illustrate the capricious nature of hot flashes. I had 10 and a half weeks of horrible hot flashes and no period. "This is it," I thought. "These things will go on for a few years, my period will stop, and—if I don't end up in an insane asylum first—so will the hot flashes." All of a sudden, on a Sunday while I was at a medical convention in Atlanta, the hot flashes stopped, and I found myself wondering what had happened. I'm sure if I had started a new treatment, or had been on a placebo in a study, I would have thought happily, "I'm not in the placebo group, and this blessed treatment works!" Since this wasn't the case, I just whispered a prayer of devout gratitude to my guardian angel. Four weeks later, my period was back, and of course that was why the flashes had stopped.)

Clonidine, which has been used for years as an antihypertensive and only recently as a treatment for hot flashes, reduced hot flashes by about 15 percent more than the placebo in the NCCTG study. However, there were a lot of side effects: fatigue, nausea, irritability, headache, and dizziness. The group then looked at Megace, a progestin used to treat breast cancer. They found an 80 percent reduction of hot flashes, and there were no side effects. But this was a short study, and there's no way of knowing whether it will prove safe in the long run. Some researchers are concerned about using progestins, particularly in women with breast cancer, because many breast cancers have progesterone receptors.

The Mayo Clinic study also found that 800 international units of vitamin E taken daily statistically decreased hot flashes. But the statistics boiled down to an average of one hot flash per woman per day—which may not help much. They also did a pilot study looking at a new antidepressant called danlafaxine (Effexor). They found that low doses, in addition to helping alleviate depression, decreased hot flashes by 50 percent. Prozac has also been shown to help. This might be especially helpful to women whose symptoms include both hot flashes and depression. The same group studied an isoflavone pill and found no effect on hot flashes. Whether this contradicts previous studies or just means that soy powder is better than a pill is not clear.

As a flashing woman myself I think there is one key component to getting through this temporary disruption in life—a sense of humor. If you can laugh at yourself and revel in this change you will, as the saying goes, turn the hot flashes into power surges.

Vaginal Dryness

Vaginal dryness as a result of vaginal atrophy is the most distressing and least talked about symptom of menopause. It occurs in about

20 percent of women, sometimes transiently and other times permanently. Sexual activity, including masturbation, reduces vaginal atrophy. The problem is that if you're sore from vaginal dryness, you don't want to have sex, and if you don't have sex, your vaginal dryness gets worse—a classic catch 22. There are two approaches. One is to help the immediate problem of painful intercourse. For this you can use water lubricants. They don't cure the basic condition, but they can help the immediate problem. KY Jelly and Astroglide are among the most frequently used. The other approach is to try to increase the vagina's own moisture. Replens, which can be purchased over the counter, will cause your vagina to absorb water and become more supple. In one study 61.5 percent of patients preferred Replens, 26.5 preferred a lubricant, and 12 percent had no preference.

Both black cohosh and soy have been reported to reduce vaginal dryness. Vitamin E capsules have been used vaginally with some success as well. (You break open the capsule and rub the vitamin E on the lining of the vagina.)

If nothing else works, you may decide to try estrogen to improve the quality of your life. In this case you want to use the smallest amount necessary and apply it to where the problem is (interestingly, estrogen by mouth often doesn't solve this problem). You can try vaginal estrogen creams. If you go that route, however, ignore the instructions on the label, which tell you to use an applicator-full. Since estrogen as a cream is well absorbed from the vagina you'll end up with blood levels that rival or are higher than what you would get with estrogen pills. All you really need is a little bit, a dab on your fingertip. If you apply it every day for two weeks, then two or three times a week, it will solve your problems. (But don't use it as a lubricant at the time of sex; it won't help that way and your male partner may grow breasts!)

There's a new product, a vaginal ring called Estring, which releases a very small amount of estrogen over a long period of time. In the first 24 hours after you've had it inserted (or inserted it yourself, like a diaphragm), you have a little spurt of estrogen; beyond that it doesn't increase hormone levels because it is low-dose and sustained-release; it is not absorbed. You keep it in for three months, then change it. It's a good last resort for women with this problem.

Sadja Greenwood, a menopause specialist, suggests another alternative, estriol cream (estriol is a very low-potency estrogen, and it can be compounded into a cream, of which you use only a little bit). Greenwood also recommends 1–2 percent testosterone cream vaginally, which she says will increase sex drive. I'm a little nervous about testosterone in general because there is preliminary evidence that it may increase breast cancer, but if you're going to use it this is probably the safest way.

Insomnia, Mood Swings, and Fuzzy Thinking

Although insomnia is often related to night sweats it is also true that you don't sleep as well when your hormones are awry. Some easy things can help. Keep your bedroom cool, exercise (but earlier in the day; if you exercise right before going to bed it will keep you awake), avoid caffeine and liquor, take warm baths or showers, increase soy intake, have cereal and milk products at bedtime, and, again, take black cohosh (an herb which has been well studied in Germany).

To counter mood swings and anxiety, try using the relaxation response (see Chapter 22), exercise (including yoga), having a plant- rather than meat-based diet, going to a psychotherapist, and finding creative outlets. Kava kava has been shown to be helpful as has St. John's wort.

For fuzzy thinking, try gingko biloba. Soy also seems to help. Other possibilities are exercise, low-fat diet, nonsteroidal anti-inflammatories (Motrin), and vitamin E. The best thing to do for your brain is use it— with work, study, crossword puzzles, reading, and card games. A recent study showed that people who stayed socially active had less cognitive decline with age. Remember, menopausal symptoms do not last forever. On average their duration is about two to three years off and on. The best approach to both symptom relief and prevention is to live a healthy lifestyle.

32

When Cancer Comes Back

We know you have a recurrence when we find that breast cancer cells have reappeared in the area around the breast (local or regional recurrence) or in other areas of the body (metastasis). For the most part, these are the microscopic cells that presumably got out before your diagnosis and found a niche elsewhere in your body. The cells can get out through the bloodstream or the lymphatic system, where they can remain dormant for years. And then something happens to wake them up (see Fig. 13-18). If we could figure out what puts these cells to sleep and then what wakes them up, we'd be a long way toward eliminating breast cancer.

One way to conceptualize it is to say that the radiation or chemotherapy has killed some cells and injured others, knocking them out; then after a long while the ones that survived recover and begin doubling again. Another possibility is that the cells that were not killed were put to sleep by tamoxifen or chemical menopause and are now awakening.

Being diagnosed with any kind of recurrence can be devastating. The process of psychosocial adjustment will start all over again; trusting your body may take longer when you've been doubly betrayed by it. All the feelings you experienced the first time around are back, much worse because now you not only don't trust your body but you begin to wonder about your doctors and treatment in general. It's important to discuss these feelings with your caregivers or to get new ones if, after talking with them, you no longer feel you are part of a team that you have confidence in. In addition, you'll want to get support and help from friends and family, counselors, therapists, and support groups.

The kinds of support groups that are available vary widely, depending on where you are. It may be that the only groups available are general cancer groups. These can be very helpful, but most women with breast cancer find breast cancer groups more helpful. In big cities you might want to search out groups for women with recurrences, or, if your disease has metastasized, for women with metastases alone. There are advantages to all three. Barbara Kalinowski, a clinical nurse specialist, co-led both a first-diagnosis group and a recurrence group which went on for a number of years. In the recurrence group, the women all faced similar issues for three years, but after a time the dynamics changed as the women with metastases began to worsen. "The women who are sick are very happy for the women who are getting better, and the women who are getting better are very supportive of the women who are sick." One of the women who was well had lunch with one of the others whose metastasis was worsening. Jackie Onassis had just died, and the sick woman said she wanted white and pink flowers at her funeral, the way Jackie had. The next week the other woman sent her a gorgeous bouquet of white and pink flowers, with a note saying, "You don't have to wait until you die for your flowers."

At the same time, Kalinowski says, women with metastatic cancer have more in common with each other as the illness progresses, and she would like to do a separate group for such women. For those who can't find a support group for women with metastatic disease nearby there are many choices on the website SusanLoveMD.com.

In order to best deal with your recurrence, you need to know more about the nature of breast cancer recurrences. In the rest of this chapter we'll discuss the types of recurrences and their symptoms. In the next chapter we'll discuss the treatments.

LOCAL AND REGIONAL RECURRENCE

There are several ways cancer comes back in the breast and node area, and they mean different things. Most commonly, it shows up in the area of the original cancer. If you've had a wide excision and radiation, it may come back in the breast itself (Fig. 32–1), and this is called local recurrence. In this case, we see it not as a spread but as leftover cancer

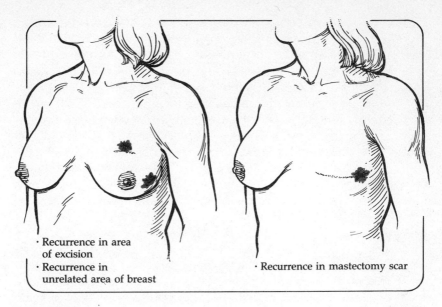

· Recurrence in area
of excision
· Recurrence in
unrelated area of breast

· Recurrence in mastectomy scar

FIGURE 32-1

inadequately treated in the first place (see Chapter 23 for a discussion of why and how this happens). We are just beginning to get some data on the significance of these recurrences and to develop a reasonable way of treating them. Studies of women who have had this kind of reappearance of cancer in the breast show that their likelihood of dying of the disease is not much greater than that of women at the same stage of disease who have had mastectomies and whose cancer has not recurred in their breasts.[1]

What kind of disease recurs is important in terms of prognosis. If the recurrence is precancer (see Chapter 16), it's most likely left over and just needs to be cleaned up with further surgery. On the other hand, if the recurrence is invasive, it may have had a second opportunity to spread. In addition, women with invasive local recurrences generally have more aggressive disease. Therefore it may well be worth adding systemic therapy to the local treatment.[2] This remains unresolved at this time, but I would encourage anyone with an invasive local recurrence to seek an opinion on getting chemotherapy or tamoxifen as well as local treatments.

The first step to take if a local recurrence is detected is to do the tests (see Chapter 21) to make sure there is no sign of cancer anywhere else in the body: bone scan, chest x ray, and liver blood tests. If the tests are normal (and they usually are) then we have to figure out what's best to do to eradicate the tumor from the breast. Usually in these cases we do a mastectomy, since the less drastic surgery and radiation didn't take care of it before. (In France they're experimenting with just doing another wide excision; so far we don't know how effective that will turn out to be.) Some doctors have argued against lumpectomy and radiation as a primary treatment on the theory that if you get a recurrence and need a mastectomy, the radiation means you can't get a reconstruction. But it isn't true. What is true is that you often can't have reconstruction with an expander (see Chapter 26), because the radiated skin can't tolerate being stretched out the way normal skin can. But expanders aren't the only form of reconstruction—or even, for that matter, the best one. The flap, as we discussed in Chapter 26, is better on a number of levels, and in this case it actually can be beneficial, because it brings new skin to the area.

There's something else we call a "local recurrence" that actually isn't a local recurrence at all—it's a new cancer in the breast. This typically occurs many years after the original cancer and in an entirely different area of the breast. Its pathology is often different—lobular instead of ductal, for example. These second cancers are not too common, but they remain possible as long as you have your breast. Though they are often counted as recurrences in the statistics for breast conservation, they have a different meaning. They should be treated as completely new cancers, much as with second cancers in the opposite breast. Most often the local treatment will be a mastectomy, since you can only receive radiation therapy once to a particular area. The addition of chemotherapy and/or tamoxifen will depend on the size and biomarkers of the tumor (see Chapter 20) .

You can also get a local recurrence in the scar or chest wall after a mastectomy. Actually the term "chest wall" is inaccurate here, because it implies that the cancer is in the muscle or bone. But usually such a recurrence appears in the skin and fat sitting where the breast was before; only rarely does it include the muscle (see Fig. 32-1). This can happen in one of two ways. The cancer can be in leftover breast tissue, since the surgeon was unable to get all that tissue out during your mastectomy. This is very similar to a recurrence after lumpectomy and radiation. It's residual, rather than metastatic. In this situation, we usually cut out the recurrence and perhaps radiate the chest wall, and you'll probably be fine. This type of chest wall recurrence is relatively uncommon.

The other, more common type of recurrence appears not in residual breast tissue, but in the scar. The cancer has spread through the bloodstream or lymphatic channels into the scar. This kind of recurrence is more serious because it often reflects microscopic cells elsewhere in the body. In 70 to 80 percent of those cases, the women will show an obvious metastasis elsewhere within two years.[3] Because of this, the doctor might then want to add systemic therapy to the surgery and radiation. A recent randomized controlled study from Europe has shown that adding tamoxifen to local excision and radiation for a postmastectomy recurrence significantly improved the five-year disease-free survival.[4] Unfortunately we can't always distinguish between the two kinds of recurrences that occur after mastectomy.

A local recurrence after mastectomy will usually show up as a pea-sized lump in your scar or under your skin. Sometimes it's in the skin itself, and is red and raised. It's usually so subtle the surgeon is likely to think at first that it's just a stitch that got left in after the operation. Then it gets bigger, and you need to get it biopsied. That can be done under local anesthesia, since the area is numb. Reconstruction rarely if ever hides a recurrence. With implants the recurrences are in front of the implant. With a flap the recurrences are not in the flap (tissue from the abdomen) but along the edge of the old breast skin.[5]

To a certain degree we can predict which women will have a local recurrence. They are the ones whose initial cancer was particularly severe: women with inflammatory breast cancer, with cancer cells in the lymphatics of the skin or of the breast, with a big tumor, or with many positive nodes. For these women we will suggest radiation therapy to the chest wall after a mastectomy to try and prevent this distressing type of recurrence. High-dose chemotherapy with stem cell rescue has been shown to be no better than standard chemotherapy, but it has taught us a lesson about the need for radiation. The initial studies of high-dose chemotherapy were done with mastectomy as the only local therapy. To the surprise of the investigators, many of the women had local recurrences in their scars in spite of all of the drugs and surgery.[6] Maybe it's harder for chemotherapy to get to the scar. Subsequent studies requiring radiation after mastectomy showed fewer local problems.

The treatments for a local recurrence are also local. Most commonly the lesion will be removed surgically and followed by radiation therapy to the chest wall if the woman has not previously had radiation. Occasionally even larger lesions will be surgically removed, including sections of rib and breastbone. Although this approach has not been shown to increase survival, it can improve the quality of life. Some newer approaches include photodynamic therapy (PDT).[7] A woman with a local recurrence is given a photosensitizing material that localizes in the skin nodules. A special laser light that is absorbed only by nodules containing the photosensitizer is then applied. This selectively destroys the nodules. This approach is most successful when there are a small number of nodules.

On occasion, women will have extensive local recurrences after mastectomy, with many nodules in the skin. They will ultimately merge together and act almost like a coat of armor across your chest and even into the back and the other breast. At this point we call it *en cuirasse,* a French word meaning "in casing." Other women can have large masses of tumor on their chest wall that weep and bleed. Both of these situations are rare but they're very distressing because you are watching the cancer grow on the outside. There must be a different mutation for this type of local recurrence than for distant metastasis, because these women usually do not have extensive disease in the rest of their body for a long time. Unfortunately we haven't a good therapy for this situation. Surgery cannot cut out enough tissue to clear it, and radiation therapy is limited in extent as well. Some have tried hyperthermia (very high heat) in an attempt to burn off the tumor, but its effect has also been limited. Sometimes chemotherapy will give some relief, but not always. These cases are very upsetting for the doctor and patient and we are still searching for the right approach to their treatment.

A *regional* recurrence is one in the lymph nodes under the arm or above the collarbone. Now that we are taking out fewer lymph nodes from the axilla (see Chapter 25), a cancerous node could be left behind. This is rare, occurring in about 2 percent of breast cancers. Further treatment to this area with either surgery or radiation often takes care of the problem, although systemic therapy is considered as well. Regional recurrence in lymph nodes elsewhere, such as the neck or above the collarbone, has a more serious implication, since it is more likely to reflect spread of the tumor through the bloodstream. Akin to local recurrence following mastectomy, it usually warrants a more aggressive approach.[8]

As physicians we tend to downplay local and regional recurrences because they are not as life threatening as metastatic disease can be. Nonetheless, for the patient they can be devastating. When a woman gets a local recurrence she finds it much harder than she did the first time not to think of herself as doomed. She gave it her best shot and it didn't work—how can she trust any treatment again? This became obvious to me when we first set up our support group for women with metastatic disease at the Faulkner Breast Centre. I wanted to exclude women with local recurrences because I thought their situation wasn't serious enough for this group. My coworkers and patients convinced me that this was not true, and they turned out to be right. The overwhelming feelings are the same. Barbara Kalinowski describes the difficulties women with recurrences have even around other women with breast cancer. "They find themselves being 'polite' in mixed groups. One woman was talking about having just had her sixth chemotherapy treatment, and the woman next to her said, 'Oh, good, you're almost through!' And she didn't have the heart to tell her this was her second time around." When a woman has gone through the tough round of surgery, radiation, and chemotherapy and has tried to put it behind her, knowing she'll have to go through it all over again can be overwhelming.

DISTANT RECURRENCE (METASTATIC DISEASE)

As hard as it is to face a local recurrence, metastatic disease can be even more devastating. There are the same feelings that go with any recurrence, compounded by the knowledge that the chance of cure is slim. Here you need to face the fact that you are not immortal and to find the way to create the best quality of life for yourself in the time you have, and, at the same time, maintain hope.

As we mentioned in Chapter 21, when breast cancer shows up in your lungs, liver, or bones, it's still breast cancer—not lung or liver or bone cancer. We can usually tell which it is by looking at it under the microscope. When a cancer spreads to a different organ, it's known as metastasis.

It's important here to differentiate "metastatic" from "micro-metastatic." "Micrometastases" is the term we use when we discuss the likelihood of small cancer cells remaining in the rest of the body at the time of an initial treatment. They are cells that we presume are there, but that are so small we can't detect them. We believe that such spread, if it exists, can often be cured (see Chapter 28). But when we talk about metastatic disease itself, we mean cancer cells that we can detect on an x ray or scan, not simply that we think are probably there. At the time we're writing this book, nothing that we know of can guarantee a cure of metastatic breast cancer. However, new therapies are being developed all the time.

The average survival of women with metastatic breast cancer from the time of the first appearance of the metastasis is between two and three and a half years, according to most studies. But 25 to 35 percent of patients live five years, and about 10 percent live more than 10 years. And 1 or 2 percent are cured.[9] There are cases in the medical literature like the woman who had metastases throughout her bones, had hormone treatment, and was well 24 years later.[10] I wish we could take credit for such rare and wonderful occurrences, but we have no idea what causes the cure in any of them. It could be a miracle, or good luck, or an extraordinary immune system. Or it could be that the cells just go on lying dormant for an abnormally long time.

There are many factors that can help predict who will live a long time, but they're not absolute. One is the length of time between your original diagnosis and your metastasis. If the metastasis shows up six months after your diagnosis, it suggests that you have a much more aggressive cancer than if it's six years after your diagnosis.

Another factor is the aggressiveness of your original tumor. Still another is whether or not your tumor was sensitive to hormones. We also look at how many places it's metastasized to—if there's only one, or if you have multiple organs involved. Where it recurs is also a consideration. Metastasis to the bone or the scar is less serious than metastasis to the lung or liver.

All this is just statistics. What happens to an individual woman may or may not conform to the norm. I've had patients with metastatic disease who have far outlived the most optimistic prognosis. I had one patient who, while she was getting her adjuvant chemotherapy, developed lung metastasis. That means she had hardly any disease-free interval, and the cancer seemed resistant to chemo. Statistically, she should have been dead within months. She was treated hormonally and the cancer disappeared for two years. It came back at that point and another treatment made it disappear for another two years. When it came back that time we gave another hormone. Ten years after her initial diagnosis, she died of breast cancer. When she was diagnosed she had an eight-year-old son, and she was able to raise him almost into adulthood. So we can't accurately predict the course of any individual's illness. This is true of initial disease, and metastatic disease is even more unpredictable.

Usually I find that women who have just finished breast cancer treatments don't want to think about the possibility of its spreading. They're busy dealing with the healing process and a metastasis is too painful to think about. But of course it's always somewhere in the back of a woman's mind. Usually about a year after her initial treatments the patient will start asking me what the symptoms of metastasis are. (This is an observation, by the way—not a guideline. If you want to know right away, or two months later, talk to your doctor. There's nothing particularly brave about toughing it out when you're worried. Every woman's pace is different.)

In medical school, we used to be taught that we shouldn't tell people who had been treated for cancer what to look for if they were worried about recurrences, because they'd start imagining that they had every symptom we told them about. I've never liked that idea. It doesn't soothe people at all; it just means they'll be afraid of everything, instead of a few specific things. When you've had cancer, you're acutely aware of your body, and any symptom you ever had—or never noticed before—can take on new, terrifying significance for you. Anything unexpected in your body has you petrified. Inevitably, this will mean a lot of fear over symptoms that turn out to be harmless. But if you know that the symptoms of breast cancer metastasis are usually bone pain, shortness of breath, lack of appetite and weight loss, and neurological symptoms like pain or weakness or headaches, there are at least limits to your fear. You'll probably be frightened when anything resembling those symptoms comes up, even if it turns out to be nothing but a tension headache or a mild flu. But at least you won't be terrified by a sore spot on your big toe or an unexpected weight gain. Knowing what symptoms to look for reduces fear; it doesn't increase it.

Most women whose breast cancer has metastasized don't show any symptoms until the disease is quite extensive. It isn't a case of years and years of terrible suffering, the way TV melodrama likes to show it.

Like other cancers, breast cancer can spread anywhere, but it's more likely to show up in some places than in others—most commonly lungs, liver, and bones. Why this is we don't know. There's a lot of research being done about it, and perhaps one day we'll have a better understanding of it. It must be that the environment of certain organs is more conducive to growth for this type of cancer cell.

In a quarter of the cases, the bones are the first site where metastatic disease is detected. This is true partly because it's more common there than in other places, and partly because it creates definite symptoms. Even if it first appears elsewhere, as the disease progresses it usually reaches the bone at some stage.

Metastasis to the bone is usually diagnosed when the patient experiences pain. Sometimes it's hard to know if the pain is ordinary low back pain or some other disease, like arthritis. Usually the pain you get with breast cancer in the bones is fairly constant and generally doesn't improve over time. With arthritis, you wake up in the morning and feel stiff, but get better as you move around during the day. With some muscular problems that cause bone pain, the more you do the worse the pain gets. But the pain from cancer is steady, and usually remains even at night, when you're not doing anything. The pain is probably caused by the cancer taking up room in the bone and pressing on it, and so sometimes it can get worse in different positions: if you're standing up on the bone you might be compressing it more and causing more pain than if you're lying down. If you have pain that lasts for more than a week or two and doesn't seem to be going away, and isn't like whatever pains have been familiar to you in your life, you should get it checked out.

We usually check bone pain by doing a bone scan. This is a radioactive test, which I've described in Chapter 21. It's not very specific, because it can be positive for a lot of different conditions, but it's quite accurate for showing when there's cancer.

If the bone scan is suspicious or suggestive, the next step is an x ray. If there's metastasis, this will show one of two things: either lytic lesions, which are holes where the cancer has eaten away the bones, or blastic lesions, which are an increase of bone where the growth factor of the cancer has caused the bone to get more dense. CAT scans and MRI, described in Chapter 10, can also be used to diagnosis cancer in specific bones.

Most of the time if you're diagnosed with a bone metastasis, the major treatment will be geared toward alleviating the symptoms. If it's just one spot in one bone and the rest of your bones are okay, we can use radiation on that one spot. It will kill the tumor cells, shrink the tumor, and give you relief. If there are several different spots in your bones that are causing pain, and we can't radiate them all, we'd probably begin with some form of systemic therapy.

A bisphosphonate, the same kind of drug used for osteoporosis, has been found to be useful in treating bone metastasis. Pamidronate, or Aredia, has been found not only to help treat known bone metastases but to prevent future ones and to significantly reduce pain.

The thing we worry about most in women with cancer in their bones is the possibility of fractures. If the cancer eats away enough bone, the bone will no longer be able to hold you up. Then you can get what's called a "pathological fracture," so named because it's caused not by a blow from outside—you've tripped on the stairs and the bone has been banged against the wood—but by something wrong in the bone itself (Fig. 32-2). It's similar to osteoporosis in that it doesn't take

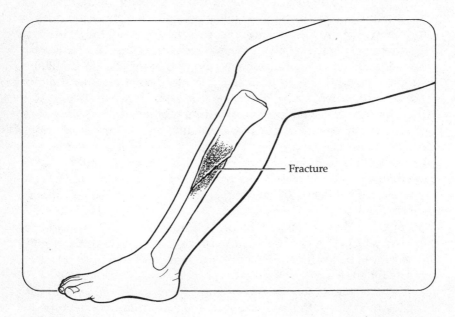

Fracture

FIGURE 32-2

very much to cause this fracture, because the bone is so weakened. So a slight pressure that usually wouldn't even cause a bruise triggers the fracture. (It's different from osteoporosis, however, in that it doesn't affect all your bones.)

One of the ways we deal with this is by trying to predict ahead of time which bones are likely to fracture, so we can help prevent it. The doctor will pay a lot of attention to what particular bones are involved. The ones to worry most about are the ones that hold you up—your leg or hip bones. The upper arm can also fracture, but it's less likely because you don't put as much constant pressure on it. You can also get a fracture in your spine. If we can see on the x rays that a bone in a critical place has metastatic disease that would be a risk for a fracture, we can do surgery ahead of time—pin the hip or stabilize the bone. Again, the idea is to keep you stabilized and functional, with as high a quality of life as possible for as long a time as possible.

New treatments for pain caused by bone metastasis are strontium and samarium. These are radioactive particles that are injected intravenously and taken up by the bone. The radioactivity can then act directly on the metastasis. These are worth asking about if you have diffuse bone disease and pain not helped adequately by Aredia.[11]

We also see breast cancer metastasis fairly often in the lungs (Fig. 32-3). Usually the symptoms for that are shortness of breath and a chronic cough. Sixty to 70 percent of patients who die of breast cancer eventually have it in their lungs. The lungs are the only site of metastasis in about 21 percent of cases. There are a couple of different ways it can form in the lungs. One is in nodules—usually several—that show up on a chest x ray. If the chest x ray shows only one nodule, we can't tell if it's lung cancer or a breast cancer spread. So we do a needle biopsy or a full biopsy to find out. (Lung cancer usually starts in just one spot, but any other cancer that has spread to the lung through the bloodstream or lymphatic channels is likely to hit multiple spots in the lung.)

If your breast cancer has spread to your lungs, you may experience shortness of breath on less exertion than normal. It can be fairly subtle. It comes on slowly, since the cancer has to have used up a lot of your lungs before you get short of breath.

Another form of metastasis in the lung is called lymphangitic spread. Here the cancer spreads along the lymphatics, and so instead of being nodules it's a fine pattern throughout the lung. That's subtler and harder to detect on a chest x ray. It too will ultimately give you shortness of breath, since it takes up room and scars the lungs, making them less able to expand and contract and to bring oxygen into your bloodstream.

The third way it can show is through fluid in the lung. That usually indicates spread in the lining around the lung rather than in the lung itself. (The lung sits in a sack with a smooth lining around it, so that it

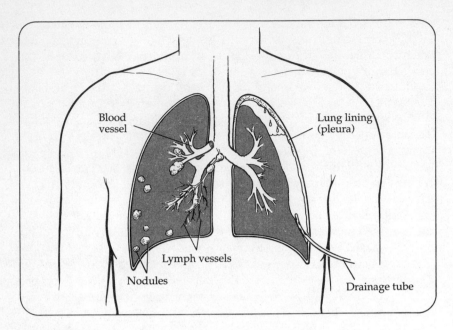

Blood vessel

Lung lining (pleura)

Lymph vessels

Nodules

Drainage tube

FIGURE 32-3

can move without sticking to your chest wall.) The cancer creates fluid around the lung (effusion), and the fluid causes the lung to collapse partially (see Fig. 32-3). Here again, you'll experience shortness of breath. Usually breast cancer in the lungs doesn't cause pain.

If we think your cancer may have metastasized to your lung, we do a chest x ray. If the x ray doesn't show nodules, fluid, or any of the other signs, we can still do a CAT scan.

The treatment for lymphangitic and nodule symptoms is chemotherapy, because we want to make breathing easier quickly. Steroids such as prednisone can also help relieve symptoms. Nodules in the lungs can be treated with hormonal therapy or chemotherapy, depending on how extensive the nodules are and whether the cancer is likely to improve with hormonal therapies.

Fluid in the lung can be treated by sticking a needle into the chest and draining the fluid. This works immediately, but only temporarily. Often the fluid comes right back again. In order to prevent the reaccumulation of fluid, we need to fasten the lining of the lung to the lung. When I was in medical school we used to do an operation, open up the chest, take a piece of gauze and rub it against the lung to irritate the spot. That got it red and raw and made it stick together and create a scar, so there was no room for fluid. A less invasive approach is to drain the fluid out through a tube and then put in some material that will scar up the lining of the sack. Tetracycline, a common antibiotic, tends to work. However, often an effective hormonal therapy or chemotherapy will keep the fluid in the lung from reaccumulating, at least for a while. Eventually, many women with recurrent pleural effusions do receive the scarring procedure and chest tube drainage.

The liver is the third most common site for metastases. Again, this can be subtle. The symptoms occur because the cancer takes up a lot of room in the liver, and that takes some time to happen. About two thirds of women who die of breast cancer have it in their liver, and about a quarter have it initially. The symptoms are common—weight loss, anorexia (loss of appetite), gastrointestinal symptoms, and pain or discomfort under your right rib cage. You may have some pain: if you do, it would be in the right upper quadrant, because it comes from the liver capsule being stretched out.

A diagnosis of liver metastasis is often suspected from blood tests. We can also do a CAT scan or an ultrasound. The major treatment for extensive liver disease is chemotherapy, although hormonal therapy can work well on smaller metastases. Hormone treatments don't work very well here. In some kinds of cancer, like colon cancer, liver metastasis can be single, and thus can sometimes be cut out. But with breast cancer there is usually more than one spot involved and surgery becomes impossible. In the rare exceptions when there is only one spot, we can surgically remove part of the liver to relieve symptoms. There are also new techniques for one or two liver metastases which involve putting hot (hyperthermia) or cold (cryosurgery) probes into the tumors and burning or freezing them. This can help the obvious spots but must be followed with systemic therapy to control the rest of the micrometastatic liver disease. Sometimes when patients have a lot of pain we radiate the liver to shrink it. At one time we were working on putting chemotherapy directly into the liver, by inserting a catheter into the artery that went into the liver, thinking that would be a more direct treatment of the metastases. But we really get just as good a response with less drastic and more comfortable forms of chemotherapy, so we don't do this much anymore.

Less common, but very serious, are neurological metastases. Breast cancer can spread to the brain and the spinal cord. It's still fairly uncommon—about 6 percent. Our adjuvant chemotherapy does not get into the brain as effectively as it does into the rest of the body. Because of this, we are seeing brain metastases with a somewhat greater frequency as systemic adjuvant therapies have become better at eradicating disease outside the brain. Predictably, the most common symptom is headache. I almost hate to say that, since most people get a lot of headaches during their lives, and I'm afraid any reader with breast cancer who gets a tension headache will be terrified. But if the headache doesn't go away in a reasonable time, check it out. In some patients it's the kind of headache that occurs with a brain tumor. It begins early in the morning before you get out of bed, then improves as the day goes on, but then gets worse and worse over time. Ultimately you also have drowsiness and nausea. It usually comes on slowly, over a period of weeks.

Behavior or mental changes are sometimes, though rarely, caused by the tumor. You can have weakness or unsteadiness in walking, or seizures. It can resemble a stroke: you suddenly can't talk, or part of your body is suddenly very weak, or you can't see out of one eye. Those kinds of symptoms come from a blocking of a portion of your brain, which the cancer growth can cause. The best way to diagnosis it is through CAT scan or MRI. About half the patients will have one lesion; the other half will have several. The treatment is usually radiation, which shrinks the metastasis. As with liver metastasis, if there's only one lesion, surgery might work. You'll also be put on steroids—dexamethasone or prednisone—right away, to reduce the swelling of the brain. Since the brain sits within a hard bony shell (the skull) there isn't much room for swelling before important structures are injured. If you're having seizures, you'll also be put on anti-seizure medication. Chemotherapy and hormonal therapies don't work very well on brain metastasis.

Another kind of brain metastasis you can get is a form of meningitis called *carcinomitis meningitis.* It affects the lining of the brain rather than the brain itself. It causes headaches and stiff neck and sometimes confusion, the way any form of meningitis does. In that situation the treatment is to operate and put a little reservoir into the lining of the brain so as to insert chemotherapy directly into the spinal fluid that bathes the brain. Radiation can also be used. Unfortunately, the therapies for carcinomitis meningitis don't work very well so some oncologists talk to their patients about not doing them.

Metastasis to the spinal cord is also very serious. The tumor can push on the spinal cord and cause paralysis. Sometimes this happens because the bone metastasis is in the vertebrae, and pushes against the spinal cord as it grows out of the bone into the spinal canal (Fig. 32-4). Sometimes the tumor grows directly in the spinal cord itself. Before the paralysis, however, there are earlier symptoms—pain, weakness, sensory loss, and disturbances of the bowel or bladder. Pain is the most common—85 to 90 percent of patients with spinal cord metastasis have pain. It may be the only symptom for months. The problem is that if you have cancer only in the bones and the back, you'll also have pain. So we have to be able to differentiate, or at least be extremely alert, to be certain that the patient with bone metastasis in her back isn't on the verge of spinal cord compression. Most of the pain is aching and con-

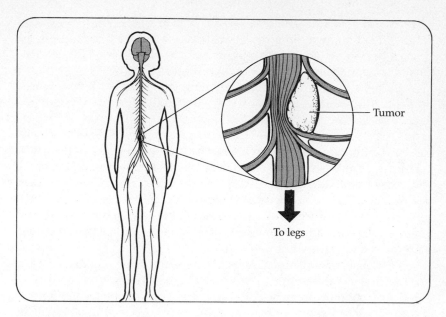

Tumor

To legs

FIGURE 32-4

tinuous. Its onset is gradual and it gets worse over time; it often becomes severe as it pushes on the spinal cord. And it's very localized:
you feel it exactly on the spot where the tumor is. There is another kind
of pain that goes downward the way sciatica does, when a disk compresses the nerves and goes down your leg, getting worse if you cough
or sneeze. You might also feel pain in your shoulder or back from spinal cord compression. Seventy-five percent of patients with metastasis
to the spinal cord have weakness in their muscles from the tumor
pushing against the nerves and about 5 percent will have spots of
numbness. Anyone with metastatic breast cancer who has unrelenting
pain in one spot, and any neurological symptoms, should be concerned. If you have no other signs of metastasis, it probably isn't spinal
cord compression, since that's rarely the first sign of metastatic disease,
although it can be. The way we diagnose it is with CAT scan or MRI.
We used to do a myelogram, in which dye is injected into the spinal
column, but we rarely do that anymore. The treatment is generally
emergency surgery if there is any evidence of nerve damage, muscle
weakness, or a large tumor pressing on the spinal cord. And, if it's one
spot, we may be able to remove the tumor and decompress the spinal
cord. Alternatively, the treatment could be emergency radiation; it is
one of the few instances in which radiation is used as an emergency
treatment. The radiation shrinks the tumor and steroids prevent the
spinal cord from swelling.

Breast cancer can also metastasize to the eye, though again it's rarely the first place breast cancer spreads. The first symptoms are double or blurred vision. It's diagnosed by CAT scan or MRI. It's also treated with radiation, which can often prevent loss of vision.

Another area is bone marrow. The main symptom is anemia, caused by a decrease in the number of red blood cells, and the white blood cells and platelets can also be decreased. Though it sounds grim, metastasis to the bone marrow actually responds very well to treatment, either with hormones or with chemotherapy. I have one patient who had breast cancer in one breast, did fine, and then got breast cancer in the other breast several years later. She decided to have mastectomy and reconstruction. Right before surgery her blood count was a little low. So we went ahead with the surgery, but we also did a bone marrow biopsy and found it had metastasized. We put her on tamoxifen, and she did well for six or seven years.

Breast cancer in all its manifestations is an unpredictable disease. These are general descriptions. As I write this many women come to mind who didn't follow the rules. Use this information to help understand your own situation and ask questions. Your situation will be unique to you no matter what happens.

TAKING CARE OF YOURSELF EMOTIONALLY

David Spiegel's study of women with metastatic disease who joined support groups (see Chapter 29) shows the importance of the mind-body connection. Not only did the women who participated in a support group live twice as long as those who did not, they also had a better quality of life.[12] A diagnosis of metastatic disease is a time to reorder your life and pay attention to what is most important to you. You may not be able to change things, but you can improve how you deal with them.

Spiegel tells the story of a woman who had always wanted to write poetry and started after her diagnosis of metastatic disease. She had a book of her poems published before her death. One of my own patients, Susan Shapiro, was very distressed with the lack of analysis of breast cancer from a feminist political perspective. She wrote an article in the local feminist paper and called a meeting. From this she started the Women's Community Cancer Project in Boston a few months before she died. I'm certain she would be happy to know her work sparked a national movement which continues today (see Chapter 34).

A diagnosis of recurrence or metastasis will remind you that you do not have control over your body. But you certainly do have control over your mind, emotions, and spirit. This is a good time to revisit some of the complementary treatments such as visualization, self-hypnosis, and imagery (see Chapter 29). And find a doctor you can talk to and who will listen to you. Shop around if you have to. If you are in a small town and/or have an insurance plan with limited choice, then schedule an appointment with your oncologist so that you can talk about what you need, as well as what he or she expects from you. (See Appendix D for the patient's and doctor's rights.) You need to know as accurately as possible what to expect from your condition and your treatments so that you can plan. Ask for the information you need and tell your doctor if there are things you would rather not know. As in any relationship, frank communication about your needs will go far toward having them met.

There are two main fears that accompany a diagnosis of recurrent breast cancer: pain and death. Pain is certainly not inevitable. Pain control has finally gone mainstream in the United States. There are pain centers, and many methods have been developed to deal with pain without clouding your mind and ruining your life (see Chapter 33).

Not everyone dies from a recurrence or metastatic breast cancer but it is certainly a possibility. David Spiegel's book *Living Beyond Limits*[13] is invaluable in addressing the needs of the heart and soul in the face of terminal illness. You may not be able to avoid death but you can control how you want to handle it. One of my patients was a great denier. From the first moment of her diagnosis she refused to let her cancer interfere with her life. Once she had metastatic disease this pattern continued. She continued to hurl herself through life: physically active, sailing, traveling, and enjoying herself. My first reaction was to be a little critical of her inability to face the reality of the situation, until I realized that she *had* faced it. She knew exactly what she was doing and was determined to take control of whatever time she had left. She slipped into a coma on her sailboat among friends and died as she wanted, where she wanted, in control to the end.

WHEN TO STOP TREATMENT

Often people ask their doctor, "How long have I got to live?" I'd never answer that—not because I wanted to withhold information from my patient, but because I simply didn't know. There are statistical likelihoods, but they do not tell what will happen to each individual. There are patients who, according to the statistics, should die in about four months and they live four years; there are others who should last four years and die in four months. I'm always amazed at the variations. One of my patients had a small cancer and negative nodes with what should have been a good prognosis, but when she finished her radiation we discovered the cancer had metastasized to her lungs, and she died in three months. It often works the other way. Another patient, a

Chinese woman who spoke no English, had a cancer that was very bad, and I privately thought she wouldn't live very long. I had to talk to her through her sons, who kept trying to get me to say how long she had. I wouldn't tell them. It's a good thing, because seven years later, she's still alive. Sometimes I think she's lived so long because she didn't know she was supposed to die.

At the same time, it's important for your doctor to be honest with you. I think it's sensible to say to a patient who has asked for a frank response, "This is serious, but we don't know how long you'll live until we see how you respond to treatment. You'll probably eventually die of breast cancer, and you probably won't live another 40 years, so you may want to plan your life with that in mind." If you insist on more specific predictions, a doctor may quote statistics—but you should always be reminded that there are exceptions to statistics. If 99 out of 100 patients in your condition die within a year, 1 out of 100 doesn't—and there's no reason to assume you won't be that one.

Eventually, however, there comes the hardest part. We've tried all the available treatments, and we know that you don't have much longer. Even then, we don't know if it's days or weeks, and there is still the possibility of a miracle. But there's a point at which you're clearly dying, and you have a right to know that. It used to be the prevailing belief that it was better not to tell patients they were dying. But this sets up an unhealthy climate of denial. Often you'll sense it yourself, but since no one else wants to talk about it you pretend it's okay in order to spare them, and they pretend it's okay in order to spare you. Such denial can keep you from finishing up your business—clearing up relationships, saying good-bye, saying the things you won't get another chance to say to the people you love, giving them the chance to say those things to you. I think doctors make a great error in denying death: we tend to look at it too much as a defeat, and to get caught up in our own denial, at the patient's expense.

While you're still feeling fairly well, you might want to talk with your doctor, and with your family members or friends, about how you want to die when the time comes. Do you want to be kept alive at all costs, or not? Do you want to die at home, or in the hospital?

Often people die in either a hospital or a nursing home, and many think of that as an inevitability. But it isn't, and it's important to consider whether it might be better for you to die either in your own home or in the home of a loved one. For many people this is the best option, particularly if there are people among their loved ones able to become full-time caregivers. Dying at home offers more control over your surroundings, and more likelihood that you will die with loved ones around you. If this is an option you want to explore, there are many hospice programs that can help you.

For some women and their families, this is not possible. If it makes more sense for you to die in a hospital, there is much you and your loved ones can do to assure that the environment is as comfortable as possible. Many hospitals have hospice rooms for dying patients, and even those that don't can be made homelike. You will want to discuss your wishes with the caregivers there, to be sure they are willing and prepared to follow them.

There are other issues you'll want to look into—perhaps even before you have decided that it's time to stop fighting your illness. When the time comes—whether that's in a few months or in 10 years—do you want to be heavily medicated or as alert as possible? No way is universally better, but one way might be better for you. If your wishes are clearly known—especially if they can be documented in a living will—you might be able to prevent those tragic situations in which doctors and family members are fighting over whether to keep you on a life-support system.

A living will is only part of a larger plan, called an "advance directive." This is a set of written instructions that comprise both a living will and a health care proxy. The living will spells out what medical treatment you do and don't want if the time arrives when you are unable to verbalize your own decisions. A health care proxy specifies a particular person whom you authorize to make decisions about your care when you no longer can.

Living wills vary from state to state, and in some cases you may need to add information to your living will. As Dr. Daniel Tobin writes in *Peaceful Dying*, the language of the typical living will may not be specific enough.[14] If the document merely says you don't want life-prolonging measures if you have an "incurable or irreversible condition," your doctor may define such a condition differently than you would. So you might want to add a specific "do-not-resuscitate" to your living will, and other additions concerning artificial nutrition and hydration. To do this means you need to spend some time thinking about what you *do* want when the time comes. Do you want to be tube fed? Do you want to be given antibiotics to fight infections, or do you want to allow your body to let you die from the infection rather than to continue for a short time and die of your cancer? These things may not be fun to think about, but they're important.

Betsy Carpenter, a long-time speaker and activist around issues of advance directives, emphatically agrees. You may or may not want life-extending treatment at some point, and you have a right to make those decisions. But it's important to make those decisions before you reach the point where you can no longer speak for yourself. Like Dr. Tobin, she stresses the importance of talking with your family and friends in advance, discussing the options open to you and how you feel about them, and listening respectfully to the feelings of your loved ones. Your illness and your ultimate death will affect those who love you deeply, and it's important to involve them in your decision-making process. Understanding your feelings and sharing their own with you will make it far less likely that they'll want to go against your wishes when the time comes.

In deciding what you do and don't want, Carpenter advises, think about four areas in particular. What are your fears? Most people fear pain, loss of control, inappropriate prolongation of life, and becoming a burden to loved ones. Each of these fears should be explored fully, in terms of what is reasonable to think may happen and in terms of your own emotions.

Pick out your health care proxy carefully, she says, and spell out who you *don't* want involved in making health care decisions for you as well. "This doesn't have to be hostile," she says. "You can write, 'although I dearly love my son Jim, I don't wish him to have any part in decision-making around my care.'" The agent you choose should be not only someone you love, but someone you fully trust to honor your wishes, and someone who knows you well enough to make decisions that you haven't spelled out, in ways that you would want. "For example," she says, "my husband is my proxy-agent, and he knows that I wouldn't want my life artificially prolonged. But suppose my daughter, who lives in London, wasn't here when I went into a coma. He might be certain that it was important for her to see me living and breathing one last time. So he might decide to keep me on life support for 24 hours until she could get back home. And he would know that, loving her, I would also want this for her." Because of such contingencies, she adds, while your living will should be specific, it shouldn't be too specific to preclude your agent from making judgments in such unforeseen circumstances. You may want to write out a declaration of precedence: "If a conflict arises between my list and my agent's decision, I give precedent to my agent over my own written word."

If there is someone you don't want even visiting you when you're dying, this too should be spelled out, says Carpenter, in a Priority of Visitation Statement. Such documents are important even for those not facing imminent death, she says. Healthy people are sometimes injured in accidents and are suddenly no longer able to verbalize their wishes.

These questions are important for every one of us to consider, since none of us is immortal, and death can come for anyone at any time. Of course, you may live another 10 or 20 years anyway—but you haven't lost anything by having those discussions, and you might even have gained a little peace of mind.

33

Metastatic Disease:
Treatments

The treatment approaches to metastatic disease are different from the approaches to primary breast cancer. As we said in Chapter 32, with metastatic cancer there isn't a reliable method of cure. Our goal is two-fold. First, we want to prolong your survival as much as possible.

Hormonal therapies, immunotherapies, and even chemotherapy have been demonstrated to induce remissions that on average last about one year, but can last as long as 10 years. Some of the newer treatments for metastatic breast cancer are being shown to improve women's overall survival, compared to some of the older chemotherapy and hormonal options. Recent studies of the new aromatase inhibitors, which block the production of estrogen in women's bodies, show improved survival compared to an older, standard therapy, Megace.[1] The new antibody therapy Herceptin and the taxanes paclitaxel (Taxol) and docetaxel (Taxotere) improve patient's survival compared with older chemotherapy regimens.[2] As this book went to press some of the antiangiogenesis drugs (especially when combined with low-dose continuous chemotherapy) were showing promise in mice and people.[3] This is certainly an important first step and we hope the beginning of a new era in the treatment of metastatic disease.

Second, we want to control your symptoms and make you feel better. Some people will say, "If I have metastatic disease I don't want any therapy—it will just make me suffer more." However, some of the best tools we have for improving quality of life are surgery, radiation therapy, hormonal therapy, and chemotherapy—the same tools we use to treat initial cancer. This may come as a surprise to many readers, especially in terms of chemotherapy. For many, the very word conjures up images of violent and debilitating nausea. But in fact, with metastatic cancer, chemotherapy and hormone therapy can actually alleviate much suffering. As we discussed in the last chapter, a woman with metastatic breast cancer can experience severe discomfort as the disease progresses—pain in her bones, shortness of breath, or weakness and lethargy. By shrinking the tumor that creates these symptoms, therapy can make her feel dramatically better. That's not a small accomplishment. Death is inevitable at some point, though most of us prefer to think that point is always years away. But more than death itself most people fear a life of prolonged, enfeebling illness, one that is too painful to enjoy and causes them to become a burden on those they love.

One of the things most difficult for patients with metastatic cancer is having no clear idea of what to expect—how long they will live and how much pain they are likely to be in. Two things are important to consider. One is dealing with your own emotions, through counseling, a support group, religion—whatever works best for you. (We discussed this at length in Chapters 22 and 32.) The other important thing is to get as much information as your doctor has about the probable progress of your illness and what it entails. Some doctors are very uncomfortable with death; they see their job as fighting even the thought of death until the last minute, and therefore they deal with your fear of dying by pretending it won't happen. Sometimes doctors try to deal with the patient's fear by using every kind of therapy as rapidly and in as great a dose as possible, to try to ward off the inevitable. Often the patient herself goes along with this approach. But it's as dangerous as the opposite extreme of shying away from any treatment at all. In this chapter I want to discuss more sensibly what treatments are available for metastatic disease and what you should expect from them.

During and after your treatment for metastatic disease you'll be followed with the staging tests—bone scan, chest x ray, and blood tests—as well as a few other tests such as CAT scans. These will help to determine if you're indeed responding to treatment (see Chapters 21 and 32).

We speak about two kinds of responses to treatment for metastatic breast cancer—partial and complete. A partial response is when the tumor volume regresses by at least 50 percent, and a complete response means it regresses so far that we can no longer detect it. For us to measure a response like this you need to have what's called "measurable disease." We have to be able to see it clearly enough measure it.

We can't always do that. If you have a nodule of cancer in your lungs, we can take x rays to determine how well it's gone down. But pain from bone metastasis is harder to measure. We know that treatments are working because your pain is reduced, but that isn't a scientific measurement: we can't say your pain went away 50 percent or 38 percent. So some symptoms are easier than others to measure, and we don't always get an exact estimate of your response.

For the doctor planning the most effective treatment, the job is to figure out what the symptoms are and match the treatment, with the least toxicity possible.

HORMONAL (ENDOCRINE) TREATMENTS

We've known for a long time that breast cancer in women is often an endocrine disease—the endocrine glands are the ones that make hormones. We can test the cancer when the tumor is first removed and tell if it's sensitive to hormones by doing the estrogen receptor test described in Chapter 20.

In women who have metastatic disease and a tumor that's sensitive to hormones, using endocrine treatments first often makes more sense than chemotherapy. When a patient has responded to one hormone therapy, we know she's likely to respond to a second and possibly a third one, so we use them serially.

The first hormonal treatment devised was used in premenopausal women and consisted of oophorectomy—which meant surgically removing the ovaries. Now we can either do this surgically or use drugs (ablation). In menstruating women who are estrogen receptor positive, the response to oophorectomy is 35 percent. An additional 25 percent will have improvement in their symptoms and a prolonged period of stable disease.

Of course, removing the ovaries puts you into immediate menopause, complete with mood swings and hot flashes. But it also can almost immediately relieve your metastatic breast cancer symptoms, often by the time you leave the hospital. This approach was out of fashion temporarily with the introduction of chemotherapy, but it has resumed an important place in the treatment of metastatic disease with the introduction of several new drugs that can turn off the ovaries' ability to make estrogen and can be just the right treatment for a woman with bone metastasis and an estrogen receptor positive tumor.

Whether we remove the ovaries or inactivate them with drugs, the treatment is effective. Reversible menopause can be induced by using some of the GnRH agonists such as Lupron or Zoladex (see Chapter 28), which block FSH and LH and stop your periods. Another way to block estrogen is to block the receptor that it fits into in the cell in the breast. This is the way antiestrogens such as tamoxifen and toremifene work. They can be used in both premenopausal and postmenopausal women whose tumors are sensitive to estrogen. If you were on tamoxifen in the past and then stopped, it's worth trying again to treat your metastatic disease. On the other hand, if the metastasis began while you were on tamoxifen, you're probably resistant and should try something else.

In women who are postmenopausal (whether by chemotherapy or naturally) estrogen is principally made by the enzyme aromatase, which converts testosterone and androstenedione to estrogen. This enzyme is found in the adrenal glands, fat, muscle, and breast tissue itself. The first aromatase inhibitor used was aminoglutethimide, but that caused a problem by also blocking the adrenal glands' production of other hormones. The most recent aromatase inhibitors—anastrozole (Arimidex), letrazole (Femara), and exemestane (Aromasin)—are much less toxic than aminoglutethimide and have very good response rates. They are currently the drugs of choice once a tumor becomes resistant to tamoxifen. The aromatase inhibitors are well tolerated and have been shown to improve women's overall survival compared to the standard hormonal therapy Megace.

Megace is a kind of progestin. Its biggest side effect is increased appetite, which leads to weight gain. This occurs in about half the patients, and they gain somewhere between 10 and 20 pounds. Twelve percent of women gain more than 30 pounds. (In fact, Megace is so likely to cause weight gain that they tried using it in treating people with AIDS and other wasting diseases.) Megace works for about 20 to 30 percent of women and is now generally used after the aromatase inhibitors.

Since antiestrogens work, some doctors have been looking at the possibility of using antiprogesterones as well. The most well known antiprogesterone is RU486, which is used outside the U.S. for abortions. There's been a very small study showing that some breast cancers do respond to antiprogesterones. But the response rate is a disappointing 10–18 percent. Provera has also been used as a progestin therapy, but again has only modest activity.[4]

You might think that if all these different hormones work separately they'd work even better together. Initial studies did not show much benefit, but trials of aromatase inhibitors and tamoxifen together are now going on. Patients who respond to one therapy are more likely to respond to the next one. Once a woman stops responding to hormones she still has the option of chemotherapy.

Some women will experience a phenomenon called "flare" with hormonal treatment of metastatic breast cancer. What this means is that within the first month of therapy there is an exacerbation of the patient's disease. It actually indicates a good prognosis. Typically it occurs with someone who has bone metastasis and is put on tamoxifen. Suddenly her pain is worse than ever. But then she's back to normal soon after. We think this happens because tamoxifen can actually work initially as a weak estrogen in some women, stimulating their cancer, before it starts to function as an antiestrogen. But it's good to know about because flare can be very scary.

When you look at the overall effectiveness of all the hormonal treatments you'll see that it's about 40 percent. But it doesn't work out equally for all women: if your tumor is strongly estrogen and progesterone receptor positive, you'll have a 60 percent response rate. That means in over half the cases symptoms are alleviated for a significant amount of time. Women with lower levels of estrogen (ER) and progesterone (PR) have a lower response rate, but it is still significant. Only twenty percent of women whose breast cancers are truly ER and PR negative by modern tumor-staining techniques have no chance of benefiting from hormonal therapy.

Usually the effects of endocrine treatments last for about 12–18 months, but many women stay in remission for 2–5 years, and some are free of disease for as long as 10 years. The 24-year survivor mentioned in the previous chapter was treated with hormonal therapies only. A widely held belief among medical oncologists is that chemotherapy works faster than hormonal therapy in reversing symptoms. One reason for this belief may be that chemotherapy often results in faster tumor shrinkage, as seen on x rays. Another reason may be that patients who respond to endocrine therapy are usually those with the more slowly growing disease. There is probably a relationship between the rate at which the disease grows and the rate at which it disappears. However, endocrine treatment is important; patients can have dramatic relief of bone pain within a day or two.

When the tumor does show up again, sometimes just stopping the drug can give a secondary response. We think this is because the antiestrogen tamoxifen can sometimes actually stimulate tumor growth over time; therefore, stopping tamoxifen can halt the growth of the tumor cells again.

As always, I urge all readers to consider participating in a clinical trial or at least finding out which trials they are eligible for (see Chapter 12). For premenopausal women not participating in a trial, at UCLA we try either tamoxifen or goserelin first. If that works, we stay with it until the symptoms recur and then go on to Megace or one of the other hormonal treatments. With postmenopausal women we start with tamoxifen (since removing the ovaries of a postmenopausal woman doesn't change much); if that works for a time the next step is tamoxifen withdrawal, then anastrozole, then halotestin (a male hormone), and finally chemotherapy. If a woman was on tamoxifen adjuvant therapy at the time of her metastasis we would start with anastrozole for postmenopausal women and goserelin (Zoladex) for premenopausal women. Only when a woman stops responding to hormones do we go on to chemotherapy.

The woman with metastatic breast cancer whose tumor is sensitive to hormones is comparatively lucky, because she has more avenues of treatment that are less toxic than does the woman whose tumor is resistant to hormonal influence. As we said earlier, however, even some women with hormone receptor negative tumors may respond to hormone therapy. This is because the older methods of measuring ER and PR were somewhat inaccurate and women whose cancer was called negative were actually low positive. Most oncologists feel that any woman with any degree of ER or PR positivity, however small, should be given treatment with hormonal therapy at some time during the course of her metastatic disease. All women with metastasis should question their medical oncologist about the possibility of hormonal treatment. Some medical oncologists are better trained in giving chemotherapy than endocrine therapy, and they derive a greater financial profit from it as well. It just may not occur to them to try a hormonal maneuver first unless you bring it up. Certainly the best quality of life is likely to be associated with less toxic but successful hormonal treatments.

CHEMOTHERAPY

For the women whose tumors are not responsive to hormone therapy, the alternative is chemotherapy. The percentage of patients who develop an objective response (at least 50 percent shrinkage in tumor volume) to chemotherapy is generally about twice that of patients who have an objective response with hormone therapy. The percentage of patients who respond at least partially to the commonly used single-agent chemotherapy treatments is 20 to 59 percent, and about 10–15 percent will have a complete response—their tumors will totally vanish by x-ray examination for 6 to 12 months. Usually it takes around six weeks for the response to occur, although patients' symptoms generally improve within a few weeks. The duration of the response is between 5 and 13 months. The maximum duration that we've so far found is over 180 months—which means, in effect, that it's over 10 years and thus could be called a cure. (Unfortunately, this length of survival is very rare.) The average survival of the responders is 15 to 42 months. It is generally less for women whose cancers are resistant to chemotherapy. So chemotherapy, like hormone therapy, can help you to live with symptom improvement for anywhere between one and four years, and there's a small chance it can give you 10 or more years of quality life.

More than 80 cytotoxic drugs—drugs that kill cells—have been tested. Of these, about 10 are used commonly in breast cancer treatment. Interestingly, breast cancer creates the kind of tumor that is responsive to the greatest array of drugs—most other cancers don't respond to as many chemicals. The standard drugs are the same ones we discussed in Chapter 28 in terms of adjuvant treatment: cyclophosphamide (Cytoxan) (C), methotrexate (M), 5-fluorouracil (F), Adriamycin (A), epirubicin (E), and paclitaxel or docetaxel (T). These drugs have the highest antitumor activity among all the patients studied, and only limited cross-resistance.

What is used depends very much on what was used at the time of diagnosis of metastatic disease. If you already had CMF then Adriamycin might be tried. If you had Adriamycin when you were diagnosed then paclitaxel or docetaxel might be the next choice. Fortunately there are other drugs as well. These include capecitabine (Xeloda), mitoxantrone (Novantrone), vinorelbine (Navelbine), and gemcitabine (Gemzar), all of which have documented antitumor activity in breast cancer.

Each drug has limitations. With Adriamycin, we can give only a certain dosage, and then it becomes toxic to the heart. Once you've reached that point you can't ever use it again. Some of the other drugs you can take indefinitely.

In the past, we used the drugs together in chemotherapy, which we don't do in hormonal therapy. Now we know there's often no great advantage to giving the drugs together, as opposed to one at a time, as treatment for metastatic disease. As we discussed in Chapter 28, chemotherapy acts at different points in the cell's cycle. Theoretically, when we give the chemotherapy we kill a certain fraction of the existing cancer cells. Though in reality you have millions of cancer cells, for the sake of simplicity let's say that you have a thousand. On the first hit of chemotherapy drugs we kill 200. Then there are 800 cells left. We wait three weeks, during which some grow back. When you hit the next cycle, you have 900; the chemo kills another 150 and you're down to 750. We keep doing this, and hopefully we get you down to a small enough number that your immune system can fight them effectively for a time. We'll never be able to kill them all off, unfortunately, but we can get a lot. This is an effective way to help improve patients' symptoms. The cells don't all divide at the same time—one group divides now; another group divides the day after tomorrow. An interesting new approach, metronomic chemotherapy, involves giving very low dose chemotherapy continuously. This has been found to block angiogenesis, and has shown good results in mice and some people.

Many of the chemotherapy drugs produce the standard side effects—vomiting and bone marrow suppression, etc.—and when the drugs are combined they tend to be worse. For this reason, giving one chemotherapy drug at a time can significantly reduce side effects without sacrificing anything in a woman's overall survival. As I mentioned in Chapter 28, there are now terrific antinausea drugs that have almost eliminated this problem. Most drugs involve some hair loss. Several have a very low potential to cause leukemia down the road. Since you're dealing with metastatic breast cancer, though, that's not a reason to eliminate them. Most will decrease your white cell count. Attempts have been made to test the tumor cells against a variety of drugs in a test tube to predict the right drug or combination of drugs. Although it sounds like a great idea, it hasn't worked in practice as well as we would like.

While cancer cells can build up resistance to a particular drug, this is not always the case. Sometimes we'll treat metastatic cancer with a drug and get a response; the disease recurs and we use the same drug again, and again it works. It always amazes me how often we find a drug that doesn't work for the majority of patients but turns out to be exactly what one particular person needs. I had one patient with horrible lumps all over her chest. We treated her with just about everything, including experimental drugs, and nothing seemed to work. Then we went back and tried straight 5-fluorouracil, which usually works only modestly in breast cancer—and everything disappeared. So we sometimes can't predict what the right drug is for a particular person, and if you have metastatic disease, you need to keep that in mind. You may feel discouraged if particular drugs don't seem to be working, especially if they're the standard breast cancer drugs. But you never know when we'll hit on the one that will alleviate your symptoms.

Once we've found a drug that works, we generally continue it for a long time. How long a time is something doctors disagree on. There are two philosophies. One is that we'll get about as much response as we're going to get in about six months, so we should give the chemo for six months and then stop. The other philosophy is to give it continuously until the patient becomes resistant to it, and then move on to something else. There are arguments for both schools. Most of the studies suggest improved quality of life and better symptom control with continuous therapy, but again this might not be best for every woman. It's something you should discuss with your doctor and be clear about before you start treatments.

You would think that combining chemotherapy and hormonal therapy might work better than either one alone. But it doesn't work that way. In women with hormonally sensitive tumors, adding chemotherapy to hormones doesn't increase the disease-free or overall survival. However, chemotherapy works just as well after a hormonal therapy has been used.

Any woman with metastatic disease needs to investigate the available clinical trials. New drugs and/or new combinations of drugs and biologic agents are being tested all of the time and may be the best choice for someone with metastatic disease (see Chapter 32). It's important to talk with your doctor and get clear, precise information about what drugs are best for you, how long and in what sequence you can take them, and what their side effects are.

For a while it was popular to use high-dose chemotherapy with stem cell rescue to treat metastatic disease. As discussed in Chapter 23, we now have two randomized controlled studies examining its use in women with metastasis and neither has shown a benefit over standard chemotherapy. Although there's always a temptation to go for what appears to be the most aggressive therapy, in this case the benefit isn't worth the increased side effects for most women. I would not recommend a stem cell transplant outside of a clinical trial.

IMMUNOTHERAPY

We have always dreamt that somehow we could find something distinctive about the cancer cell and develop an antibody to it. We would then give the antibody, kill or control all of the cancer cells, and do little or no harm to the rest of the body. With Herceptin we have the first of that model. About 30 percent of women with breast cancer have too many copies of the Her-2 neu oncogene. This particular oncogene tells the cell to grow: harder, stronger, and longer. Herceptin is an antibody to that oncogene, which blocks it in its tracks.

In the spring of 1999 researchers reported on two multicenter trials of Herceptin in metastatic disease.[5] In one study women with metastatic disease and overexpression of Her-2 neu were given Herceptin. In the other study women with metastasis and Her-2 neu overexpression were randomized to get either Adriamycin or Taxol in conjunction with Herceptin or chemotherapy alone. One hundred and sixty-nine women got the antibody and chemotherapy and the same number got chemotherapy alone. The ones who received chemotherapy alone had a 32.6 percent response rate. This means that the tumor shrunk. On the other hand, remission, which gives the person some more time, isn't that rare. This response rate lasted five months. The women with chemotherapy and Her-2 neu antibodies had a greater response rate (52 percent) and it lasted longer (eight months). Most important, women's overall survival was improved by an average of five months with the addition of Herceptin. The study of Herceptin alone showed a 15 percent response rate, with the responses lasting an average of nine months.

That five-month improvement may not look impressive on the surface. But remember, these are people with the worst disease. It may suggest that, when it's ready to be used in earlier stages, it can have a more dramatic effect. Any woman with metastatic disease should have her tumor tested for Her-2 neu overexpression. If she is positive, Herceptin is a reasonable choice.

Other forms of immunotherapy such as vaccines are also being tested. Although we commonly think of a vaccine as prevention, such as the one used for polio or measles, it can also be used in treatment. These vaccines are made by training immune cells to hone in on a certain target found on breast cancer cells. It sounds great, but there are problems that have prevented it from being effective as of yet. For one thing, not every cancer cell is the same. This means that a vaccine against one element such as Her-2 will kill only the cells that express it, leaving the others behind. Vaccines for metastatic breast cancer are being tested in clinical trials and may be useful in the near future.

BISPHOSPHONATES

Most of the treatments we have discussed involve killing or controlling the cancer cell. The other approach is to alter the tissue that the cancer is trying to grow in. Pamidronate (Aredia) is a bisphosphonate, a drug that blocks the resorption (breakdown) of bone. It has been shown to be very effective in treating bone metastasis. When there is cancer in the bone there is an increase in the resorption, which is one of the reasons the bone gets weaker and often fractures. Several studies have shown that giving women pamidronate will decrease not only the resorption of the bone but also the number of new bone metastases that develop and the incidence of bone fractures.[6] In one study there was a suggestion that it also decreased other sites of metastatic disease, although this has not been confirmed yet by other studies. It certainly is worth taking for any woman with bone metastasis. Other bisphosphonates such as alendronate (Fosamax), commonly used to treat osteoporosis, have not been tried yet.

OTHER TREATMENTS

I've been talking about systemic therapies so far, but sometimes local treatment is called for. There are certain kinds of metastatic disease that respond best to local treatments because they're really local problems.

Radiation, for example, works best if the cancer has spread to your eye. Spinal cord involvement with impending bone fracture (in which your bone is so weakened that it is about to break)—another kind of local problem, where the one spot can be treated—also lends itself well to radiation. For impending bone fractures following spinal cord compression, surgical treatment is often needed to stabilize the bone prior to radiation.

Radiation for metastatic cancer is the same as for initial breast cancer, but the treatment is for a different purpose—to alleviate pain or other symptoms. It usually takes a couple of weeks before the pain noticeably lessens.

The timing is somewhat different too. There are usually 10 to 15 treatments, spread over two and a half to four weeks. A smaller dose of radiation is used. While a primary radiation treatment to your breast might use 6,000 centigrays of radiation over six and a half weeks, with 180 centigrays per treatment, the treatment for someone with, for example, bone metastasis in the hip might use 3,000 centigrays over 10 treatments of 300 centigrays each.

Surgery, as we mentioned in Chapter 32, is best if there is one spot in the lung or brain, for example, of a woman who has had a reasonably long interval between primary diagnosis and development of metastatic disease. If the cancer has recurred in several places, however, systemic treatment is best.

PAIN CONTROL

In terms of palliation—getting rid of symptoms so you feel better—treatments of the cancer itself aren't the only options. We've come an enormous way in pain control. So if, for example, you're in severe pain because of bone metastasis, we now have ways of putting a catheter in the space along the spinal cord and dripping continuous low-dose morphine in to get rid of all the pain. Administered this way, it won't affect your mind the way it would if administered systemically. This won't cure you, but in your last three or four months of life, when systemic therapy is no longer working, it can give you quality time and reduce or eliminate suffering. Yet there's a whole specialty now on pain control—that includes psychiatrists, anesthesiologists, and internists. We have acquired a lot of knowledge about chronic pain and how to deal with it. Anybody who has chronic pain because of metastatic cancer and isn't getting relief should ask to be referred to a pain unit. Sometimes oncologists and people who work on cancer are so focused on treating and curing the disease that they forget about these ancillary things that can make an enormous difference in a patient's life. So ask to see a pain specialist; it may mean having to travel to the local medical school, but it can make a big difference to you.

EXPERIMENTAL TREATMENTS

Throughout this book I've been encouraging women to participate in phase three clinical trials (see Chapters 12 and 32)—trials of drugs or treatments that have been tested in earlier phases and shown not to harm the patient. There is a trickier area to consider with metastatic cancer, and that is phase one or two trials. These are much earlier stages in the testing of a drug, designed to determine first the toxicity of a possibly useful drug, and then whether it works.

Since you now know that, unlike in the case of your first diagnosis, traditional treatments offer only a very slim chance of cure, an experimental treatment may be worth considering. Generally there is no harm in trying an innovative new therapy and postponing treatment with other standard therapies.

When is the best time to become involved in an experimental trial? Classically, people do it when nothing else has helped and they've run out of options. The problem is that by the time you run out of options you're least likely to be able to respond to the new treatment: you have no resources left. So the best time may be when you have been diagnosed with metastatic disease but are feeling well. You have a chest x ray or bone scan that shows a lesion but you actually have modest symptoms. At this stage, there's no rush to use chemotherapy or hormonal therapy since, as we said earlier, there's no evidence that treating with chemo earlier will give you better survival odds than waiting until you have symptoms; however, it is a good time to try something experimental. You have an opportunity to see if it works, and then if it doesn't you can still get the usual chemotherapy if symptoms worsen.

These kinds of treatments will not be routinely offered by your doctor, unless it's a doctor who is working on the experiments. The best way to find out about them is to go to your local cancer center and see what they're involved in. You can also call the Physician Data Query (PDQ) at the National Cancer Institute (1–800–4-CANCER), which is a computerized searching system. They will print out for you a list of every clinical trial that you're eligible for, either in your own geographical area or in the whole United States if you're willing and able to travel, or you can check cancertrials.nci.nih.gov or clinical trials.gov on the Internet.

I think this is really worthwhile. It's a gamble, but sometimes the gamble pays off. For example, the women who first participated in the tests for docetaxel or Taxol had a remarkable response lasting 18 months to two years.

There are exciting new experiments being worked on for metastatic disease. One example is antiangiogenesis drugs. Angiogenesis is the cancer's attempt to develop new blood vessels to support its growth. With drugs that block this function, the cancer theoretically will not be able to get enough nourishment from its inadequate blood vessels and will die. Clinical trials are going on with this category of drugs.

The best quality of life is not having any symptoms from your cancer. But only you can decide what price in toxicity you are willing to pay. Some women want to try everything new and others don't. Don't let yourself be pushed by your doctor or family. Decide in your own heart what the best approach is for you.

34

The Politics of Breast Cancer

Breast cancer has certainly come out of the closet. There are three-day walks, mountain climbs, Races for the Cure, bike rides, art exhibits, lobby days, gala fund-raisers, and pink ribbons. Few women are embarrassed to admit they have had breast cancer and all are aware of the advances we have made. With all this publicity and public support it's easy to forget that this awareness is a relatively new phenomenon. The first edition of this book made no mention of the politics of the disease: there were none. The second edition chronicled its birth. And some day soon we will be able to rest on our laurels because politics will not be necessary. Until that day I think it is very important that we continue to remember and record our recent history. For those of you who have been a part of it—read it with pride. For those who are just joining this sisterhood—know that you stand with many strong women before you.

The politics of breast cancer had its forerunners 50 years ago. In 1952 the American Cancer Society started the Reach to Recovery program. This was a group of women helping women: survivors of breast cancer helping newly diagnosed women. Members of Reach to Recovery, all of whom had had mastectomies, would visit a patient in the hospital and reassure her that there was life after mastectomy. They were, and continue to be, a wonderful resource for women with breast cancer.

From there, support groups for women with breast cancer evolved. Women sat together and talked about their experiences and their feelings. It was tremendously helpful for these people to learn they were not alone. Others shared their feelings about their disease, which was shrouded in so much mystery and fear.

All this underlined the fact that there was little psychosocial support from the medical profession—you had to get it from somewhere else. And since it continued to be something hidden from public view, there still remained an aura of something shameful and disreputable about it.

The next big step came in the 1970s when Shirley Temple Black, Betty Ford, and Happy Rockefeller told the world they had breast cancer. Their openness began to create an environment in which breast cancer could be looked at as a dangerous disease that needed to be addressed by public institutions, rather than a private and shameful secret. There was a dramatic increase in the number of women in America who got mammograms, and in the number of breast cancers diagnosed.

Those were the days of the one-step procedure. You'd go in for the

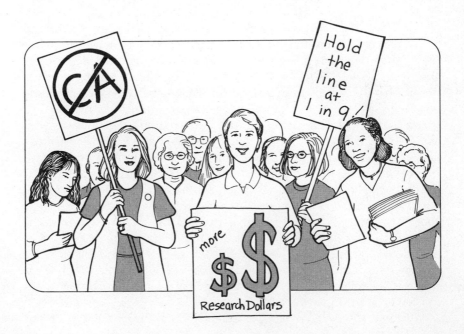

biopsy; it would be done under general anesthetic; and, if the lump was positive, your breast would be immediately removed.

In 1977 Rose Kushner, a writer with breast cancer, wrote a terribly important book entitled *Why Me?* It ushered in the two-step procedure. Kushner saw no reason for a woman to have to decide whether to have a mastectomy before she even knew whether she had breast cancer. She argued passionately that it was important for the woman to have her biopsy, learn if she had cancer, and then, if she did, decide what avenue to pursue. Doctors were still working on the erroneous assumption that time was everything: if they didn't get the cancer out the instant they found it, it would spread and kill the patient. Kushner had done enough research to realize that wasn't the case—that a few weeks between diagnosis and treatment wouldn't do any medical harm, and would do a great deal of emotional good. She pushed for the two-step procedure, and her book influenced large numbers of women to demand it for themselves.

Another force on the horizon at that time was Nancy Brinker. Brinker's sister, Susan G. Komen, was diagnosed with breast cancer in 1977 and died in 1980. In 1983 Brinker founded the Susan G. Komen Breast Cancer Foundation, which is based in Dallas, Texas. Ironically, she herself got breast cancer soon afterwards. Since the mid-1980s they've been working to raise money for research and for making mammograms available to more women. They organize the yearly Race for the Cure, which takes place in a number of cities.

For a long time that was pretty much all that was going on around breast cancer. Then in the late 1980s, almost spontaneously in different parts of the country, a number of political women's cancer groups sprang up. One was in the Boston area, started by a patient of mine, Susan Shapiro, who had breast cancer. When she was diagnosed she began to search for anyone working on the political issues around women and cancer, and she couldn't find anything. Yet she was passionately convinced that there were political implications to cancer, and particularly to women's cancers. She wrote an article in the feminist newspaper *Sojourner,* called "Cancer as a Feminist Issue," and at the end of it she announced a meeting at the Cambridge Women's Center. A lot of women showed up, women who had been as frustrated as she by the lack of political response to their disease. They formed the Women's Community Cancer Project. Their scope was fairly broad. It included all cancers that women got and also the role of women as caregivers for children, spouses, and parents with cancer. Inevitably, much of the focus was on breast cancer. Shapiro died in January 1990, but the project continues to flourish.

At about the same time the Women's Community Cancer Project was beginning, the Women's Cancer Resource Center in Oakland, California, Breast Cancer Action in the bay area, and the Mary-Helen Mautner Project for Lesbians with Cancer in Washington, D.C., got under way. All of these groups were aware of the work the AIDS movement had been doing. For the first time we were seeing people with a killer disease aggressively demanding more money for research, changes in insurance bias, and job protection. Women with breast cancer took note of that—particularly those women who had been part of the feminist movement. They were geared, as were the gay activists with AIDS, to the idea of identifying oppression and confronting it politically.

At the time these groups were emerging, I was finishing work on the first edition of this book. As I went on my book tour, talking with women, I began to realize how deep women's anger was, and how ready they were to do something. The key moment for me was in Salt Lake City in June 1990, when I gave a talk for 600 women. It was the middle of the afternoon, during the week, and the audience was mostly older women. It was a pretty long talk, and at the end I said, "We don't know the answers, and I don't know what we have to do to make President Bush wake up and do something about breast cancer. Maybe we should march topless to the White House." I was making a wisecrack, hoping to end a somber talk with a little lightness.

I got a great response, and afterwards women came up to me asking when the march was, how they could sign up for it, and what they could do to help organize it. I realized that, throughout the country, this issue touched all kinds of women, and that they were all fed up with the fact that this virtual epidemic was being ignored. I saw that it wasn't just in the big centers like San Francisco and Boston and Washington, D.C., where I'd have expected to see political movements springing up. It was everywhere—everywhere women were ready to fight for attention to breast cancer.

I felt that we needed to have some sort of national organization to give these women the hook they needed to begin organizing. I spoke to Susan Hester of the Mautner Project, Amy Langer of NABCO (the National Coalition of Breast Cancer Organizations), and Nancy Brinker of the Komen Foundation about the idea. We all were enthusiastic, and the result was a planning meeting. The initial groups involved included Y-ME (Y-ME National Breast Cancer Organization), the Women's Community Cancer Project, Breast Cancer Action, Cancer Care, and Canact from New York. Then we called an open meeting, to be held in Washington, and wrote to every women's group we knew of.

We had no idea who'd show up. On the day of the meeting the room was packed. There were representatives from all kinds of groups; the American Cancer Society and the American Jewish Congress were there. So was the Human Rights Campaign Fund, a big gay and lesbian group. There were members of breast cancer support groups from all around the country—such as Arm in Arm from Baltimore, the Linda Creed group from Philadelphia, and Share from New York. Overall there were about 100 or so individuals representing 75 organizations. We were overwhelmed, and we started the National Breast Cancer Coalition on the spot. Out of that meeting came the first Board of the Coalition.

Amy Langer of NABCO chaired the initial meetings until bylaws and officers could be chosen. A year later Fran Visco, a lawyer from Philadelphia who had had breast cancer in her late 30s, became the first elected president, and remains the president today. Our first action, in the fall of 1991, was a project we called "Do the Write Thing." We wanted to collect and deliver to Washington 175,000 letters, representing the 175,000 women who would be diagnosed with breast cancer that year, and we wanted the number of letters from each state to match the number of women in that state who would get breast cancer. We managed to identify groups in each state who could work with us. In October we ended up with 600,000 letters—it was an enormous response. We delivered them to the White House. The guards just stood there; nobody would help us lift the boxes. All these women who'd had mastectomies were lifting heavy boxes of letters onto the conveyer belt.

We were all certain that the letters would just be dumped into the shredder. We were afraid that our first action had been a flop. But in reality, we had succeeded in a number of ways. For one thing, we had organized in such a way that we had a group in every state. That meant a large and potentially powerful organization. For another, even if the White House ignored us, the members of Congress didn't. When we started lobbying for increased research money they granted us $43 million more, raising the 1993 appropriation to $132 million. That was a small triumph.

We held hearings to determine how much research money was really needed, and it was one of the first times scientists and activists interested in breast cancer had met together. This created an interesting coalition. As a result of the hearings we decided we needed $433 million for breast cancer research. The total budget at the time was $93 million. So we started lobbying for $300 million more, armed with our report based on the scientists' testimony.

At first the reaction was overwhelmingly negative. Everybody in Congress kept saying there was no money and it would be impossible to come up with anything like another $300 million. But we kept at it, and when the politicians told us there wasn't any more money, we said, "Well, you found money for the Savings and Loan bailout. You found money for the Gulf War. We think you can find this money too, if you really decide it's important that women are dying." We testified at the Senate, and at the House. We lobbied, we sent faxes, and we called. But despite support from many Congress members we couldn't figure out how to get enough money.

Then Senator Tom Harkin noticed that, amazingly, in the past there actually had been some money for breast cancer in the Defense Department—$25 million spent on mammogram machines for the army. At our urging he decided to try and increase that to $210 million, which, added to an increase in the NIH funding, would bring the total to $300 million.

The Defense Department people were so worried that the firewall between the domestic budget and the defense budget might be breached that they agreed to have a breast cancer research program within the Department of Defense.

So there was $210 million in the Department of Defense budget and the extra $100 million in the NCI budget. That was the $300 million more we had gone after. Against all odds, we had succeeded. Part of it was being in the right place at the right time. But most of it was the enormous amount of work all the women in the coalition and around the country had put in. Overnight we had an enormous amount of clout and were well recognized for a group that had just begun.

We were ready to move on to our next step. It was one thing to raise money, but we wanted to have a say in how it was spent. We wanted women from our groups, women with breast cancer, to be involved in the decision-making panels on review boards for grants, on the National Cancer Advisory Board, and in all the decision making. We started lobbying for that, and our next major project was to deliver 2.6 million signatures to the White House in October 1993 to represent the 2.6 million women living with breast cancer at the time—1.6 million who knew they had breast cancer, and 1 million who were yet to be diagnosed. We mobilized around the country collecting signatures, and we delivered our 2.6 million signatures to President Clinton on October 18. As a measure of how far we'd come from October 1991, this time we were welcomed in the East Room, where Fran Visco and I shared the stage with both Hillary and Bill Clinton, along with Secretary of Health and Human Services Donna Shalala. The room was filled with 200 of our people. It was an awesome moment.

And President Clinton followed up. In December we had a meeting to set national strategy—a meeting of activists, politicians, scientists, doctors, laypeople, and businesspeople. We came up with a National Action Plan. In each one of the subgroups working on this plan there was one of our activist members. We were at the table and we were changing the policy of business as usual around breast cancer.

Being with the scientists, talking and working with them, the activists were able to learn that the answers aren't always easy, that scientists have to work months and years to come up with one useful discovery. The scientists saw that the activists weren't shrill, uninformed troublemakers but intelligent, concerned people fighting to save their own and others' lives.

One of the reasons we wanted the money from the Department of Defense was to attract new people, to get researchers working on new aspects of breast cancer. And it worked. When the $210 million was made available by the Department of Defense, they got 2,400 grant applications. Many of these were from people who had never done breast cancer research before.

Our goals remain the same. We want access for all women to high-quality screening and treatment for breast cancer. In the year 2000 this means we are lobbying to make sure that underserved women who are diagnosed with breast cancer through free mammograms provided by the Center for Disease Control program will also have access to treatment. We want influence for women with breast cancer. Through Project LEAD, a program that brings scientists together for a weekend to teach advocates the basics of breast cancer research, we are currently training activists to be effective advocates and to contribute when they get a seat at the table. And we are fighting for research into the cause of breast cancer, how to prevent it and how to cure it. The increase in environmental research as well as in basic research is in part in response to our efforts. We want to attract more basic research, rather than focus all our energies on how to treat existing disease. We need both, of course, but ultimately the goal is to stop the cancer before a woman gets it in the first place.

I've learned through this that you really can affect how the government acts. A small group of committed people can do a lot. So few people let their feelings be known that the people who do it, and who do it vociferously, get an undue amount of power. We didn't have any money—not like the gun lobby or the tobacco industry. But we were organized.

Our movement continues to grow. Many of the women in the coalition have never been involved in political action before. Now they find themselves working side by side with the baby boomers who marched in the '60s and learned the value of political protest and who now are confronting breast cancer, realizing that, like civil rights and war resistance and the early women's movement issues, breast cancer research needs to be fought for.

The current breast cancer political movement is moving into a new phase. It's becoming international. The National Breast Cancer Coalition has held two international conferences in Brussels and is helping nascent politic groups get started in Eastern Europe and Africa. The Komen Foundation has held Races for the Cure in Italy, Germany, and Argentina and is spreading its message of empowerment. Women all over the world are learning that this is more than a personal issue.

The issues that are being addressed have broadened as well. The NBCC is involved in setting the standards for quality breast care; and the Komen Foundation has funded a large project with the American Society for Clinical Oncology to identify the level of care that is currently being delivered. All of the political groups have taken up the cause of clinical trial enrollment and are helping to educate women about the benefits of participating in trials. Breast cancer politics have matured beyond pink ribbons and shower cards.

The demand for prevention and research, however, has remained core to our work. This is an issue we can all agree on and one we all have to fight for. We can't afford to be good girls any longer. We can't let this disease pass on to another generation. Our lives and the lives of our daughters depend on it.

As I continue to speak around the country, I always finish my talks with an anecdote about my daughter, Katie. Although she is no longer four years old and her future aspirations have changed, this story has become a symbol to many women of what this movement is all about.

In 1993, at the Los Angeles Breast Cancer Coalition "War Mammorial," created by artist Melanie Winter, 1,300 white plastic casts of women's torsos were set on a hill. From a distance they looked like graves, but up close they showed the variety of women's bodies: large breasts, small breasts, some with mastectomies, and some with implants. Katie was walking around trying to figure out which breasts she wanted when she grew up. Then she turned serious.

"Are these the graves of women with breast cancer?" she asked.

"No, these women are all alive," I told her. "But some women do die from breast cancer."

"Well, you're trying to stop that, aren't you, Mommy?"

"Yes, Katie, I would like to stop breast cancer before you grow up."

She thought about that a minute. "What if you die first?" she asked.

"I'd like to stop breast cancer before I die," I replied.

She thought again, then turned to me and said, "If there is breast cancer left after you die it's a big problem. Because I'm not going to be a breast surgeon. I'm going to be a ballerina."

Well, Katie doesn't have to worry—she can go ahead and be a ballerina, or anything else she wants to be. And she won't be haunted, as so many women are now, by the fear of getting breast cancer. As long as we keep fighting, the discoveries we're making, buttressed by the political activism that lets the scientists and the government know we won't let up until we've ended breast cancer, will bring about her wish. That's what keeps me going. Twenty years from now, a comfortable retiree with no more breast cancer to worry about, I can sit in the audience waiting for the curtain to rise, and watch my beautiful, healthy daughter pirouette across the stage.

APPENDICES

A

Drugs Used for Systemic Treatment of Breast Cancer

This list of drugs is not meant to be exhaustive. Check with your oncologist about your specific drugs. Unusual signs and symptoms should be reported to your doctor immediately.

I. CHEMOTHERAPY

capecitabine (Xeloda)   oral
   Use: for metastatic disease resistant to anthracyclines and Taxol
   Method of action: converted to 5-FU in body; prevents DNA and RNA synthesis
   Adverse effects: nausea, diarrhea, tingling hands and feet, fatigue, anemia, reduced immunity

cyclophosphamide (Cytoxan)   IV or oral
   Use: primary therapy and metastatic disease
   Method of action: interferes with tumor cell growth

Adverse effects: temporary or permanent infertility, hair loss, cystitis, immune suppression

docetaxel (Taxotere)   IV
   Use: locally advanced or metastatic disease after failure of first treatment
   Method of action: inhibits cell division
   Adverse effects: fluid retention, suppressed immunity, hair loss, loss of feeling in hands and feet

doxorubicin (Adriamycin, Rubex) IV
    Use: primary therapy and metastatic disease
    Method of action: inhibits DNA synthesis
    Adverse effects: nausea, hair loss, immune suppression, may cause heart damage, increased risk of leukemia

epirubicin (Ellence) IV
    Use: primary therapy and metastatic disease
    Method of action: inhibits DNA synthesis
    Adverse effects: nausea, hair loss, immune suppression, may be less toxic to heart than doxorubicin, increased risk of leukemia

etoposide (VePesid) oral
    Use: metastatic disease
    Method of action: stops cell division
    Adverse effects: immune suppression, nausea, diarrhea

5-Fluorouracil (5-FU) IV
    Use: primary and metastatic disease
    Method of action: prevents DNA and RNA synthesis
    Adverse effects: nausea, diarrhea, tingling hands and feet, fatigue, anemia, reduced immunity, less hair loss than other drugs

methotrexate IV
    Use: primary and metastatic disease
    Method of action: interferes with DNA synthesis and repair
    Adverse effects: immune suppression, nausea, gastrointestinal distress, flu-like symptoms

mitoxantrone (Novantrone) IV
    Use: metastatic disease; may be less effective than doxorubicin and epirubicin
    Method of action: inhibits DNA synthesis
    Adverse effects: nausea, hair loss, immune suppression, may cause heart damage, increased risk of leukemia

mitomycin C (Mutamycin) IV
    Use: metastatic disease
    Method of action: inhibits DNA synthesis
    Adverse effects: nausea, hair loss, immune suppression, may cause heart damage, increased risk of leukemia

paclitaxel (Taxol) IV
    Use: metastatic disease
    Method of action: inhibits cell division
    Adverse effects: fluid retention, suppressed immunity, hair loss, loss of feeling in hands, feet

trastuzumab (Herceptin) IV
    Use: metastatic disease in patients who overexpress HER2 neu
    Method of action: blocks HER2, a growth factor receptor, to inhibit tumor cell growth
    Adverse effects: anemia, immune suppression, flulike symptoms

vinblastine (Velban) IV
    Use: metastatic disease
    Method of action: inhibits cell division
    Adverse effects: nausea, diarrhea, tingling hands and feet, fatigue, anemia, reduced immunity

vinorelbine (Navelbine) IV
    Use: metastatic disease
    Method of action: inhibits cell division
    Adverse effects: Nausea, diarrhea, tingling hands and feet, fatigue, anemia, reduced immunity

II. HORMONAL THERAPY

anastrozole (Arimidex)   oral
Use: for advanced breast cancer in postmenopausal women whose disease has progressed after tamoxifen treatment
Method of action: inhibits production of aromatase—an enzyme that converts precursor hormones to estrogen in the breast
Adverse effects: hot flashes, nausea, diarrhea

exemestrone (Aromasin)   oral
Use: for advanced breast cancer in postmenopausal women with estrogen receptor positive tumors
Method of action: inactivates aromatase
Adverse effects: hot flashes, nausea, fatigue

goserelin (Zoladex) IV
Use: advanced breast cancer, primarily in premenopausal women
Method of action: blocks release of luteinizing hormone and follicle stimulating hormone to shut down ovaries
Adverse effects: hot flashes, vaginal dryness

letrozole (Femara)   oral
Use: for advanced breast cancer in postmenopausal women with estrogen receptor positive tumors
Method of action: non-steroidal aromatase inhibitor which blocks production of estrogen
Adverse effects: nausea, vomiting, fatigue

megestrol acetate (Megace)   oral
Use: Advanced breast cancer in women whose disease has progressed after tamoxifen treatment
Method of action: uncertain; may prevent estrogen from reaching tumor
Schedule: 40-mg tablet, 4 times a day
Adverse effects: weight gain, PMS-like effects, increased risk of blood clots

tamoxifen (Nolvadex)   oral
Use: breast-cancer prevention and treatment of primary and metastatic disease
Method of action: selective estrogen receptor modulator (SERM) that blocks estrogen in breast but not in uterus
Adverse effects: hot flashes, vaginal dryness, increased risk of blood clots, endometrial cancer

toremifene citrate (Fareston)   oral
Use: metastatic disease in postmenopausal women with ER-positive tumors
Method of action: selective estrogen receptor modulator (SERM) that blocks estrogen in breast
Adverse effects: hot flashes, vaginal dryness, increased risk of blood clots; risk of endometrial cancer still unknown

B

Resources, References, and Additional Reading

The most up to date resource is my website, www.SusanLoveMD.com. For those of you who are not yet on the Internet I have provided this appendix. It has been culled from my own experience as well as from many other sources and is by no means exhaustive. Although I believe each listing is helpful, I am not personally familiar with every one and welcome feedback, comments, and additions that readers may have. These can be sent to PO Box 846, Pacific Palisades, California 90272. Much of the appendix is reprinted with permission from, and thanks to, the annual resource guide published by the National Alliance of Breast Cancer Organizations (NABCO).

BREASTFEEDING

La Leche League International, 1400 N. Meacham Road, Schaumburg, IL 60173-4048. (847) 519-7730 or www.lalecheleague.org. *Best source of support and information about breast feeding.*

www.breastfeeding.com *is a comprehensive website for information, support, national list of lactation counselors and shopping.*

Margot Edwards, "A Working Mother Can Breastfeed When . . . " Penny-press Inc. 1100 23rd Ave. East, Seattle, WA 98112.

Marsha Walker, Jeanne Watson Driscoll, "Expressing, Storing and Transporting Breastmilk." Pamphlet available from Lactation Associates, Educators and Consultants to Health Care Professionals, 254 Conant Road, Weston, MA 02193. (617) 893-3553.

La Leche League International, *The Womanly Art of Breastfeeding* third edition (New York: New American Library, 1991). *A very supportive book.*

Ruth Lawrence, *Breastfeeding: A Guide for the Medical Profession,* fifth edition (St. Louis: Mosby 1998). *Written by a professor of pediatrics, this is a good source of scientific information as well as practical advice about breastfeeding.*

PLASTIC SURGERY

American Society of Plastic and Reconstructive Surgeons, 444 East Algonquin Road, Arlington Heights, IL 60005. (312) 228-9900 or (800) 635-0635 (referral message tape). *Will provide written information and mail a list of certified reconstructive surgeons by geographical area after caller provides details on above (800) message tape.*

Command Trust Network, Inc. *The Breast Implant Information Network.* For information, call (800) 887-6828; for attorney settlement information, call (513) 651-9770. *A network established to provide assistance and information to women with or considering implants.*

"Breast Implants: An Information Update" (US Food and Drug Administration). *Information on silicone and saline implants for reconstruction and augmentation.* Call (800) 532-4440 or www.fda.gov/oca/breastimplants/bitac.html

"Silicone Breast Implants: Why has Science been Ignored?" (1996) Prepared for American Council on Science and Health by Michael Fumento, order from ACSH, 1995 Broadway, 2nd floor, New York, NY 10023-5860. (212) 362-7044.

Marcia Angell, *Science on Trial: The Clash of Medical Evidence and the Law in the Breast Implant Case.* (New York: Norton, 1996). Examines litigation and scientific studies following 1992 FDA ban on silicone implants.

Karen Berger and John Bostwick, *What Women Want to Know about Breast Implants.* (St. Louis: Quality Medical Pub, 1998). (800) 348-7808. *Highlights from their larger book: A Woman's Decision: Breast Care, Treatment & Reconstruction* (St. Martin's Press,1998). *Very good on reconstruction.*

Nancy Bruning, *Breast Implants: Everything You Need to Know* (Alameda, CA: Hunter House, 1995). Paperback. *Valuable resource for any woman considering breast implants or for those who already have implants.*

Amy J. Goldrich, *Command Trust Network's Introduction to the Legal System* (1992). Available for $18 from Command Trust Network, 256 South Linden Drive, Beverly Hills, CA 90212. (310) 556-1738. *Reference booklet for women with implants who are pursuing lawsuits against implant manufacturers.*

John B. Tebbets. *The Best Breast: The Ultimate, Discriminating Woman's Guide to Breast Augmentation* (CosmetXpertise, 1999). Hardcover.

COMMON PROBLEMS OF THE BREAST

American College of Surgeons, 55 East Erie Street, Chicago, IL 60611. (312) 664-4050. *Will provide names of certified surgeons specializing in breast surgery by geographical area.*

"Questions and Answers about Breast Calcifications"(P199, 1995). Fact sheet, NCI. (800) 4-CANCER.

"Understanding Breast Changes: A Health Guide for All Women" (P051, 1998). Booklet from NCI. (800) 4-CANCER.*Explains how to evaluate breast lumps and other normal breast changes that often occur and are confused with breast cancer. It is for all asymptomatic women.*

"Stereotactic core needle biopsy of the breast" (Fisher Imaging Corp, 1993). *Video describes the procedure.* 28 minutes. Single copies free from marketing department (800) 825-8257.

"When you can't feel it—needle localization and breast biopsy" (Beth Israel Medical Center, NY, 1991). *Video describes the procedure.* 16 minutes, $15. To order, call (212) 420-2069.

Kerry A. McGuinn, *The Informed Woman's Guide to Breast Health* (Palo Alto: Bull Publishing, 1992). Paperback. *A thorough review of breast lumps and benign conditions.*

Kirby I. Bland, Edward M. Copeland (Eds.), *The Breast: Comprehensive Management of Benign and Malignant Diseases* (WB Saunders, 1998). *Textbook.*

Cushman Haagensen, (Ed.), *Diseases of the Breast* third edition (Philadelphia: Saunders 1986). *This textbook is the ultimate reference for benign breast tumors. However, his approach to breast cancer is dated.*

Judy C. Kneece, RN, OCN, *Solving the Mystery of Breast Pain* (EduCare Publishing, 1996). $7.95 plus $4.50 shipping. *This handbook provides straightforward answers to many questions about breast pain.* EduCare Publishing, P.O. Box 280305, Columbia, SC 29228. (800) 849-9271.

Judy C. Kneece, *Solving the Mystery of Breast Discharge* (EduCare Publishing, 1996) $7.95 plus $4.50 shipping. *This handbook provides straightforward answers to many questions about breast discharge.* EduCare Publishing, P.O. Box 280305, Columbia, SC 29228. (800) 849-9271.

GENETICS, RISKS, PREVENTION, AND DETECTION OF BREAST CANCER

Genetics, Risk, and Prevention

The Family Cancer Risk Counseling and Genetic Testing Directory (found on CancerNet, NCI's website: http://cancernet.nci.nih.gov/wwwprot/genetic/genesrch.shtml). *Offers a listing of cancer risk counseling resources and genetic testing providers across the country. The Directory is searchable by name, city, state, country, and type of cancer or cancer gene.*

FORCE (www.facingourrisk.org). *Groups organized around women who are at high risk for breast and ovarian cancer especially those with BRCA1 or 2.*

National Society of Genetic Counselors (www.nsgc.org). *To find a genetic counselor to help you understand your risks and explore your options.*

The Alliance of Genetic Support Groups (www.geneticalliance.org).

The National Cancer Institute's Breast Cancer Risk Assessment Tool. *The "Risk Disk" (September 1998) is free from the NCI and serves as an interactive patient education tool to help assess an individual's risk of developing breast cancer.* NCI, (800) 4-CANCER.

National Women's Health Network, "Hearts, Bones, Hot Flashes and Hormones" (2000). $1. National Women's Health Network, 514 10th St NW Suite 400, Washington, DC 20004. (202) 347-1140. *An excellent review of the current state of knowledge about postmenopausal hormone therapy.*

Committee on the Relationship Between Oral Contraceptives and Breast Cancer, Institute of Medicine, "Oral Contraceptives and Breast Cancer" (Washington, DC: National Academy Press, 1991).

"Cancer and Genetics: Answering Your Patients' Questions." *Booklet produced jointly by the American Cancer Society and PRR, Inc which answers patients' questions about inherited cancer syndromes, identifies individuals and families that may be at higher than average risk due to alterations in cancer susceptibility genes, and familiarizes the reader with the social and clinical implications of decisions to seek genetic testing.* American Cancer Society. (800) ACS-2345.

"Cancer Facts Questions and Answers: The Breast Cancer Prevention Trial" (1998). *This fact sheet answers common questions about The Breast Cancer Prevention Trial including its design, results and significance for women.* Available at no charge from the National Cancer Institute. (800) 4-CANCER.

"DES Exposure: Questions and Answers for Mothers, Daughters and Sons" (1990). DES Action, Oakland, CA 94612. (800) DES-9288. *Authoritative booklet.* 20 pages, $2.50. *They also have free literature on DES.*

"Diet Nutrition and Cancer Prevention: A Guide to Food Choices" (87–2878) National Cancer Institute. *This booklet describes what is known about diet nutrition and cancer prevention.*

"Understanding Breast Changes: A Health Guide for All Women." (97–3536, 1997). *Booklet explains various type of breast changes that women experience and outlines methods that doctors use to distinguish between benign changes and cancer.* NCI's CIS, (800) 4-CANCER.

"Understanding Gene Testing" (97–3905, 1997). *This easy-to-understand guide provides readers with basic information and addresses issues raised when considering testing under managed care.* 30 pages. Order from NCI's CIS, (800) 4-CANCER.

"Understanding Genetics of Breast Cancer for Jewish Women." (American Jewish Congress and Hadassah, 1997). *As follow-up to the First Leadership Conference on Jewish Women's Health Issues, this brochure was compiled to answer questions about hereditary risk of breast cancer and deciding if genetic testing is right for you.* Available by calling the Hadassah Health Education Department, (212) 303-80094.

"Genetic Testing for Cancer Risk: It's Your Choice" (National Action Plan on Breast Cancer). *Hosted by Cokie Roberts, this video gives an overview of the risks and benefits of being tested for genetic susceptibility to breast and ovarian cancer.* Companion brochure available. 14 minutes. A free copy of the tape can be obtained from NCI, (800) 4-CANCER.

"Testing for Hereditary Risk of Breast and Ovarian Cancer—Is it right for you?" (MY8447, Myriad Genetics 1999) a video from Myriad, a for-profit company marketing gene testing, designed to answer questions and suggest topics to be discussed with a physician or counselor. Order by calling (800) 469-7423 or visit www.myriad.com.

Nancy C. Baker, *Relative Risk: Living with a Family History of Breast Cancer* (New York: Viking, 1991). *Discusses risk factors as well as women's reactions to being at "increased risk."*

Kevin Davies and Michael White, *Breakthrough: The Race to Find the Breast Cancer Gene* (New York: John Wiley, 1996). *A history of the discovery of the BRCA1 gene, including information on current treatments and future research directions.*

Patricia T. Kelly, *Assessing Your True Risk of Breast Cancer* (New York: Henry Holt, 2000). *Her latest book tells you how to calculate your own personal risk.*

M. Margaret Kemeny and Paula Dranov, *Breast Cancer and Ovarian Cancer: Beating the Odds* (Reading, MA: Addison-Wesley, 1992). *Reviews risk factors.*

Earl Mindell, *Earl Mindell's Vitamin Bible* (New York: Warner, 1994).

Prevention Magazine (Ed.), *The Complete Book of Cancer Prevention: Foods, Lifestyle and Medical Care to Keep You Healthy.*

Carol Rinzler, *Estrogen and Breast Cancer: A Warning to Women.* (Order from BCA Bookstore, 1280 Columbus Avenue, Suite 204, San Francisco, CA 94133.)

Basil Stoll (Ed.), *Reducing Breast Cancer Risk in Women* (Norwell, MA: Kluwer Academic Publishers, 1995). *Review of what is currently known about prevention, limited as it is.*

Laurie Tarkan, *My Mother's Breast; Daughters Face their Mothers' Cancer* (Taylor Publishing, 1999). Paperback.

Detection

Agency for Health Care Policy and Research, "Quality Determinants of Mammography". *Guidelines for consumers and health care professionals on what is necessary for the best possible test.* For a copy of the consumer or professional guidelines, call (800) 358-9295.

National Consortium of Breast Centers, c/o Barbara Rabinowitz, RN, MSW, ACSW, Comprehensive Breast Center, Robert Wood Johnson Medical School , One Robert Wood Johnson Place, CN19, New Brunswick, NJ 08903-0019. *Will send you a list of breast centers throughout the country registered with them. Many are diagnostic only and others are involved in both diagnosis and treatment.*

"The Older You Get, The More You Need a Mammogram" (5020, 1993). (800) ACS-2345.

"Questions and Answers About Choosing a Mammography Facility" (94–3228, 1994). This four-page brochure should accompany "Are You Age 50 or Over? A Mammogram Could Save Your Life" from NCI. (800) 4-CANCER.

CANCER IN GENERAL

American Cancer Society, (800) ACS-2345 or www.cancer.org. *National toll-free hotline provides information on all forms of cancer, and referrals for the ACS-sponsored "Reach to Recovery" program.*

AMC Cancer Research Center's Cancer Information Line, 1600 Pierce St, Denver CO 80214. (800) 525-3777. *Professional cancer counselors provide answers to questions about cancer, support and advice and will mail instructive free publications upon request. Equipped for deaf and hearing impaired callers.*

Cancer Information Service of the National Cancer Institute (www.nci.nih.gov). This information service can be reached toll-free at (800) 4-CANCER. *They give information and direction through their national and regional network on all aspects of cancer. Spanish-speaking staff members are available on request.*

Cancer Information Service of the Canadian Cancer Society. *Information service in English and French.* For calls from Canada only (888) 939-3333, or www.cancer.ca

Cancer Care, Inc. (800) 813-HOPE or www.cancercare.org. *Support services, education, information, referrals and financial assistance.*

Vital Options TeleSupport Cancer Network, the GroupRoom Radio Talk Show, PO Box 19233, Encino CA 91416-9233. (818) 788-5225. *A weekly syndicated call-in cancer talk show linking callers with other patients, long-term survivors, family members, physicians, researchers and therapists experienced in working with cancer issues.*

BREAST CANCER IN GENERAL

Community Breast Health Project (www.med.Stanford.EDU:80/CBHP). *One of the first community breast cancer resource centers. Information from Ellen Mahoney, MD (founder and breast surgeon).*

Department of Defense Decision Guide (www.bcdg.org). *An interactive guide through the decisions a newly diagnosed woman needs to make.*

Faces of Hope (www.facesofhope.net). *Nationally recognized not-for-profit educational breast cancer program that focuses on the importance of early detection and prevention. The program features a portable photo exhibit of breast cancer survivors.*

ibreast (www.ibreast.com). Website of Dr. Marisa Weiss, radiation oncologist, and author of *Living Beyond Breast Cancer.*

Mothers Supporting Daughters with Breast Cancer (www.mothersdaughters.org). *MSDBC is a national nonprofit organization co-founded by a mother and her daughter. The support services provided by this organization are designed to help mothers who have daughters battling breast cancer.*

National Action Plan on Breast Cancer (www.napbc.org): *The National Action Plan is a public private partnership which sprung out of the demands of advocates.*

SusanLoveMD.com (www.susanlovemd.com). *Provides breast cancer content, personal guidance, chats and community for baby boomer women.*

MAMM Magazine *covers issues helpful to women who have been diagnosed with breast and reproductive cancer, their partners and their families. Published ten times a year.* Subscription, $17.95 per year. Contact MAMM Magazine, 349 West 12th Street, New York, NY 10014-1796, (888) 901-MAMM or subscription@mamm.com.

Judges and Lawyers Breast Cancer Alert, 50 King Street, Suite 6D, New York, NY 10014. *Confidential hotline for judges, lawyers and law students who have been diagnosed with breast cancer.*

National Alliance of Breast Cancer Organizations (NABCO), 9 East 37th Street, 10th Floor, New York, NY 10016. (888) 80-NABCO; (212) 719-0154 or www.nabco.org. *Membership organization is a central source of information about breast cancer and provides up-to-date information packets. Their Annual Resource List is available for $5; guide to Regional Support Groups is available for $2 from their office, or free at* www.nabco.org.

National Breast Cancer Coalition, 1707 L Street NW, Suite 1060, Washington, DC 20036, (202) 296-7477 or www.natlbcc.org. *Coalition of over 500 groups involves women with the disease and those who care about them in changing public policy as it relates to progress against breast cancer. The NBCC welcomes individuals and organizations as members.*

Susan G. Komen Breast Cancer Foundation, Occidental Tower, 5005 LBJ Freeway, Suite 370, Dallas, TX 75244. (800) I'M AWARE, (972) 855-1600, or www.breastcancerinfo.com. *Largest private funder of breast cancer research in the U.S. as well as organizers of Races for the Cure.*

Women's Information Network Against Breast Cancer (WIN ABC) 19325 East Navilla Place, Covina, CA 91723, (626) 332-2255, or www.winabc.org. *National non-profit organization offering resources, peer support and referral sources through telephone counseling, mail support and community outreach.*

Y-ME National Breast Cancer Organization, 212 West Van Buren Street, Chicago, IL 60607. *Provides support and counseling through their national toll-free hotline, (800) 221-2141 (24 hours; Spanish language line, (800) 986-9505);* www.y-me.org. *Trained peer counselors are matched by background and experience to callers whenever possible. Y-ME offers information on establishing local support programs, and has 23 chapters nationwide. Y-ME also has a hotline for men whose partners have had breast cancer.*

YWCA Encore Plus Program ENCOREplus, (800) 95-EPLUS or www.ywca. org. *Provides early detection, outreach, education, post-diagnostic support and exercise services to all women.*

Inflammatory Breast Cancer (www.ibcsupport.org). *Good information regarding the relatively rare inflammatory breast cancer.*

Lymphedema Network (www.lymphnet.org). *Support for all kinds of lymphedema although that caused by breast cancer surgery is the most prominent.*

Male Breast Cancer (interact.withus.com/interact/mbc/). Information on male breast cancer.

Young Survivor Coalition (www.youngsurvival.org). Young breast cancer survivors.

Pregnant with Cancer Support Group P.O. Box 1243, Buffalo, NY 14220, (800) 743-6724 ext. 308 or www.pregnantwithcancer.org. *For women who are facing a diagnosis of cancer while pregnant, this group will match a new patient with someone who once faced cancer while pregnant.*

"Breast Cancer Facts and Figures 1999/2000" (American Cancer Society). *A booklet containing statistics including incidence, survival and trends.* Order from American Cancer Society (800) ACS-2345 or www.cancer.org.

"A Helping Hand—The Resource Guide for People with Cancer" (Cancer Care, Inc., 1997). Cancer Care, (800) 813-HOPE, or www.cancercare.org.

"If You've Thought about Breast Cancer," Rose Kushner Breast Cancer Advisory Center, (Summer 1998 edition). *Updated general pamphlet on breast cancer detection and treatment, including definitions and resources.* Order multiple copies from The Rose Kushner Breast Cancer Advisory Center, PO Box 224, Kensington, MD 20895, (301) 949-2531. Single copies free of charge from Y-ME.

"Understanding Breast Cancer Treatment" (July 1998). *This booklet contains lists of questions that will help a patient talk to her doctor about breast cancer. Topics covered include: early detection, diagnosis, treatment, adjuvant therapy, and reconstruction.* 72 pages. NCI's CIS, (800) 4-CANCER or rex.nci.nih.gov.

"What You Need to Know about Breast Cancer" (98–1556, August 1998). *NCI's most comprehensive pamphlet on breast cancer, this updated booklet covers symptoms, diagnosis, treatment, emotional issues and questions to ask your doctor.* Includes an index of terms. 44 pages. NCI's CIS, (800) 4-CANCER or rex.nci. nih.gov. (Note: A 1999 version is expected to be available mid-year).

"Your Breast Cancer Treatment Handbook," by Judy C. Kneece, RN, OCN (EduCare Publishing, 1998). *This easy to use book contains useful information about managing treatment decisions and addresses sensitive emotional issues in an insightful manner.* 210 pages. EduCare Publishing, P.O. Box 280505, Columbia, SC 29228, (800) 849-9271 or www.cancerhelp.com/ed.

"Initial Discovery and Diagnosis," (1999). Video. *In this first of a planned series of 12 videos for breast cancer patients, seven breast cancer survivors share how they learned of their breast cancer diagnosis and how they learned to cope with their disease. Also includes a resource guide.* 15 minutes, $15.00. Contact Woman to Woman, (877) 85-WOMAN or www.womantowomanvideos.org.

Roberta Altman and Michael J. Sarg, *The Cancer Dictionary* (NY: Facts on File, 1992). *Includes acronyms for chemotherapy protocols and simple anatomical illustrations.* Order from Facts on File (800) 322-8755.

Larry and Valerie Althouse, *You Can Save Your Breast: One Woman's Experience with Radiation Therapy* (New York: WW Norton, 1982).

Suzanne W. Braddock, et al., *Straight Talk About Breast Cancer: From Diagnosis to Recovery: A Guide for the Entire Family* (Addicus Books, 1996). Paperback.

Linda Brown Harris, *Breast Cancer Handbook: A Basic Guide for Gathering Information, Understanding the Diagnosis, and Choosing the Treatment* (1992). *A great booklet on breast cancer with many questions you should pose to your doctors.* Melpomene Institute for Women's Health Research, 1010 University Avenue, St. Paul, MN 55104 (612) 642-1951.

Yashar Hirshaut, Peter Pressman. *Breast Cancer: The Complete Guide.* (Bantam Books, 1997). Paperback. *An easy-to-follow resource written by an oncologist and a surgeon.*

Vladimir Lange, *Be A Survivor: Your Guide to Breast Cancer Treatment* (Lange Productions, 1998). *Has great graphics.*

Kathy LaTour, *The Breast Cancer Companion* (NY: William Morrow & Co, 1994). *Guidebook offers useful tips, insights of 75 survivors and background information about advocacy and politics of breast cancer.*

John Link. *The Breast Cancer Survival Manual: A Step-by-Step Guide for the Woman with Newly Diagnosed Cancer* (Owl Books, 2000). Paperback. *Another step-by-step guide by a medical oncologist.*

Rosie O'Donnell and Deborah Axelrod with Tracy C. Semler, *Bosom Buddies: Lessons and Laughter on Breast Health and Cancer* (Warner Books, 1999). *Answers frequently asked questions about breast cancer in an easy-to-read manner.*

Swirsky and Barbara Balaban, *The Breast Cancer Handbook: Taking Control After You've Found a Lump 2nd edition* (NY: Power Publications, 1998). *Easy to read guide takes you step-by-step through diagnosis and treatment.*

M. J. Silverstein, editor. *Ductal Carcinoma in Situ of the Breast.* (Baltimore, MD: Williams, and Wilkins, 1997).

J. R. Harris, S. Hellman, I. C. Henderson, D. W. Kinne, *Breast Diseases* (Philadelphia, Lippincott 1991). *Medical textbook with a very comprehensive treatment of breast cancer.*

EMOTIONAL ASPECTS

Wellness Community-National, 35 East 7th Street, Cincinnati,OH 45242. (888) 793-WELL; www.wellness-community.org. *Started in California with many centers across the country, its facilities provide free psychosocial care to cancer patients and their families.*

The Wellness Community, 1235 Fifth Street, Santa Monica CA 90401. (310) 393-1415. *Extensive support and education programs which encourage emotional recovery and a feeling of wellness.*

Cancer Care, Inc. and the National Cancer Care Foundation, 1180 Avenue of the Americas, New York NY 10036. (800) 813-HOPE, www.cancercare.org. *A social service agency which helps patients and their families cope with the impact of cancer. Direct services are limited to the greater New York area but callers will be referred to similar assistance available in their areas.*

Cancer Hope Network, 2 North Road, Suite A, Chester, NH 07930, 877-HOPENET. *Offers one-on-one support to cancer patients and their families undergoing cancer treatment from trained volunteers who have survived cancer.*

The Cancer Wellness Center/The Barbara Kassel Brotman House. *Offers free emotional support on its 24-hour hotline and through support groups, relaxation groups, educational workshops and library.* 215 Revere Drive, Northbrook, IL 50062. (708) 509-9595.

Gilda's Club, 195 W. Houston Street, New York, NY 10014. (212) 647-9700. *A free, nonprofit program where people with cancer and their families and friends join with others to build social and emotional support as a supplement to medical care in a nonresidential, home-like setting.* Twenty-five locations nationwide.

The National Self-Help Clearinghouse, c/o Graduate School and University Center of City University of New York, 33 West 42 Street, Room 620N, New York, NY 10036. *Will refer written inquiries to regional self-help services.*

Reach to Recovery Program of the American Cancer Society. *Trained volunteers visit newly-diagnosed patients.* (800) ACS-2345.

Coping Magazine. *A bi-monthly magazine for cancer patients and survivors.* Subscription $18/year. Media America, Inc., 2019 North Carothers, Franklin, TN 37064. (615) 790-2400 (copingmag@aol.com).

"Actions People with Cancer Can Take to Join with their Physicians in the Fight for Recovery." *Brochure free of charge from Wellness Community,* 2716 Ocean Park Blvd, Santa Monica CA 90405 (310) 314-2555.

"Breast Cancer and Sexuality" (Cancer Care, NY, 1998*). Booklet on sexuality, intimacy and menopausal symptoms.* Free from (800) 813-HOPE or www. cancercare.org.

"For Single Women with Breast Cancer" (1994). *Y-ME booklet offers practical guidance and emotional support for women without partners or those who live alone.* Single copies available free; (800) 221-2141.

"Facing Forward: A Guide for Cancer Survivors" (9302424, 1992). *Addresses the special needs of cancer survivors and their families.* 43 pages. NCI (800) 4-CANCER.

"Taking Time: Support for People with Cancer and the People Who Care About Them," (National Cancer Institute, P126, 1996). *Booklet addresses the feelings and concerns of others in similar situations and how they have coped.* 68 pages. Call NCI's CIS, (800) 4-CANCER.

"Talking with your Doctor" (American Cancer Society, 4638-CC, 1997 edition). *Suggestions for effective doctor/patient communication.* Six pages. Call the ACS, (800) ACS-2345.

"Teamwork: The Cancer Patients' Guide to Talking with Your Doctor" (National Coalition for Cancer Survivorship, $3.00 for members of the NCCS, $4.00 for non-members). *Useful suggestions on how to best begin and maintain a working relationship with a physician.* 32 pages. Contact NCCS, 1010 Wayne Avenue, 5th Floor, Silver Spring, MD 20910, (888) 937-6227 or www.cansearch.org.

Anne Fogelsanger, *See Yourself Well: For People with Cancer* (Brooklyn, NY: Equinox). Audiocassette, $10.95. *May be helpful to use while under treatment.*

Barbara Bergholz and Eva Shaw, *Diana's Gift.* (La Jolla, CA: Gentle Winds Press, 1992).

Helene Davis, *Chemo-poet and Other Poems.* (Cambridge, MA: Alice James Books, 1989).

Wendy Schlessel Harpham, *Diagnosis Cancer: Your Guide Through the First Few Months* (NY: W. W. Norton, 1992). *Guide for newly-diagnosed cancer patients, written by an internist who is also a cancer survivor.*

Danette G. Kauffman, *Surviving Cancer* (Washington, D.C.: Acropolis Books, 1989). *A practical guide to experiencing cancer and its treatment, with an emphasis on lists of resources for managing the medical, emotional and financial aspects of this disease.*

Ronnie Kaye, *Spinning Straw into Gold: Your Emotional Recovery from Breast Cancer* (NY: Fireside, 1991). Paperback. *Excellent guide to the emotional aspects of this disease from a psychologist who is also a survivor.*

L. LeShan, *Cancer as a Turning Point: A Handbook for People with Cancer, Their Families and Health Professionals.* (NY: E.P. Dutton, 1989).

Leatrice Lifshitz, *Her Soul Beneath the Bone: Women's Poetry on Breast Cancer.* (Urbana: University of Illinois, 1988).

Raymond A. Moody, M.D., *The Light Beyond: New Explorations by the Author of Life After Life* (Bantam, 1988).

Susan Nessim and Judith Ellis, *Cancervive: The Challenge of Life After Cancer* (Boston: Houghton Mifflin, 1992, $8.95). *Addresses the practical and emotional issues faced by cancer survivors such as insurance, relationships, infertility and long-term side effects of treament.*

Hester Hill Schnipper, Joan Feinberg Berns. *Woman to Woman: A Handbook for Women Newly Diagnosed with Breast Cancer.* (Wholecare Paperback, 1999).

Midge Stocker, editor, *Confronting Cancer, Constructing Change: New Perspectives on Women and Cancer. Essays confronting cancer myths.*

Rebecca Zuckweiler. *Living in the Postmastectomy Body: Learning to Live in and Love Your Body Again.* (Andrews McMeel Publishing, 1998). Paperback. *The author, a nurse and psychotherapist who had a double mastectomy, focuses on regaining confidence in your body.*

Practical Advice: Complements to Breast Cancer Therapy—Treating the Body and Soul

— Retreats and getaways designed for cancer survivors are increasingly available. Casting for Recovery offers weekend retreats that teach survivors how to fly-fish and focus on emotional and physical well-being. Contact Casting for Recovery, (888) 553-3500 or cfrprogram@aol.com.

— The Colorado Outward Bound School offers a course specifically for women surviving cancer, (888) 837-5204. Healing Adventures sponsors outdoor adventures for people challenged by cancer, and for their friends and families, (510) 237-8291. Wilderness Bay Wellness Foundation designs and delivers therapeutic wilderness programs for female cancer patients and survivors, (773) 334-0809.

— Women in Nature is an annual outdoor adventure in northern Minnesota for cancer survivors, (612) 520-1704. Life Choices Wellness Center seven day retreat includes meditation and empowerment activities, (800) 439-0083. Two other programs are Summits-Inner Mountain Wilderness Education Center, (907) 766-2074, lifechoices@lewcenter.com, and Expedition Inspiration at (208) 726-6456 or www.expeditioninspiration.org.

FAMILIES AND CHILDREN

Caringkids (http://oncolink.upenn.edu/forms/listserv.html). *Internet support group for children who know someone who is ill; monitored, open forum where children may exchange information, share their feelings and make friends with other children dealing with similar issues.*

Helping Children Cope Program of Cancer Care, Inc. (800) 813-HOPE or www.cancercare.org. *Offers support groups and telephone counseling for children whose parent has cancer.*

Kids Count Too *is a six session program of the American Cancer Society for preschool through teenage children who are coping with a parent's cancer.* To find the program nearest you, contact the ACS, (800) ACS-2345 or www.cancer.org.

Kids Konnected, 27071 Cabot Road, Suite 102, Laguna Hills, CA 92653. (800) 899-2866. *Provides friendship, education, understanding and support to kids who have a parent with cancer.*

The National Family Caregivers Association, ⅀ National Family Counseling Assn, 10400 Connecticut Avenue #500, Kensington, MD 20895-3944, (800) 896-3650 or www.nfcacares.org. *Offers information, education, support, public awareness and advocacy to address the common needs of family caregivers.*

"It Helps to Have Friends" (American Cancer Society, 4654.00). *A pamphlet for families with a parent who has cancer.* Call the ACS, (800) ACS-2345.

"Helping Children Cope When a Parent Has Cancer," 12 pages. American Cancer Society. *A booklet to help you help your children.*

"Handbook for Mothers Supporting Daughters with Breast Cancer" (1999). 26 pages. Contact Mothers Supporting Daughters with Breast Cancer, 21710 Bayshore Road, Chestertown, MD 21620-4401, (410) 778-1982, msdbc@dmv.com or www.mothersdaughters.org.

"A Shared Purpose: A Guide for Daughters Whose Mothers Have Advanced Breast Cancer." (Cancer Care, 1998). *Answers questions about advanced breast cancer, and addresses feelings and emotions that mothers and daughters may face.* 18 pages. Contact Cancer Care, (800) 813-HOPE or www.cancercare.org.

"Journaling Through the Storm" and "Silver Linings: The Other Side of Cancer" (Oncology Nursing Press, 1998). Companion volumes: an illustrated journal that invites the patient and her family to chronicle events, thoughts and feelings; and a collection of inspirational essays and poems. Contact ONS Customer Service, (412) 921-7373, customer.service@ons.org or www.ons.org.

"Taking Time: Support for the People with Cancer and the People Who Care About Them" (92–2059) National Cancer Institute. *Booklet for persons with cancer and their families.* 69 pages. NCI (800) 4-CANCER.

"When Someone in Your Family Has Cancer" (National Cancer Institute, P619, 1995). *Written for the young person whose parent has cancer, this booklet describes what cancer is, its treatment, and its emotional impact on family relationships. Includes a glossary of cancer-related terms.* 28 pages. Call the NCI's CIS, (800) 4-CANCER

Books for Parents

"My Mom Has Breast Cancer: A Guide for Families" Video (1996). *A KIDS-COPE, Inc. video for parents and children about coping with a mother's breast cancer diagnosis. Structured as interviews with six breast cancer survivors and their young children.* Contact KIDSCOPE, 3400 Peachtree Road, Suite 703, Atlanta, GA 30326, (404) 233-0001 or www.kidscope.org.

"Talking About Cancer: A Parent's Guide to Helping Children Cope" Video (Fox Chase Cancer Center). *A videotape that helps parents with cancer explain their diagnosis to their children,* 18 minutes. Call the Fox Chase Cancer Center, (888) FOX-CHASE.

Kathleen McCue, MA, CCLS with Ron Bonn, *How to Help Children Through a Parent's Serious Illness* (NY: St. Martin's Press, 1994). *Explains a child's special needs when a parent is seriously ill. Provides guidelines, advice, and real-life examples to help parents and other caregivers help children during this stressful time.*

Elizabeth Winthrop and illustrated by Betsy Lewin, *Promises* (NY: Clarion Books, 2000). *Book addresses the range of emotions that children can experience when a parent has cancer*

Books for Children

Claire Blake, Eliza Blanchard, and Kathy Parkinson, *The Paper Chain* (Health Press, 1998). *For children ages three to eight, this book relays the emotions of two young boys whose Mom has breast cancer.* 32 pages. Bookstores or call Health Press, (800) 643-BOOK.

Pat Brack and Ben Brack, *Moms Don't Get Sick* (Aberdeen, SD: Melius Publishing, 1990). *One woman's story as told through her eyes and those of her ten year old son. Excellent for women with children.*

Christine Clifford, *Our Family Has Cancer Too!* (Duluth, MN: Pfeifer-Hamilton Pubs, 1997). *For children ages five to 14, this book talks about one child's struggle to understand and cope with his mother's cancer.* Illustrated with cartoons. 64

pages. Bookstores or contact The Cancer Club, 6533 Limerick Drive, Edina, MN 55439, (800) 586-9062 or www.cancerclub.com.

Judylaine Fine, *Afraid to Ask, A Book for Families to Share About Cancer* (NY: Lothrop, Lee and Shepard Books, 1986).

Wendy S. Harpham, *When a Parent has Cancer: A Guide to Caring for Your Children* with *Becky and The Worry Cup.* (Harper Collins Publishers, 1997). The author, a lymphoma survivor, presents sensitive and practical advice to help children understand and cope with a parent's diagnosis of cancer. An illustrated children's book is included that tells the poignant story of Becky, a seven-year-old girl and her experiences with her mother's cancer.

H. Elizabeth King, *Kemoshark* (1995). *A colorfully illustrated booklet to help children understand chemotherapy when their parent is undergoing treatment.* 14 pages. Contact KIDSCOPE, 3399 Peachtree Road, Suite 2020, Atlanta, GA 30326, (404) 233-0001 or www.kidscope.org.

Sherry Kohlenberg, *Sammy's Mommy Has Cancer* (NY: Magination Press, 1993). *The author, who was diagnosed with breast cancer when she was 34 and her son was 18 months old, offers parents a thoughtful and sensitive way to explain breast cancer to a child.* (800) 374-2721 or www.maginationpress.com.

Laura Numeroff and Wendy S. Harpham, *Kid's Talk – Kids Speak Out About Breast Cancer* (Samsung Telecommunications America and Sprint PCS, 1999). *For children aged ten and younger, short stories told by children about living with a mother with breast cancer.* Call the Susan G. Komen Foundation, (800) I'M-AWARE.

Carolyn Stearns Parkinson, *My Mommy Has Cancer.* (TN: Cope/Coping Books).

Deborah Weinstein-Stern, *Mira's Month* ($5.00). *When the author's breast cancer recurred, she wrote this book for her four year old daughter.* 38 pages. Contact the Blood and Marrow Transplant Information Network, 2900 Skokie Valley Road, Suite B, Highland Park, IL 60035, (888) 597-7674.

HUSBANDS AND PARTNERS

The Well Spouse Foundation, 30 East 40th Street, P.H., New York, NY 10016, (800) 838-0879 or www.wellspouse.org. *A national, non-profit membership organization which gives support to husbands, wives and partners of the chronically ill and/ or disabled. Support groups and a bi-monthly newsletter are available.*

Y-ME National Breast Cancer Organization has trained male volunteers who provide support and counseling to other male partners of women with breast cancer through their national toll-free hotline, (800) 221-2141 (9:00 am to 5:00 pm CST, Monday through Friday).

"Sexuality and Cancer: For the Woman Who has Cancer, and Her Partner" (1999 edition) 64 pages American Cancer Society. *A booklet which gives information about cancer and sexuality in areas that might concern the patient and her partner.* ACS (800) ACS-2345.

"When the Woman You Love Has Breast Cancer" (Y-ME, 1994). *A booklet that helps partners give emotional support to their loved ones.* Single copies available free, bulk orders available on request. Call Y-ME, (800) 221-2141 or www.y-me.org.

"The Breast Cancer Companion Tapes: Diagnosis and Decision-Making/ The Male Perspective." (1994, two tapes, $35.00 each). *Offers couples two separate videotapes, one for the patient and one for her partner and includes insight into how other couples have dealt with the medical and emotional issues surrounding a breast cancer diagnosis.* 30 minutes each. Contact the Breast Cancer Companion Tapes, P.O. Box 141182, Dallas, TX 75214.

Larry T. Eiler. *When the Woman You Love Has Breast Cancer* (Queen Bee Publishing, Ann Arbor, MI, 1994*). Issues faced by a man whose wife or friend has the disease, suggesting steps he can take to be supportive.* Queen Bee Publishing, 900 Victors Way, Suite 180, Ann Arbor, MI 48108, (734) 761-3399.

Judy C. Kneece. *Helping Your Mate Face Breast Cancer: Tips for Becoming an Effective Support Partner for the One You Love During the Breast Cancer Experience* (Edu Care, Inc., 1999). Paperback. *Offers helpful suggestions on coping strategies and how to support the physical and emotional recovery of a partner.*

Andy Murcia and Bob Stewart, *Man to Man: When the Woman You Love has Breast Cancer* (NY: St. Martin's Press, 1990).

Leslie R. Schover, *Sexuality and Fertility After Cancer,* (John Wiley and Sons, Inc., New York, NY, 1997). Paperback. *Explains how treatment may emotionally and physically interfere with male and female sexual function and fertility.*

Bruce Sokol, et al. *Breast Cancer: A Husband's Story.* (Crane Hill Publishing, 1997). Paperback.

Lesbians

The Lesbian Community Cancer Project 4753 North Broadway, Suite 602, Chicago, IL 60640-4907, (773) 561-4662 or www.iccp.org. *Gives support, information, education, advocacy, and direct services to lesbians and women living with cancer and their families.*

The Mautner Project for Lesbians with Cancer, 1707 L Street NW, Suite 500, Washington, DC 20036, (202) 332-5536, mautner@mautnerproject.org or www.mautnerproject.org *A volunteer organization dedicated to helping lesbians with cancer, as well as their partners, and caregivers.* The pamphlet, "Lesbians and Cancer," provides early detection information; available at no cost in English or Spanish.

The National Lesbian and Gay Health Association, (202) 939-7880, nlgha@aol.com or www.nlgha.org. *Provides general health information and resources, including cancer.*

Seattle Lesbian Cancer Project, 1122 E. Pike Street, #1333, Seattle WA 98122 (206) 286-0166. *Grassroots organization provides advocacy, education and referrals, with an emphasis on the medically underserved.*

Wendy's Hope: Reaching Out to Lesbians with Cancer and Other Life-Threatening Diseases. City of Hope, 1055 Wilshire Blvd, 12th Floor, Los Angeles CA (310) 798-9085 or corewellness.com. *Offers education, assistance and support groups.*

Sandra Butler and Barbara Rosenblum, *Cancer In Two Voices.* (Spinsters Book Company, MN, 1996, expanded edition*). A particularly moving and honest account of the authors' identity as Jewish women and as lesbians as they live with advanced breast cancer.*

"Cancer in Two Voices" Video complements the book described above. (16mm/video, rental $140/$90, plus $22.00 shipping; VHS $275.00, plus $15.00 shipping). 43 minutes. Contact Women Make Movies, Sales and Rental Department, 462 Broadway, Suite 500-C, New York, NY 10013 or (212) 925-0606.

Roz Perry, *Rose Penski* (Tallahassee, FL: Naiad Press). *A novel about a lesbian and her lover going through diagnosis and initial treatment of breast cancer.*

PERSONAL STORIES

SHOW ME: A Photo Collection of Breast Cancer Survivors' Lumpectomies, Mastectomies, Reconstructions and Thoughts on Body Image. *Fantastic resource created by a Breast Cancer Support Group which shows what your body will look like after different surgeries.* Order from Penn State Geisinger Health System Women's Center, Box 850, Code H306, Hershey PA 17033, (717) 531-5867 or view at SusanLoveMD.com.

"Victories: Three Women Triumph over Breast Disease," (MBM Communications, San Francisco, CA 1989). *Videotape of three personal stories (mastectomy/ reconstruction, benign disease, lumpectomy/chemo/RT, recurrence). Includes group discussions, husband/wife counseling and mammography.* To order call (415) 642-0460. 23 minutes, $195.00/$45.00 rental.

"Not Alone—Women Coping with Breast Cancer." (Adelphi Oncology Support Program, Garden City, NJ, Fall 1988). *Filmed during actual sessions, a group of breast cancer patients accompanied by a social worker discuss their concerns and offer mutual support.* 22 minute video, $150.00. Order from Adelphi (516) 877-4444.

"Voices of Healing: You're Not Alone—Conversations with breast cancer survivors and those who love them" (Voice Arts Publishing, Madison, WI, 1998). *This two hour audiotape package narrates the experiences and insights of breast cancer survivors, their partners and children. Covers physical, emotional, social and spiritual aspects of the disease $17.95 To order, call (800) 261-1705.*

"Cathy Saved Her Life" (1989). *Videotape of televised story of Cathy Masamitsu, an ABC "Home Show" staff member who had breast cancer.* 90 minutes, $7.50. Order from Woody Fraser Productions, PO Box 7548, Burbank, CA 91510-7548.

Elizabeth Berg. *Talk Before Sleep.* (New York: Dell, 1997). Paperback. *A fictional account of how a group of women face the diagnosis of breast cancer in one of their friends.*

Judy Brady, *One in Three: Women with Cancer Confront an Epidemic* (Pittsburgh: Clei's Press, 1991). *Collection of essays by women involved in grassroots cancer activism.*

Nancy Brinker with Catherine McEvily Harris, *The Race is Run One Step at a Time: My Personal Struggle and Everywoman's Guide to Taking Charge of Breast Cancer* (NY: Simon & Schuster, 1990). *Also available on audio cassette, account of the battle against breast cancer by the author and her sister, Susan Komen.*

Sue Buchanan. *I'm Alive and the Doctor's Dead: Surviving Cancer with Your Sense of Humor and Your Sexuality Intact.* (Zondervan Publishing House, 1998). Paperback.

Rita Busch (editor), et al. *Can You Come Here Where I Am? The Poetry and Prose of Seven Breast Cancer Survivors.* (E M Pr Paperback, 1998).

Donna Cederberg, Daria Davidson, Joy Edwards, Carol Hebestreit, Betsy Lambert, Amy Langer, Cathy Masamitsu, Sally Snodgrass, Carol Stack and Carol Washington, *Breast Cancer? Let Me Check my Schedule.* (Vancouver, WA: Innovative Medical Education Consortium, 1994). *Ten professional women share their wisdom and experience about living with breast cancer.* Order from IMEC, 500 W. 8th Street, Suite 100A, Vancouver, WA 98660.

Kathlyn Conway. *Ordinary Life: A Memoir of Illness.* (W.H. Freeman and Company, New York, NY, 1997). *Written by a psychotherapist, this book details the author's struggle through her breast cancer diagnosis and treatment.*

Linda Dackman, *Up Front: Sex and the Post-Mastectomy Woman* (NY: Viking, 1990). *A personal account, with frank details about the intimate challenges faced by a single woman in her 30's.*

Laura Evans, *The Climb of My Life.* (Harper San Francisco, 1996). *The author traces her experience from the time she was diagnosed with breast cancer in 1990 to 1995, when she led sixteen other breast cancer survivors in a climb to the summit of the highest mountain in the Western Hemisphere.*

Gayle Feldman, *You Don't Have to Be Your Mother* (NY: W.W. Norton, 1994). *Courageous account of a 40 year old, pregnant woman's struggle to deal with breast cancer and to come to terms with the death of her mother, who died of breast cancer.*

Nora Feller and Marcia Stevens Sherrill, *Portraits of Hope.* (NY: Smithmark Publishers, 1998). *Fifty-two inspirational survivors are profiled by Ms. Sherrill and their color portraits are photographed by Ms. Feller. The two-volume set includes a journal for thoughts and notes.*

Robert C. Fore, EdD and Rorie E. Fore, RN. *Survivor's Guide to Breast Cancer.* (Macon, GA: Smyth & Helwys Pub,1998) *A couple's story of faith, love and hope, it describes their experience with Rorie's diagnosis of breast cancer.*

Andrea Gabbard. *No Mountain Too High: A Triumph Over Breast Cancer: The Story of the Women of Expedition Inspiration.* (Seal Press, 1998). Paperback.

Amy Gross and Dee Ito, *Women Talk about Breast Surgery, from diagnosis to recovery* (NY: Clarkson Potter, 1990). *Women's stories describing the range of situations and treatments. Better for its support aspects than the accuracy of the medical information.*

Judy Hart, *Love, Judy - Letters of Hope and Healing for Women with Breast Cancer.* (Berkeley, CA: Conari Press, 1993).

Lois Tschetter Hjelmstad, *Fine Black Lines: Reflections on Facing Cancer, Fear and Loneliness.* (Mulberrry Hill Press, 1993). Paperback.

Carolyn Ingram, et al. *The Not-So-Scary Breast Cancer Book: Two Sisters' Guide from Discovery to Recovery.* (Impact Publication, 1999). Paperback.

Deborah Kahane, *No Less a Woman, Ten Women Shatter the Myths about Breast Cancer* (Prentice Hall Press, 1990). *A cross-section of women with breast cancer tell their own stories.*

Jane Lazarre, *Wet Earth and Dreams: A Narrative of Grief and Recovery.* (Duke University Press, 1998). *Moving cancer journal.*

Audre Lorde, *The Cancer Journals* (San Francisco: Aunt Lute Books, 1980). *Reflections on her breast cancer by an extraordinary black, Lesbian poet.* Available from Aunt Lute Books (415) 558-8116.

Christina Middlebrook. *Seeing the Crab: A Memoir of Dying Before I Do.* (NY: Doubleday, 1998). Paperback.

Jacque Miller, *The Lopsided Gal - The Humor, Blessings and Trials of Breast Cancer.* (Colorado: Parker Printing, 1987).

Musa Mayer, *Examining Myself: One Woman's Story of Breast Cancer Treatment and Recovery* (Winchester, MA: Faber and Faber, 1993). *Exploration of the emotional aspects of disease and recovery. Faber and Faber is donating a portion of the book's proceeds to the National Breast Cancer Coalition.*

Madeleine Meldin, *The Tender Bud: A Physician's Journal Through Breast Cancer* (Hillsdale, NJ: Analytic Press, 1993). *Written from the point of view of a psychiatrist attempting to keep her professional life intact during breast cancer treatment.*

Deena Metzger, *Tree* (Oakland, CA: Wingbow Press, 1983). *Written by the woman pictured in the well-known poster of an exultant woman with a mastectomy and a tattoo of a tree on her scar.* The poster can be obtained from Tree, PO Box 186, Topanga, CA 90290.

Cynthia Ploski. *Conversations with My Healers—My Journey to Wellness from Breast Cancer.* (Council Oak Books, Tulsa, OK 74210, 1995). Paperback. *Upbeat personal narratives offer help and hope to those facing breast cancer.*

Margit Esser Porter (Editor). *Hope is Contagious: The Breast Cancer Treatment Survival Handbook.* (Fireside, 1997). Paperback. *Collection of quotes from women who responded to a questionnaire on how to cope with breast cancer treatment.*

Hilda Raz (Editor). *Living on the Margins: Women Writers on Breast Cancer* (Persea Books, 1999).

Katherine Russell Rich, *The Red Devil: To Hell with Cancer—And Back* (NY: Crown Books, 1999). *This woman has been through every imaginable breast cancer treatment and tells the tale with great wit.*

Allie Fair Sawyer and Norma Suzette Jones, *Journey: A Breast Cancer Survival Guide* (Alexander, NC: WorldComm Press, 1992). *Authors share their personal experiences.*

Lillie Shockney, *Breast Cancer Survivors' Club: A Nurse's Experience.* (Windsor House, 1999). Paperback.

Melissa Springer, *A Tribe of Warrior Women: Breast Cancer Survivors.* (Crane Hill, 1996). *Contains photographs and personal vignettes of 32 breast cancer survivors.*

Claudia Sternbach. *Now Breathe: A Very Personal Journey Through Breast Cancer.* (Whiteaker Press, 1999). Paperback.

Barbara Stone, *Cancer as Initiation: Surviving the Fire: A Guide for Living with Cancer for Patient, Provider, Spouse, Family or Friend.* (Open Court Publishing, 1994). Paperback.

Carolyn Walter and Julienne Oklay, *Breast Cancer in the Life Course: Women's Experiences* (Springer, 1991).

Ken Wilber, *Grace and Grit: Spirituality and Healing in the Life and Death of Treya Killam Wilber* (Boston: Shambala, 1993).

Susan Winn, *Chemo and Lunch: One Woman's Triumph Over Hereditary Breast Cancer* (Fithian Press, 1990).

Juliet Wittman, *Breast Cancer Journal: A Century of Petals* (Golden, CO: Fulcrum Publishing, 1993). Paperback. *Well-written, honest, personal story by a journalist.*

Ina Yalof. *Straight from the Heart: Letters of Hope and Inspiration from Survivors of Breast Cancer* (NY: Kensington Books, 1996). *Women from all walks of life discuss their experiences with breast cancer.*

NOTE: Several other notable personal stories are out of print but can be found in libraries, including: *Getting Better: Conversations with Myself and Other Friends,* by Anne Hargrave; *Life Wish* by Jill Ireland; *My Breast: One Woman's Cancer Story* by Joyce Wadler; *Of Tears and Triumps: The Family Victory That Has Inspired Thousands of Cancer Patients,* by Georgia and Bud Photopulos; and *Exploding into Life* by Dorothea Lynch.

TREATMENT OPTIONS

Cancerfax. *This service allows access to NCI's Physician's Data Query (PDQ) system (see entry below) via fax machine, 24 hours/day, 7 days/week, at no charge. Two versions of the treatment are available: one for health care professionals and the other for lay people. Information is also available in Spanish.* For information and list of necessary codes, call (301) 402-5874 or call (800) 4-CANCER or on the web, cancernet.nci.nih.gov (no 'www' is needed).

PDQ (Physician Data Query). *The cancer information database of NCI, providing prognostic, stage and treatment information and more than 1,500 clinical trials that are open to patient accrual. Access by computer equipped with a modem, and by fax (see above).* For more information, call NCI at (800) 4-CANCER.

CANHELP. *Will research patient's treatment options (including alternative therapies) based on your medical records. A personalized 10–15 page packet will be mailed within seven working days for $400.00.* Contact CANHELP, 3111 Paradise Bay Road, Port Ludlow, WA 98365-9771 (206) 437-2291.

National Comprehensive Cancer Network (www.nccn.org). *Provides accepted treatment guidelines for breast cancer care.* 50 Huntingdon Pike, Suite 200; Rockledge PA 19046. (215) 728-4788; patient information service (888) 909-NCCN.

NIH Consensus Conference Statement: Treatment of Early Stage Breast Cancer (June, 1990, Vol. 8, No. 6). *Still the current standard, the treatment recommendations of the expert panel convened by the National Institutes of Health.* On the web: www.odp.od.nih.gov/consensus.

International Cancer Alliance (ICA), 4853 Cordell Avenue, Suite 11, Bethesda MD 20814. (800) I-CARE-61. *Provides a free Cancer Therapy Review that includes information on a specific type of cancer (description, detection and staging, treatment, diagnostic tests and clinical trials). Cancer Breakthroughs report is sent quarterly.*

Surgery

"Mastectomy: A Treatment for Breast Cancer" (87–658 8/87) 24 pages. National Cancer Institute. *Information about different types of breast surgery.*

"Standards for Breast-Conservation Treatment" (3405, 1992). ACS booklet, call (800) ACS-2345.

"The Surgical Management of Primary Breast Cancer" (3493, 1991). ACS booklet, call (800) ACS-2345.

Rosalind Dolores Benedet, *Healing: A Woman's Recovery Guide to Recovery After Mastectomy* (San Francisco: R. Benedet Publishing, 1993). *Guide to postoperative care after a mastectomy.* To order, send $10 plus $1 shipping to R. Benedet Publishing, 220 Montgomery Street Penthouse #2, San Francisco, CA 94104.

Radiation

"Radiation Therapy: A Treatment For Early Stage Breast Cancer" (87–659 9/1987). 20 pages. National Cancer Institute, (800) 4-CANCER. *This booklet discusses the treatment and side effects of primary radiation therapy.*

"Radiation Therapy and You: A Guide to Self-Help During Treatment" (97–2227, 1997). 52 pages National Cancer Institute, (800) 4-CANCER. *Written for the patient receiving radiation.*

"The Role of Radiation Therapy in the Management of Primary Breast Cancer" (3492, 1991). ACS booklet, (800) ACS-2345.

Systemic Therapy

American Society of Clinical Oncology (ASCO), 435 North Michigan Avenue, Suite 1717 Chicago, IL 60611. (312) 644-0828. *Will mail to medical professionals a list of member oncologists by geographical area.*

"Chemotherapy and You: A Guide to Self-Help During Treatment" (97–1136, 1997). *A question-and-answer booklet, including glossary and guide to side-effects.* 56 pages. NCI (800) 4-CANCER.

"Chemotherapy: *Your* Weapon Against Cancer" (1998 edition). *Explanation of the benefits and side effects of chemo.* One copy free from The Chemotherapy Foundation, 183 Madison Ave, Suite 403, NY, NY 10016. (212) 213-9292.

"Chemotherapy: What it is, How it Helps" (1990, 4512). *Brief introduction to chemotherapy.* (800) ACS-2345.

Community Clinical Oncology Program ("CCOP") (April 1993, updated periodically). *List of the 48 medical centers in 36 states and Puerto Rico selected by NCI to participate in newest clinical protocols and to accrue patients to clinical trials.* (800) 4-CANCER.

"Coping with the Side Effects of Chemotherapy" (1992). 19 page booklet. Order from Wyeth-Ayerst (800) 395-9938.

"Helping Yourself During Chemotherapy: 4 steps for Patients" (94–3701, 1994). *Easy-to-read brochure suggests four steps to follow during chemo.* NCI (800) 4-CANCER.

"Questions and Answers About Tamoxifen" (1994). *Fact sheet on tamoxifen (Nolvadex) and its side effects.* 4 pages. NCI (800) 4-CANCER.

"The Role of Chemotherapy in the Management of Primary Breast Cancer" (3356, 1991). Booklet from ACS (800) ACS-2345.

Robert Bazell. *HER-2: The Making of Herceptin, A Revolutionary Treatment for Breast Cancer.* (NY: Random House, 1998). *Written by NBC's chief science correspondent, the story of Genentech's Herceptin , the first gene-based therapy for breast cancer.*

Nancy Bruning, *Coping with Chemotherapy* (Ballantine Books, 1993). *Overview of medical and emotional effects of chemotherapy.*

Michael W. DeGregorio, Valeria J. Wiebe, *Tamoxifen and Breast Cancer.* (Yale University Press, 1999). Paperback.

Marylin J. Dodd, *Managing the Side effects of Chemotherapy and Radiation Therapy: A Guide for Patients and their Families.* (UCSF Nursing Press, 3rd edition, 1996). *Suggestions for managing each side effect.* Order from UCSF Nursing Press, 521 Parnassus Ave, Room N535C, San Francisco, CA 94143 (415) 476-4992.

V. Craig Jordan, et al. *Tamoxifen for the Treatment and Prevention of Breast Cancer.* (Publisher Research and Representation, 1999).

John F. Kessler MD, et al. *Tamoxifen: New Hope in the Fight Against Breast Cancer.* (Wholecare Mass Market Paperback, 1999).

Judith McKay, and Nancee Hirano, *The Chemotherapy and Radiation Survival Guide.* (Oakland: New Harbinger Pub, 1998). *Written by two oncology nurses about physical and psychological issues.* Call (800) 748-6273 or www.newharbinger.com

Joyce Slayton-Mitchell, *Winning the Chemo Battle* (NY: WW Norton, 1991). *Personal and account of chemotherapy treatment from a woman who has "been there."*

National Bone Marrow Transplant Link. 20411 West 12 Mile Road #108, Southfield MI 48076 (9–00) LINK-BMT or http://comnet.org/nbmtlink. *Information clearinghouse on bone marrow transplants which also links patients or family with former patients or family.*

Blood and Marrow Transplant Newsletter, Blood and Marrow Transplant Information Network, 2900 Skokie Valley Road, Suite B, Highland Park, IL 60035, (888) 597-7674, (847) 433-4599 (fax) or www.bmtnews.org. *Quarterly newsletter for patients who have had or who are considering bone marrow, peripheral stem cell or cord blood transplantation; also attorney referral service to help resolve insurance problems.*

COMPLEMENTARY AND ALTERNATIVE THERAPIES

The Alternative Medicine Homepage (www.pitt.edu/~cbw/altm.html). *Links to information sources about complementary and alternative therapies.*

The National Center for Complementary and Alternative Medicine (http://nccam.nih.gov). *Good place to research alternatives scientifically.*

The Osher Center for Integrative Medicine (www.ucsf.edu/ocim.research/breastcancer.html). *University of California San Francisco Center studying alternatives in women with breast cancer.*

The Rosenthal Center for Complementary and Alternative Medicine (www.cpmcnet.columbia.edu/dept/rosenthal/women.html). *Columbia University's center does research on alternatives and women's health.*

American Botanical Council/HerbalGram (www.herbalgram.org*). Herbal information on the internet.*

Herbal Research Foundation (http://sunsite.unc.edu/herbs.hrinfo.html).

IBIS, Interactive BodyMind Information System *(www.teleport.com/~ibis). Everything you want to know about the alternative options for any one disease.*

The Cancer Club, 6533 Limerick Drive, Edina, MN 55439. (800) 586-9062, www.cancerclub.com. *Markets humorous and helpful products including a quarterly newsletter, books and videos.*

Center for Mind-Body Medicine, 5225 Connecticut Ave NW, Suite 414, Washington DC 20015 or www.cmbm.org. *A leader in promoting complementary cancer care (treatments that combine standard treatments with alternative approaches).*

The Institute for the Advancement of Health, 16 East 53rd Street, New York, NY 10022. (212) 832-8282. *A national organization devoted to promoted awareness of mind body health interactions. Supplies information on behavioral techniques to promote comfort and health.*

National Center for Complementary and Alternative Medicine, NIH. *Investigates alternative medical treatments, offers information packages.* NCCAM Clearinghouse, Box 8218, Silver Spring, MD 20907. (888) 644-6226, http://nccam.nih.gov.

The Planetree Health Resource Center. *A non-profit, consumer-oriented resource for health information, including materials on relaxation and visualization techniques.* Write or call for a catalogue and price list: 2040 Webster Street, San Francisco, CA 95115. (415) 923-3680.

"Unproven Methods of Cancer Management"(3028 /88) American Cancer Society. *The local Division Offices have statements providing details on each of 27 treatment methods listed in this brochure.*

The National Council Against Health Fraud. Call the Council's Resource Center (800) 821-6671 or write to Dr. John Renner, Consumer Health Information Research Institute, 3521 Broadway, Kansas City, MO 64111.

German Commission E Monograph. Translated and made available by the American Botanical Council. (PO Box 201660, Austin, TX 78720). *This is the German government's analysis of indication and safety of commonly used herbs.*

Harold H. Benjamin, *The Wellness Community Guide to Fighting for Recovery (revised and expanded edition of From Victim to Victor)* (NY: Putnam, 1995).

Herbert Benson, *The Relaxation Response* (NY: Avon Books, 1985).

John Boik. *Natural Compounds in Cancer Therapy.* (Princeton, MN: Oregon Medical Press, 2000). *Thoroughly reviews the potential of selected natural compounds in cancer treatment, including mechanisms of action, activity, pharmacology, and toxicology.*

Joan Borysenko, *Minding the Body, Mending the Mind* (Menlo Park: Addison Wesley, 1987).

Christine Clifford, illustrated by Jack Lindstrom, *Not Now...I'm Having a No Hair Day: Humor and Healing for People with Cancer* (Pfeifer-Hamilton, Duluth, MN, 1996, $9.95). *Author shows how the power of laughter and positive thinking can promote recovery and growth.* Contact The Cancer Club, 6533 Limerick Drive, Edina, MN 55439, (800) 586-9062 or www.cancerclub.com.

Norman Cousins, *The Healing Heart* (NY: Avon Books 1983).

Norman Cousins, *Anatomy of An Illness* (NY: Bantam Books, 1986).

Linda Dackman, *Affirmations, Meditations, and Encouragements for Women Living with Breast Cancer* (San Francisco: Harper, 1992). *Uses quotes and anecdotes to provide insight into the process.*

Larry Dossey, M.D., *Healing Words: The Power of Prayer and the Practice of Medicine* (San Francisco: Harper-Collins, 1993).

Ron Falcone, Lynn Sonberg. *Natural Medicine for Breast Cancer.* (Dell, 1997). Paperback. *Includes herbal and other alternative remedies for fatigue, loss of appetite, nausea and liver toxicity due to breast cancer treatment.*

Neil Fiore, *The Road Back To Health* (NY: Bantam Books 1984). *Good explanation on how to make your own visualization tapes, by a psychologist and former cancer patient. Book is out of print but may be found in some libraries.*

Anne Fogelsanger," See Yourself Well: For People with Cancer" (Brooklyn: Equinox, 1994). *Audiocassette provides series of mental exercises to encourage relaxation.*

The Humor Project. *A resource for humorous materials; free catalogue available. Quarterly magazine, Laughing Matters, available for $16/year. Conferences are held on using humor to cope with illness.* 110 Spring Street, Saratoga Springs, NY 12866-3397. (518) 587-8770.

Jon Kabat-Zinn, *Full Catastrophe Living: Using the Wisdom of Your Body and Mind to Face Stress, Pain and Illness* (Delta Press, 1990).

Michael Lerner, *Choices in Healing: Integrating the Best of Conventional and Complementary Approaches to Cancer* (Cambridge, MA: MIT Press, 1994). *A wonderful book on ways to integrate alternative approaches to traditional medicine.*

Ellen Michaud and Editors of *Prevention Magazine, Fighting Disease: The Complete Guide to Natural Immune Power.*

Ralph Moss, *Cancer Therapy: The Independent Consumer's Guide to Non-Toxic Treatment and Prevention* (NY: Equinox Press, 1992). *Discusses nearly 100 non-toxic modes of cancer prevention and treatment.*

Bill Moyers, *Healing and the Mind* (NY: Doubleday, 1993).

P.C. Roud, *Making Miracles: An Exploration into the Dynamics of Self-Healing* (NY: Warner Books, 1990).

Ellen Schaplowsky, Nan Lu. *Traditional Chinese Medicine: A Woman's Guide to Healing from Breast Cancer.* (Avon Books, 1999).

Bernie Siegel, M.D., *Love Medicine and Miracles* (NY: Perennial Library, 1987 $8.95). *Promotes visualization, meditation, discussion and positive thinking.*

David Spiegel, *Living Beyond Limits: New Hope and Help for Facing Life-Threatening Illness* (NY: Times Books, 1993).

Susan Weed. *Breast Cancer? Breast Health! The Wise Woman Way.* (Ash Tree Publication, 1997). Paperback.

Honora Lee Wolfe, Bob Flaws. *Better Breast Health Naturally with Chinese Medicine.* (Blue Poppy Press, 1998).

LIVING WITH BREAST CANCER

The National Coalition for Cancer Survivorship (NCCS), 1010 Wayne Avenue, Suite 505, Silver Spring, MD 20910, (877) 622-7937 or www.cansearch.org. *Raises awareness of cancer survivorship through its publications, quarterly newsletter, education to eliminate the stigma of cancer, and advocacy for insurance, employment, and legal rights.*

National Cancer Survivors Day Foundation, PO Box 682285, Franklin TN 37068-2285 (615) 794-3006 or www.ncsdf.org. *National Cancer Survivors Day is America's nationwide, annual celebration of life for cancer survivors, their families, friends and oncology teams, celebrated on the first Sunday in June each year.*

"Facing Forward: A Guide for Cancer Survivors," (NCI, P119, 1994*). Booklet focuses on maintaining physical health, emotions, managing insurance and employment.* Call NCI's CIS 9800) 4-CANCER.

Karen M Hassey, "Pregnancy and Parenthood After Treatment for Breast Cancer" *Oncology Nursing Forum,* Vol. 15 (4): 439–444, 1988. *You will probably have to get this from a hospital or medical library. A very good review of all that has been published on the subject.*

"The Cancer Survivor's Toolbox," *a self-learning audio program also available in Spanish and Chinese.* Free to survivors and professionals, call (877) TOOLS-4-U.

Susan Kuner, et al. *Speak the Language of Healing: Living with Breast Cancer Without Going to War.* (Conari Press, 1999). Paperback.

Carolyn Runowicz and Donna Haupt, *To Be Alive: A Woman's Guide to a Full Life After Cancer* (New York: Henry Holt, 1996). *Written by an oncologist and breast cancer survivor.*

Marisa C. Weiss, Ellen Weiss. *Living Beyond Breast Cancer: A Survivor's Guide for When Treatment Ends and the Rest of your Life Begins.* (New York: Times Books, 1998). Paperback.

Appearance and Comfort

"Look Good . . . Feel Better" is a public service program from the Cosmetic, Toilet and Fragrance Association Foundation in partnership with ACS and the National Cosmetology Association. *It is designed to help women recovering from cancer deal with changes in their appearance resulting from cancer treatment. The program's print and videotape materials are designed for both patients and health professionals.* Call (800) 395-LOOK or your local ACS office.

"Look Good . . . Feel Better: Caring for Yourself Inside and Out." (CTFA Foundation, 1988). *The LGFB Program's video for cancer patients undergoing chemotherapy and radiation therapy. Women discuss their experiences, and beauty professionals review ways to look and feel better during treatment, including makeup, nail care and wigs.* 16 minutes. Order from CTFA (800) 395-LOOK.

Practical Advice: How To Find Post-Mastectomy Products

— Prostheses. The lingerie areas in some department stores employ professionals who will fit you with a prosthesis and a bra to wear with it. Smaller lingerie boutiques in major cities often perform this function as well—check your local yellow pages under "Lingerie" or "Brassieres," or in larger cities, under "Breast Prosthesis." Prostheses may also be ordered from selected surgical supply stores, often listed under "Surgical Appliances and Supplies." Temporary prostheses can be ordered by mail. Women who cannot afford a prosthesis may wish to contact the Y-ME Prosthesis Bank (see listing below).

— Bathing suits and lingerie. Contact the sources mentioned above. In addition, a number of specialty boutiques sell clothing with post-mastectomy needs in mind, although there is not yet a national chain. Consult your yellow pages under "lingerie."

If you have difficulty locating a local retailer, contact the Reach to Recovery volunteer at your American Cancer Society office, call a local breast cancer support group, or contact the social work department of your hospital.

Becoming, Inc. *is a catalog of clothes and prostheses where 2% of profits go to breast cancer programs.* (800) 980-9085.

Breast Cancer Resource Center of the Princeton YWCA *offers free wigs and prostheses to women in need.* Paul Robeson Place, Princeton, NJ 08540. (609) 252-2003.

"Buyer's Guide to Wigs and Hairpieces". Two page summary from Ruth L. Weintraub, Inc., 420 Madison Avenue, Suite 406, NY 10017 (212) 838-1333.

Camp Health Care *offers breast forms and lingerie.* (800) 788-2267.

Charming with Dignity. *Supplies fashion-designed turbans and the "Softee Comfort Form" prosthesis for use immediately following breast surgery. Call for catalog.* 112 West 34 Street, Suite 1617, NY 10120. (800) 477-8188.

External Reconstruction Technology, Inc. *The "Third Alternative" is a non-surgical procedure that sculpts a breast from a cast of your body and then colors it to match your skin tone.* 4535 Benner Street, Philadelphia, PA 19135. (215) 333-8424.

Hat & Soul. *Sells hats by mail order.* (719) 991-HATS or e-mail tahmed@ix. netcom.com.

Intimate Image. *Offers full line of prostheses, lymphedema sleeves, lingerie.* (888) 848-7965.

ISA Designs. *Line of headware.* For catalog call (888) ISA-HATS.

Ladies' First Choice. *Post-breast surgery boutique, medicare accepted, newsletter published. Mail orders accepted.* 6465 Sunnyside Road SE, Salem, OR 97306. (503) 363-3940 or (800) 300-3940.

Ladies' First, Inc. Wholesale manufacturer of Softee Comfort form and mastectomy lingerie. *Accepts Medicare.* For provider near you (800) 497-8285 or www.wvi.com/ladies1.

Lady Grace Stores. *Chain of post-breast surgery stores with locations in Massachusetts, New Hampshire, Florida and Maine. Mail orders and Medicare accepted; they publish a newsletter.* (800) 922-0504.

Lands' End. *Five different styles of specially designed mastectomy swimwear.* Order a catalog from (800) 356-4444.

New Beginnings. *Post-mastectomy fashion service that takes phone orders.* 1556 Third Avenue, Room 603, NY 10128 (212) 369-6630.

Schwartz' Intimate Apparel. *Post-surgery boutique. Phone orders, Medicaid and Medicare accepted.* 108 Skokie Blvd., Wilmette, IL 60091 (708) 251-1118.

"TLC" is a catalog created by the American Cancer Society. *Medicare reimbursement available.* For catalog, call (800) 850-9445.

Y-ME Prosthesis and Wig Bank. *Y-ME maintains a prosthesis and wig bank for women with financial need. If the appropriate size is available, Y-ME will mail anywhere in the country for a nominal handling fee.* (800) 221-2141.

"Beauty of Control" (1995) with Jill Eikenberry, *videotape created by Laurie Feldman about cosmetic and emotional side effects of treatment.* Medical Video Productions, 450 North New Ballas Rd, Suite 266, St. Louis MO 63141 (800) 822-3100.

"Best Look Forward" (Graduate Hospital, 1991). *Videotape in which a makeup artist and hairdresser give advice and demonstrations, including on eyebrows and lashes.* 30 minutes, $45.00. Order from The Graduate Hospital Cancer Program, 1840 South Street, Philadelphia, PA 19146 or call Eileen Murphy at (215) 893-7298.

"Maintaining a Positive Image with Breast Cancer Surgery." *Videotape covering prosthetic, lingerie and swimsuit choices following breast cancer surgery.* $19.95 plus $2 postage. Johanna's on Call to Mend Esteem, 199 New Scotland Avenue, Albany, NY 122208. (518) 482-4178.

"Maintaining a Positive Image with Hair Loss and Cancer Therapy." *Videotape providing useful tips for maintaining self-esteem during treatment.* $19.95 plus $2 postage. Johanna's on Call to Mend Esteem, 199 New Scotland Avenue, Albany, NY 122208. (518) 482-4178.

Reconstruction

"Breast Reconstruction Following Mastectomy" American Society of Plastic and Reconstructive Surgeons 444 East Algonquin Road, Arlington Heights, Il 60005. (312) 228 9900. *For referrals call the Society's message tape at (800) 635-0635.*

RENU Breast Reconstruction Counseling. Einstein Medical Center, Philadelphia (215) 456-7387. *A support program staffed by trained volunteers who have had post-mastectomy reconstruction. Hot-line counseling and written materials are available.*

"A Sense of Balance: Breast Reconstruction." $29.95 videotape. To order call (617) 732-3379. *An interactive videotape developed by the staff at the Breast Evaluation Center of the Dana Farber Cancer Institute to inform about the pros and cons of various types of reconstruction.*

"Breast Reconstruction After Mastectomy" (1991, 4630). *Describes types of surgery with photographs and drawings and answers commonly asked questions.* 20 pages. ACS (800) ACS-2345.

Marilyn Snyder, *An Informed Decision: Understanding Breast Reconstruction.* (NY: M. Evans/Little, Brown, 1989). Paperback $12.95. *An informative mixture of one woman's account and clearly presented illustrated information about breast reconstruction after mastectomy.*

Lymphedema

The National Lymphedema Network and Network Hotline, 2211 Post Street, Suite 404, San Francisco, CA 94115. (800) 541-3259; nln@lymphnet.org; www.lymphnet.org.. *Nonprofit organization that provides patients and professionals with information about prevention and treatment of this complication of lymph node surgery. Call hotline for referrals for medical treatment, physical therapy, general information and support in your area. They will send an information packet.*

Breast Cancer Physical Therapy Center, 1905 Spruce Street, Philadelphia, PA 19103. *Provide a booklet on exercises to help manage lymphedema.* Cost is $8.95 which includes shipping.

Jeannie Burt, et al. *Lymphedema: A Breast Cancer Patient's Guide to Prevention and Healing.* (Hunter House, 2000). Paperback. *Covers preventing lymphedema, and reducing lymphedema through professional therapy and self-massage.*

Joan Swirsky and Diane Sackett Nannary. *Coping with Lymphedema.* (Garden City Park, NY: Avery, 1998). *Practical guide to understanding, treating and living with lymphedema.* (800) 548-5757 x123.

Diet

American Institute for Cancer Research, 1759 R Street NW, Washington DC 20009. *Provides information on cancer and nutrition, publishes a newsletter and cookbooks, offers a hotline for nutrition-related cancer inquiries.* (800) 843-8114, www. aicr.org.

"Eating Hints for Cancer Patients" (98–2079, 1998). *Suggestions and recipes.* NCI 4-CANCER.

Saundra N. Aker and Polly Lennsen, *A Guide to Good Nutrition During and After Chemotherapy and Radiation* (3rd edition, 1988). *Practical approach to nutrition.* Order from The Fred Hutchinson Cancer Research Center Clinical Nutrition Program, 1124 Columbia Street, Room E211, Seattle, WA 98104. (206) 667-4834.

Daniel W. Nixon, *The Cancer Recovery Eating Plan: The Right Foods to Help Fuel Your Recovery* (NY: Random House, 1996). Paperback. *Includes a three-month eating plan and recipes.*

Donna Weihofen, Christina Marino, *The Cancer Survival Cookbook* (Minneapolis, MN: Chronimed Pub, 1997). Paperback. *Nourishing recipes and advice on overcoming eating problems.* Bookstores or (800) 848-2793.

Exercise

The YWCA ENCOREplus Program. *Designed to provide supportive discussion and rehabilitative exercise for women who have been treated for breast cancer.* Call your local YWCA for more information, or contact the YWCA Office of Women's Health Initiatives, 624 9th Street, NW, Washington, DC 20001. (202) 628-3636.

"Beginning Ballet for the Post-Mastectomy Woman" (First Position Productions, 1990). *Videotape of a class of women who have had mastectomies.* 50 minutes, $39.95. First Position Productions, Star Route Box 472, Sausalito, CA 94965. (415) 381-9034.

"Better than Before Fitness." *Video with exercises designed to restore muscle tone and range of motion.* 50 minutes, $49.95 plus $5.95 shipping. Order from (800) 488-8354 or www.breastfit.com.

"Focus on Healing Through Movement & Dance" (Sherry LeBed Davis/Albert Einstein Medical Center, PA). Movement program and 14-day plan for breast cancer survivors of all ages and fitness levels. Video $29.75 plus tax and shipping (800) 366-6038 or www.enhancementinc.com.

"Get Up and Go: After Breast Surgery." (ACS/University of Michigan, Oak Park, MI, 21989). Order from *Health Tapes Inc.*, (888) 225-5486. *Total body exercises demonstrated by five women who have had a mastectomy, lumpectomy or reconstructive surgery. Increasingly challenging levels.* 60 minutes, $39.95.

"One Move at a Time: Exercise for Women Recovering from Breast Cancer" (Minneapolis: Green Light Productions, 1996). *Video with simple, gentle exercise.* $19.95 plus $4.45 shipping. Order from The Cancer Club, 6533 Limerick Drive, Edina, MN 55439, (800) 586-9062, or www.cancerclub.com.

Stretch Exercise Program (1988). *An eight-week exercise/support program for women who have had surgery for breast cancer. Manual, video materials and sessions offered free through volunteer services.* Call the Alabama Division of the ACS (205) 879-2242.

MENOPAUSE

Menomaven (www.menomaven.com): *Source of a wonderful set of cards for sorting through menopause.*

Powersurge (www.dearest.com). *One of the first, and the best source of information for menopausal women.*

National Women's Health Network, 1325 G Street NW, Washington, DC 20005. *Written packets and booklets on many aspects of women's health, including menopause, benign and malignant breast diseases.*

Women's Health Initiative. 1-800-54-WOMEN. *This is the first controlled, national study to look at postmenopausal women and their health including hormone replacement therapy, diet, calcium and exercise. If we do not participate, we will never know the answers. Call to find the center closest to you.*

Women's Health in Midlife (www.cw.bc.ca/womens/midlife/). *The Women's Health in Midlife Project (W.H.I.M.) is a provincial initiative designed to help women make informed choices about managing key midlife health issues through health education and community action.*

Sandra Coney, *The Menopause Industry: How the Medical Establishment Exploits Women* (Alameida, CA: Hunter House, 1994). *May be ordered by calling 1-800 266-5592. This book describes the most accurate view of menopause I have seen. It will wake you up.*

Paula Brown Doress, Diana Laskin Siegel, and The Midlife and Older Women Book Project, *Ourselves, Growing Older* (New York: Simon and Schuster, 1987). *Good overview of midlife and beyond, written in cooperation with the Boston Women's Health Book Collective.*

Paula Brown Dranov, *Estrogen: Is it Right for You? A Thorough Factual Guide to Help You Decide.* (New York: Simon and Schuster, 1993). *A short, balanced book on the pros and cons of hormone therapy.*

Sadja Greenwood, M.D., *Menopause Naturally: Preparing for the Second Half of Life* (San Francisco: Volcano Press, 1989). *Good discussion of menopause without hormone replacement therapy, and the dangers of hormonal replacement.*

Dee Ito, *Without Estrogen: Natural Remedies for Menopause and Beyond* (New York: Random House, 1995). Paperback.

Carol Laudau, Michele G. Cyr and Anne W. Moulton, *The Complete Book of Menopause* (New York: Berkeley, 1992). *Written by two gynecologists and a psychologist, this book is a good overall guide to menopause in all of its aspects. It sticks to traditional medicine and lifestyle issues and doesn't discuss alternative therapies.*

Susan M. Love, *Dr. Susan Love's Hormone Book: Making Informed Choices About Menopause.* (New York: Times Books, 1998). Paperback.

Janine O'Leary Cobb, *Understanding Menopause: Answers and Advice for Women in the Prime of Life.* (New York: Penguin, 1993). *A very good and friendly book by the editor of the newsletter: 'A Friend Indeed.'*

Susan Perry and Katherine A. O'Hanlan, *Natural Menopause: The Complete Guide to a Woman's Most Misunderstood Passage.* (Reading, MA: Addison-Wesley, 1992). *A good guide to all of the aspects of menopause with a friendly balanced approach (doesn't include alternatives).*

Richard J. Santen, Margaret Borwhat, Sarah Gleason, *Menopause* (Bethesda: The Hormone Foundation, 1998). *Summary of a 1997 meeting that discussed postmenopausal hormone deficiency after breast cancer.* For a free copy, call The Hormone Foundation (800) HORMONE or www.hormone.org.

Ann M. Voda. *Menopause, Me, and You: The Sound of Women Pausing.* (Binghamton, New York: Haworth Press, 1997*). A wonderful book of women's experiences. It is especially strong in describing women's experiences of bleeding.*

Ann M. Voda, Margaret Dennerstein, and S.R. O'Donnell, *Changing Perspective on Menopause.* (Austin: University of Texas Press, 1982). *Menopause from an anthropological, literary, psychological, and physiological perspective.*

Honora Lee Wolfe. *Menopause: A Second Spring* (Boulder, CO: Blue Poppy, 1985*). A good overview of traditional Chinese medicine and how it views menopause.*

RECURRENCE AND METASTASIS

Free Wishes (www.agingwithdignity.org). *An online living will that is legal in 33 states and DC. Website includes advice on establishing a surrogate, advance directives, is free of charge.*

Choice in Dying, 200 Varick Street, New York, New York 10014 (800) 989-WILL. *A nonprofit educational organization which distributes the living will, a document that records a patient's wishes during treatment and in regard to terminal care.*

Hospice Resources: National Hospice Organization, 1901 North Moore Street, Suite 901, Arlington, VA 22209 (800) 658-8898 or www.nho.org. *Will provide a directory of hospice programs by state.*

Hospice Foundation of America, 2001 S Street NW, Suite 300, Washington DC 20009. (202) 638-5419 or www.hospicefoundation.org.

Hospice Link, 190 Westbrook Road, Essex CT 06426-0713. (800) 331 1620 or (203) 767-1620 in Alaska and Connecticut.

Royal Victoria Hospital Palliative Care Service, 687 Pine Avenue West, Montreal QC H3A 1A1 (514) 843-1542. *An independent national organization of groups providing palliative care and hospice in Canada.*

"After Breast Cancer: A Guide to Follow Up Care" (87–2400) National Cancer Institute. 11 pages. *Considers the importance of follow up, signs of recurrence and the physical and emotional effects of having had breast cancer.*

"Advanced Cancer: Living Each Day" (85–856) National Cancer Institute 30 pages. *A booklet written to make living with advanced cancer easier."*Caring for the Patient with Cancer at Home: A Guide for Patients and Families" (4656-PS 1988 edition) 40 pages. *A guidebook providing detailed helpful information on how to care for the patient at home.*

"I Still Buy Green Bananas: Living with Hope, Living with Breast Cancer" (Y-ME, 1997). *Practical advice and personal stories.* Single copies from Y-ME (800) 221-2141.

"Managing Cancer Pain" (1994). *Still current, consumer booklet details US Government's Agency for Health Care Policy guidelines for treating cancer pain.* Order from AHCPR Publications Clearinghouse (800) 358-9295.

"Questions and Answers about Pain Control: A Guide for People with Cancer and Their Families" (4518-PS, 1995). *Discusses pain control using both medical and non-medical methods.* 76 pages. ACS (800) ACS-2345 or NCI (800) 4-CANCER.

"When Cancer Recurs: Meeting the Challenge Again" (96–2709, 1996). *Booklet details the different types of recurrence, types of treatment.* 30 pages. NCI (800) 4-CANCER.

"On with Life," 1999 edition is NABCO's updated video about living with advanced breast cancer. Order free of charge from NABCO (888) 80-NABCO or nabcoinfo@aol.com.

Marcia Lattanzi-Licht with John Mahoney and Galen Miller. *The Hospice Choice: In Pursuit of a Peaceful Death.* (Fireside, 1998). *Coping with dying and providing comfort care rather than curative treatment.*

Musa Mayer, Linda Lamb (Editor). *Advanced Breast Cancer: A Guide to Living with Metastatic Disease,* 2nd edition (patient-centered guides). (O'Reilly & Associates, 1998). Paperback. *Updated, retitled edition of 1997 Holding Tight, Letting Go, is excellent.*

FINANCIAL AID, INSURANCE AND EMPLOYMENT

The viatical industry, which can provide a breast cancer patient with a portion of her life insurance benefits before death, has grown to more than 50 companies nationwide. For more information, contact your insurance company.

Airlifeline (800) 446 1231(eww.airlifeline.org). *A free, nationwide service that flies qualified patients to treatment centers nationwide.*

The American Federation of Clinical Oncologic Societies *has identified 15 basic criteria for choosing a health insurance plan to ensure coverage of high quality cancer care.* Available at www.asco.org.

American Preferred Prescription (800) 227-1195; Bio Logics (800) 850-4306; Community Prescription Service (800) 842-0502; Managed Rx Plans (800) 799-8765 and Medi-Express RX (800) 873-9773 *are services that ship medications by mail. Each has different policies regarding insurance and payment.*

The Breast Health Access for Women with Disabilities Project, Alta Bates Medical Center, Dept. of Rehabilitation, 2001 Dwight Way, Berkeley CA 94704 (510) 204-4866. *Provides direct services and public and professional education for this population.*

HealthAllies.com will help you negotiate your medical bills.

ICI Pharmaceutical Nolvadex (Tamoxifen) Patient Assistance Program, Manager Professional Services, ICI Pharmaceuticals, Division of ICI Americas Inc, Wilmington Delaware 19897. (800)-456-5678. *Provides tamoxifen to patients with financial need. Write for an application.*

American Association of Retired People (AARP) Pharmacy Service. Catalog Dept., Box 19229, Alexandria , VA 22320. *Members can use their non-profit service to save on prescriptions delivered by mail. Good for tamoxifen (Novaldex). Write for free catalog.*

Corporate Angel Network Inc (CAN), Westchester County Airport, Building 1, White Plains, New York 10604 (914) 328-1313 (www.corpangelnetwork. org). *A nationwide program designed to give patients with cancer the use of available seats on corporate aircraft to get to and from recognized treatment centers. There is no cost or any financial need requirement.*

Mission Air Transportation Network (Canada), 77 Bloor Street West, Suite 1711, Toronto, ON M5S 3A1 (416) 924-9333. *Same as above.*

National Cancer Institute, Bethesda, Maryland 20892-4200. (800) 638-6694. *Patients who are treated here as part of a clinical study receive their treatment free and may be housed free of charge at the hospital facilities of the NCI.*

Practical Advice: Pharmaceutical Company Breast Cancer Patient Assistance Programs

One of the most common concerns of women with breast cancer is obtaining adequate reimbursement for treatment, especially when drug therapy is ongoing. Some necessary drugs and treatments are not covered by Medicare and insurance plans—an unneeded frustration at a difficult and overwhelming time. The following is a listing of selected company reimbursement assistance programs for oncology-related products.

These programs are best accessed by a physician or nurse on the breast cancer patient's behalf. Eligibility requirements and application procedures vary with each program. Programs also vary by type of assistance, including reimbursement counseling, assistance with filing claims, appeal of denied claims and enrollment in State and Federal health insurance programs. Some companies offer free products for women who are uninsured and can demonstrate financial need. Since programs change, check the website of the Pharmaceutical Research and Manufacturers of America (PhRMA) at www.phrma.org for updates.

Adria Laboratories
ADRIA Pt. Assist Plan
Columbus OH
(614) 764-8100
Adriamycin, Vincristine, Vinblastine

ALZA Pharmaceuticals
ALZA Oncology Connection Program
(800) 609-1083
Doxil (liposomal doxorubicin)

Amgen, Inc.
Amgen SAFETYNET® Program
(800) 272-9376
Epogen (epoetin alfa),
Neupogen (filgrastim)

AstraZeneca Pharmaceuticals
Patient Assistance Program
(800) 424-3727
Nolvadex (tamoxifen citrate),
Arimidex (anastrozole),
Zoladex (goserelin)

Aventis Pharmaceuticals
Aventis Oncology Program (PACT)
Providing Access to Chemotherapy
(800) 996-6626
Taxotere (docetaxel)

Bristol-Myers Squibb
Oncology/Immunology
Patient Assistance Program
(800) 332-2056
BCNU (carmustine),
Cisplatin (plastinol),
Cytoxan (cyclophosphamide),
Megace (megestrol),
Taxol (paclitaxel)

Genentech, Inc.
Uninsured Pt Assist Prgrm
(800) 879-4747
Herceceptin (trastuzumab)

Glaxo Wellcome,Inc.
Pt Assistance Program
(800) 722-9294

Wellcovorin (leucovorin),
Navelbine (vinorelbine tartrate)

Immunex Reimbursement Hotline
(800) 321-4669
Leucovorin Calcium (leucovorin),
Leukine (sargramostim),
methotrexate,
Novantrone (mitoxantrone)

Eli Lilly Oncology
Lilly Cares
(800) 545-6962
Velban (vinblastine),
Oncovin (vincristine)

Merck and Co., Inc.
The Merck Patient Assistance Program
(800) 994-2111
Decadron (dexamethasone)

Novartis Pharmaceuticals
Novartis Pt Asst Program
(800) 257-3273
Aredia (pamidronate disodium),
Femara (letrozole)

Ortho Biotech, Inc.
Procritline™
(800) 553-3851
Procrit (epoetin alfa)

Pharmacia Oncology
RxMAP Prescription Medication Assistance Program
(800) 242-7014
Adriamycin (doxorubicin),
Provera/Depo-Provera
(medroxyprogesterone),
Zinecard (dexrazoxane)

Roche Laboratories, Inc.
Roche Medical Needs Program
(800) 443-6676
Xeloda (capecitabine),
5-FU (fluorouracil)

Roxane Laboratories, Inc.
Patient Assistance Program
(800) 274-8651
Roxanol (morphine),
Roxicodone (oxycodone)

Schering Laboratories/
Key Pharmaceuticals
Commitment to Care

(800) 656-9485
Fareston (toremifine)

SmithKline Beecham Oncology
Access to Care Program
(800) 546-0420
Kytril (granisetron hydrochloride)

Insurance and Employment

Information and Counseling about Cancer and the Workplace. Phyllis Stein, Radcliffe Career Services, Radcliffe College 10 Garden Street, Cambridge Mass 02138 (617) 495-8631; and Barbara Lazarus, Associate Provost for Academic Programs, Carnegie Mellon University, Pittsburg, PA 15213 (412) 268 6994.

Patient Advocate Foundation (PAF) 780 Pilot House Drive, Suite 100C, Newport News, VA 23606. (800) 532-5274. *Provides patient education relative to managed care terminology and policy issues thrt may affect coverage, legal intervention services, and counseling to resolve job and insurance problems.*

The Job Accommodation Network *provides information on employee's rights under the Americans with Disabilities Act.* Call (800) ADA-WORK.

The National Insurance Consumer Helpline *answers consumer questions, offers problem-solving support and printed materials on life and property casualty insurance.* (800) 942-4242.

"Cancer Treatments Your Insurance Should Cover" (April 1995). Brochure you can order from Association of Community Cancer Centers, 11600 Nebel St, Suite 201, Rockville MD 20852 (301) 984-9496.

"What You Should Know About Health Insurance" (731,7/87)"What You Should Know About Disability Insurance" (733 10/87) Health Insurance Association of America, 1025 Connecticut Avenue, NW, Washington, DC 20004-3998. (202) 223-7780.

"Cancer: Your Job, Insurance and the Law (4585-ps /87) 6 pages. American Cancer Society. *Summarizes cancer patients' legal rights regarding insurance and employment.*

"The Americans with Disabilities Act: Protection for Cancer Patients Against Employment Discrimination" (4585, 1993). *Brochure defines the ADA law by describing employment rights of the cancer patient.* ACS (800) ACS-2345.

"Cancer. Your Job, Insurance and the Law" (4585-PS, 1987). *Summarizes cancer patients' legal rights; gives complaint procedure instructions.* 6 pages. ACS (800) ACS-2345.

"The Consumer's Guide to Disability Insurance" (1995). *A comprehensive guide to understanding disability insurance.* Health Insurance Assn of America (HIAA) (202) 824-1600.

"The Consumer's Guide to Long-Term Care Insurance (1995). HIAA, (202) 824-1600.

The Consumer's Guide to Medicare Supplement Insurance" (1995). *Instructions on using private insurance to supplement Medicare for maximum coverage.* HIAA (202) 824-1600.

"The Managed Care Answer Guide" (1997). *Reference handbook for cancer patients insured by managed care plans.* Consumer publication of the Patient Advocate Foundation (757) 873-6668.

"State Laws Relating to Breast Cancer" (CDC, March 1998). *The Centers for Disease Control and Prevention's summary of statutes across the country related to breast cancer.* Available from the CDC at (770) 488-4751 or www.cdc.gov.

"Surviving the Legal Challenges: A Resource Guide for Women with Breast Cancer" (California Women's Law Center, 1998). *Useful, 85 page reference on women's legal rights.* Free. (213) 637-9900 or www.cwlc.org.

"What Cancer Survivors Need to Know About Health Insurance" (1995). *Provides clear understanding of health insurance and how to receive maximum reimbursement on claims.* 37 pages. Single copies available free from National Coalition for Cancer Survivorship at (888) 937-6227. *The NCCS also publishes A Cancer Survivor's Almanac which contains useful information about insurance coverage.*

Charles B. Inlander and Eugene I. Pavalon, *Your Medical Rights.*

CLINICAL TRIALS

NCI Cancer trials (cancertrials.nci.nih.gov). *This is a listing of all cancer clinical trials.*

Center Watch: Clinical Trials Listing Service (www.centerwatch.com): *Lists all kinds of trials, not just breast cancer.*

National Surgical Adjuvant Breast and Bowel Project (www.nsabp.pitt. edu). *The group responsible for most of the breast cancer clinical trials including the tamoxifen prevention trial, STAR trial and lumpectomy and radiation trial.* 3550 Terrace Street Room 914, Pittsburgh, PA 15261 (412) 648-9720. *Will let you know of physicians participating in their trials in your area.*

Other regional websites include Eastern Clinical Oncology Group at ecog.dfci.Harvard.edu, Southwest Oncology Group at www.oo.saci.org and the CALGB at www-calgb.uchicago.edu.

Community Clinical Oncology Program (CCOP). (April 1993, updated periodically). National Cancer Institute (800 4-CANCER). *Network of 48 medical centers in 36 states and Puerto Rico that have been selected by the National Cancer Institute to participate in the introduction of the newest clinical protocols and to accrue patients to clinical trials.*

"Pharmaceutical Frontiers: Research on Breast Cancer" (1993). *Brochure providing overview of the latest research options. Lists the approved medications used in treating breast cancer and the drugs in clinical trials.* One copy free from Editor,

Pharmaceutical Frontiers, Pharmaceutical Manufacturer's Association, 1100 Fifteenth Street NW, Washington, DC 20005.

"Patient to Patient: Cancer Clinical Trials and You" (NIH No. V112). *15-minute videotape provides simple information.* NCI's CIS (800) 4-CANCER.

"Taking Part in Clinical Trials: What Cancer Patients Need to Know" (98–1998). *Booklet for patients considering participating in cancer treatment trials, includes glossary, also available in Spanish.* NCI's CIS (800) 4-CANCER.

POLITICS

Breast Cancer Advocacy Sites on the Internet

National

National Breast Cancer Coalition (www.natlbcc.org): *The national advocacy group (I am one of the founders) responsible for increasing breast cancer funding to $900 million. Good source of advocacy opportunities.*

Sister's Network (www.sistersnetworkinc.org). *Sisters Network is the first nationwide African-American breast cancer survivors organization targeting African-American Women.*

Local Advocacy Groups

(This is a selection; check susanlovemd.com or the NBCC for others in your area.)

Breast Cancer Action (www.bcaction.org): *San Francisco group which aims to influence policy changes necessary to end the breast cancer epidemic.*

Florida Breast Cancer Coalition (www.bellsouthbuzz.com): *Grassroots organization advocating for increased funding for breast cancer research. Member of the NBCC.*

Georgia Breast Cancer Coalition (www.gabcc.org): *Provides Georgians with an organizational platform from which to educate the public and increase research funding to eradicate breast cancer. Member of NBCC.*

Huntington Breast Cancer Action Coalition (www.hbac.org): *New York group dedicated to promoting and providing breast cancer awareness, education and advocacy, involvement and support. Member of NBCC.*

Linda Creed Breast Cancer Foundation (www.libertynet.org/lcbf/lcbf. html): *Philadelphia group committed to empowering women and their families to practice breast health, foster the healing process and establish a public agenda for prevention and cure. Member of NBCC.*

Massachusetts Breast Cancer Coalition (www.mbcc.org): *Aims to stop breast cancer epidemic through activism, advocacy and education, our goal is the cure, prevention and ultimate eradication of breast cancer.*

SHARE: Self-Help for Women with Breast and Ovarian Cancer (www. sharecancersupport.org): *New York advocacy group with hotlines in English and Spanish. Aims to provide people with breast or ovarian cancer with opportunities to be more in control of their lives during and after diagnosis.*

International Breast Cancer Advocacy

Brustkrebs-Initiative, Hilfe zur Brusthgesundheit (www.brustkrebs.net): *A German language Breast Cancer Activism site.*

Canadian Breast Cancer Foundation (www.cbcf.org): *Supports the advancement of breast cancer research, diagnosis and treatment.*

Europa Donna (www.oncoweb.com/edonna): *European Breast Cancer Coalition.*

Practical Advice: How to Get Involved with Breast Cancer Organizations

Political Advocacy. Although each person can become active through contacting local and national elected officials, the most effective way to bring about change can be by taking part in a national movement. The National Breast Cancer Coalition was formed in 1991 to involve women with the disease and those who care about them in changing public policy as it relates to progress against breast cancer. The NBCC's goals include expanding breast cancer research funding; improving access to screening, diagnosis and treatment for all women, and increasing the degree of influence of survivors in guiding research, trials and medical policy. The NBCC welcomes individuals and organizations as members. Many of the NBCC's members are local Coalitions in more than 40 states. A list of current state coordinators can be obtained by calling the NBCC: National Breast Cancer Coalition, 1707 L Street NW, Suite 1060, Washington, DC 20036 (202) 296-7477, (202) 265-6854 (fax) or www.natlbcc.org.

Roberta Altman, *Waking Up, Fighting Back: The Politics of Breast Cancer* (Little, Brown, 1996). *A journalist's survey of the issues and controversies of the breast cancer advocacy movement.*

Anne Kasper and Susan Ferguson, *Breast Cancer: Society Constructs an Epidemic* (New York: St. Martin's Press, 2000).

Ellen Leopold, *A Darker Ribbon: Breast Cancer, Women, and Their Doctors in the Twentieth Century* (Beacon Press, 1999).

Karen Stabiner, *To Dance with the Devil: The New War on Breast Cancer* (Dell, 1998). Paperback.

Virginia M. Soffa, *The Journey Beyond Breast Cancer: From the Personal to the Political.*

C

NCI-designated Cancer Centers Listed by State (http://www.nci.nih.gov/cancercenters/centerslist.html)

Alabama

Albert F. LoBuglio, M.D.
Director, UAB Comprehensive
  Cancer Center
University of Alabama at
  Birmingham
1824 Sixth Avenue South, Room
  237
Birmingham, Alabama 35293-3300
Tel: 205/934-5077
Fax: 205/975-7428
(Comprehensive Cancer Center)

Arizona

Daniel D. Von Hoff, M.D.
Director, Arizona Cancer Center
University of Arizona
1501 North Campbell Avenue
Tucson, Arizona 85724
Tel: 520/626-7925
Fax: 520/626-2284
(Comprehensive Cancer Center)

California

John S. Kovach, M.D.
Director, Cancer Research Center
Beckman Research Institute, City of
  Hope
Needleman Bldg., Room 204
1500 East Duarte Road
Duarte, California 91010
Tel: 626/301-8164
Fax: 323/865-0102
(Comprehensive Cancer Center)

Walter Eckhart, Ph.D.
Director, Cancer Center
Salk Institute
10010 North Torrey Pines Road
La Jolla, California 92037
Tel: 858/453-4100 X1386
Fax: 858/457-4765
(Cancer Center)

Erkki Ruoslahti, M.D.
President & CEO
The Burnham Institute

10901 North Torrey Pines Road
La Jolla, California 92037
Tel: 858/455-6480 X3209
Fax: 858/646-3198
(Cancer Center)

David Tarin, M.D., Ph.D.
Director, UCSD Cancer Center
University of California at San Diego
9500 Gilman Drive
La Jolla, California 92093-0658
Tel: 858/822-1222
Fax: 858/822-0207
(Clinical Cancer Center)

Judith C. Gasson, Ph.D.
Director, Jonsson Comprehensive
  Cancer Center
University of California Los Angeles
  Factor Building, Room 8-684
10833 Le Conte Avenue
Los Angeles, California 90095-1781
Tel: 310/825-5268
Fax: 310/206-5553
(Comprehensive Cancer Center)

Peter A. Jones, Ph.D.
Director, USC/Norris
  Comprehensive Cancer Center
University of Southern California
1441 Eastlake Avenue,
Rm. 815, MS #83
Los Angeles, California 90033
Tel: 323/865-0816
Fax: 323/865-0102
(Comprehensive Cancer Center)

Frank L. Meyskens, Jr., M.D.
Director, Chao Family
  Comprehensive Cancer Center
University of California at Irvine
101 The City Drive
Building. 23, Rt. 81, Room 406
Orange, California 92868
Tel: 714/456-6310
Fax: 714/456-2240
(Comprehensive Cancer Center)

Frank McCormick, Ph.D.
Director, UCSF Cancer Center &
  Cancer Research Institute
University of California San
  Francisco
2340 Sutter Street, Box 0128

San Francisco, California 94115-0128
Tel: 415/502-1710
Fax: 415/502-1712
(Comprehensive Cancer Center)

Colorado

Paul A. Bunn, Jr., M.D.
Director, University of Colorado
  Cancer Center
University of Colorado Health
  Science Center
4200 East 9th Avenue, Box B188
Denver, Colorado 80262
Tel: 303/315-3007
Fax: 303/315-3304
(Comprehensive Cancer Center)

Connecticut

Vincent T. DeVita, Jr., M.D.
Director, Yale Cancer Center
Yale University School of Medicine
333 Cedar Street, Box 208028
New Haven, Connecticut 06520-8028
Tel: 203/785-4371
Fax: 203/785-4116
(Comprehensive Cancer Center)

District of Columbia

Marc E. Lippman, M.D.
Director, Lombardi Cancer Research
  Center
Georgetown University Medical
  Center 3800 Reservoir Road, N.W.
Washington, DC 20007
Tel: 202/687-2110
Fax: 202/687-6402
(Comprehensive Cancer Center)

Florida

John C. Ruckdeschel, M.D.
Center Director & CEO
H.Lee Moffitt Cancer Center &
  Research Institute at the University
  of South Florida
12902 Magnolia Drive
Tampa, Florida 33612-9497
Tel: 813/979-7265
Fax: 813/979-3919
(Clinical Cancer Center)

Hawaii

Carl-Wilhem Vogel, M.D., Ph.D.
Director, Cancer Research Center of
   Hawaii
University of Hawaii at Manoa
1236 Lauhala Street
Honolulu, Hawaii 96813
Tel: 808/586-3013
Fax: 808/586-3052
(Clinical Cancer Center)

Illinois

Nicholas J. Vogelzang, M.D.
Director, Cancer Research Center
University of Chicago Cancer
   Research Center
South Maryland Avenue, MC 1140
Chicago, Illinois 60637-1470
Tel: 773/702-6180
Fax: 773/702-9311
(Comprehensive Cancer Center)

Steven Rosen, M.D.
Director, Robert H. Lurie Cancer
   Center
Northwestern University
303 East Chicago Avenue
Olson Pavilion 8250
Chicago, Illinois 60611
Tel: 312/908-5250
Fax: 312/908-1372
(Comprehensive Cancer Center)

Indiana

Richard F. Borch, M.D., Ph.D.
Director, Purdue University Cancer
   Center
Hansen Life Sciences Research
   Building
South University Street
West Lafayette, Indiana 47907-1524
Tel: 765/494-9129
Fax: 765/494-9193
(Cancer Center)

Stephen D. Williams, M.D.
Director, Indiana University Cancer
   Center
Indiana Cancer Pavilion
535 Barnhill Drive, Room 455
Indianapolis, Indiana 46202-5289

Tel: 317/278-0070
Fax: 317/278-0074
(Clinical Cancer Center)

Maine

Kenneth Paigen, Ph.D.
Director, The Jackson Laboratory
600 Main Street
Bar Harbor, Maine 04609-0800
Tel: 207/288-6041
Fax: 207/288-6044
(Cancer Center)

Maryland

Martin D. Abeloff, M.D.
Director, Johns Hopkins Oncology
   Center
North Wolfe Street, Room 157
Baltimore, Maryland 21287-8943
Tel: 410/955-8822
Fax: 410/955-6787
(Comprehensive Cancer Center)

Massachusetts

David G. Nathan, M.D.
President, Cancer Center
Dana-Farber Cancer Institute
44 Binney Street, Rm. 1828
Boston, Massachusetts 02115
Tel: 617/632-2155
Fax: 617/632-2161
(Comprehensive Cancer Center)

Richard O. Hynes, Ph.D.
Director & Professor of Biology
Center for Cancer Research
Massachusetts Institute of
   Technology
77 Massachusetts Avenue,
Room E17-110
Cambridge, Massachusetts 02139-
   4307
Tel: 617/253-6422
Fax: 617/253-8357
(Cancer Center)

Michigan

Max S. Wicha, M.D.
Director, Comprehensive Cancer
   Center

University of Michigan 6302 CGC/
0942
1500 East Medical Center Drive
Ann Arbor, Michigan 48109-0942
Tel: 734/936-1831
Fax: 734/615-3947
(Comprehensive Cancer Center)

William P. Peters, M.D., Ph.D.
Director & Chief Executive Officer
Barbara Ann Karmanos Cancer
Institute
Wayne State University
Operating the Meyer L. Prentis
Comprehensive
Cancer Center of Metropolitan
Detroit
4100 John R. Street
Detroit, Michigan 48201-1379
Tel: 313/993-7777
Fax: 313/993-7165
(Comprehensive Cancer Center)

Minnesota

John H. Kersey, M.D.
Director, University of Minnesota
Cancer Center
Box 806, 420 Delaware Street, S.E.
Minneapolis, Minnesota 55455
Tel: 612/624-8484
Fax: 612/626-3069
(Comprehensive Cancer Center)

Franklyn G. Prendergast, M.D., Ph.D.
Director, Mayo Clinic Cancer Center
Mayo Foundation
200 First Street, S.W.
Rochester, Minnesota 55905
Tel: 507/284-3753
Fax: 507/284-9349
(Comprehensive Cancer Center)

Nebraska

Kenneth H. Cowan, M.D., Ph.D.
Director, University of Nebraska
Medical Center/
Eppley Cancer Center
600 South 42nd Street
Omaha, Nebraska 68198-6805
Tel: 402/559-7081
Fax: 402/559-4651
(Cancer Center)

New Hampshire

E. Robert Greenberg, M.D.
Director, Norris Cotton Cancer
Center
Dartmouth-Hitchcock Medical
Center
One Medical Center Drive, Hinman
Box 7920
Lebanon, New Hampshire 03756-
0001
Tel: 603/650-6300
Fax: 603/650-6333
(Comprehensive Cancer Center)

New Jersey

William N. Hait, M.D., Ph.D.
Director, The Cancer Institute of New
Jersey
Robert Wood Johnson Medical
School
195 Little Albany Street, Room 2002B
New Brunswick, New Jersey 08901
Tel: 732/235-8064
Fax: 732/235-8094
(Clinical Cancer Center)

New York

I. David Goldman, M.D.
Director, Cancer Research Center
Albert Einstein College of Medicine
Chanin Building, Room 209
1300 Morris Park Avenue
Bronx, New York 10461
Tel: 718/430-2302
Fax: 718/430-8550
(Comprehensive Cancer Center)

David C. Hohn, M.D.
President & CEO, Roswell Park
Cancer Institute
Elm & Carlton Streets
Buffalo, New York 14263-0001
Tel: 716/845-2389
Fax: 716/845-7609
(Comprehensive Cancer Center)

Bruce W. Stillman, Ph.D.
Director, Cold Spring Harbor
Laboratory
P.O. Box 100
Cold Spring Harbor, New York 11724

Tel: 516/367-8383
Fax: 516/367-8879
(Cancer Center)

Franco M. Muggia, M.D.
Director, Kaplan Cancer Center
New York University Medical Center
550 First Avenue
New York, New York 10016
Tel: 212/263-6485
Fax: 212/263-8210
(Comprehensive Cancer Center)

Paul A. Marks, M.D.
President, Memorial Sloan-Kettering
    Cancer Center
1275 York Avenue
New York, New York 10021
Tel: 212/639-6561
Fax: 212/717-3299
(Comprehensive Cancer Center)

Daniel W. Nixon, M.D.
President, American Health
    Foundation
320 East 43rd Street
New York, New York 10017
Tel: 212/953-1900
Fax: 212/687-2339
(Cancer Center)

Karen H. Antman, M.D.
Director, Herbert Irving
    Comprehensive Cancer Center;
    College of Physicians & Surgeons
Columbia University
177 Fort Washington Avenue
6th Floor, Room 435
New York, New York 10032
Tel: 212/305-8602
Fax: 212/305-3035
(Comprehensive Cancer Center)

North Carolina

H. Shelton Earp, M.D.
Lineberger Professor of Cancer
    Research & Director, UNC
    Lineberger Comprehensive Cancer
    Center
University of North Carolina Chapel
    Hill School of Medicine, CB-7295
102 West Drive

Chapel Hill, North Carolina 27599-
    7295
Tel: 919/966-3036
Fax: 919/966-3015
(Comprehensive Cancer Center)

O. Michael Colvin, M.D.
Director, Duke Comprehensive
    Cancer Center
Duke University Medical Center Box
    3843
Durham, North Carolina 27710
Tel: 919/684-5613
Fax: 919/684-5653
(Comprehensive Cancer Center)

Frank M. Torti, M.D.
Director, Comprehensive Cancer
    Center
Wake Forest University
Bowman Gray School of Medicine
Medical Center Boulevard
Winston-Salem, North Carolina
    27157-1082
Tel: 336/716-7971
Fax: 336/716-0293
(Comprehensive Cancer Center)

Ohio

James K. V. Willson, M.D.
Director, Ireland Cancer Center
Case Western Reserve University and
    University Hospitals of Cleveland
11100 Euclid Ave., Wearn 151
Cleveland, Ohio 44106-5065
Tel: 216/844-8562
Fax: 216/844-7832
(Comprehensive Cancer Center)

Clara D. Bloomfield, M.D.
Director, Comprehensive Cancer
    Center
Arthur G. James Cancer Hospital
Ohio State University A455 Staring
    Loving Hall
300 West 10th Avenue
Columbus, Ohio 43210-1240
Tel: 614/293-7518
Fax: 614/293-7520
(Comprehensive Cancer Center)

Oregon

Grover C. Bagby, Jr., M.D.
Director, Oregon Cancer Center
Oregon Health Sciences University
3181 S.W. Sam Jackson Park Rd.,
    CR145
Portland, Oregon 97201-3098
Tel: 503/494-1617
Fax: 503/494-7086
(Clinical Cancer Center)

Pennsylvannia

John H. Glick, M.D.
Director, University of Pennsylvania
    Cancer Center
16th Floor Penn Tower
3400 Spruce Street
Philadelphia, Pennsylvania 19104-
    4283
Tel: 215/662-6065
Fax: 215/349-5325
(Comprehensive Cancer Center)

Giovanni Rovera, M.D.
Director, The Wistar Institute
3601 Spruce Street
Philadelphia, Pennsylvania 19104-
    4268
Tel: 215/898-3926
Fax: 215/573-2097
(Cancer Center)

Robert C. Young, M.D.
President, Fox Chase Cancer Center
7701 Burholme Avenue
Philadelphia, Pennsylvania 19111
Tel: 215/728-2781
Fax: 215/728-2571
(Comprehensive Cancer Center)

Carlo M. Croce, M.D.
Director, Kimmel Cancer Center
Thomas Jefferson University
233 South 10th Street
BLSB, Room 1050
Philadelphia, Pennsylvania 19107-
    5799
Tel: 215/503-4645
Fax: 215/923-3528
(Clinical Cancer Center)

Ronald B. Herberman, M.D.
Director, University of Pittsburgh
    Cancer Institute
3471 Fifth Avenue, Suite 201
Pittsburgh, Pennsylvania 15213-3305
Tel: 412/692-4670
Fax: 412/692-4665
(Comprehensive Cancer Center)

Tennessee

Arthur W. Nienhuis, M.D.
Director, St. Jude Children's Research
    Hospital
332 North Lauderdale
P.O. Box 318
Memphis, Tennessee 38105-2794
Tel: 901/495-3301
Fax: 901/525-2720
(Clinical Cancer Center)

Harold L. Moses, M.D.
Director, Vanderbilt Cancer Center
Vanderbilt University Medical
    Research Building II
Nashville, Tennessee 37232-6838
Tel: 615/936-1782
Fax: 615/936-1790
(Clinical Cancer Center)

Texas

John Mendelsohn, M.D.
President, University of Texas
M.D. Anderson Cancer Center
1515 Holcombe Boulevard, Box 91
Houston, Texas 77030
Tel: 713/792-6000
Fax: 713/799-2210
(Comprehensive Cancer Center)

Charles A. Coltman, Jr., M.D.
Director, San Antonio Cancer
    Institute
8122 Datapoint Drive, Suite 600
San Antonio, Texas 78229-3264
Tel: 210/616-5580
Fax: 210/692-9823
(Comprehensive Cancer Center)

Utah

Stephen M. Prescott, M.D.
Director, Huntsman Cancer Institute

University of Utah
15 North 2030 East, Rm 7410
Salt Lake City, Utah 84112-5330 .
Tel: 801/581-4330
Fax: 801/585-3833
(Clinical Cancer Center)

Vermont

David W. Yandell, Sc.D.
Director, Vermont Cancer Center
University of Vermont Medical
    Alumni Bldg
Burlington, Vermont 05405
Tel: 802/656-4414
Fax: 802/656-8788
(Comprehensive Cancer Center)

Virginia

Charles E. Myers, Jr., M.D.
Director, Cancer Center
University of Virginia,
Health Sciences Center Hospital Box
    334
Charlottesville, Virginia 22908
Tel: 804/924-2562
Fax: 804/982-0918
(Clinical Cancer Center)

Gordon D. Ginder, M.D.
Professor of Medicine & Director
Massey Cancer Center
Virginia Commonwealth University
P.O. Box 980037
Richmond, Virginia 23298-0037
Tel: 804/828-0450
Fax: 804/828-8453
(Clinical Cancer Center)

Washington

Leland H. Hartwell, Ph.D.
President & Director
Fred Hutchinson Cancer Research
    Center
1100 Fairview Avenue, North
P.O. Box 19024, D1060
Seattle, Washington 98104-1024
Tel: 206/667-4305
Fax: 206/667-5268
(Comprehensive Cancer Center)

Wisconsin

John E. Niederhuber, M.D.
Director, Comprehensive Cancer
    Center
University of Wisconsin
600 Highland Ave., Rm. K4/610
Madison, Wisconsin 53792-0001
Tel: 608/263-8610
Fax: 608/263-8613
(Comprehensive Cancer Center)

Norman R. Drinkwater, Ph.D.
Director, McArdle Laboratory for
    Cancer Research
University of Wisconsin 1400
University Avenue, Room 1009
Madison, Wisconsin 53706-1599
Tel: 608/262-2177 or 7992
Fax: 608/262-2824
(Cancer Center)

Types of Centers:

Cancer Centers: 10
Clinical Cancer Centers: 12
Comprehensive Cancer Centers: 37
Total: 59

D

The Wellness Community
Physician /Patient Statement[1]

In 1990, six prominent Los Angeles oncologists met with the staff of the Wellness Community, over a period of six months, to answer the question, "What can cancer patients expect from their oncologists?" The question was considered important since they believed that the relationship between the patient and the physician can affect the course of the illness. After many meetings they arrived at *The Wellness Community Patient/Oncologist Statement*. They then tested the *Statement* with their patients and found that a great majority of their patients had confidence in their physician and considered their relationship "excellent." However, there was agreement among patients that the issues considered in the *Statement* were important to a continuation of such "excellent" relationships. The *Statement* below was then published in the UCLA Jonsson Comprehensive Cancer Center Bulletin and is given by physicians to their patients.

The effective treatment of serious illness requires a considerable effort by both the patient and the physician. A clear understanding by both of us as to what each of us can realistically and reasonably expect of the other will do much to enhance the outlook. I am giving this "statement" to you as one step in making our relationship as effective and productive as possible. It might be helpful if you would read this statement and, if you think it appropriate, discuss it with me. As your physician, I will make every effort to:

1. Provide you with the care most likely to be beneficial to you.
2. Inform and educate you about your situation, and the various treatment al-

1. Reprinted with the kind permission of The Wellness Community

ternatives. How detailed an explanation is given will be dependent upon your specific desires.

3. Encourage you to ask questions about your illness and its treatment and to answer your questions as clearly as possible. I will also attempt to answer the questions asked by your family; however, my primary responsibility is to you, and I will discuss your medical situation only with those people authorized by you.

4. Remain aware that all major decisions about the course of your care shall be made by you. However, I will accept the responsibility for making certain decisions if you want me to.

5. Assist you to obtain other professional opinions if you desire, or if I believe it to be in your best interests.

6. Relate to you as one competent adult to another, always attempting to consider your emotional, social and psychological needs as well as your physical needs.

7. Spend a reasonable amount of time with you on each return visit unless required by something urgent to do otherwise, and give you my undivided attention during that time.

8. Honor all appointment times unless required by something urgent to do otherwise.

9. Return phone calls as promptly as possible, especially those you indicate are urgent.

10. Make available test results promptly if you desire such reports and I will indicate to you, at the time the test is given, when you can expect the results and who you should call to get them.

11. Provide you with any information you request concerning my professional training, experience, philosophy and fees.

12. Respect your desire to try treatment that might not be conventionally accepted. However, I will give you my honest opinion about such unconventional treatments.

13. Maintain my active support and attention throughout the course of the illness.

I hope that you as the patient will make every effort to:

1. Comply with our agreed-upon treatment plan.
2. Be as candid as possible with me about what you need and expect from me.
3. Inform me if you desire another professional opinion.
4. Inform me of all forms of therapy you are involved with.
5. Honor all appointment times unless required by something urgent to do otherwise.
6. Be as considerate as possible of my need to adhere to a schedule to see other patients.
7. Attempt to make all phone calls to me during the working hours. Call on nights and weekends only when absolutely necessary.
8. Attempt to coordinate the requests of your family and confidantes, so that I do not have to answer the same questions about you to several different persons.

Notes

1. THE BREAST AND ITS DEVELOPMENT

1. Cooper A. *On the Anatomy of the Breast.* London: Orme, Green, Brown and Longmans, 1840.

2. Petrakis N. Personal communication. 1999.

3. Ayalah D, Weinstock IJ. *Breasts*, vol. 1. New York: Summit Books, 1979.

4. Stanway A, Stanway P. *The Breast.* London: Granada Publishing Ltd., 1982.

5. New England Research Institute. Women and their health in Massachusetts. Final report 1991. Watertown, MA, 1991.

6. Sluijmer AV, Heineman MJ, DeJong FH, Evers JL. Endocrine activity of the postmenopausal ovary: The effects of pituitary down-regulation and oophorectomy. *Journal of Clinical Endocrinology and Metabolism* 1995; 80:2163–2167.

7. Ushiroyama T, Sugimoto O. Endocrine function of the peri- and postmenlopausal ovary. *Hormone Research* 1995; 44:64–68.

8. Hreshchyshyn MM, Hopkins A, Zylstra S, Anbar M. Effects of natural menopause, hysterectomy, and oophorectomy on lumbar spine and femoral neck bone densities. *Obstetrics and Gynecology* 1988; 72:631.

9. Ayalah and Weinstock, *Breasts.*

10. Robinson JE, Short RV. Changes in breast sensitivity at puberty, during the menstrual cycle, and at parturition. *British Medical Journal* 1977; 1:1188.

2. GETTING ACQUAINTED WITH YOUR BREASTS

1. Kash K, Holland J, Halper M, et al. Psychological distress and surveillance behaviors of women with a family history of breast cancer. *Journal of the National Cancer Institute* 1992; 84:24.

3. BREAST FEEDING

1. American Academy of Pediatrics. *Pediatrics* 1997; 100(6):1035–1039.
2. Roberts KL, Reiter M, Schuster D. A comparison of chilled and room temperature cabbage leaves in treating breast engorgement. *Journal of Human Lactation* 1995; 11:191–194.
3. Guinee VF, Olsson H, Moller T, et al. Effect of pregnancy on prognosis for young women with breast cancer. *Lancet* 1994; 343:1587.
4. Petrek J. Breast cancer during pregnancy. *Cancer Supplement* 1994; 74(1):518–27.
5. Semple JL, Lugowski SJ, Baines CJ, Smith DC, McHugh A. Breast milk contamination and silicone implants: Preliminary results using silicon as a proxy measurement for silicone. *Plastic Reconstructive Surgery* 1998; 102:528–533.
6. Enger SM, Ross RK, Paganini-Hill A, Bernstein L. Breastfeeding experience and breast cancer risk among postmenopausal women. *Cancer Epidemiology, Biomarkers & Prevention* 1998; 7(May):365–369.
7. Newcomb PA, Storer BE, Longnecker MP, et al. Lactation and a reduced risk of premenopausal breast cancer. *New England Journal of Medicine* 1994; 330(2):81.
8. Newcomb PA, Weiss NS, Storer BE, Scholes D, Young BE, Voigt LF. Breast self-examination in relation to the occurrence of advanced breast cancer. *Journal of the National Cancer Institute* 1991; 83(4):260.
9. Little RE, Anderson KW, Irvin CH, et al. Maternal alcohol use during breast feeding and infant mental and motor development at one year. *New England Journal of Medicine* 1989; 321:425.

4. VARIATIONS IN DEVELOPMENT

1. Stanway A, Stanway P. *The Breast.* London: Granada Publishing Ltd., 1982.

5. PLASTIC SURGERY

1. Letterman G, Schurter MA. A history of mammoplasty with emphasis on correction of ptosis and macromastia. In: Goldwyn R, ed. *Plastic and Reconstructive Surgery of the Breast.* Boston: Little, Brown, 1976; 361.
2. Hatcher C, Brooks L, Love C. Breast cancer and silicone implants: Psychological consequences for women. *Journal of the National Cancer Institute* 1993; 85(17):1361.
3. Sanchez-Guerrero J, Colditz GA, Karlson EW, Hunter DJ, Speizer FE, Liang MH. Silicone breast implants and the risk of connective-tissue diseases and symptoms. *New England Journal of Medicine* 1995; 332(25):1666–70.
4. Duffy MJ, Woods JE. Health risks of failed silicone gel breast implants: a 30-year clinical experience. *Plastic Reconstructive Surgery* 1994; 94(2):295–9.
5. Merkatz RB, Bagley GP, McCarthy EJ. A qualitative analysis of self-reported expe-

riences among women encountering difficulties with silicone breast implants. *Journal of Women's Health* 1993; 2(2):105.

6. Silverstein MJ, Gierson ED, Gamagami P, Handel N, Waisman JR. Breast cancer diagnosis and prognosis in women augmented with silicone gel-filled implants. *Cancer* 1990; 66(July 1):97.

7. Noone RB. A review of the possible health implications of silicone breast implants. *Cancer* 1997; 79(9):1747–1756.

8. Silverman BS, Brown SL, Bright RA, et al. A critical assessment of the relationship between silicone implants and connective tissue diseases (a review). *Regul Toxicology Pharmacology* 1996; 23(1 Pt 1):74–85.

9. Deapen DM, Brody GS. Augmentation mammaplasty and breast cancer: a 5-year update of the Los Angeles study. *Plastic Reconstructive Surgery* 1992; 89(4):660–5.

10. Berkel H, Birdsell DC, Jenkins H. Breast augmentation: a risk factor for breast cancer? *New England Journal of Medicine* 1992; 326(25):1649–53.

11. Heuston JT. Unilateral agenesis and hypoplasia: Difficulties and suggestions. In: R G, ed. *Plastic and Reconstructive Surgery of the Breast*. Boston: Little, Brown, 1976; 361.

12. Gifford S. Emotional attitudes toward cosmetic breast surgery: Loss and restitution of the 'ideal' self. In: Goldwyn R, ed. *Plastic and Reconstructive Surgery of the Breast*. Boston: Little, Brown, 1976; 117.

6. BREAST PAIN AND THE MYTH OF FIBROCYSTIC DISEASE

1. Boyd NF, Lockwood GA, Byng JW, Tritchler DL, Yaffe MJ. Mammographic densities and breast cancer risk. *Cancer Epidemiology, Biomarkers & Prevention* 1998; 7(December):1133–1144.

2. Cancer Committee of the American College of Pathologists. Is "fibrocystic" disease of the breast precancerous? *Archives of Pathology and Laboratory Medicine* 1986; 110:173.

3. Preece PE, Hughes LE, Mansel RE, et al. Clinical syndromes of mastalgia. *Lancet* 1976; 2:670.

4. Mansel RE. Breast pain. *British Medical Journal* 1994; 309(1 October):866–868.

5. Sitruk-Ware R, Sterkers N, Mauvais-Jarvis P. Benign breast disease I: Hormonal investigation. *Obstetrics and Gynecology* 1979; 53:457.

6. Watt-Boolsen S, Ryegaard R, Blichert-Toft M. Primary periareolar abscess in the nonlactating breast: Risk of recurrence. *American Journal of Surgery* 1987; 153:571.

7. Kumar S, Mansel RE, Hughes LE, et al. Prolactin response to thyrotropin-releasing hormone stimulation and dopaminergic inhibition in benign breast disease. *Cancer* 1984; 53:1311.

8. Ayres J, Gidwani G. The 'luteal breast:' Hormonal and sonographic investigations of benign breast disease in patients with cyclic mastalgia. *Fertility and Sterility* 1983; 40:779.

9. Wren BG. The breast and the menopause. *Bailliere's Clinical Obstetrics and Gynaecology* 1996; 10(3):433–447.

10. Barros AC, Mottola J, Ruiz CA, Borges MN, Pinotti JA. Reassurance in the treatment of mastalgia. *The Breast Journal* 1999; 5(3):162–165.

11. Page JK, Mansel RE, Hughes SE. Clinical experience of drug treatments for mastalgia. *Lancet* 1985; 2:373.

12. Steinbrunn BS, Zera RT, Rodriguez JL. Mastalgia: Tailoring treatment to type of breast pain. *Postgraduate Medicine* 1997; 102(5):183–198.

13. Greenblatt RB, Dmowsky WP, Mahesh VB, et al. Clinical studies with an anti-gonadotropin-Danazol. *Fertility and Sterility* 1971; 22:102.

14. Mansel RE, Dogliotti L. European multicentre trial of bromocriptine in cyclical mastalgia. *Lancet* 1990; 335:190.

15. Fentiman IS, Caleffi M, Brame K, et al. Double-blind controlled trial of tamoxifen therapy for mastalgia. *Lancet* 1986; 1:287.

16. Steinbrunn et al. Mastalgia.

17. Hamed H, Chaudary MA, Caleffi M, Fentiman IS. LHRH analogues for treatment of recurrent and refractory mastalgia. *Annual Review College of Surg England* 1990; 72(4):221–224.

18. Boyd N, McGuire V, Shannon P, et al. Effect of low-fat high carbohydrate diet on symptoms of cyclical mastopathy. *Lancet* 1988; 2(8603):128.

19. Ghent WR, Eskin BA, Low DA, al. e. Iodine replacement in fibrocystic disease of the breast. *Canadian Journal of Surgery* 1993; 36(453).

20. LeBan MM, Meerscharet JR, Taylor RS. Breast pain: A symptom of cervical radiculopathy. *Archives of Physical Medicine and Rehabilitation* 1979; 60:315.

21. Page et al. Clinical Experience of drug treatments for mastalgia.

22. Maddox PR, Harrison BJ, Mansel RE, al. e. Non-cyclical mastalgia: an improved classification and treatment. *British Journal of Surgery* 1989; 76(9):901–904.

23. Preece et al. Clinical syndromes of mastalgia.

7. BREAST INFECTIONS AND NIPPLE PROBLEMS

1. Thomsen AC, Espersen MD, Maigaard S. Course and treatment of milk stasis, noninfectious inflammation of the breast and infectious mastitis in nursing women. *American Journal of Obstetrics and Gynecology* 1984; 149:492.

2. Meguid MM, Oler A, Numann PJ, Khan S. Pathogenesis-based treatment of recurring subareolar breast abscesses. *Surgery* 1995; 118:775–782.

3. Maier WP, Berger A, Derrick BM. Periareolar abscess in the nonlactating breast. *American Journal of Obstetrics and Gynecology* 1982; 149:492.

4. Sartorius O. Personal communication.

5. Watt-Boolsen S, Ryegaard R, Blichert-Toft M. Primary periareolar abscess in the nonlactating breast: Risk of recurrence. *American Journal of Surgery* 1987; 153:571.

6. Love SM, Schnitt SJ, Connolly JL, Shirley RL. Benign breast diseases. In: Harris JR, Hellman S, Henderson IC, Kinne DW, eds. *Breast Diseases*. Philadelphia: J. B. Lippincott, 1987; 22.

8. LUMPS AND LUMPINESS

1. Tabar L, Pentek Z, Dean PB. The diagnostic and therapeutic value of breast cyst puncture and pneumocystography. *Radiology* 1981; 14:1659.

2. Herrman JB. Mammary cancer subsequent to aspiration of cysts in the breast. *Annals of Surgery* 1971; 173:40.

3. Haagensen CD. The relationship of gross cystic disease of the breast and carcinoma. *Annals of Surgery* 1977; 185:375.

4. Dupont WD, Page DL. Risk factors for breast cancer in women with proliferative breast disease. *New England Journal of Medicine* 1985; 312:146.

5. Haagenson CD. *Diseases of the Breast*. Philadelphia, PA: W. B. Saunders, 1996.

6. Greenberg R, Skornick Y, Kaplan O. Management of breast fibroadenomas. *Journal of General Internal Medicine* 1998; 13(Sept):640–645.

7. Dupont WD, Page DL, Parl FF, et al. Long-term risk of breast cancer in women with fibroadenoma. *New England Journal of Medicine* 1994; 331(1):10.

9. MAMMOGRAPHY

1. Bailar JC. Mammography: A contrary view. *Annals of Internal Medicine* 1976; 84:77.

2. Sadowski N. Personal communication 1988.

3. Kornguth P, Rimer B, Conaway M, et al. Impact of patient-controlled compression on the mammography experience. *Radiology* 1993; 186(1):99.

4. Homer MJ. Nonpalpable breast microcalcifications: Frequency, management, and results of incisional biopsy. *Radiology* 1992; 185:411.

5. Berend ME, Sullivan DC, Kornguth PJ, et al. The natural history of mammographic calcifications subjected to interval follow-up. *Archives of Surgery* 1992; 127(November):1309.

6. Stomper P, Kopans D, Sadowski N, et al. Is mammograph painful? A multicenter patient survey. *Archives of Internal Medicine* 1988; 148(3):521.

10. OTHER IMAGING TECHNIQUES

1. Parker SH, Lovin JD, Jobe WE, et al. Stereotactic breast biopsy with a biopsy gun. *Radiology* 1990; 176(Sept.):741.

2. Petro J, Klein S, Niazi Z, Salzberg C, Byrne D. Evaluation of ultrasound as a tool in the follow-up of patients with breast implants: A preliminary, prospective study. *Annals of Plastic Surgery* 1994; 32(6):580.

3. Peters-Engl C, Medl M, Mirau M, et al. Color-coded and spectral Doppler flow in breast carcinomas—Relationship with the tumor microvasculature. *Breast Cancer Research and Treatment* 1998; 47:83–89.

4. Waxman ADR, L, Memsic LD, Foster CE, et al. Thallium scintigraphy in the evaluation of mass abnormalities of the breast. *Journal of Nuclear Medicine* 1993; 34:18.

5. Akashi-Tanaka S, Fukutomi T, Miyakawa K, Uchiyama N, Tsuda H. Diagnostic value of contrast-enhanced computed tomography for diagnosing the intraductal component of breast cancer. *Breast Cancer Research and Treatment* 1998; 49:79–86.

6. Randal J. Researchers test hi-tech bra for detecting breast cancer. *Journal of the National Cancer Institute* 1997; 89(19):1400–1401.

11. BIOPSY

1. Layfield LJ, Parkinson B, Wong J, Guiliano AE, Bassett LW. Mammographically guided fine-needle aspiration biopsy of nonpalpable breast lesions. *Cancer* 1991; 68:2007.

2. Martelli G, Pilotti S, de Yoldi GC, et al. Diagnostic efficacy of physical examination, mammography, fine needle aspiration, cytology (triple-test) in solid breast lumps: An analysis of 1708 cases. *Tumori* 1990; 76:476.

3. Pass HA. Stereotactic biopsy of breast cancer. PPO Updates (*Principles & Practice of Oncology*) 1998; 12(12):1–7.

4. Martelli et al. Diagnostic efficacy.

12. UNDERSTANDING STUDIES AND CLINICAL TRIALS

1. Cummings SR, Eckert S, Krueger KA, Grady D, Powles TJ, et al. The effect of raloxifene on risk of breast cancer in postmenopausal women: Results from the MORE trial. *Journal of the American Medical Association* 1999; 281(23):2189–2197.

2. Colditz GA, Hankinson SE, Hunter DJ, et al. The use of estrogens and progestins and the risk of breast cancer in postmenopausal women. *New England Journal of Medicine* 1995; 332:1589–1593.

3. Stanford JL, Weiss NS, Voight LF, Dahling JR, Habel LA, Rosing M. Combined estrogen and progestin hormone replacement therapy in relation to risk of breast cancer. *Journal of the American Medical Association* 1995; 274:37–142.

4. Mitchell S. MDs urged not to be unduly influenced by reported increase in CHD with HRT. *Reuter's* 2000 (April 7).

5. Herrington D. Reported at the American College of Cardiology Meeting, March, 2000.

13. THE MOLECULAR BIOLOGY OF BREAST CANCER

1. Hoagland M, Dodson B. *The Way Life Works.* New York: Times Books, 1998.

2. Ibid.

3. Weaver VM, Peterson OW, Wang F, et al. Reversion of the malignant phenotype of human breast cells in three-dimensional culture and in vivo by integrin blocking antibodies. *The Journal of Cell Biology* 1997; 137(1):231–245.

4. O'Reilly MS, Holmgren L, Shing Y, et al. Angiostatin: A novel angiogenesis inhibitor that mediates the suppression of metastases by a Lewis lung carcinoma. *Cell* 1994; 79(2):315–328.

5. Reynolds T. Researchers slowly unveil where cancer cells hide. *Journal of the National Cancer Institute* 1998; 90(22):1690–1691.

6. Kuiper GG, Enmark E, Pelto-Huikko M, Nillson S, Gustafsson JA. Cloning of a novel receptor expressed in rat prostate and ovary. *Proceedings of National Academy of Sciences U.S.A.* 1996; 93(12):5925–5930.

7. Groshong SD, Owen GI, Grimison B, et al. Biphasic regulation of breast cancer cell growth by progesterone: Role of the cyclin-dependent kinase inhibitors, p21 and p27 (Kip l). *Molecular Endocrinology* 1997; 11(11):1593–1607.

14. RISK FACTORS: GENETIC AND HORMONAL

1. Newell GR, Vogel VG. Personal risk factors: What do they mean? *Cancer* 1988; 62:1695.

2. Cuzick J. Women at high risk of breast cancer. *Reviews on Endocrine-Related Cancer* 1987; 25:5.

3. Miller AB. Epidemiology and prevention. In: Harris JR, Hellman S, Henderson IC, Kinne DW, eds. *Breast Diseases.* Philadelphia: J.B. Lippincott, 1987.

4. Seidman H, Stellman SD, Mushinski MH. A different perspective on breast cancer risk factors: Some implications of the nonattributable risk. *CA: A Cancer Journal for Clinicians* 1982; 32:301.

5. Willett WC, Stampfer MJ, Colditz GA, Rosner BA, Hennekens CJ, Speizer FE. Moderate alcohol consumption and the risk of breast cancer. *New England Journal of Medicine* 1980; 316:1174.

6. Eley JW, Hill HA, Chen VW, et al. Racial differences in survival from breast cancer. Results of the National Cancer Institute Black/White Cancer Survival Study. *Journal of the American Medical Association* 1994; 272(12):947.

7. Kelsey JL, Berkowitz GS. Breast cancer epidemiology. *Cancer Research* 1988; 48:5615.

8. Haynes S: Prevention and early detection of breast cancer in lesbians. National Gay and Lesbian Health Education Conference 1992.

9. Lynch HT, Albano WA, Heieck JJ, et al. Genetics, biomarkers, and control of breast cancer: A review. *Cancer, Genetics, and Cytogenetics* 1984; 13:43.

10. Easton DF, Bishop DT, Ford D, Crockford GP, Consortium BCL. Genetic linkage analysis in familial breast and ovarian cancer: Results from 214 families. *American Journal of Human Genetics* 1993; 52:678.

11. Shattuck-Eidens D, Oliphant A, McClure M, at al. BRCA1 sequence analysis in women at high risk for susceptiblity mutations:risk factor analysis and implications for genetic testing. *Journal of the American Medical Association* 1997; 278:1242.

12. Struewing JP, Abehovich D, Peretz T, et al. The carrier frequency of nazi Jewish individuals [See comments; published erratum appears in *Nat Genet* 1996; 12(1):110}. *Nat Genet* 1995; 11:198.

13. Bergthorsson JT, Johannsdottir J, Jonasdottir A, et al. Chromosome imbalance at the 3p14 region in human breast tumors: High frequency in patients with inherited predisposition due to BRCA2. *European Journal of Cancer* 1998; 34(1):1544.

14. Dorum A, Moller P, Kamsteeg EJ, et al. A BRCA1 founder mutation, identified with haplotype analysis, allowing genotype/phenotype determination and predictive testing. *European Journal of Cancer* 1997; 33:2390

15. Iglehart JD, Miron A, Rimer BK, Winer EP, Berry D, Shildkraut JM. Overestimation of hereditary breast cancer risk. *Annals of Surgery* 1998; 228(3):375–384.

16. Ibid.

17. Newman B, Mu H, Butler LM, Millikan RC, Moorman PG, King M-C. Frequency of breast cancer attributable to BRCA1 in a population-based series of American women. *Journal of the American Medical Association* 1998; 279:915–921.

18. Peto J, Collins N, Barfoot R, Seal S, Warren W, Rahman N, Easton DF, Evans C, Deacon J, Stratton MR. Prevalence of BCA1 and BRCA2 gene mutations in patients with early-onset breast cancer. *Journal of the National Cancer Institute* 1999; 91(11):943-9.

19. Shattuck-Eidens D, Oliphant A, McClure M, at al. BRCA1 sequence analysis in women at high risk for susceptiblity mutations:risk factor analysis and implications for genetic testing. *Journal of the American Medical Association* 1997; 278:1242. (op cit).

20. Frank TS, Manley SA, Olopade OI, et al. Sequence analysis of BRCA1 and BRCA2: Correlation of mutations with family history and ovarian cancer risk. *Journal of Clinical Oncology* 1998; 16:2417.

21. MacMahon B, Cole P, Brown J. Etiology of human breast cancer: A review. *Journal of the National Cancer Institute* 1973; 50:21.

22. Rosenberg L, Palmer JR, Kaufman DW, Strom BL, Schottenfeld D, Shapiro S. Breast cancer in relation to the occurrence and time of induced and spontaneous abortion. *American Journal of Epidemiology* 1988; 127:981.

23. Dahling JR, Malone KE, Voigt LF, White E, Weiss NS. Risk of breast cancer among young women: Relationship to induced abortion. *Journal of the National Cancer Institute* 1994; 86(21):1584.

24. Henderson BE, Ross RK, Judd HL, Krailo MD, Pike MC. Do regular ovulatory cycles increase breast cancer risk? *Cancer* 1985; 56:1206.

25. Olsson H, Ranstam J, Olsson ML. The number of menstrual cycles prior to the first full-term pregnancy an important risk factor of breast cancer? *Acta Oncologica* 1987; 26:387.

26. Bernstein L, Yuan JM, Ross RK, et al. Serum hormone levels in pre-menopausal Chinese women in Shanghai and white women in Los Angeles: Results from two breast cancer case-control studies. *Cancer Causes and Control* 1990; 1:51.

27. Ibid.

28. Yuan J, Yu MC. Risk factors for breast cancer in Chinese women in Shanghai. *Cancer Research* 1988; 48:1949.

29. Anonymous. Breast feeding and the risk of breast cancer in young women. United Kingdom National Case-Control Study Group. *British Medical Journal* 1993; 307(6895):17.

15. RISK FACTORS: EXTERNAL

1. Holmes MD, Hunter DJ, Colditz GA, et al. Association of dietary intake of fat and fatty acids with risk of breast cancer. *Journal of the American Medical Association* 1999; 281(10):914–920.

2. Goldin BR, Adlercreutz H, Gorbach SL, et al. Estrogen excretion patterns and plasma levels in vegetarian and omnivorous women. *New England Journal of Medicine* 1982; 307:1542.

3. Berkel H, Birdsell D, Jenkins H. Breast augmentation: A risk factor for breast cancer? *New England Journal of Medicine* 1992; 326(25):1649.

4. Rohan TE, Howe GR, Friedenreich CM, Jain M, Miller AB. Dietary fiber, vitamins A, C, and E, and risk of breast cancer: A cohort study. *Cancer Causes and Control* 1993; 4:29.

5. Willett WC, Stampfer MJ, Colditz GA, Rosner BA, Hennekens CJ, Speizer FE. Moderate alcohol consumption and the risk of breast cancer. *New England Journal of Medicine* 1980; 316:1174.

6. Yood MU, Johnson CC, Blount A, et al. Race and differences in breast cancer survival in a managed care population. *Journal of the National Cancer Institute* 1999; 91(17):1487–1491.

7. Tokunaga M, Land CE, Yamamoto T, et al. Breast cancer among atomic bomb survivors. In: Boice JD, Jr., Fraumeni JF, Jr., eds. *Radiation Carcinogenesis Epidemiology and Biological Significance,* vol. 45. New York: Raven Press, 1984.

8. Tokunaga M, Land CE, Tokuoka S, et al. Incidence of female breast cancer among atomic bomb survivors, 1950–1985. *Radiation Research* 1994; 138:209–223.

9. Land C. Epidemiology of radiation induced breast cancer NAPBC Breast Cancer Etiology Working Group Workshop on Medical Ionizing of Radiation and Human Breast Cancer 1997.

10. Miller AB, Howe GR, Sherman GJ, et al. Mortality from breast cancer after irradiation during fluoroscopic examinations in patients being treated for tuberculosis. *New England Journal of Medicine* 1989; 321:1285.

11. Mettler FA, Hempelmann LH, Dutton AM, Pifer JW, Toyooka ET, Ames WR. Breast neoplasma in women treated with x rays for acute postpartum mastitis. A pilot study. *Journal of the National Cancer Institute* 1969; 43:803.

12. Hoffman DA, Lonstein JE, Morin MM, et al. Breast cancer in women with scoliosis exposed to multiple diagnostic x rays. *Journal of the National Cancer Institute* 1989; 81:1307.

13. Simon N. Breast cancer induced by radiation. Relation to mammography and treatment of acne. *Journal of the American Medical Association* 1977; 237(8):789.

14. Hildreth NG, Shore RE, Dvoretsky PM. The risk of breast cancer after irradiation of the thymus in infancy. *New England Journal of Medicine* 1989; 321:1281.

15. Boice JD, Day NE, Anderson A, et al. Second cancer following radiation treatment for cervical cancer. An international collaboration among cancer registries. *Journal of the National Cancer Institute* 1985; 74:955.

16. Tucker MA, Coleman CN, Cox RS, et al. Risk of second cancers after treatment for Hodgkin's disease. *New England Journal of Medicine* 1988; 318:76.

17. Li FP, Corkery J, Vawter G, et al. Breast carcinoma after cancer therapy in childhood. *Cancer* 1983; 51:521.

18. Rosenberg L, Miller DR, Kaufman DW, et al. Breast cancer and oral contraceptive use. *American Journal of Epidemiology* 1984; 119:167.

19. Kelsey JL, Fischer DB, Holford TR, et al. Exogenous estrogens and other factors in the epidemiology of breast cancer. *Journal of the National Cancer Institute* 1981; 55:327.

20. Bernstein L, Ross R, Henderson B. Relationship of hormone use to cancer risk. Monograph of the National Cancer Institute 1992; 12:137.

21. Greenberg ER, Barnes AB, Resseguie L, et al. Breast cancer in mothers given diethylstilbestrol in pregnancy. *New England Journal of Medicine* 1984; 311:1393.

22. Kelsey JL, Berkowitz GS. Breast cancer epidemiology. *Cancer Research* 1988; 48:5615.

23. Stone L. *The Family, Sex, and Marriage.* New York: Harper and Row, 1979.

24. Hale JR. *Renaissance Europe.* Berkeley, CA: University of California Press, 1971.

25. Fraser A. *The Weaker Vessel.* New York: Vintage, 1984.

26. Grady D, Rubin SM, Petitti DB, et al. Hormone therapy to prevent disease and prolong life in postmenopausal women. *Annals of Internal Medicine* 1992; 117(12):1016.

27. Ettinger B. Overview of estrogen replacement therapy: A historical perspective. Society for Experimental Biology and Medicine 1998; 217:2–5.

28. Hulley S, Grady D, Bush T, et al. Randomized trial of estrogen plus progestin for secondary prevention of coronary heart disease in postmenopausal women. Heart and Estrogen/progestin Replacement Study (HERS) Research Group. *Journal of the American Medical Association* 1998; 280(7):605–613.

29. Herrington D. HRT does not prevent heart disease progression. American College of Cardiology Meeting, Anaheim, CA, March 2000.

30. Mitchell S. MDs urged not to be unduly influenced by reported increase in CHD with HRT. *Reuter's* April 7, 2000.

31. Ettinger B, Friedman GD, Bush T, Quesenberry CP, Jr. Reduced mortality associated with long-term postmenopausal estrogen therapy. *Obstetrics and Gynecology* 1996; 87(1):6–12.

32. Schairer C, Lubin J, Troisi R, Sturgeon S, Brinton L, Hoover R. Menopausal estrogen and estrogen-progestin replacement therapy and breast cancer risk. *Journal of the American Medical Association* 2000; 283(4):485–491.

33. The Writing Group for the PEPI Trial. Effects of estrogen or estrogen/progestin regimens on heart disease risk factors in postmenopausal women: The postmenopausal estrogen/progestin interventions (PEPI) trial. *Journal of the American Medical Association* 1995; 273(3):199.

34. Brinton LA, Brogan DR, Coates RJ, Swanson CA, Potischman N, Stanford JL. Breast cancer risk among women under 55 years of age by joint effects of usage of oral contraceptives and hormone replacement therapy. *Menopause* 1998; 5(3):145–151.

35. Whittemore AS. The risk of ovarian cancer after treatment for infertility. *New England Journal of Medicine* 1994; 331(12):805.

36. Wolff MS, Weston A. Breast cancer risk and environmental exposures. *Environmental Health Perspectives* 1997; 105(Supplement 4):891–895.

37. Wolff MS, Toniolo PG, Lee EW, Rivera M, Dubin N. Blood levels of organo-

chlorine residues and risk of breast cancer. *Journal of the National Cancer Institute* 1993; 85:648.

38. Krieger N, Wolff MS, Hiatt RA, Rivera M, Vogelman J, Orentreich N. Breast cancer and serum organochlorines: A prospective study among white, black and Asian women. *Journal of the National Cancer Institute* 1994; 86(8):589.

39. Ibid.

40. Hunter DJ, Hankinson SE, Larden F, et al. Plasma organochlorine levels and the risk of breast cancer. *New England Journal of Medicine* 1997; 337:1253–1258.

41. van't Veer P, Lobbezoo IE, Martin-Moreno JM, et al. DDT and postmenopausal breast cancer in Europe: Case control study. *British Medical Journal* 1997; 315:81–85.

42. Lopez-Carillo L, Blair A, Lopez-Cervantes M, et al. Dicholorodiphenyltrichloroethane serum levels and breast cancer risk: A case control study from Mexico. *Cancer Research* 1997; 57:3728–3732.

43. Hunter DJ, Hankinson SE, Larden F, et al. Plasma organochlorine levels and the risk of breast cancer. *New England Journal of Medicine* 1997; 337:1253–1258. (OP CIT #40)

44. Wang J, Inskip PD, Bioce JDJ. Cancer incidence among medical diagnostic xray workers in China 1950 to 1985. *International Journal of Cancer* 1990; 45:889–895.

45. Vaughan TL, Lee JA, Strader CH. Breast cancer incidence of a nuclear facility: Demonstration of a morbidity surveillance system. *Health Phys* 1993; 64:349–354.

46. Pukkala E, Auvinen A, Wahberg G. Incidence of cancer among Finnish airline attendants. *British Medical Journal* 1995; 311:649–952.

47. Boice JDJ, Mandel JS, Doody MM. Breast cancer among radiologic technologists. *Journal of theAmerican Medical Association* 1995; 274:394–401.

48. Goss PE, Sierra S. Current perspectives on radiation induced breast cancer. *Journal of Clinical Oncology;* 16:338–347.

49. Demers PA, Thomas DB, Rosenblatt KA, et al. Occupational exposure to electromagnetic fields and breast cancer in men. *American Journal of Epidemiology* 1991; 134(4):340.

50. Stevens RG, Davis S. The melatonin hypothesis: Electric power and breast cancer. *Environmental Health Perspectives* 1996; 104(Supplement 1):135–140.

51. Bartsch C, Bartsch H, Buchberger A, et al. Serial transplants of DMBA-induced mammary tumors in Fischer rats as a model system for human breast cancer. VI. The role of different forms of tumor-associated stress for the regulation of pineal melatonin secretion. *Oncology* 1999; 56(2):169–176

52. Graham C: EMF effects on melatonin in humans NAPBC Etiology Working Group Workshop on Electromagnetic Fields, Light at Night and Human Breast Cancer 1997.

53. Ibid.

54. Loomis DP, Savitz DA, Ananth CV. Breast cancer mortality among female electrical workers in the United States. Journal of the National Cancer Institute 1994; 86(12):921. *Environmental Health Perspectives* 1996; 104(Supplement 1):135–140.

16. PRECANCEROUS CONDITIONS

1. Davis HH, Simons M, Davis JB. Cystic disease of the breast relationship to cancer. *Cancer* 1974; 17:957.

2. Dupont WD, Page DL. Risk factors for breast cancer in women with proliferative breast disease. *New England Journal of Medicine* 1985; 312:146.

3. Fisher B, Costantino JP, Wickerham DL, Redmond CK, Kavanah M, et al. Tamoxifen for prevention of breast cancer: Report of the National Surgical Adjuvant

Breast and Bowel Project P-1 study. *Journal of the National Cancer Institute* 1998; 90(18):1371–1388.

4. Haagensen CD, Lane N, Lattes R, et al. Lobular neoplasia (so-called lobular carcinoma in situ) of the breast. *Cancer* 1978; 42:737.

5. Wheeler JEW, Enterline HT, Rosenman JM, et al. Lobular carcinoma in situ of the breast: Long-term follow-up. *Cancer* 1974; 34:554.

6. Anderson JA. Lobular carcinoma in situ: A long-term follow-up in 52 cases. *Acta Pathology and Microbiology of Scandinavia* (A) 1974; 82:519.

7. Rosen PP, Lieberman PH, Braun DW. Lobular carcinoma of the breast. *American Journal of Surgical Pathology* 1987; 2:225.

8. Alpers CE, Wellings SR. The prevalence of carcinoma in situ in normal and cancer-associated breasts. *Human Pathology* 1985; 16:796.

9. Nielsen M, Jensen J, Andersen J. Precancerous and cancerous breast lesions during lifetime and at autopsy. *Cancer* 1984; 54:612.

10. Betsill WL, Rosen PP, Lieberman PH, et al. Intraductal carcinoma: Long-term follow-up after treatment by biopsy alone. *Journal of the American Medical Association* 1978; 239:1863.

11. Page DL, Dupont WD. Intraductal carcinoma of the breast. *Cancer* 1982; 49:751.

12. Silverstein MJ, Lagios MD, Craig PH, et al. A prognostic index for ductal carcinoma in situ. *Cancer* 1996; 77:2267–2274.

13. Sternlicht MD, Kadeshian P, Shao Z-M, Safarians S, Barsky SH. The human myoepithelial cell is a natural tumor suppressor. *Clinical Cancer Research* 1997; 3:1949–1958.

14. Gupta SK, Douglas-Jones AG, Fenn N, Morgan JM, Mansel RE. The clinical behavior of breast carcinoma is probably determined at the preinvasive stage (ductal carcinoma in situ). *Cancer* 1997; 80(9):1740–1745.

15. Anastassiades O, Iakovou E, Stavridou N, Gogas J, Karameris A. Multicentricity in breast cancer: A study of 366 cases. *American Journal of Clinical Pathology* 1993; 99(3):238.

16. Rosen P, Fracchia A, Urban J, et al. "Residual" mammary carcinoma following simulated partial mastectomy. *Cancer* 1975; 35:739.

17. Holland R, Hendriks J, Verberek A, et al. Extent, distribution and mammographic/histological correlations of breast ductal carcinoma in situ. *Lancet* 1990; 335:519.

18. Noguchi S, Motomura K, Inaji H, Imaoka S, Koyama H. Clonal analysis of predominantly intraductal carcinoma and precancerous lesions of the breast by means of polymerase chain reaction. *Cancer Research* 1994; 54(April 1):1849–1853.

19. Fisher B, Costantino J, Redmond C, et al. Lumpectomy compared with lumpectomy and radiation therapy for the treatment of intraductal breast cancer. *New England Journal of Medicine* 1993; 328(22):1581.

20. Silverstein MJ, Lagios MD, Groshen S, Waisman JR, Lewinsky BS, et al. The influence of margin width on local control of ductal carcinoma in situ of the breast. *The New England Journal of Medicine* 1999; 340(19):1455–1461.

21. Fisher B, Dignam J, Wolmark N, Wickerham DL, Fisher ER, et al. Tamoxifen in treatment of intraductal breast cancer: National Surgical Adjuvant Breast and Bowel Project B-24 randomized controlled trial. *Lancet* 1999; 353(June 12):1993–2000.

22. Finkelstein SD, Sayegh R, Thompson WR. Late recurrence of ductal carcinoma in situ at the cutaneous end of surgical drainage following total mastectomy. *American Surgeon* 1993; 59(July):410.

23. Fisher DE, Schnitt SJ, Christian R, Harris JR, Henderson IC. Chest wall recurrence of ductal carcinoma in situ of the breast after mastectomy. *Cancer* 1993; 71(10):3025.

24. Silverstein M, Waisman J, Gamagami P, et al. Intraductal carcinoma of the breast (208 cases). Clinical factors influencing treatment choice. *Cancer* 1990; 66(1):102.

17. THE INTRADUCTAL APPROACH—A BREAST PAP SMEAR?

1. Leborgne R. Intraductal biopsy of certain pathologic processes of the breast. *Surgery* 1946; 19:47-54.

2. Papanicolaou GN, Holmquist DG, Bader GM, Falk EA. Exfoliative cytology of the human mammary gland and its value in the diagnosis of cancer and other diseases of the breast. *Cancer* 1958; II(2):377-409.

3. Buehring GC. Screening for breast atypias using exfoliative cytology. *Cancer* 1979; 43(5): 1788–99.

4. Sartorius OW, Smith HS, Morris P, Benedict D, Friesen L. Cytologic evaluation of breast fluid in the detection of breast disease. *Journal of the National Cancer Institute* 1977; 67:277–284.

5. Wrensch MR, Petrakis NL, King EB, et al. Breast cancer incidence in women with abnormal cytology in nipple aspirates of breast fluid. *American Journal of Epidemiology* 1992; 135:130–141.

6. Sauter E, Ross E, Daly M, et al. Nipple aspirate fluid: A promising non-invasive method to identify cellular markers of breast cancer risk. *British Journal of Cancer* 1997; 76(4):494–501.

7. Fabian C, Zalles C, Kamel S, et al. Correlation of breast tissue biomarkers with hyperplasia and dysplasia in fine-needle aspirates (FNAs) of women at high and low risk for breast cancer. Proceedings of Annual Meeting of American Association of Cancer Researchers 1994; 35(A1703).

8. Papanicolaou et al. Exfoliative cytology of the human mammary gland.

18. PREVENTION

1. Miller AB. Epidemiology and prevention. In: Harris JR, Hellman S, Henderson IC, Kinne DW, eds. *Breast Diseases*. Philadelphia: J.B. Lippincott, 1987.

2. Bernstein L, Henderson BE, Hanisch R, Sullivan-Halley J, Ross RK. Physical exercise activity and reduced risk of breast cancer in young women. *Journal of the National Cancer Institute* 1994; 86:1403.

3. Bernstein L, Ross RK, Lobo RA, Hanisch R, Krailo MD, Henderson BE. The effects of moderate physical activity on menstrual cycle patterns in adolescence: Implications for breast cancer prevention. *British Journal of Cancer* 1987; 55:681.

4. Thune I, Brenn T, Lund E, Gaard M. Physical activity and the risk of breast cancer. *New England Journal of Medicine* 1997; 336:1269–1275.

5. Frisch RE, Wyshak G, Albright N, et al. Lower lifetime occurrence of breast cancer and cancer of the reproductive system among former college athletes. *American Journal of Clinical Nutrition* 1987; 45:328.

6. Spicer DV, Pike MC, Pike A, Rude R, Shoupe D, Richardson J. Pilot trial of a gonadotropin hormone agonist with replacement hormones as a prototype contraceptive to prevent breast cancer. *Contraception* 1993; 47:427.

7. Spicer D, Ursin G, Parisky YR, et al. Changes in mammographic densities induced by a hormonal contraceptive designed to reduce breast cancer risk. *Journal of the National Cancer Institute* 1994; 86(6):431.

8. Fisher B, Costantino JP, Wickerham DL, Redmond CK, Kavanah M, et al. Tamoxifen for prevention of breast cancer: Report of the National Surgical Adjuvant Breast and Bowel Project P-1 study. *Journal of the National Cancer Institute* 1998; 90(18):1371–1388.

9. Gail MH, Brinton LA, Byar DP, et al. Projecting individualized probabilities of developing breast cancer for white females who are examined annually. *Journal of the National Cancer Institute* 1989; 81(24):1879–1886.

10. Gail M, Costantino JP, Bryant J, et al. Weighing the risks and benefits of tamoxifen treatment for preventing breast cancer. *Journal of the National Cancer Institute* 1999; 91:1829–1846.

11. Powles TJ. Status of antiestrogen breast cancer prevention trials. Oncology 1998; 12(3(Supplement 5)):28–31.

12. Veronesi U, Maisonneuve P, Costa A, et al. Prevention of breast cancer with tamoxifen: Preliminary findings from the Italian randomized trial among hysterectomized women. *Lancet* 1998; 352:93–97.

13. Cummings SR, Eckert S, Krueger KA, Grady D, Powles TJ, et al. The effect of raloxifene on risk of breast cancer in postmenopausal women: Results from the MORE trial. *Journal of the American Medical Association* 1999; 281(23):2189–2197.

14. Chlebowski RT, Collyar DE, Somerfield MR, Pfister DG. American Society of Clinical Oncology technology assessment on breast cancer risk reduction strategies: tamoxifen and raloxifene. *Journal of Clinical Oncology* 1999; 17(6):1939–1955.

15. Veronesi U, DePalo G, Costa A. Chemoprevention of breast cancer with retinoids. NCI Monographs 1992; 12:93.

16. Veronesi U, DePalo G, et al. Randomized trial of fenretinide to prevent second breast malignancy in women with early breast cancer. *Journal of the National Cancer Institute* 1999; 91:1847–1856.

17. Temple W, Lindsay R, Magi E, Urbanski S. Technical considerations for prophylactic mastectomy in patients at high risk for breast cancer. *American Journal of Surgery* 1991; 161(4):413.

18. Hartmann LC, Schaid DJ, Woods JE, Crotty TP, et al. Efficacy of bilateral prophylactic mastectomy in women with a family history of breast cancer. *New England Journal of Medicine* 1999; 340(2):77–84.

19. Eisen A, Weber BL. Prophylactic mastectomy - the price of fear (editorial). *New England Journal of Medicine* 1999; 340(2):137–138.

20. Rebbeck TR, Levin AM, Eisen A, Snyder C, Watson P, Cannon-Albright L, Issacs C, Olopade O, Garber JE, Godwin AK, Daly MB, Narod SA, Neuhasen SL, Lynch HT, Weber BL. Breast cancer risk after bilateral prophylactic oophorectomy in BRCA1 mutation carriers. *Journal of the National Cancer Institute* 1999; 91(17):1475-9.

21. Schrag D, Kuntz KM, Garber JE, et al. Decision analysis - Effects of prophylactic mastectomy and oophorectomy on life expectancy among women with BRCA1 or BRCA2 mutations. *New England Journal of Medicine* 1997; 336(20):1465–1471.

19. SCREENING

1. Thomas DB, Gao DL, Self SG, et al. Randomized trial of breast self-examination in Shanghai: Methodology and preliminary results. *Journal of the National Cancer Institute* 1997; 89:355–365.

2 Ibid.

3. Baines CJ. Reflections on breast self-examination. *Journal of the National Cancer Organization* 1997; 89:339–340.

4. Wolfe JN. Breast cancer screening. *Breast Cancer Research and Treatment* 1991; 18:S89.

5. Senie R, Rosen P, Lesser M, Kinne D. Breast self-examination and medical examination related to breast cancer stage. *American Journal of Public Health* 1981; 71:583.

6. Anon. UK trial of early detection of breast cancer group: First results on mortality reduction in the UK trial of early detection of breast cancer. *Lancet* 1988; ii:411.

7. Shapiro S, Venet W, Strax P, et al. Ten-to-fourteen-year effects of screening on breast cancer mortality. *Journal of the National Cancer Institute* 1982; 69:349.

8. Ibid.

9. Shapiro S. Periodic screening for breast cancer: the HIP Randomized Controlled Trial (Health Insurance Plan). *Journal of the National Cancer Institute* 1997; 22:27–30.

10. Miller A, Baines C, To T, Wall C. Canadian National Breast Screening Study: 2. Breast cancer detection and death rates among women aged 50–59 years. *Canadian Medical Association Journal* 1992; 147(10):1477.

11. Fletcher SW, Black W, Harris R, Rimer BK, Shapiro S. Report of the international workshop for screening for breast cancer. *Journal of the National Cancer Institute* 1993; 85(20):1644.

12. National Institutes of Health. Consensus Development Statement: Breast cancer screening for women ages 40–49 1997(January 21–23).

13. Kerlikowske K, Grady D, et al. Effect of age, breast density, and family history on the sensitivity of first screening mammography. *Journal of the American Medical Association* 1996; 276:33–38.

14. Kopans DB. NBSS Revisited-Again (response). *Journal of the National Cancer Institute* 1993; 85(21):1774.

20. DIAGNOSIS AND TYPES OF CANCER

1. Fisher ER, Sass R, Fisher B. Biological considerations regarding the one- and two-step procedures in the management of patients with invasive carcinoma of the breast. *Surgery, Gynecology, and Obstetrics* 1985; 161:245.

2. Dixon JM, Anderson TJ, Page DL, et al. Infiltrating lobular carcinoma of the breast: An evaluation of the incidence and consequence of bilateral disease. *British Journal of Surgery* 1983; 70:513.

3. Gotteland M, May E, May-Levin F, Contesso G, Delarue JC, Mouriesse H. Estrogen receptors (ER) in human breast cancer. *Cancer* 1994; 74(3):864.

4. Ewers SV, Attewell R, Baldetorp B, et al. Prognostic significance of flow cytometric DNA analysis and estrogen receptor content in breast carcinomas—a 10-year survival study. *Breast Cancer Research and Treatment* 1992; 24:115.

5. Slamon D, Godolphin W, Jones L, et al. Studies of the Her-2/neu proto-oncogene in human breast and ovarian cancer. *Science* 1989; 244(4905):707.

6. Cobleigh MA, Vogel CL, Tripathy D, et al. Multinational study of the efficacy and safety of humanized anti-Her-2 monoclonal antibody in women who have Her-2 Over-expressing metastatic breast cancer that has progressed after chemotherapy for metastatic disease. *Journal of Clinical* 1999; 17:2639–2648.

7. Mass RD, Sanders C, Kasian C, et al. The concordance between the clinical trial assay (CTA) and fluorescence in situ hybridization (FISH) in the Herceptin pivotal trials. Proceedings of the American Society of Clinical Oncologists 2000; 19:75a Abstract 291.

8. Wong WW, Vijayakumar S, Weichselbaum RR. Prognostic indicators in node-negative early stage breast cancer. *American Journal of Medicine* 1992; 92:539.

21. STAGING: HOW WE GUESS IF YOUR CANCER HAS SPREAD

1. Ciatto S, Pacini P, Azzini V, et al. Preoperative staging of primary breast cancer: A multicentric study. *Cancer* 1988; 61(5):1038.

2. Haagensen C. *Diseases of the Breast.* Philadelphia: Saunders, 1971.

3. Wong WW, Vijayakumar S, Weichselbaum RR. Prognostic indicators in node-negative early stage breast cancer. *American Journal of Medicine* 1992; 92:539.

4. Lorde A. *A Burst of Light.* New York: Firebrand Books, 1988.

22. FEARS, FEELINGS, AND WAYS TO COPE

1. Rollin B. *First, You Cry.* New York: New American Library, 1976.

2. Kushner R. *Alternatives.* Cambridge, MA: Kensington Press, 1984.

3. Peters-Golden H. Breast cancer: Varied perceptions of social support in the illness experience. *Social Science Medicine* 1982; 16:483.

4. Kaspar A. Telephone interview.

5. Taylor SE, Lichtman RR, Wood JV. Attributions, beliefs about control and adjustment to breast cancer. *Journal of Perspectives on Sociology and Psychology* 1984; 46:489.

6. Ibid.

7. Wellisch DK, Gritz ER, Schain W, Wang HJ, Siau J. Psychological functioning of daughters of breast cancer patients. Part II: Characterizing the distressed daughter of the breast cancer patient. *Psychosomatics* 1992; 33(2):171.

8. Lichtman RR, Taylor SE, et al. Relations with children after breast cancer: The mother-daughter relationship at risk. *Journal of Psychosociology and Oncology* 1984; 2:1.

23. TREATMENT OPTIONS: AN OVERVIEW

1. Veronesi U. Randomized trials comparing conservative techniques with conventional surgery: An overview. In: Tobias JS, Peckham MJ, eds. *Primary Management of Breast Cancer: Alternatives to Mastectomy Management of Malignant Disease Series.* London: E. Arnold; 1985.

2. Fisher B, Anderson S, Redmond CK, Wolmark N, Wickerham DL, Cronin WM. Reanalysis and results after 12 years of follow-up in a randomized clinical trial comparing total mastectomy with lumpectomy with or without irradiation in the treatment of breast cancer. *New England Journal of Medicine* 1995; 333(22):1456–1661.

3. Schnitt SJ, Abner A, Gelman R, et al. The relationship between microscopic margins of resection and the risk of local recurrence in patients with breast cancer treated with breast conserving surgery and radiotherapy. *Cancer* 1994;74:1746.

4. Fisher B, Anderson S, Redmond CK, et al.

5. Schnitt SJ, Pierce S, Gelman R, et al. A prospective study of conservative surgery alone in the treatment of selected patients with Stage I breast cancer. *Cancer* 1996;77:1094–1100.

6. Wolmark N, Dignam J, Margolese R, Wickerham DL, Fisher B. The role of radiotherapy and tamoxifen in the managment of node negative invasive breast cancer <1 cm treated with lumpectomy: Preliminary results of NSABP Protocol B-21. *Proceedings of ASCO* 2000; 19(Abstract 271).

7. Overgaard M, Jensen M-B, Overgaard J, et al. Randomized controlled trial evaluating postoperative radiotherapy in high-risk post-menopausal breast cancer patients given tamoxifen: Report from the Danish Breast Cancer cooperative Group DBCG 82c Trial. *Lancet* 1999; 353:1641.

8. Ragaz J, Jackson SM, Le N, et al. Adjuvant radiotherapy and chemotherapy in node-positive premenopausal women with breast cancer. *New England Journal of Medicine* 1997;337:956.

9. Silverstein MJ, Gierson ED, Waisman JR, Senofsky GM, Colburn WJ, Gamagami P. Axillary lymph node dissection for T1a breast carcinoma: Is it indicated? *Cancer* 1994;73:664.

10. Giuliano AE, Jones RC, Brennan M, Statman R. Sentinel lymphadenectomy in breast cancer. *Journal of Clinical Oncology* 1997;5:2345–2350.

11. Krag DN, Weaver OJ, Alex JC, Fairbank JT. Surgical resection and radiolocalization of the sentinel node in breast cancer using a gamma probe. *Surgical Oncology* 1993;2:335.

12. Cox CE, Haddad F, Cox JM, et al. Lymphatic mapping in the treatment of breast cancer. *Oncology* 1998; 12:1283.

13. Morton DL. Interoperative lymphatic mapping and sentinel lymphadenectomy: Community standard care or clinical investigation? *Cancer* 1997; 3:341.

14. Cox CE, Pendas S, Cox JM, et al. Guidelines for sentinal node biopsy and lymphatic mapping of patients with breast cancer. *Annals of Surgery* 1998; 227(5):645–653.

15. Hagen A, Hrushesky WJM. Menstrual timing of breast cancer surgery. *American Journal of Surgery* 1998;104:245–261.

16. Hrushesky WJM, Bluming AZ, Gruber SA, Sothern RB. Menstrual influence on surgical cure of breast cancer. *Lancet* 1989;2:949.

17. Ratajczak HV, Sothern RB, Hrushesky WJM. Estrous influence on surgical cure of a mouse breast cancer. *Journal of Experimental Medicine* 1988;168:73–83.

18. Cooper LS, Gikett CE, Patel NK, Barnes DM, Fentiman IS. Survival of premenopausal breast carcinoma patients in relation to menstrual cycle timing of surgery and estrogen receptor/progesterone receptor status of the primary tumor. *Cancer* 1999;86:2053–2058.

19. Heer K, Kumar H, Speirs V, Greenman J, et al. Vascular endothelial growth factor in premenopausal cancer-indicator of the best time for breast cancer surgery? *British Journal of Cancer* 1998;78:1203–1207.

20. Bonadonna G, Valagussa VE, Rossi A, et al. Ten-year experience with CMF-based adjuvant chemotherapy in resectable breast cancer. *Breast Cancer Research and Treatment* 1985;5:95.

21. Wolmark N, Fisher B. Adjuvant chemotherapy in Stage II breast cancer: An overview of the NSABP clinical trials. *Breast Cancer Research Treatment* 1983; 3(Supplement):S19.

22. Early Breast Cancer Collaborative Trialists' Group, 1988.

23. Early Breast Cancer Collaborative Trialists' Group. Polychemotherapy for early breast cancer: An overview of the randomized trials. *The Lancet* 1998; 352(Sept 19):930–942.

24. Rajagopal S, Goodman PJ, Tannock IF. Adjuvant chemotherapy for breast cancer: Discordance between physicians' perception of benefit and the results of clinical trials. *Journal of Clinical Oncology* 1994;12:1296.

25. Paik S. Bryant J, Park C, Fisher B, et al. erbB-2 and response to doxorubicin in patients with axillary lymph node-positive, hormone receptor-negative breast cancer. *Journal of the National Cancer Institute* 1998; 90(18):1361–1370.

26. Demetri GD, Berry D, Norton L, et al. Clinical outcomes of node-positive breast

cancer patients treated with dose-intensified Adriamycin/cyclophosphamide (AC) followed by Taxol (T) as adjuvant systemic chemotherapy (CALGB 9141) Meeting abstract). *Proceedings of the Annual Meeting of the Society of Clinical Oncology* 1997; 16(A503).

27. Peters WP, Berry D, Vrendenburgh JJ, et al. Five year follow up of high dose combination alkylating agents with ABMT as consolidation after standard dose CF for primary breast cancer involving >10 axillary lymph nodes. (Duke/CALGB 8782). *Proceedings of American Society of Clinical Oncology* 1995; 14:317.

28. Peters WP, CALGB, et al. A prospective randomized comparison of two doses of combination alkylating agents (AA) as consolidation after CAF in high-risk primary breast cancer involving ten or more axillary lymph nodes: Preliminary results of CALGB 9082/SWOG 9114/NCIC MA-13. *Proceedings of American Society of Clinical Oncology* 1999; May.

29. Scandinavian Breast Cancer Study Group. Results from a randomized adjuvant breast cancer study with high-dose chemotherapy with CTCb supported by autologous bone marrow stem cells versus dose escalated and tailored FEC therapy. *Proceedings of American Society of Clinical Oncology* 1999; May.

30. Stadtmauer EA, ECOG, et al.. Phase III randomized trial of high-dose chemotherapy (HDC) and stem cell support (SCT) shows no difference in overall survival or severe toxicity compared to maintenance chemotherapy with cyclophosphomide, methotrexate and 5-Fluorouracil (CMF) for women with metastatic breast cancer who are responding to conventional induction chemotherapy: The Philadelphia Intergroup Study. *Proceedings of American Society of Clinical Oncology* 1999; May.

31. Bezwoda WR, et al., Randomized controlled trial of high dose chemotherapy (HD-CNVp) vs standard dose (CAF) chemotherapy for high risk surgically treated primary breast cancer. *Proceedings of American Society of Clinical Oncology* 1999; May.

32. Cobleigh MA, Vogel CL, Tripathy NJ, et al. Efficacy and safety of Herceptin (humanized anti-HER-2 antibody) as a single agent in 222 women with HER-2 overexpression who relapsed following chemotherapy for metastatic breast cancer [Abstract 376]. Proceedings of the American Society of Clinical Oncology 1998; 16:376.

33. Slamon D, Leyland-Jones B, Shak S, Paton V, Bajamonde A, et al.. Addition of Herceptin (humanized anti-HER2 antibody) to first line chemotherapy for HER2 overexpressing metastatic breast cancer (HER2+/MBC) markedly increases anticancer activity: A randomized, multinational controlled Phase III trial *Proceedings ASCO* 1998; 17:98a.

34. Vogel CL, Cobleigh MA, Tripathy D, et al.: Efficacy and safety of Herceptin (Trustuzumab, humanized anti-HER-2 antibody) as a single agent in first-line treatment of HER-2 overexpressing metastatic breast cancer (HER-2+/mBC) [Abstract 23]. *21st Annual Sant Antonio Breast Cancer Symposium* 1998.

35. Recht A, Come SE, Henderson IC, et al. The sequencing of chemotherapy and radiation therapy after conservative surgery for patients with early-stage breast cancer. *New England Journal of Medicine* 1996;334:1356.

36. Fisher B, Brown A, Mamounas E, et al. Effect of preoperative chemotherapy on local-regional disease in women with operable breast cancer: Findings from National Surgical Adjuvant Breast and Bowel Project B-18. *Journal of Clinical Oncology* 1997; 15:2483.

37. Cortazar P, Johnson BE. Review of the efficacy of individualized chemotherapy selected by in vitro drug sensitivity testing for patients with cancer. *Journal of Clinical Oncology* 1999; 17:1625–1631.

38. Early Breast Cancer Collaborative Trialists' Group. Effects of adjuvant tamoxifen and of cytotoxic therapy on mortality in early breast cancer: An overview of 61 randomized trials among 28,896 women. *New England Journal of Medicine* 1988;319:1681.

39. Taylor CW, Green S, Dalton WS, et al. Multicenter randomized clinical trial of goserelin versus surgical ovariectomy in premenopausal patients with receptor posi-

tive metastatic breast cancer: an intergroup study. *Journal of Clinical Oncology* 1998; 16:994.

40. Bonadonna G, Valagussa VE, Rossi A, et al. Ten-year experience with CMF-based adjuvant chemotherapy in resectable breast cancer. *Breast Cancer Research and Treatment* 1985;5:95.

41. Butta A, MacLennan K, Flanders KC, et al. Induction of transforming growth factor beta 1 in human breast cancer in vivo following tamoxifen treatment. *Cancer Research* 1992;52:4261.

42. Fisher B, Dignam J, Bryant J et al. Five versus more than five years of tamoxifen therapy for breast cancer patients with negative lymph nodes and estrogen receptor-positive tumors. 1996.

43. Peto, R. Five years of tamoxifen—or more? [Editorial; comment]. *Journal of the National Cancer Institute* 1996; 88(24):1791–1793.

44. Jordan VC, Fritz NF, Langan-Fahey S, Thompson M, Tormey DC. Alteration of endocrine parameters in premenopausal women with breast cancer during long term adjuvant therapy with tamoxifen as the single agent. *Journal of the National Cancer Institute* 1991; 83(20):1488.

45. Early Breast Cancer Trialists' Collaborative Group. Tamoxifen for early breast cancer: An overview of the randomized trials. *The Lancet* 1998;351:1451–1467.

46. Hutchins L, Green S, Ravdin P, et al. CMF versus CAF + / - tamoxifen in high-risk node-negative breast cancer patients and a natural history follow-up study in low risk node-negative patients: Update of tamoxifen results. *Breast Cancer Research and Treatment* 1999;57:25.

47. Bernstein L, Deapen D, Cerhan JR, et al. Tamoxifen therapy for breast cancer and endometrial cancer risk. *Journal of the National Cancer Institute* 1999; 91(19):1654–1662.

48. Hutchins L, Green S, Ravdin P, et al.

49. Fisher B, Anderson S, Wolmark N, Tan-Chiu E. Chemotherapy with or without tamoxifen for patients with ER negative breast cancer and negative nodes: Results from NSAPB B23. Proceedings of ASCO, 2000; 19(Abstract 277):72a.

50. Osborne, C. Recent Changes in the Adjuvant Treatment of Breast Cancer. Presented at Breast Cancer: Perspectives on Data and Developments Satellite, December 11, 1999, San Antonio, Tex.

51. Fisher B, Digman J, Wolmark N, DeCillis A, Emir B, Wickerham DL, Bryant J, Dimitrov NV, Abramson N, Atkins JN, Shibata H, Deschenen L, Margolese RG. Tamoxifen and chemotherapy for lymph node negative, estrogen receptor positive breast cancer. *Journal of the National Cancer Institute* 1997; 89(22):1673-82.

52. Ejlertsen B, Dombernowsky P, Mouridsen HT et al. Comparable effect of ovarian ablation (OA) and CMF chemotherapy in premenopausal hormone receptor positive breast cancer patients (PRP). *Proceedings of ASCO* 1999; 18:66a.

53. Davidson N, O'Neill A, Vukov A et al. Effect of chemohormonal therapy in premenopausal, node (+), receptor (+) breast cancer: An Eastern Cooperative Oncology Group Phase III Intergroup Trial (E5188, INT-0101). *Proceedings of ASCO* 1999;18:67a.

24. SPECIAL CASES

1. Hortobagyi GN, Blumenschein GR, Spanos W, et al. Multimodal treatment of locally advanced breast cancer. Cancer 1983; 51:763.

2. Perez CA, Graham ML, Taylor ME, et al. Management of locally advanced carcinoma of the breast I. *Noninflammatory. Cancer Supplement* 1994; 74(1):453.

3. Chang S, Buzdar AU, Hursting SD. Inflammatory breast cancer and body mass index. *Journal of Clinical Oncology* 1998; 16(12):3731–3735.

4. Ashikari R, Rosen PP, Urban JA, et al. Breast cancer presenting as an axillary mass. *Annals of Surgery* 1976; 183:415.

5. Feigenberg Z, Zer M, Dintsman M. Axillary metastases from an unknown primary source: A diagnostic and therapeutic approach. *Israeli Journal of Medical Science* 1976; 12:1153.

6. van Ooijen B, Bontenbal M, Henzen-Logmans SC, Koper PC. Axillary nodal metastases from an occult primary consistent with breast carcinoma. *British Journal of Surgery* 1993; 80(10):1299.

7. Lagios MD, Westdahl PR, Rose MR, et al. Paget's disease of the nipple. *Cancer* 1984; 54:545.

8. Kister SJ, Haagensen CD. Paget's disease of the breast. *American Journal of Surgery* 1970; 119:606.

9. Lagios, et al., 1984.

10. Malak G, Tapolcsanyi L. Characteristics of Paget's carcinoma of the nipple and problems of its negligence. *Oncology* 1974; 30:278.

11. Haagensen CD. *Diseases of the Breast.* Philadelphia: W. B. Saunders, 1975.

12. Bartoli C, Zurridas C, Veronesi P, et al. Small sized phyllodes tumor of the breast. *European Journal of Surgical Oncology* 1990; 16:215–219.

13. Salvadori B, Greco M, Galluzzo D, et al. Surgery for malignant mesenchymal tumors of the breast: A series of 31 cases. *Tumori* 1982; 68:325–329.

14. Guinee VF, Olsson H, Moller T, et al. Effect of pregnancy on prognosis for young women with breast cancer. *Lancet* 1994; 343:1587.

15. Lambe M, Hsieh CC, Trichopoulos D, Ekbom A, Pavia M, Adami HO. Transient increase in the risk of breast cancer after giving birth. *New England Journal of Medicine* 1994; 331(1):5.

16. Dixon JM, Sainsbury JRC, Rodger A. Breast cancer: Treatment of elderly patients and uncommon conditions. *British Medical Journal* 1994; 309:1292–1295.

17. Thompson WD. Genetic epidemiology of breast cancer. *Cancer* 1994; 74:279.

18. Henderson IC, Patek AJ. Are breast cancers in young women qualitatively distinct? *The Lancet* 1997; 349:1488–1489.

19. McCormick B. Selection criteria for breast conservation: The impact of young and old age and collagen vascular disease. *Cancer* 1994; 74:430.

20. Lee CG, McCormick B, Mazumdar M, Vetto J, Borgen PI. Infiltrating breast carcinoma in patients age 30 years and younger: Long term outcome for life, relapse, and second primary tumors. *International Journal of Radiation, Oncology, Biology, and Physics* 1992; 23:969.

21. Silliman RA, Balducci L, Goodwin JS, Holmes FF, Leventhal EA. Breast cancer care in old age: What we know, don't know, and do. *Journal of the National Cancer Institute* 1993; 85(3):190.

22. Horobin JM, Preece PE, Dewar JA, Wood RAB, Cuschieri A. Long-term follow-up of elderly patients with locoregional breast cancer treated with tamoxifen alone. *British Journal of Surgery* 1991; 78(January):213.

23. Bates T, Riley DL, Houghton J, Fallowfield L, Baum M. Breast cancer in elderly women: A Cancer Research Campaign trial comparing treatment with tamoxifen and optimal surgery with tamoxifen alone. *British Journal of Surgery* 1991; 78(May):591.

24. Lambe et al., 1994.

25. Guinee, VF, et al., 1994.

26. Petrek JA. Childbearing issues in breast carcinoma survivors. *Cancer* 1997; 79(7):1271–1278.

27. Deapen MD, Pike MC, Casagrande JT, et al. The relationship between breast cancer and augmentation mammoplasty: An epidemiologic study. *Plastic and Reconstructive Surgery* 1986; 77:361.

28. Jacobson GM, Sause WT, Thomson JW, Plenk HP. Breast irradiation following silicone gel implants. *International Journal of Radiation, Oncology, Biology and Physics* 1986; 12(5):835.

29. Schwartz RM, Newell RB, Hauch JF, et al. A study of familial male breast carcinoma and a second report. *Cancer* 1980; 46:2629.

30. Jackson AW, et al. Carcinoma of the male breast in association with the Klinefelter syndrome. *British Medical Journal* 1965; 1:223.

31. Campbell JH, Cummins SD. Metastases simulating mammary cancer in prostatic carcinoma under estrogenic therapy. *Cancer* 1951; 4:303.

32. Hittmair AP, Lininger RA, Tavassoli FA. Ductal carcinoma in situ (DCIS) in the male breast. *Cancer 1998*; 83(10):2139–2149.

25. SURGERY

1. Lanzafame RJ, McCormick CJ, Rogers DW, et al. Mechanisms of the reduction of tumor recurrence with the carbon dioxide laser in experimental mammary tumors. *Surgery, Gynecology and Obstetrics* 1988; 67:493.

2. Silen W, Matory WE, Love SM. *Atlas of Techniques in Breast Surgery.* Philadelphia: Lippincott-Raven, 1996.

3. Troyan S. Personal communication.

4. Silen et al., 1996.

5. Rosen PP, Lesser MT, Kinne DW, et al. Discontinuous or "skip" metastases in breast carcinoma: Analysis of 1,228 axillary dissections. Annals of Surgery 1983; 197:276.

6. Siegel BM, Mayzel KA, Love SM. Level I and II axillary dissection in the treatment of early-stage breast cancer. *Archives of Surgery* 1990; 125:1144.

7. Lorde A. *The Cancer Journals.* New York: Spinsters, 1980.

26. PROSTHESIS AND RECONSTRUCTION

1. Metzger D. *Tree & The Woman Who Slept with Men to Take the War Out of Them.* Oakland, CA: Wingbow Press, 1983.

2. Rollin B. *First, You Cry.* New York: New American Library, 1976.

3. Kushner R. *Why Me?* Cambridge, MA: Kensington Press, 1982.

4. Johnson CH, van Heerden JA, Donohue JH, et al. Oncological aspects of immediate breast reconstruction following mastectomy for malignancy. *Archives of Surgery* 1989; 124:819.

27. RADIATION THERAPY

1. Cuzick J, Stewart H, Peto R, et al. Overview of randomized trials of postoperative adjuvant radiotherapy in breast cancer. *Cancer Treatment Report* 1987; 71:15.

2. Whelan TJ, Mackenzie RG, Levine M, et al. A randomized trial comparing two fractionation schedules for breast irradiation postlumpectomy in node-negative breast cancer. Proceedings of American Society of Clinical Oncology 2000; 19.

3. Kurtz JM, Amalric R, Brandone H, et al. Contralateral breast cancer and other second malignancies in patients treated by breast-conserving therapy with radiation. *International Journal of Radiation, Oncology, Biology, and Physics* 1987; 15:277.

28. SYSTEMIC TREATMENTS

1. Bonadonna G, Valagussa VE, Rossi A, et al. Ten-year experience with CMF-based adjuvant chemotherapy in resectable breast cancer. *Breast Cancer Research and Treatment* 1985; 5:95.

2. ASCO. American Society of Clinical Oncology recommendations for the use of hematopoetic colony stimulating factors: Evidence-based clinical practice guidelines. *Journal of Clinical Oncology* 1994; 12:247.

3. Denmark-Wahnefried W, Winer EP, Rimer BK. Why women gain weight with adjuvant chemotherapy for breast cancer. *Journal of Clinical Oncology* 1993; 11(7):1418.

4. Goodwin PJ, Ennis M, Pritchard KI, Trudeau M, Hood N. Risk of menopause during the first year after breast cancer diagnosisis. *Journal of Clinical Oncology* 1999; 17(8):2365–2370.

5. Bines J, Oleske DM, Cobleigh MA. Ovarian function in premenopausal women treated with adjuvant chemotherapy for breast cancer. *Journal of Clinical Oncology* 1996; 14(5):1718–1729.

6. Cobleigh MA, Bines J, Harris D, LaFollette S, Lincoln ST, Walter JM. Amenorrhea following adjuvant chemotherapy for breast cancer. *Proceedings of the American Society of Clinical Oncology* 1995; 14:115.

7. Bryce CJ, Shenkier T, Gelmon K, Trevisan C, Olivitto I. Menstrual disruption in premenopausal breast cancer patients receiving CMF (V) vs AC adjuvant chemotherapy. *Breast Cancer Research and Treatment* 1998; 50:284.

8. Montz FJ, Wolff A, Cambone JC. Gonadal protection and fecundity rates in cyclophosamide-treated rats. *Cancer Research* 1991; 51:2124.

9. Ataya K, Rao LV, Lawrence E, Kimmel R. Luteinizing hormone releasing hormone agonist inhibits cyclophosamide induced ovarian follicular depletion in rhesus monkeys. *Biology of Reproduction* 1995; 52:365.

10. Fisher B, Rockette H, Fisher ER, et al. Leukemia in breast cancer patients following adjuvant chemotherapy or postoperative radiation: The NSABP experience. *Journal of Clinical Oncology* 1985; 3:1640.

11. Klewer SE, Goldberg SJ, Donnerstein RL, Berg RA, Hutter JJ, Jr. Dobutamine stress echocardiography: A sensitive indicator of diminished myocardial function in asymptomatic doxirubin-treated long-term survivors of childhood cancer. *Journal of the American College of Cardiologists* 1992; 19(2):394.

12. Lucca, Gianni. Abstract #255. *American Society of Clinical Oncology* 1999.

13. Siegel BS. *Love, Medicine and Miracles*. New York: Harper & Row; 1986.

14. Loprinski CL, Dugler J, Sloan JA, et al. Venlafaxine alleviates hot flashes: an NCCTG Trial. Abstract 4, Proceedings of ASCO, Volume 19, 2000.

15. Saphner T, Tormey DC, Gray R. Venous and arterial thrombosis in patients who received adjuvant therapy for breast cancer. *Journal of Clinical Oncology* 1991; 9(2):286.

16. Fisher ER, Fisher B, Wickerham DL, Costantino JP, Redmond C. Response: Endometrial cancer in tamoxifen-treated breast cancer patients: findings from the National Surgical Adjuvant Breast and Bowel Project (NSABP) B-14. *Journal of the National Cancer Institute* 1994; 86(16):1253.

17. Bernstein L, Deapen D, Cerhan JR, et al. Tamoxifen therapy for breast cancer and endometrial cancer risk. *Journal of the National Cancer Institute* 1999; 91(19):1654–1662.

18. Bertelli G, Venturini M, Del Mastro L, et al. Tamoxifen and the endometrium: Findings of pelvic untrasound examination and endometrial bioppsy in asymptomatic breast cancer patients. *Breast Cancer Research and Treatment* 1998; 47(1):41–46.

19. Caleffi M, Fentiman IS, Clark GM, et al. Effect of tamoxifen on oestrogen binding,

lipid and lipoprotein concentrations and blood clotting parameters in premenopausal women with breast pain. *Journal of Endocrinology* 1988; 119(2):335.

20. Kristensen B, Ejlertsen B, Dalgaard P, et al. Tamoxifen and bone metabolism in postmenopausal low-risk breast cancer patients: A randomized study. *Journal of Clinical Oncology* 1994; 12(5):992.

21. Ibid.

22. Budzar AU, Marcus C, Holmes F, Hug V, Hortobagyi G. Phase II evaluation of Ly156758 in metastatic breast cancer. *Oncology* 1988; 45(5):344–345.

23. Gradishar WJ, Glusman JE, Vogel CL, et al. Raloxifene HCl: A new endocrine agent is active in estrogen receptor positive metastatic breast cancer. *Breast Cancer Research and Treatment* 1997; 46(53(abst no 209)).

29. COMPLEMENTARY AND ALTERNATIVE TREATMENT

1. Lee MM, Lin SS, Wrensch MR, Adler SR, Eisenberg D. Alternative therapies used by women with breast cancer in four ethnic populations. *Journal of the National Cancer Institute* 2000; 92:42–47.

2. Cassileth BR, Lusk EJ, Strouse TB, et al. Contemporary unorthodox treatments in cancer medicine: A study of patients, treatments and practitioners. *Annals of Internal Medicine* 1984; 101:105–112.

3. Cousins N. *Anatomy of an Illness.* New York: Bantam Books; 1979.

4. Spiegel D, Bloom JR, Kraemer HC, Gottheil E. Effect of psychosocial treatment on survival of patients with metastatic breast cancer. *Lancet* 1989; 2:888.

5. Fawzy FI, Fawzy NW, Hyun CS, et al. Malignant melanoma: Effects of an early structured psychiatric intervention, coping, and affective state on recurrence and survival six years later. *Archives of General Psychiatry* 1993; 50:681.

6. Duckro P, Magaletta PR. The effect of prayer on physical health: Experimental evidence. *Journal of Health and Religion.*

7. Dossey L. Healing Words: *The Healing Power of Prayer.* San Francisco: Harper, 1993.

8. Simonton OC, Matthews S, Creighton JL. *Getting Well Again.* New York: Bantam Books, 1992.

9. Cousins, 1979.

10. Ibid.

11. Benson H. *Beyond the Relaxation Response.* New York: Berkley Books, 1985.

12. Mella DL. *The Lengendary and Practical Use of Gems and Stones.* Albuquerque, NM: Domel, 1979.

13. Kushi M. *The Cancer Prevention Diet.* New York: St. Martin's Press, 1983.

14. Cassileth BR. Evaluating complementary and alternative therapies for cancer patients. *CA-A Cancer Journal for Clinicians* 1999; 49:362–375.

15. DiPaola RS, Zhang H, Lamberg GH, et al. Clinical biological activity of an estrogenic herbal combination (PC-SPES) in prostate cancer. *New England Journal of Medicine* 1998; 339:785–791.

16. Sun AS, Ostadal O, Ryznar V, et al. Phase I/II study of stage III and IV non-small cell lung cancer patients taking a specific dietary supplement. *Nutrition and Cancer* 1999; 34:62–69.

17. Kennedy D. Food and Drug Administration's warning on laetrile.

18. Gonzalez NJ, Isaacs LL. Evaluation of pancreatic protoleolytic enzyme treatment of adenocarcinoma of the pancreas with nutrition and detoxification support. *Nutrition and Cancer* 1999; 33:117–124.

19. Bruzynski SR, Kubove E. Initial clinical study with antineoplaston A2 injections in cancer patients with five years' follow-up. *Drugs Exper Clinical Research* 1987; 13:1–11.

20. Green S. Antineoplastons: An unproven cancer therapy. *Journal of the American Medical Association* 1992; 267:2924–2928.

21. Harrison LE, Wojciechowicz DC, Brennan MF, Paty PB. Phenylacetate inhibits isoprenoid biosynthesis and suppresses growth of human pancreatic carcinoma. *Surgery* 1998; 124:541–550.

22. Miller DR, Anderson GT, Stark JJ, et al. Phase I/II trial of the safety and efficacy of shark cartilage in the treatment of advanced cancer. *Journal of Clinical Oncology* 1998; 16:3649–3655.

23. Trull L. *The CanCell Controversy: Why is a possible cure for cancer being suppressed?* Norfolk, VA: Hampton Roads, 1993.

24. Lorde A. *A Burst of Light.* New York: Firebrand Books, 1988.

30. LIFE AFTER BREAST CANCER

1. Robbins GF, Berg JW. Bilateral primary breast cancers: A prospective clinical pathological study. *Cancer* 1964; 17:1501.

2. Haagensen CD, Lane N, Bodian C. Coexisting lobular neoplasia and carcinoma of the breast. *Cancer* 1983; 51:1468.

3. Anon. Impact of follow-up testing on survival and health related quality of life in breast cancer patients. A multicenter randomized controlled trial. The GIVO Investigators. *Journal of the American Medical Association* 1994; 271(20):1587.

4. Stierer M, Rosen HR. Influence of early diagnosis on prognosis of recurrent breast cancer. *Cancer* 1989; 64:1128.

5. Kitzinger S. *Woman's Experience of Sex.* New York: G. P. Putnam's Sons, 1983.

6. Wellisch DK, Jamison KR, Pasnau RO. Psychosocial aspects of mastectomy. II. The man's perspective. *American Journal of Psychiatry* 1978; 135:543.

7. Baider L, Kaplan-DeNour A. Couples' reactions and adjustments to mastectomy: A preliminary report. *International Journal of Psychiatry and Medicine* 1984; 14:265.

8. Ganz PA, Rowland JH, Desmond K, et al. Life after breast cancer: Understanding women's health related quality of life and sexual functioning. *Journal of Clinical Oncology* 1998; 16:501.

9. Tasmuth T, Kataja M, Blomqvist C, von Smitten K, Kalso E. Treatment-related factors predisposing to chronic pain in patients with breast cancer—a multivariate approach. *Acta Oncology* 1997; 36(6):625–630.

10. Wallace MS, Wallace AM, Lee J, Kobke MK. Pain after breast surgery: A survey of 282 women. *Pain* 1996; 66(Aug):2–3.

11. Tasmuth T, Blomqvist C, Kalso E. Chronic post-treatment symptoms in patients with breast cancer operated in different surgical units. *European Journal of Surgical Oncology* 1999; 25(1).

12. Crawford JS, Simpson J, Crawford P. Myofascial release provides symptomatic relief from chest wall tenderness occasionally seen following lumpectomy and radiation in breast cancer patients [letter]. *International Journal of Radiation, Oncology, Biology and Physics* 1996; 34(5): 1188–1189.

13. Eija K, Tiina T, Pertti NJ. Amitriptyline effectively relieves neuropathic pain following treatment of breast cancer. *Pain* 1996; 64(2):293–302.

14. Petrek JA, Heelan MC. Incidence of breast carcinoma-related lymphedema. *Cancer* 1998; 83:2776.

15. Kasserollen RG. The Vodder School: The Vodder method. *Cancer* 1998; 83:2840.

16. Foldi E. The treatmentof lymphedema. *Cancer* 1998; 83:2883.

17. Casley-Smith JR, Morgan RG, Piller NB. Treatment of lymphedema of the arms and legs with 5,6-Benso(alpha)-pyrone. *New England Journal of Medicine* 1993; 329:1158.

18. Loprinzi CL, Kugler JW, Sloan JA, et al. Lack of effect of coumarin in women with lymphedema after treatment for breast cancer. *New England Journal of Medicine* 1999; 340(5):346–350.

19. Wieneke MH, Dienst ER. Neuropsychologic assessment of cognitive functioning following chemotherapy for breast cancer. *Psychooncology* 1995; 4:61.

20. Schagen SB, van Dam FSAM, Muller MJ, Boogerd W, Lindeboom J, Bruning PF. Cognitive deficits after postoperative adjuvant chemotherapy for breast carcinoma. *Cancer* 1999; 853640–650.

21. Irvine D, Vincent L, Graydon JE, Bubela N, Thompson L. The prevalence and correlates of fatigue in patients receiving treatment with chemotherapy and radiotherapy. Comparison with the fatigue experienced by healthy individuals. *Cancer Nursing* 1994; 17(5):367–378

22. Johnston E, Crawford J. The hematologic support of the cancer patient. In: Berger A, Portenoy R, Weissan D, eds. *Principles and Practice of Supportive Oncology.* Philadelphia: Lippincott-Raven, 1998; 549.

23. Friendenreich C, Courneya KS. Exercise as rehabilitation for cancer patients. *Clinical Journal of Sports Medicine* 1996; 6:237.

24. Young-McCaughon S, Sexton DL. A retrospective investigation of the relationship between aerobic exercise and quality of life in women with breast cancer. *Oncology Nursing Forum* 1991; 18:751.

25. Schwartz A. Patterns of exercise and fatigue in physically active cancer survivors. *Oncology Nursing forum* 1998; 25:485.

26. Huntington M. Weight gain in patients receiving adjuvant chemotherapy for carcinoma of the breast. *Cancer* 1985; 65:572.

27. Herbert JR, Hurley TG, Ma Y, Hampl JS. The effect of dietary exposure on recurrence and mortality in early stage breast cancer. *Breast Cancer Research and Treatment* 1998; 51:17.

28. Mignot L, et al. Breast cancer and subsequent pregnancy. *American Society of Clinical Oncology Proceedings* 1986; 5:57.

29. Peters M. The effect of pregnancy in breast cancer. *Prognostic Factors in Breast Cancer* 1968; 65.

30. El Hussein E, Tan SL. Successful in vitro fertilization and embryo transfer after treatment of invasive carcinoma of the breast. *Fettility and Sterility* 1992; 58:194.

31. Sauer MV, Paulson RJ, Lobo RA. Successful pre-embryo donation in ovarian failure after treatment for breast cancer. *Lancet* 1990; 335:723.

31. DEALING WITH MENOPAUSAL SYMPTOMS

1. Eden JA, Bush T, Nand S, Wren BG. A case-control study of combined continuous estrogen-progestin therapy among women with a personal history of breast cancer. *Menopause* 1995; 2(2):67–72.

2. DiSaia PJ, Grosen EQ, Odicio F, et al. Replacement therapy for breast cancer survivors: A pilot study. *Cancer* 1995; 76(2075–2078).

3. Xu X, Duncan AM, Merz BE, Kurzer MS. Effects of soy isoflavones on estrogen and phytoestrogen metabolism in premenopausal women. *Cancer Epidemiology Biomarkers and Prevention* 1998; 7(12):1101–1108.

4. Lu L-JW, Anderson KE, Grady JJ, Nagamani M. Effects of soya consumption for one month on steroid hormones in premenopausal women: Implications for breast cancer risk reduction. *Cancer Epidemiology, Biomarkers and Prevention* 1996; 5:63–70.

5. McMichael-Phillips DE, Harding C, Morton M, Potten CS, Bundred NJ. The effects

of soy supplementation on epithelial proliferation in the normal human breast. *American Journal of Clinical Nutrition* 1998; 68(Suppl):1431S-1436S.

6. Petrakis NL, Barnes S, King EB, et al. Stimulatory influence of soy protein isolate on breast secretion in pre- and postmenopausal women. *Cancer Epidemiology, Biomarkers and Prevention* 1996; 5:785–794.

7. Shao Z-M, Wu J, Shen Z-Z, Barsky SH. Genistein exerts multiple suppressive effects on human breast carcinoma cells. *Cancer Research* 1998; 58:4851–4857.

8. Ito A, Goto T, Okamoto T, Yamada K, Roy G. A combined effect of tamoxifen (TAM) and miso for the development of mammary tumors induced with MNU in SD rats. *Proceedings of the American Association for Cancer Research* 1996; 37(March).

9. Albertazzi P, Pansini F, Bonaccorsi G, Zanotti L, Forini E, De Aloysio D. The effects of dietary soy supplementation on hot flushes. *Obstetrics and Gynecology* 1998; 91(1):6–11.

10. Potter SM, Baum JA, Teng H, Stillman RJ, Shay NF, Erdman JWJ. Soy protein and isoflavones: Their effects on blood lipids and bone density in postmenopausal women. *American Journal of Clinical Nutrition* 1998; 68(6Suppl):1375S-1379S.

11. Goodman MT, Wilkens LR, Hankin JH, Lyu LC, Wu AH, Kolonel LN. Association of soy and fiber consumption with the risk of endometrial cancer. *American Journal of Epidemiology* 1997; 146(4):294–306.

12. Pan Y, Anthony M, Clarkson TB. Effect of estradiol and soy phytoestrogens on choline acetyltransferase and nerve growth factor mRNAs in the frontal cortex and hippocampus of female rats. *Proceedings of the Society of Experimental Biology and Medicine* 1999; 221(2):118–125.

13. Leonetti HB, Longo S, Anasti JN. Transdermal progesterone cream for vasomotor symptoms and postmenopausal bone loss. *Obstetrics and Gynecology* 1999; 94(2):225–228.

14. Ibid.

15. Riis BJ, Thomsen K, Strom V, Christiansen C. The effect of percutaneous estradiol and natural progesterone on postmenopausal bone loss. *American Journal of Obstetrics and Gynecology* 1987; 156(1):61–65.

16. Greendale GA, Reboussin BA, et al. Effects of estrogen and estrogen-progestin in mammographic parenchymal density. Postmenopausal Estrogen/Progestin Interventions (PEPI) Investigators. *Internal Medicine* 1999; 130(4 pt1):262–269.

17. Greendale GA, Reboussin BA, Hogan P, et al. Symptom relief and side effects of postmenopausal hormones: Results from the Postmenopausal Estrogen/Progestin Interventions Trial. *Obstetrics and Gynecology* 1998; 92(6):982–988.

18. Schairer C, Lubin J, Troisi R, Sturgeon S, Brinton L, Hoover R. Menopausal estrogen and estrogen-progestin replacement therapy and breast cancer risk. *Journal of the American Medical Association* 2000; 283(4):485–491.

19. Lange CA, Richer JK, Horwitz KB. Hypothesis: Progesterone primes breast cancer cells for cross-talk with proliferative or antiproliferative signals. *Molecular Endocrinology* 1999; 13(6):829–836.

20. Plu-Bureau, Le MG, et al. Progestogen use and decreased risk of breast cancer in a cohort study of premenopausal women with benign breast disease. *British Journal of Cancer* 1994; 70:270–277.

21. Powles TJ, Paterson AHG, McCloskey EV, Ashley S. Adjuvant clondronate reduces the incidence of bone metastasis in patients with primary operable breast cancer. *Proceedings of American Society of Clinical Oncology* 1998; 17(123A).

22. Ettinger B, Black DM, Mitlak BH, et al. Reduction of vertebral fracture risk in postmenopausal women with osteoporosis treated with raloxifene. *Journal of the American Medical Association* 1999; 282(7):637–645.

23. O'Brien M, Montes A, Powles TJ. Hormone replacement therapy as treatment of breast cancer—a phase II study of Org OD 14 (tibilone). *British Journal of Cancer* 1996; 73(9):1086–1088.

24. Ohta H, Komukai S, Makita K, Masuzawa T, Nozawa S. Effects of 1-year ipriflavone treatment on lumbar bone mineral density and bone metabolic markers in postrmenopausal women with low bone mass. *Hormone Research* 1999; 51(4):178–183.

25. Ettinger B, Grady D. The waning effect of postmenopausal estrogen therapy on osteoporosis. *New England Journal of Medicine* 1993; 329(16):1192–1193.

26. Ettinger B, Genant HK, Steiger P, Madvig P. Low-dosage micronized 17 beta-estradiol prevents bone loss in postmenopausal women. *American Journal of Obstetrics and Gynecology* 1992; 166(2):479–488.

27. Anon. HRT does not prevent heart disease progression report from 49th Annual Scientific Session of the American College of Cardiology in Anaheim, CA. Reuters Health, March 14, 2000.

28. Stampfer MJ, Colditz GA, Willett WC, et al. Postmenopausal estrogen therapy and cardiovascular disease: Ten years follow up from the Nurses' Health Study. *New England Journal of Medicine* 1991; 325:756–762.

29. Lieberman S. A review of the effectiveness of cimicifuga racemosa (black cohosh) for the symptoms of menopause. *Journal of Women's Health* 1998; 7(5):525–529.

30. Anon. Meeting summary, American Society for Clinical Oncology 1998.

31. Loprinzi CL, Peethambaram PP. Management of menopausal symptoms in breast cancer patients. *Annals of Medicine* 1995; 27(6):653–656

32. WHEN CANCER COMES BACK

1. Fisher B, Anderson S, Fisher ER, et al. Significance of ipsilateral breast tumour recurrence after lumpectomy. *Lancet* 1991; 338(10 August):327.

2. Ibid.

3. Toonkel LM, Fix I, Jacobson LH, Wallach CB. The significance of local recurrence of carcinoma of the breast. *International Journal of Radiaiton, Oncology, Biology, Physics* 1983; 9(1):33.

4. Borner M, Bacchi A, Goldhirsch A, et al. First isolated locoregional recurrence following mastectomy for breast cancer: Results of a phase III multicenter study comparing systemic treatment with observation after excision and radiation. *Journal of Clinical Oncology* 1994; 12:2071.

5. Slavin SA, Love SM, Goldwyn RM. Recurrent breast cancer following immediate reconstruction with myocutaneous flaps. *Plastic and Reconstructive Surgery* 1994; 93(May):1191.

6. Marks LB, Halperin EC, Prosnitz LR, et al. Post-mastectomy radiotherapy following adjuvant chemotherapy and autologous bone marrow transplantation for breast cancer patients with > 10 positive axillary lymph nodes. *International Journal of Radiation Oncology, Biology, Physics* 1992; 23(5):1021.

7. Taber SW, Fingar VH, Wieman TJ. Photodynamic therapy for palliation of chest wall recurrence in patients with breast cancer. *Journal of Surgical Oncology* 1998; 68(4):209–214

8. Recht A, Pierce S, Abner A, et al. Regional nodal failure after conservative surgery and radiotherapy for early-stage breast carcinoma. *Journal of Clinical Oncology* 1991; 9:988.

9. Clark GM, Sledge WJ, Jr., Osbourne CK, et al. Survival from first recurrence: Relative importance of prognostic factors in 1,015 breast cancer patients. *Journal of Clinical Oncology* 1987; 5:55.

10. Ibid.

11. Robinson RG, Preston DF, Baxter KG, Dusing RW, Spicer JA. Clinical experience

with strontium-89 in prostatic and breast cancer patients. *Seminars in Oncology* 1993; 20(3 Supp 2):44.

12. Spiegel D, Bloom JR, Kraemer HC, Gottheil E. Effect of psychosocial treatment on survival of patients with metastatic breast cancer. *Lancet* 1989; 2(8668):888.

13. Spiegel D. Living Beyond Limits: *New Hope and Help for Facing Life-threatening Illness.* New York: Times Book, 1993.

14. Tobin DR, with Lindsey K. *Peaceful Dying.* Reading, MA: Perseus Books, 1999.

33. METASTATIC DISEASE: TREATMENTS

1. Buzdar A, Jonat W, Howell A, et al. Anastrozole, a potent and selective aromatase inhibitor, versus megastrol acetate in postmenopausal women with advanced breast cancer: Results of overview analysis of two phase III trials. *Journal of Clinical Oncology* 1996; 14:2000.

2. Slamon D, Leyland-Jones B, Shak S, Paton V, Bajamonde A, et al.: Addition of Herceptin (humanized anti-HER2 antibody) to first line chemotherapy for HER2 over-expressing metastatic breast cancer (HER2+/MBC) markedly increases anticancer activity: A randomized, multinational controlled Phase III trial. *American Society of Clinical Oncology Proceedings* 1998; 17:98a.

3. Knerbel: Low dose chemotherapy DOD *Era of Hope June 9–11* 2000.

4. Perrault D, Eisenhauer EA, Pritchard KI, et al. Phase II study of the progesterone antagonist mifepristone in patients with untreated metastatic breast carcinoma: A National Cancer Institute of Canada Clinical Trials Group study. *Journal of Clinical Oncology* 1996; 14(10):2709–2712.

5. Shak S. Overview of the trastuzumab (Herceptin) anti-HER2 monoclonal antibody clinical program in HER2-overexpressing metastatic breast cancer. *Seminars in Oncology* 1999; 26(4(Suppl 12)):71–77.

6. Lipton A, Theriault RL, Hortobagyi GN, et al. Pamidronate prevents skeletal complications and is effective palliative treatment in women with breast carcinoma and osteolytic bone metastases: Long term follow-up of two randomized, placebo- and controlled trials. *Cancer* 2000; 88(5):1082–1090.

Glossary

abscess: Infection which has formed a pocket of pus.

adenocarcinoma: Cancer arising in gland forming tissue. Breast cancer is a type of adenocarcinoma.

adenine: A nucleotide base which pairs with thymine in forming DNA.

adjuvant chemotherapy: Anticancer drugs used in combination with surgery and/or radiation as an initial treatment before there is detectable spread, to prevent or delay recurrence.

adrenal gland: Small gland found above each kidney which secretes cortisone, adrenalin, aldosterone and many other important hormones.

alopecia: Hair loss, a common side effect of chemotherapy.

amenorrhea: Absence or stoppage of menstrual period.

amino acid: The building block of proteins.

androgen: Hormone which produces male characteristics.

angiogenesis (angiogenic): Stimulates new blood vessels to be formed.

anorexia: Loss of appetite.

apoptosis: Cell suicide.

areola: Area of pigment around the nipple.

aspiration: Putting a hypodermic needle into a tissue and drawing back on the syringe to obtain fluid or cells.

asymmetrical: Not matching.

ataxia telangectasia: Disease of the nervous system; carriers of the gene are more sensitive to radiation and have a higher risk of cancer.

atypical cell: Mild to moderately abnormal cell.

atypical hyperplasia: Cells that are not only abnormal but increased in number.

augmented: Added to such, as an augmented breast: one which has had a silicone implant added to it

autologous: From the same person. An autologous blood transfusion is blood removed and then transfused back to the same person at a later date.

axilla: Armpit.

axillary lymph nodes: Lymph nodes found in the armpit area.

axillary lymph node dissection: Surgical removal of lymph nodes found in the armpit region.

base pairs: Two nucleic acids which bind together in DNA and RNA

benign: Not cancerous.

bilateral: Involving both sides, such as both breasts.

biological response modifier: Usually natural substances such as colony stimulating factor that stimulates the bone marrow to make blood cells, that alter the body's natural response.

biopsy: Removal of tissue. This term does not indicate how *much* tissue will be removed.

bone marrow: The soft inner part of large bones that produces blood cells.

bone scan: Test to determine if there is any sign of cancer in the bones.

brachial plexus: A bundle of nerves in the armpit which go on to supply the arm

breast reconstruction: Creation of artificial breast after mastectomy by a plastic surgeon.

bromocriptine: Drug used to block the hormone prolactin.

calcifications: Small calcium deposits in the breast tissue that can be seen by mammography.

carcinoembryonic antigen (CEA): Nonspecific (not specific to cancer) blood test used to follow women with metastatic breast cancer to help determine if the treatment is working.

carcinogen: Substance that can cause cancer.

carcinoma: Cancer arising in the epithelial tissue (skin, glands, and lining of internal organs). Most cancers are carcinomas.

cell cycle: The steps a cell goes through in order to reproduce itself.

cellulitis: Infection of the soft tissues.

centigray: Measurement of radiation absorbed dose, same as a rad.

checkpoint: Point in the cell cycle where the cell's DNA is checked for mutations before it is allowed to move forward.

chemotherapy: Treatment of disease with certain chemicals. The term usually refers to *cytotoxic* drugs given for cancer treatment.

chromosome: Genes are strung together in a chromosome.

cohort study: Study of a group of people who have something in common when they are first assembled and who are then observed for a period of time to see what happens to them

colostrum: Liquid produced by the breast before the milk comes in: pre-milk.

comedo: Type of DCIS where the cells filling the duct are more aggressive looking.

comedon: Whitehead pimple.

contracture: Formation of a thick scar tissue; in the breast a contracture can form around an implant.

core biopsy: Type of needle biopsy where a small core of tissue is removed from a lump without surgery.

corpus luteum: Ovarian follicle after ovulation.

cortisol: Hormone produced by the adrenal gland.

costochondritis: Inflammation of the connection between ribs and breast bone, a type of arthritis.

cribriform: Type of DCIS where the cells filling the duct have punched out areas.

cyclical: In a cycle like the menstrual period, which is every 28 days, or chemotherapy treatment, which is periodic.

cyst: Fluid filled sac.

cystosarcoma phylloides: Unusual type of breast tumor.

cytology: Study of cells.

cytologist: One who specializes in studying cells.

cytosine: A nucleotide base which pairs with guanine in DNA.

cytotoxic: Causing the death of cells. The term usually refers to drugs used in chemotherapy.

danazol: Drug used to block hormones from the pituitary gland, used in endometriosis and rarely breast pain.

diethylstilbesterol (DES): Synthetic estrogen once used to prevent miscarriages, now shown to cause vaginal cancer in the daughters of the women who took it. DES is sometimes used to treat metastatic breast cancer.

DNA: Deoxyriboneucleic acid, the genetic code.

double helix: The structure of DNA which allows it to be easily replicated.

doubling time: Time it takes the cell population to double in number.

ductal carcinoma in situ (DCIS): Ductal cancer cells that have not grown outside of their site of origin, sometimes referred to as pre-cancer.

edema: Swelling caused by a collection of fluid in the soft tissues.

electrocautery: Instrument used in surgery to cut, coagulate or destroy tissue by heating it with an electric current.

embolus: Plug or clot of tumor cells within a blood vessel.

engorgement: Swelling with fluid, as in a breast engorged with milk.

erb B2: Another name for the HER-2 neu oncogene.

esophagus (esophageal): Organ carrying food from the mouth and the stomach.

estrogen: Female sex hormones produced by the ovaries, adrenal glands, placenta, and fat.

estrogen receptor: Protein found on some cells to which estrogen molecules will attach. If a tumor is positive for estrogen receptors, it is sensitive to hormones.

excema: Skin irritation characterized by redness and open weeping.

excisional biopsy: Taking the whole lump out.

extracellular matrix: The material which surrounds the cells.

fat necrosis: Area of dead fat usually following some form of trauma or surgery, a cause of lumps.

fibroadenoma: Benign fibrous tumor of the breast most common in young women.

fibrocystic disease: Much misused term for any benign condition of the breast.

fibroid: Benign fibrous tumor of the uterus (not in the breast).

flow cytometry: Test that measures DNA content in tumors.

fluoroscopy: Use of an x-ray machine to examine parts of the body directly rather than taking a picture and developing it, as in conventional x rays. Fluoroscopy uses more radiation than a single x ray.

follicle stimulating hormone (FSH): Hormone from the pituitary gland which stimulates the ovary.

follicles: In the ovaries, eggs encased in their developmental sacs.

frozen section: Freezing and slicing tissue to make a slide immediately for diagnosis.

frozen shoulder: Stiffness of the shoulder, which is painful and makes it hard to lift the arm over your head.

galactocele: Milk cyst sometimes found in a nursing mother's breast.

gene: A linear sequence of DNA that is required to produce a protein.

genetic: Relating to genes or inherited characteristics.

genome: All of the chromosomes that together form the genetic map.

germ line: Cells that are involved in reproduction, i.e., sperm and eggs.

ghostectomy: Removal of breast tissue in the area where there was a previous lump.

guanine: One of the base pairs that form DNA; pairs with cytosine.

gynecomastia: Swollen breast tissue in a man or boy.

hemorrhage: Bleeding.

hemangioma: A birth mark consisting of overgrowth of blood vessels.

hematoma: Collection of blood in the tissues. Hematomas may occur in the breast after surgery.

Her-2 neu: An oncogene which, when overexpressed, leads to more cell growth.

heterogeneous: Composed of many different elements. In relation to breast cancer, heterogeneous refers to the fact that there are many different types of breast cancer cells within one tumor.

homeopathy: System of therapy using very small doses of drugs, which can produce in healthy people symptoms similar to those of the disease being treated. These are believed to stimulate the immune system.

hormone: Chemical substance produced by glands in the body which enters the bloodstream and causes effects in other tissues.

hot flashes: Sudden sensations of heat and swelling associated with the menopause.

HRT: Hormone replacement therapy.

human choriogonadotropin (HCG): Hormone produced by the *corpus luteum*.

hyperplasia: Excessive growth of cells.

hypothalmus: Area at the base of the brain that controls various functions including hormone production in the pituitary.

hysterectomy: Removal of the uterus. Hysterectomy does not necessarily mean the removal of ovaries *(oophorectomy)*.

immunocytochemistry: Study of the chemistry of cells using techniques that employ immune mechanisms.

immune system: Complex system by which the body is able to protect itself from foreign invaders.

incisional biopsy: Taking a piece of the lump out.

infiltrating cancer: Cancer which can grow beyond its site of origin into neighboring tissue. Infiltrating does not imply that the cancer has already spread outside the breast. Infiltrating has the same meaning as invasive.

informed consent: Process in which the patient is fully informed of all risks and complications of a planned procedure and agrees to proceed.

in situ: In the site of. In regards to cancer, in situ refers to tumors that haven't grown beyond their site of origin and invaded neighboring tissue.

intraductal: Within the duct. Intraductal can describe a benign or malignant process.

intraductal papilloma: Benign tumor which projects like a finger from the lining of the duct.

invasive cancer: Cancers that are capable of growing beyond their site of origin and invading neighboring tissue. Invasive does not imply that the cancer is aggressive or has already spread.

lactation: Production of milk from the breast.

latissimus flap: Flap of skin and muscle taken from the back used for reconstruction after mastectomy or partial mastectomy.

lidocaine: Drug most commonly used for local anesthesia.

lobules: Parts of the breast capable of making milk.

lobular carcinoma in situ: Abnormal cells within the lobule which don't form lumps. They can serve as a marker of future cancer risk.

lobular: Having to do with the lobules of the breast.

local treatment of cancer: Treatment of the tumor only.

lumpectomy: Surgery to remove lump with small rim of normal tissue around it.

luteinizing hormone: Hormone produced by the pituitary which helps control the menstrual cycle.

lymphatic vessels: Vessels that carry lymph (tissue fluid) to and from lymph nodes.

lymphedema: Milk arm. This swelling of the arm can follow surgery to the lymph nodes under the arm. It can be temporary, or permanent and occur immediately, or any time later.

lymph nodes: Glands found throughout the body which help defend against foreign invaders such as bacteria. Lymph nodes can be a location of cancer spread.

macrophages: Blood cells that are part of the immune system.

malignant: Cancerous.

mastalgia: Pain in the breast.

mastitis: Infection of the breast. Mastitis is sometimes used loosely to refer to any benign process in the breast.

mastodynia: Pain in the breast.

mastopexy: Uplift of the breast through plastic surgery.

menarche: First menstrual period.

metastasis: Spread of cancer to another organ, usually through the blood stream.

metastasizing: Spreading to a distant site.

methylxanthine: Chemical group to which caffeine belongs.

microcalcification: Tiny calcifications in the breast tissue usually seen only on a mammogram. When clustered can be a sign of ductal carcinoma in situ.

micrometastasis: Microscopic and as yet undetectable but presumed spread of tumor cells to other organs.

micropapillary: Type of DCIS where the cells filling the duct take the form of 'finger' projections into the center.

mitosis: Cell division.

mutation: An alteration of the genetic code.

myocutaneous flap: Flap of skin and muscle and fat taken from one part of the body to fill in an empty space.

myoepithelial cells: The cells which surround the ductal lining cells and may serve to contain the cells.

necrosis: Dead tissue.

nodular: Forming little nodules.

nuclear magnetic resonance (NMR or MRI): Imaging technique using a magnet and electrical coil to transmit radio waves through the body.

nucleotide: One of the base pairs forming DNA.

observational study: A study in which a factor is observed in a group of people.

oncogene: Tumor genes are present in the body. These can be activated by carcinogens and cause cell to grow uncontrollably.

oncogenes: Altered DNA which can lead to cancerous growth.

oncology: Study of cancer.

oophorectomy: Removal of the ovaries.

osteoporosis: Softening of the bones, and bone loss, that occurs with age in some people.

oxytocin: Hormone produced by the pituitary gland, involved in lactation.

p53: A tumor suppressor gene.

palliation: Act of relieving a symptom without curing the cause.

pathologist: Doctor who specializes in examining tissue and diagnosing disease.

pectoralis major: Muscle which lies under the breast

phlebitis: Irritation of a vein.

pituitary gland: A gland located in the brain which secretes many hormones to regulate other glands in the body: the master gland.

Poland's syndrome: A congenital condition in which there is no breast development on one side of the chest.

polygenic: Relating to more than one gene.

polymastia: Literally many breasts. Existence of an extra breast or breasts.

postmenopausal: After the menopause has occurred.

Premarin: Estrogen from pregnant horses' urine that is sometimes given to women after the menopause.

progesterone: Hormone produced by the ovary involved in the normal menstrual cycle.

prognosis: Expected or probable outcome.

prolactin: Hormone produced by the pituitary that stimulates progesterone production by the ovaries and lactation.

prophylactic subcutaneous mastectomies: Removal of all breast tissue beneath the skin and nipple, to prevent future breast cancer risk.

prosthesis: Artificial substitute for an absent part of the body, as in breast prosthesis.

protein: Formed from amino acids, this is the building block of life.

protocol: Research designed to answer a hypothesis. Protocols often involve testing a specific new treatment under controlled conditions.

proto-oncogene: Normal gene controlling cell growth or turnover.

Provera: Progesterone which is sometimes given to women in combination with Premarin after menopause.

pseudolump: Breast tissue that feels like a lump but when removed proves to be normal.

ptosis: Drooping, as in breasts which hang down.

punch biopsy: A biopsy of skin done which just punches a small hole out of the skin.

quadrantectomy: Removal of a quarter of the breast.

rad: Radiation absorbed dose, same as centigray. One chest x ray equals 1/10 of a rad.

randomized: Chosen at random. In regard to a research study it means choosing the subjects to be given a particular treatment by means of a computer programmed to choose names at random.

randomized controlled study: A study in which the participants are randomized to one treatment or another.

recurrence: Return of cancer after its apparent complete disappearance.

remission: Disappearance of detectable disease.

repair endonucleases: Enzymes that can repair mutations.

RNA: Ribonucleic acid; carries the message from the DNA into the cell to make proteins.

sarcoma: Cancer arising in the connective tissue.

scoliosis: Deformity of the back bone which causes a person to bend to one side or the other.

scleroderma: An autoimmune disease which involves thickening of the skin, difficulty swallowing among other symptoms.

sebaceous: Oily, cheesy material secreted by glands in the skin.

selenium: Metallic element found in food.

SERM: Selective estrogen receptor modulator: a compound which is estrogenic in some organs and anti-estrogenic in others.

seroma: Collection of tissue fluid.

side effect: Unintentional or undesirable secondary effect of treatment.

silicone: Synthetic material used in breast implants because of its flexibility, resilience and durability.

somatic: A cell that forms the organs of the body but is not involved in reproduction.

S phase fraction: A measure of how many cells are dividing at a time; if it is high it is thought to indicate an aggressive tumor.

subareolar abscess: Infection of the glands under the nipple.

subcutaneous tissue: The tissue under the skin.

systemic treatment: Treatment involving the whole body, usually using drugs.

tamoxifen: Estrogen blocker used in treating breast cancer.

telomere: The end of a chromosome, a bit of which is clipped off every time a cell divides.

telomerase: An enzyme which reattaches the end of a chromosome when it divides.

thoracic: Concerning the chest (thorax).

thoracic nerves: Nerves in the chest area.

thoracoepigastric vein: Vein that starts under the arm and passes along the side of the breast and then down into the abdomen.

thymine: A nucleotide base which pairs with adenine in DNA formation.

titration: Systems of balancing. In chemotherapy, titration means using the largest amount of a drug possible while keeping the side effects from becoming intolerable.

trauma: Wound or injury.

triglyceride: Form in which fat is stored in the body, consisting of glycerol and three fatty acids.

tru-cut biopsy: Type of core needle biopsy where a small core of tissue is removed from a lump without surgery.

tumor: Abnormal mass of tissue. Strictly speaking a tumor can be benign or malignant.

tumor dormancy: Tumors which are present in a stable state

tumor suppressor gene: A gene that prevents cells from growing if they have a mutation.

veg-f: Vascular epidermal growth factor; a protein which stimulates new blood vessels to grow.

virginal hypertrophy: Inappropriately large breasts in a young woman.

xeroradiography: Type of mammogram taken on a xerox plate rather than x-ray film.

Index

Note: Page numbers in italics refer to illustrations in the text.

Herbal remedies (*cont.*)
 for breast pain, 88
 for cancer treatment, 510, 512
 contraindications for use, 88
 for depression and anxiety, 498, 554
 for fuzzy thinking, 554
 for hot flashes, 551
 for insomnia, 554
 for vaginal dryness, 553
Herceptin, 214, 334, 385, 480, 575, 583–584
Heredity. *See* Family history
Herrington, David, 550
HERS trial, 175, 249, 550
Hester, Susan, 591
Heuston, John T., 77
Hill, Hester, 357
Hirshfield-Bartek, Judi, 357
Hispanic women, and breast cancer incidence, 217(table)
Hoagland, Mahlon, 184–185
Hodgkin's disease, 244–245, 465
Homeopathy, 508–509, 512
Hormone receptors, 211–214, 233. *See also* Estrogen receptor negative tumors; Estrogen receptor positive tumors
Hormone receptor tests, *333–334*, 344, 390
Hormone replacement therapy, 28
 after breast cancer, 543–544
 and alcohol consumption, 252
 alternatives to, 544–548
 and birth control pills, 252–253
 and breast cancer risk, 21, 214, 247–253
 duration of use, 251
 and heart disease, 249, 550–551
 for prevention of osteoporosis, 248–249
 studies on, 174–176. *See also* Women's Health Initiative
 for symptom control, 248
 and tamoxifen, 493
 types of cancer associated with, 253
Hormones
 birth control pills. *See* Birth control pills
 and breast cancer prevention, 294–296
 and breast cancer risk, 211–214, 233–236, *235*. *See also* Hormone replacement therapy
 and breast development. *See* Breast development
 and breast feeding, *36*, 48–49
 and breast shape, 28
 and cyclical breast pain, 86–*90*
 in food, 240
 and invasive cancer, 272
 melatonin, 258
 and menopause, 18–21
 and menstruation, 16–18, *17*
 and milk production, *33–35*
 and ovaries, 19–21
 and ovulation, 16–19, *17*
 and pregnancy, 18, *36*
 for treatment of painful breasts, 88–90
 weak estrogens, 255
 witch's milk, 12, 14, 102–103
 See also Estrogen; Progesterone
Hormone therapy for breast cancer, 211–213, 389–395, 480, 491–495
 increase in symptoms at start of treatment, 578

and metastatic disease, 575–580
 See also Raloxifene; Tamoxifen
Horwitz, Katherine, 214, 547
Hot flashes, 18
 and chemotherapy, 488
 and natural progesterone cream, 547
 and tamoxifen, 492
 and zoladex, 495
 treatments for, 492, 545, 551-552
Human choriogonadotropin (HCG), 18, 254
Husbands and lovers
 feelings about woman's illness, 358–359, 526
 post-treatment issues, 524–526
Hypnosis, for breast augmentation, 56
Hypothalamus, 19
Hysterectomy, effect on breasts, 28. *See also* Oopherectomy

IBIS trial, 302
Ibuprofen, for painful breasts, 88, 90, 92
Iglehart, J. Dieil, 229
IHC. *See* Immunohistochemistry
Imagery techniques. *See* Visualization techniques
Immune system, 209
 and alternative/complementary medicine, 509
 and chemotherapy, 479–480, 482–483
 and mind-body connection, 499
 and nonlactational mastitis, 97
Immuno-augementative therapy, 509
Immunohistochemistry (IHC), 334
Immunotherapy, 480, 583–584. *See also* Herceptin
Infections, 93–101
 after a biopsy, 160–161
 after lymph node surgery, 441
 after reconstructive surgery, 450–451
 and cancer, 101
 cellulitis, 97, 533–534
 chronic subareolar abscess, 98–*100*, 289
 lactational mastitis, 94–97, *95*
 nonlactational mastitis, 97–98
 surgical removal of tissue, 97–100
 susceptibility during chemotherapy, 483
 syphilis, 101
 TB, 101
 treatments for, 95–100
 See also Inflammatory breast cancer
Infiltrating ductal carcinoma. *See* Invasive ductal cancer
Infiltrating lobular carcinoma. *See* Invasive lobular cancer
Inflammatory breast cancer, 101, 179, 342, 400–401, 411
Inframammary ridge, 5, 7, 27–*28*
Insurance coverage after illness, 539–540
Insurance coverage for breast problems
 and clinical trials, 180–181
 and "fibrocystic disease," 84
 and genetic testing, 230
 and high-dose chemotherapy with stem cell rescue, 384
 prosthesis coverage, 439, 446
Intercosalbrachial nerve, 529–530
Intervention studies. *See* Studies and clinical trials

Vaccines, 584
Vaginal discharge, 492
Vaginal dryness
    and chemotherapy, 489
    and tamoxifen, 492
    treatments for, 551–553
Variations in breast development, 51–57, *52*
    asymmetrical breasts, 56–57
    corrections for. *See* Plastic surgery
    extra breast tissue, 52–53
    extra nipples, *13*, 51–53
    and injuries to the breast bud, 53–54
    inverted nipples. *See* Inverted nipples
    lack of nipples, 53
    Poland's syndrome (undeveloped or missing
        breasts), 53, 71
    and self-image, 56–57
    very large breasts, 54–56
    very small breasts, 55–56
Vascular endothelial cell growth factor (veg-f),
    206–207
Veg-f. *See* Vascular endothelial cell growth fac-
    tor
Versed, 155
Vinorelbine, 581
Virginal hypertrophy, 54–56
Visco, Fran, 592
Visualization techniques, 500–502
    for breast augmentation, 56
    for breast pain, 88
    and chemotherapy, 487
Visual problems, 494, 568, 570
Vitamins, 175–176
    and breast cancer prevention, 239–240, 258
    and breast pain, 87
    and hot flashes, 551–552
    and osteoporosis, 548

WAVE trial, 175
Weakness, and metastatic disease, 568–569
Weight
    and breast cancer risk, 239, 292-293
    loss as a symptom of metastatic disease, 563,
        567

WELL-HART trial, 175
Wellisch, David, 356, 526
WHI. *See* Women's Health Initiative
White women
    breast cancer incidence, 217(table)–218(table),
        222, 235
    inflammatory breast cancer rate, 401
    and tamoxifen risk, *301*
Wide excision, 278, 424–425. *See also*
    Lumpectomy
Wigs, 447
Winged scapula, 433–434
WINS study, 239
Winter, Melanie, 595
Wire localization biopsy, 147–148, 153–*154*, 159,
    325
WISDOM. *See* Women's International Study of
    long-Duration Oestrogen after Menopause
Witch's milk, 12, 14, 102–103
Wolff, Mary, 254–255
Women's Cancer Resource Center, 590–591
Women's Community Cancer Project, 570, 590–
    591
Women's Health Initiative (WHI), 171–172, 175–
    176, 223, 238, 249, 251, 550
Women's International Study of long-Duration
    Oestrogen after Menopause (WISDOM),
    175
Wrensch, Margaret, 283, 289

Xeloda (capecitabane), 581
X rays, and breast cancer risk, 243–244. *See also*
    Mammography

Y-ME, 447, 591
Young women, breast cancer in, 406–409. *See
    also* Adolescence; Age
YWCA, 527

Zofran, 487
Zoladex (goserelin), 390–391, 395, 486, 495, 542,
    578, 580